Preface

This new English edition has been completely revised and updated. The pocket atlas is meant as a companion to lectures. It also serves as a valuable orientation tool for course work in microscopic anatomy. More than ever before, histology plays a very important role in medicine and biology. Therefore, the short instructive texts have been updated so that they incorporate the latest scientific findings. An understanding of micromorphological techniques is a prerequisite for the study of biochemistry, physiology and the relatively young discipline of molecular cell biology. Accordingly, cytology and histology rank high in the curriculum.

This pocket atlas does not attempt to provide a complete theoretical knowledge of histology, which may be approached using comprehensive works on cytology, histology and microscopic anatomy. It rather conveys a basic understanding of the elements in histology and the microscopic anatomy of the human body. Students of histology will value this pocket atlas as a course companion book while using microscopic techniques. The atlas will help them to recognize the crucial elements and structures in a histological image and make it easier to arrive at the correct diagnosis.

You will find 16 tables in the appendix. Students have suggested this addition. With the help of these tables, students can test their ability to recognize and interpret the relevant structures in histological images.

The intuitive layout of the current edition makes it easy to find references. Many new images have been added.

I am grateful to my colleagues of the Lübeck Institute of Anatomy for their invaluable assistance in creating this new edition. The names of my colleagues who graciously provided original images are listed in the appendix.

My secretary, Mrs. Roswitha Jönsson, was an extraordinary help to me. She took care of the final corrections to the manuscript. My thanks go to Mr. Albrecht Hauff and Dr. Wolfgang Knüppe who supervised this edition with their customary care. Special thanks also go the talented team at the Georg Thieme Verlag.

I hope that this latest edition of the pocket atlas will be a helpful guide for students of medicine, dentistry, veterinary medicine, biology and related sciences. I wish that it might open your window to the fascinating world of the smallest structures of the organism.

Lübeck, Spring of 2003 *Wolfgang Kühnel*

Contents

1 Spinal Ganglion Cells

Human and animal cells are dedicated to specialized functions within the organism, and their sizes, shapes and structures vary accordingly. *Spinal ganglion cells* are mostly pseudounipolar neurons and can be spherical, ellipsoid, or pear-shaped, with diameters between 20 and 120 µm. The round cell nuclei, up to 25 µm in size, contain little chromatin [1]. The nuclei always have a clearly visible nucleolus (2–4 µm). Glial cells form a layer around the spinal ganglion cells. Therefore, they are also called satellite cells [2]. The small round or spindle-shaped nuclei of these satellite cells stand out because they are heavily stained. There are delicate connective tissue fibers (endoneurium) and nerve fiber bundles (fascicles) [3] between the ganglion cells. In the upper right of the figure, a wide strand of connective tissue (stained blue) traverses the section (cf. Figs. 32, 66, 256, 671–674).

1 Nucleus with clearly visible nucleolus
2 Satellite cells
3 Nerve fibers
4 Capillaries
Stain: azan; magnification: × 400

2 Multipolar Neurons

Anterior horn motor cells—i.e., *motor neurons of the columna anterior* from the *spinal cord*—were obtained by careful maceration of the spinal cord and stained as a "squeeze preparation" (tissue spread out by gentle pressure). This technique makes it possible to preserve long stretches of the numerous long neurites and make them visible after staining. In a tissue section, most of the cell processes would be sheared off (see Fig. 20). In this preparation, it is hardly possible to distinguish between axons (neurites, axis cylinder) and the heavily branched dendrites. Axons extend from the nerve cell to the musculature and form synapses.

Stain: carmine red; magnification: × 80

3 Smooth Muscle Cells

The structural units of the smooth musculature are the band-shaped or spindle-shaped muscle cells, which usually occur in bundles of different sizes. Muscle cells build strong layers, e.g., in the walls of hollow organs (cf. Figs. 220–223). They can be isolated from these hollow organs by maceration with nitric acid. However, the long, extended cell processes often break off during this procedure. Dependent on their location and function in the tissue, smooth muscle cells are between 15 and 200 µm long. During pregnancy, uterine smooth muscle cells may reach a length of 1000 µm. On average, they are 5–10 µm thick. The rod-shaped nucleus is located in the cell center. When muscle cells contract, the nucleus sometimes coils or loops into the shape of a corkscrew.

Stain: carmine red; magnification: × 80

1

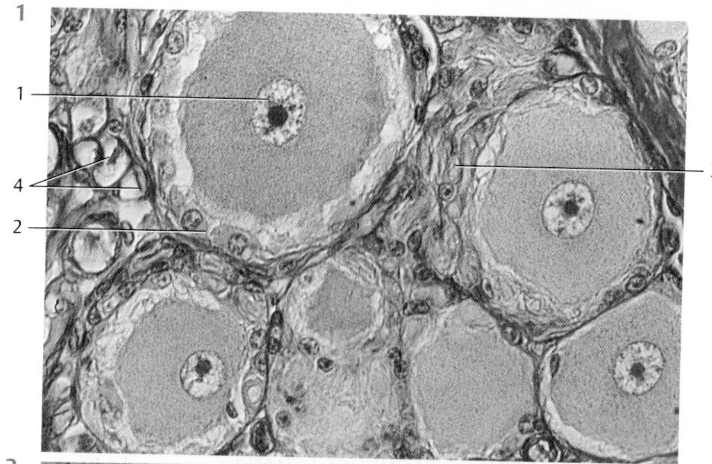

2

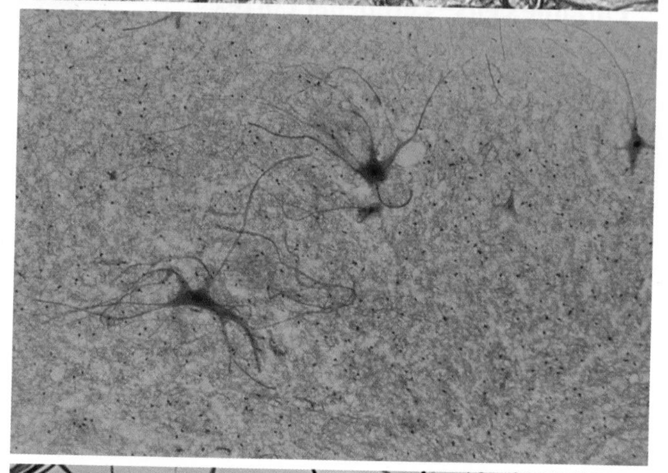

3

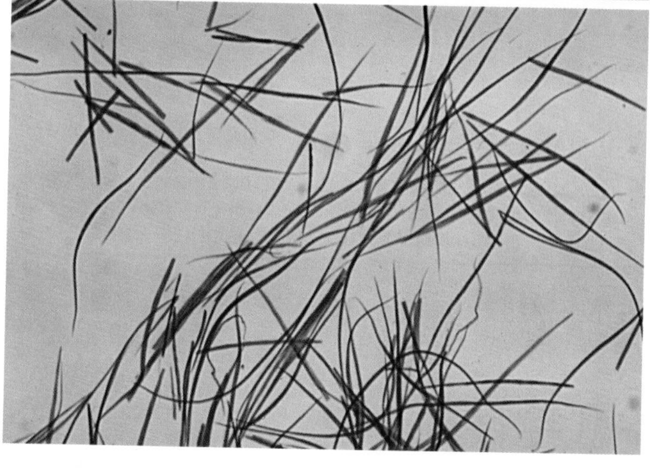

4 Fibrocytes—Fibroblasts

In connective tissue sections, the nonmotile (fixed) *fibrocytes* look like thin, spindle-shaped elements. However, their true shape can be brought out in thin whole-mount preparations. Fibrocytes are sometimes rounded, sometimes elongated, flattened cells with membranous or thorn-like processes 1. The cell processes often touch each other and form a web. Their large, mostly oval nuclei feature a delicate chromatin structure (not visible in this preparation). Here, the nuclei appear homogeneous (cf. Figs. 135–139).
Fibroblasts biosynthesize all components of the fibers and the extracellular matrix (ground substances). Fibrocytes are fibroblasts that show much lower rates of biosynthetic activity.

1 Fibrocytes with cytoplasmic processes
2 Nuclei from free connective tissue cells
Stain: Gomori silver impregnation, modified; magnification: × 650

5 Purkinje Cells—Cerebellar Cortex

Pear-shaped *Purkinje cells*, which are about 50–70 µm high and 30–35 µm wide (*cell soma, perikaryon*) 2, send out 2–3 µm thick dendrites that branch out like trellis trees. These delicate trees reach up to the cortical surface, extending their fine branches espalier-like in only one plane. The axon (*efference*) 1 spans the distance between the basal axon hillock and the cerebellar cortex. The elaborate branching can only be seen using metal impregnation (cf. Figs. 254, 681, 682).

1 Axon
2 Perikaryon
Stain: Golgi silver impregnation; magnification: × 50

6 Oocyte

Oocyte from a sea urchin ovary. Large, heavily stained *nucleolus* 2 inside a loosely structured nucleus 1. The finely granulated cytoplasm contains yolk materials. Cell organelles are not visible (cf. Figs. 542–550, 557).

1 Nucleus
2 Nucleolus
Stain: azan; magnification: × 150

7 Vegetative Ganglion Cell

Large *vegetative ganglion cell* from the *Auerbach plexus* (*plexus myentericus*) from cat duodenum. A collateral branches from the upward extending axon. The downward-pointing cell processes are dendrites. Note the large nucleus (cf. Figs. 432–437).

Stain: Cauna silver impregnation; magnification: × 650

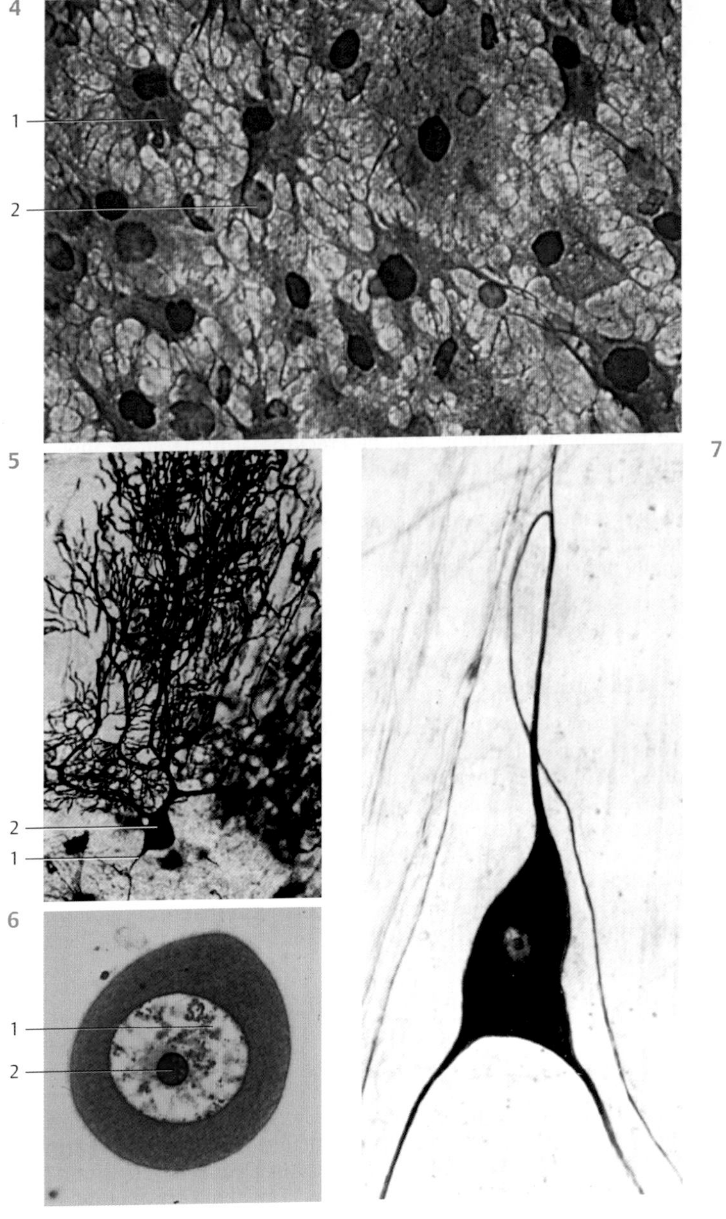
4
1
2
5
2
1
6
1
2
7

8 Cell Nucleus

The *nucleus* is the center for the genetically determined information in every eukaryotic cell. The nucleus also serves as a *command* or *logistics center* for the regulation of cell functions. There is a correlation between the geometry of the nucleus and the cell dimensions, which offers important diagnostic clues. The nucleus is usually round in polygonal and isoprismatic (cuboid) cells and ellipsoid in pseudostratified columnar cells; it has the form of a spindle in smooth muscle cells and is flattened in flat epithelial cells. In granulocytes, the nucleus has several segments. The fibrocyte in this figure is from subcutaneous connective tissue. Its elongated, irregularly lobed nucleus shows indentations and deep dells. The structural components of a nucleus are the *nuclear membrane*, the *nuclear lamina*, the *nucleoplasm*, and the *chromosomes* with the *chromatin* and the *nucleolus*. The chromatin is finely granular (*euchromatin*), but more dense near the inner nuclear membrane (*heterochromatin*). The small electron-dense patches are heterochromatin structures as well. The DNA is packaged in a much denser form in heterochromatin than in euchromatin, and heterochromatin therefore appears more heavily stained in light microscopy preparations. A nucleolus is not shown here. The cytoplasm of the fibrocyte contains mitochondria [1], osmiophilic secretory granules [2], vesicles, free ribosomes and fragments of the rough (granular) endoplasmic reticulum membranes. Collagen fibrils are cut longitudinally or across their axis [3].

Electron microscopy; magnification: × 13 000

9 Cell Nucleus

Detail section showing two secretory cells from the mucous membranes of the tuba uterina (oviduct). Their long, oval nuclei show multiple indentations of different depths. Therefore, the nucleus appears to be composed of tongues and irregular lobes in this preparation. The cytoplasm extends into the deep nuclear indentations. The distribution of the finely granular chromatin (*euchromatin*) is relatively even. Only at the inner nuclear membrane is the chromatin condensed in a fine osmiophilic line. The cytoplasm in the immediate vicinity of the nucleus contains cisternae from granular endoplasmic reticulum [1], secretory granules [2] and sporadically, small mitochondria.

Electron microscopy; magnification: × 8500

10 Cell Nucleus

Rectangular nucleus in an orbital gland cell from the water agama (lizard). The nucleus contains two strikingly large *nucleoli* [1], which are surrounded by a ring of electron-dense heterochromatin [↗]. This heterochromatin contains the genes for the *nucleolus organizer*. The heterochromatin layer along the inner nuclear membrane or the nuclear lamina shows several gaps, thus forming *nuclear pores*.

i Expanded intercellular space
→ In the lower part of the picture are two cell contacts in the form of desmosomes
Electron microscopy; magnification: × 12 000

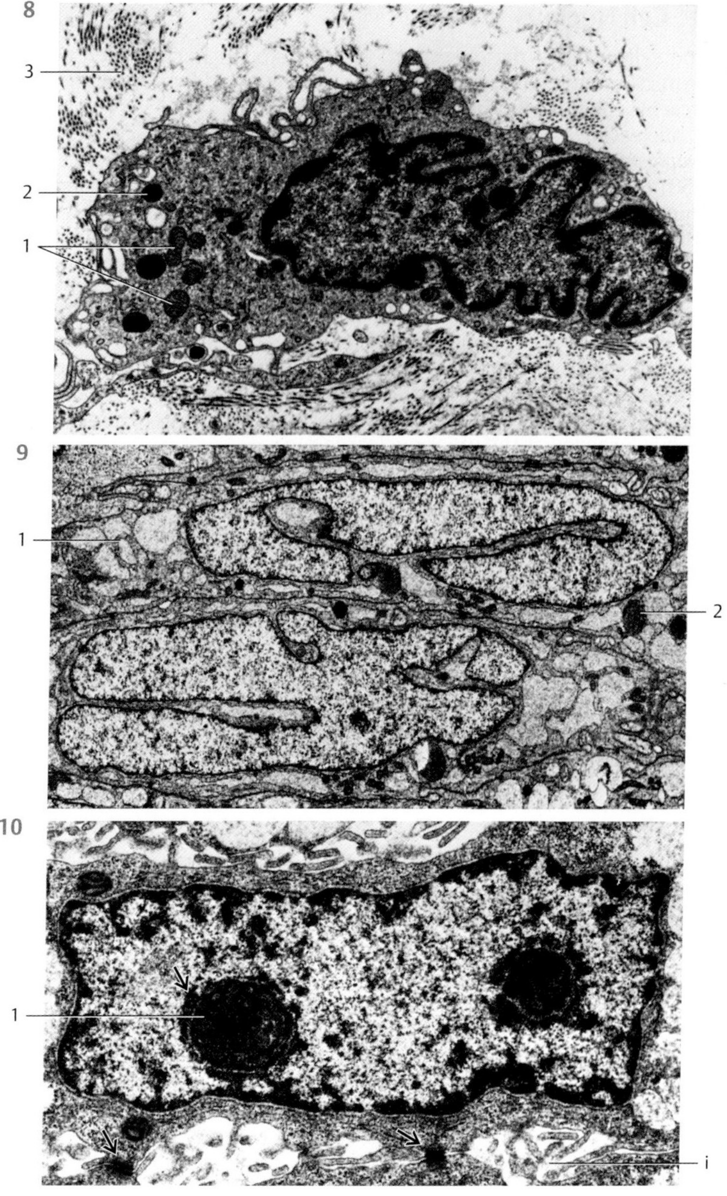
8
3
2
1
9
1
2
10
1
i

11 Cell Nucleus

Round cell nucleus (detail section) to illustrate the nuclear membrane. In light microscopy, cell nuclei are surrounded by a darkly stained line, which represents the nuclear membrane.

This nuclear membrane consists of two *cytomembranes*, which separate the *karyoplasm* from the *hyaloplasm*. Between the two membranes is the 20–50 nm wide perinuclear space, the *perinuclear cisterna* 1, which communicates with the vesicular spaces between the endoplasmic reticulum membranes. The outer nuclear membrane is confluent with the endoplasmic reticulum and shows membrane-bound ribosomes. The perinuclear cisterna is perforated by *nuclear pores* ↗ (see Fig. 12), which form *pore complexes*. Their width is about 30–50 nm, and they are covered with a diaphragm. At these covered pores, the outer and inner nuclear membrane lamellae merge. In the adjacent cytoplasm, close to the nuclear membrane, are cisternae of the granular endoplasmic reticulum 2. The inner lamella of the nuclear membrane is covered with electron-dense material. This is heterochromatin, which is localized at the inner nuclear lamina 3.

1 Perinuclear cisterna
2 Granular endoplasmic reticulum
3 Heterochromatin
Electron microscopy; magnification: × 50 000

12 Cell Nucleus

Tangential section through the surface of a cell nucleus. Note the *pores* in the nuclear membrane ↗. A look in the direction of the chromatin at the inner nuclear membrane shows a ring-shaped osmiophilic area with coarse granules. There is no heterochromatin close to the round cell pores. In the adjacent cytoplasm are mitochondria 1 and rough endoplasmic reticulum membranes 2.

1 Mitochondria
2 Granular endoplasmic reticulum
Electron microscopy; magnification: × 38 000

13 Cell Nucleus

Cell nucleus and adjacent cytoplasm from an *enterocyte* (jejunum) in a freeze-fracture plane (*cryofracture, freeze-etching*), which renders a profile view of the nuclear membranes. The view is on the inner side of the inner lamella of the inner nuclear double membrane 1. The white fracture line in this figure corresponds to the perinuclear cisterna (Fig. 11). The lower plane 2 gives a view of the inner side of the inner lamella of the outer nuclear double membrane. Note the abundance of *nuclear pores* 3, which allow the intracellular transport of materials between nucleus and cytoplasm. Note ↗ that the two nuclear membranes merge at the pore region. Above the nucleus are vesicles of various sizes and an array of Golgi membranes 4.

1 Inner lamella of the inner nuclear membrane
2 Inner lamella of the outer nuclear membrane
3 Nuclear pores
4 Area with Golgi membranes
Electron microscopy; magnification: × 22 100

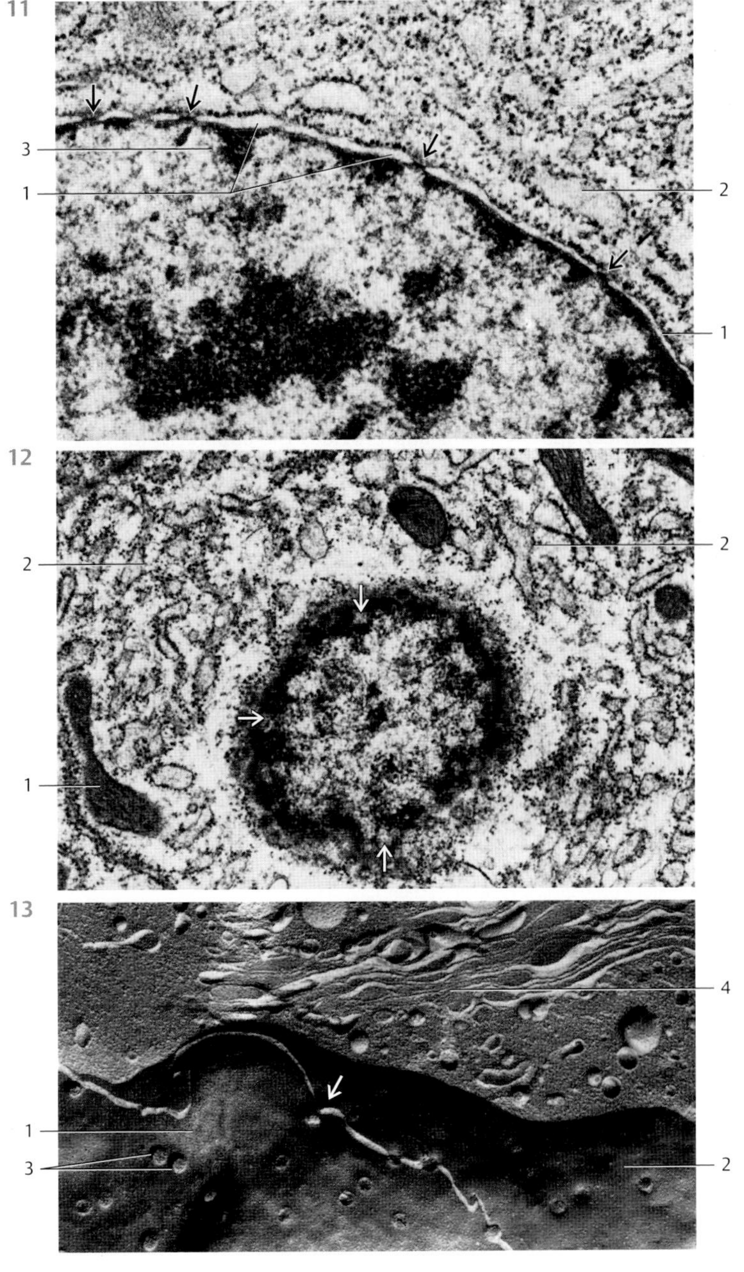
11
3
1
2
1
12
2
2
1
13
4
1
3
2

14 Mitosis and Cytokinesis

The most common type of nuclear cell division is mitosis. Mitosis yields two genetically identical daughter nuclei. It is followed by cell division (*cytokinesis*). The inactive period between active periods of cell division is called *interphase*. Nuclear division and cell division are the high points of the cell cycle. This cycle is segmented into the phases G1, S, G2 and mitosis. Mitosis is completed in six consecutive steps.
The figure on the right presents different stages of mitosis. The dividing cells were Indian muntjac fibroblasts in cell culture (*Muntiacus muntjac*).

a) Interphase. Phase between divisions. The chromatin is dispersed or forms small aggregates. It is often possible to distinguish between highly condensed chromatin, called heterochromatin, and less densely packed chromatin, called euchromatin. One or two nucleoli are routinely present.
b) Prophase. Begin of mitosis. The chromatin condenses to form chromosomal threads, which become increasingly thicker and shorter (coil stage, spirem). The nucleolus dissolves and the nuclear membrane falls apart. The nuclear spindle forms and provides the apparatus for chromosome movement. The nuclear membrane dissolves in the following prometaphase.
c) Metaphase. The chromosomes are arranged in the equatorial plane of the spindle, the metaphase plane. It now becomes apparent that there are two identical sister chromatids in each chromosome. Each chromatid has an area for the attachment to one of the spindle fibers, which extends to both spindle poles. This is the stage when karyotyping works best.
d-f) Anaphase. The two identical sister chromatids separate and move to the cell pole. Phase of the double (daughter) stars or diaster. In a later anaphase stage, a cytokinetic actin ring forms in the position of the equatorial plane.
g) Telophase. Completion of the nuclear division. The chromatids combine and form a coil. A new nuclear membrane forms, the cytoplasm divides by contracting the cytokinetic actin ring (division ring) (*cytokinesis*). A new cell wall is synthesized in the place of the cytokinetic actin ring.
h) Interphase.

Stain: DNA-specific Feulgen reaction

15 Chromosomes

Chromosomes in the metaphase of mitosis. The *centromeres* are stained with the DNA fluorescence dye DAPI blue, the *chromosome arms* are dyed red using the immunoassay for the protein pKi-67 in the “*perichromosomal layer*.” All chromosomes consist of two *chromatids*, which are connected only via centromere. The chromosome set for the mouse species CD in this figure consists of four acrocentric chromosomes (one-armed, V-shaped in this phase), chromosomes 19, X and Y, and 18 metacentric chromosomes (two-armed, X-shaped in this phase), which are the result of the centric fusion of two formerly acrocentric chromosomes.

Magnification: × 2600

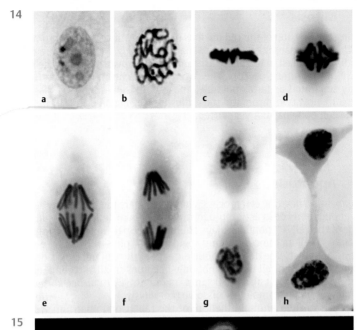

14

a b c d

e f g h

15

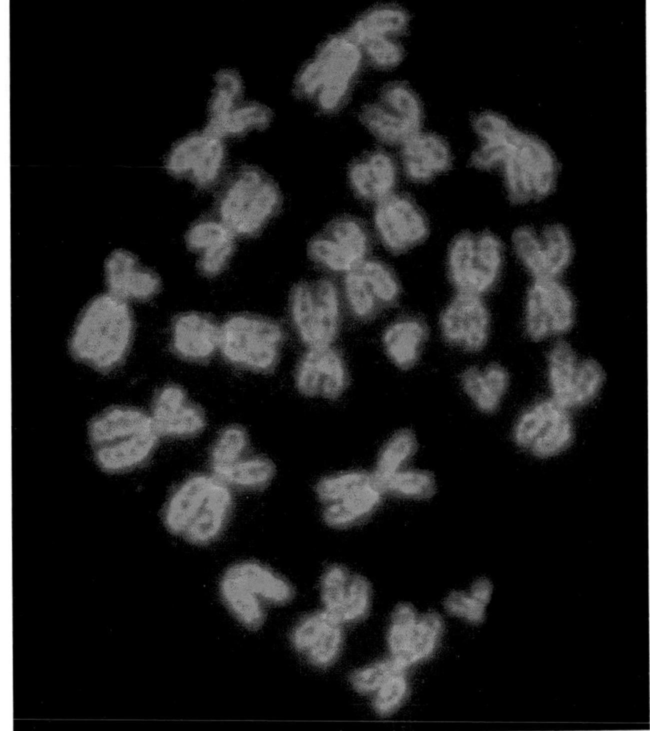

16 Mitosis

During the division of the cell nucleus of *eucytes* (mitosis), the chromosomes for the future daughter cells are separated (cf. Fig. 14). The figure shows a dividing fibroblast in the *anaphase* (ana, Greek: upward). This is the shortest phase in the mitotic process. The two daughter chromosome sets [1] are already separated as far as possible, and the division spindle is dismantled. There are now two chromatid stars (*diasters*) (cf. Fig. 14 e and f). The division of the cell body has not yet started.

1 Daughter chromosomes
Electron microscopy; magnification × 1400

17 Apoptosis

Apoptosis is a necrotic cell process. The cell triggers the process by activating the endogenous destruction program that leads to cell death ("*suicide program* of the cell"). Apoptosis plays an important part in the development of organs as well as the control and regulation of physiological regeneration. During apoptosis, the deoxyribonucleic acid of the cell nucleus is destroyed. In the process, the cell nucleus not only becomes small and condensed (*nuclear pyknosis*), but it also breaks into fragments (*extra nuclei, karyorrhexis*), which will finally completely dissolve (*karyolysis*).
Apoptosis in the cavum epithelium of the rabbit endometrium with chromatin bodies [1]. Cytoplasmic processes of a macrophage envelop part of the apoptotic cell like a horseshoe [2]. Uterine clearance [3].

1 Chromatin bodies
2 Macrophage processes
3 Uterine clearance
Electron microscopy; magnification: × 10 500

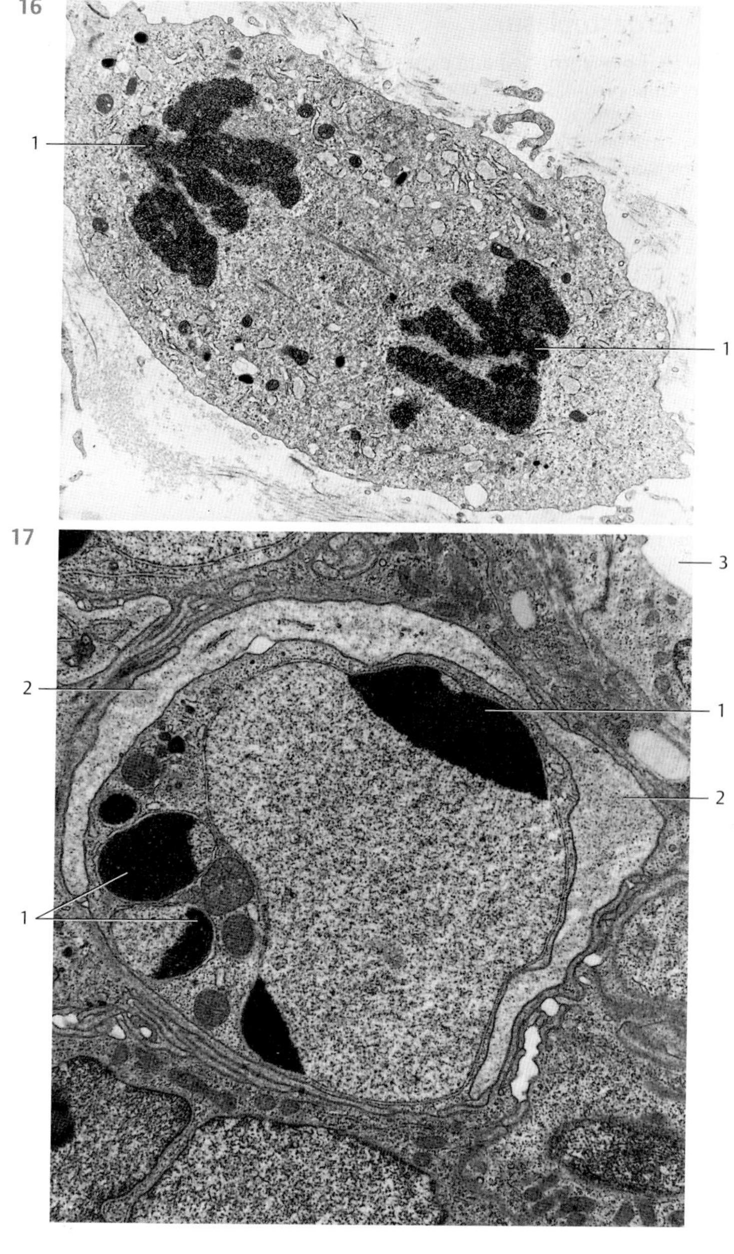
16
1
1
17
3
2
1
2
1

18 Ergastoplasm

Cells that biosynthesize and export large amounts of proteins have strongly basophilic cytoplasmic regions, which have been named *ergastoplasm* (from Greek: ergasticos = industrious, working cytoplasm). In light microscopic images, this basophilic material appears in a variety of forms. The homogeneous or banded material (*chromophilic substance*) from the basal part of highly active secretory gland cells (see Fig. 19) is very well known, and so are the smaller or larger chromophilic bodies in the cytoplasm of nerve cells (see Fig. 20). Due to their ribosome content, these cell components have a high affinity for basic dyes (e.g., hematoxylin). Electron microscopy reveals an elaborate system of densely packed granular endoplasmic reticulum (*rough ER, rER*) as the material that makes up the basophilic ergastoplasm seen in light microscopy (see Fig. 21–25).
This figure shows acini from the exocrine pancreas. These cells show pronounced basal basophilia ①. In contrast, the supranuclear and apical cytoplasmic regions are only sparsely granulated.

1 Cell regions with ergastoplasm, basal basophilia
2 Lumina of the acini
3 Blood vessels
Stain: hematoxylin-eosin; magnification × 400

19 Ergastoplasm

Basophilic cytoplasm (blue) in the basal regions of gland cells (*basal basophilia*) ① (cf. Fig. 18). The presence of ribosomes accounts for the affinity to basic dyes. The basophilic cytoplasm corresponds to the granular (rough) endoplasmic reticulum (rER) (see Figs. 21–25). The supranuclear and apical cell regions contain no ergastoplasm and therefore remain unstained. The round cell nuclei in the basal cytoplasmic region are stained light blue. Parotid gland (glandula parotidea) of the rat.

1 Cell regions with ergastoplasm, basal basophilia
2 Acini
3 Blood vessels
Stain: methylene blue, pH 3.5; nuclei are not specifically stained; magnification: × 400

20 Ergastoplasm—Nissl Bodies

The cytoplasm of multipolar neurons from the columna anterior of the spinal cord contains a dense distribution of fine or coarse bodies, which can be emphasized by staining with cresyl violet. They are called *Nissl bodies* or *Nissl substance* ① (*tigroid bodies*), after Franz Nissl (1860–1919), who discovered them. Electron microscopy identifies groups of polysomes and components of the rough (granular) endoplasmic reticulum (*ergastoplasm*) as the structures that correspond to the Nissl bodies (cf. Figs. 21–25, 250, 251).

1 Nissl bodies (substance)
2 Nucleus with nucleoli
3 Dendrites
4 Glial cell nuclei
Stain: cresyl violet; magnification: × 800

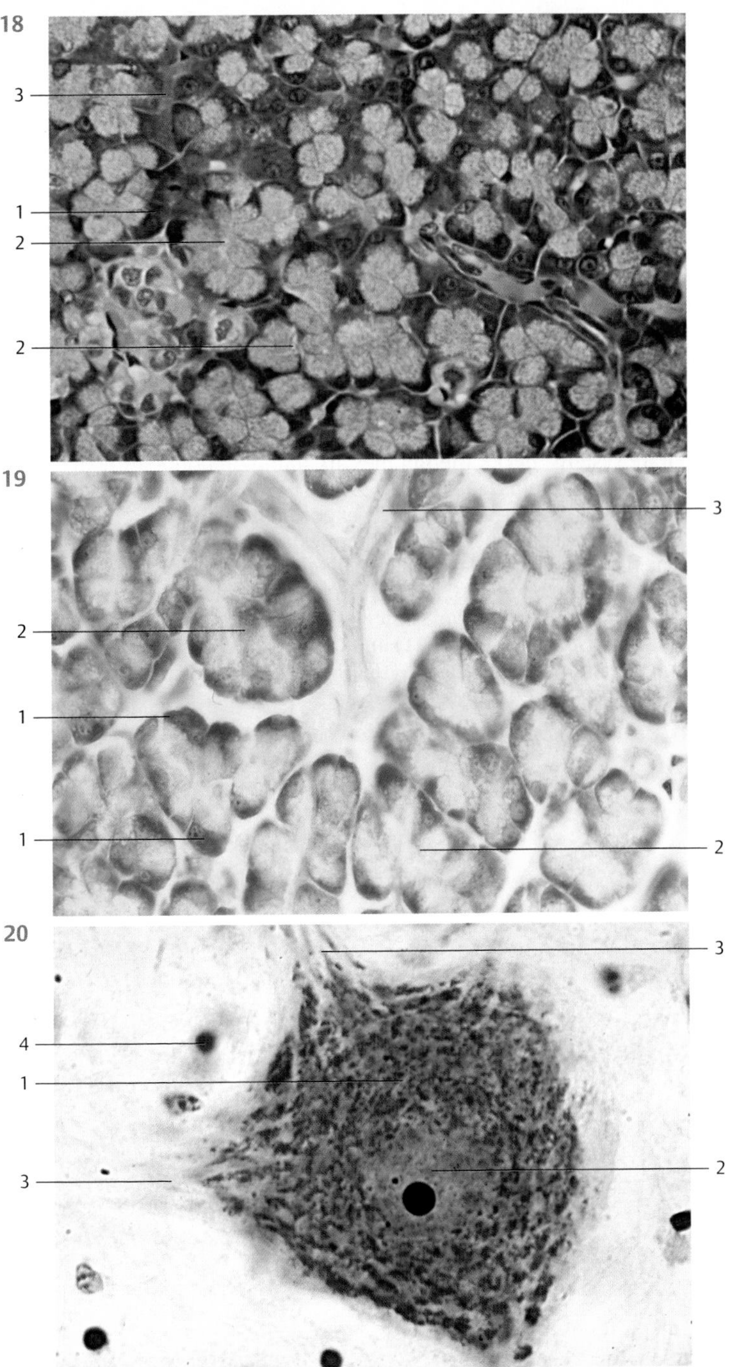
18
3
1
2
2
19
3
2
1
1
2
20
3
4
1
3
2

21 Granular (Rough) Endoplasmic Reticulum (rER)—Ergastoplasm

The *endoplasmic reticulum* (ER) is a continuous system of cell membranes, which are about 6 nm thick. Dependent on cell specialization and activity, the membranes occur in different forms, such as stacks or tubules. The ER double membranes may be smooth or have granules attached to their outer surfaces. These granules are about 25 nm in diameter and have been identified as *membrane-bound ribosomes*. Therefore, two types of ER exist: the granular or rough form (*rER, rough ER*) and the agranular or smooth form (*sER, smooth ER*).
Paired multiplanar stacks of lamellae are one characteristic forms of rER. The membranes are narrowly spaced and spread over large parts of the cell. The two associated membranes in this matrix are 40–70 nm apart. When cells assume a storage function, these membranes move away from each other and thus form *cisternae*, with a lumen that may be several hundred nanometers wide.
Elaborate systems of rER membranes are found predominantly in cells that biosynthesize proteins (see Figs. 19, 22–25). Proteins, which are synthesized on membranes of the rER, are mostly exported from the cell. They may be secreted from the cell (including hormones and digestive enzymes, etc.) or become part of intracellular vesicles (*membrane proteins*). The smooth endoplasmic reticulum (see Figs. 26–29) eluded light microscopy.
The cisternae of the endoplasmic reticulum interconnect both with the perinuclear cisternae (see Fig. 11) and the extracellular space.
This picture shows ergastoplasm (rER) from an exocrine pancreas cell, which produces digestive enzymes.

Electron microscopy; magnification: × 60 000

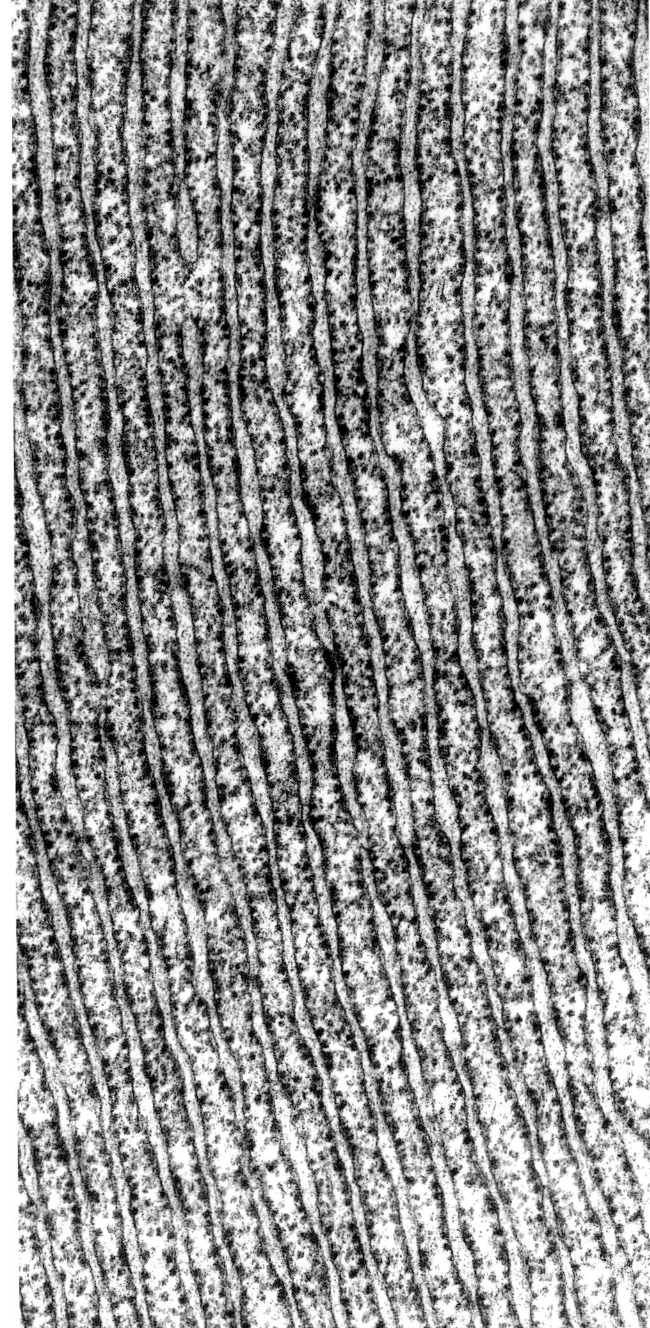

22 Granular (Rough) Endoplasmic Reticulum (rER)—Ergastoplasm

The granular endoplasmic reticulum (rER) exists not only in the form of strictly parallel-arranged membrane stacks, which are shown in Figure 21 as transections. On the contrary, dependent on the specific function of a cell, rER is found in various forms and dimensions. The transition between granular and agranular ER can be continuous.

In this figure, the *rER* presents as loosely packed stacks of cisternae with ribosomes attached to it like pearls on a string (*membrane-bound ribosomes*). The figure shows a mitochondrion of crista-type 1 between the rER cisternae. There are also free ribosomes 3 and *polysomes* 2 in rosette configuration present in the cytoplasmic matrix. Such collocations of granular ER cisternae and adjacent free ribosomes are identical to the structures that are visible after staining with basophilic dyes in light microscopy preparations (see Figs. 16, 20). Section from a rat hepatocyte.

1 Mitochondria with osmiophilic granula mitochondrialia
2 Polyribosomes
3 Free ribosomes
Electron microscopy; magnification: × 38 000

23 Granular (Rough) Endoplasmic Reticulum (rER)—Ergastoplasm

This figure shows *rER* double membranes, which are aligned in parallel and densely populated with ribosomes (*ergastoplasm*). In the bottom part of the picture, the transections are slightly curved. In some places, especially at their ends, the cisternae are distended into shapes resembling vacuoles, balloons or flasks. The *rER* content—consisting of proteins, which have all been synthesized on membrane-bound ribosomes—is frequently extracted during preparation, and therefore the rER cisternae appear empty.

However, in this section from a rat exocrine pancreatic cell, the narrow crevices as well as the large, distended cisternae show a fine granular or flocculent material. This material is the protein component of the definitive pancreatic excretion (cf. Figs. 21, 22, 26, 27, 149, 150).

The ergastoplasm—defined by the basophilic substance seen in light microscopy (see Fig. 18–20)—is not solely due to membrane-bound ribosomes. The free ribosomes and polysomes in the cytoplasm also contribute to basophilia (see Fig. 22).

1 Distended rER cisternae
Electron microscopy; magnification: × 33 500

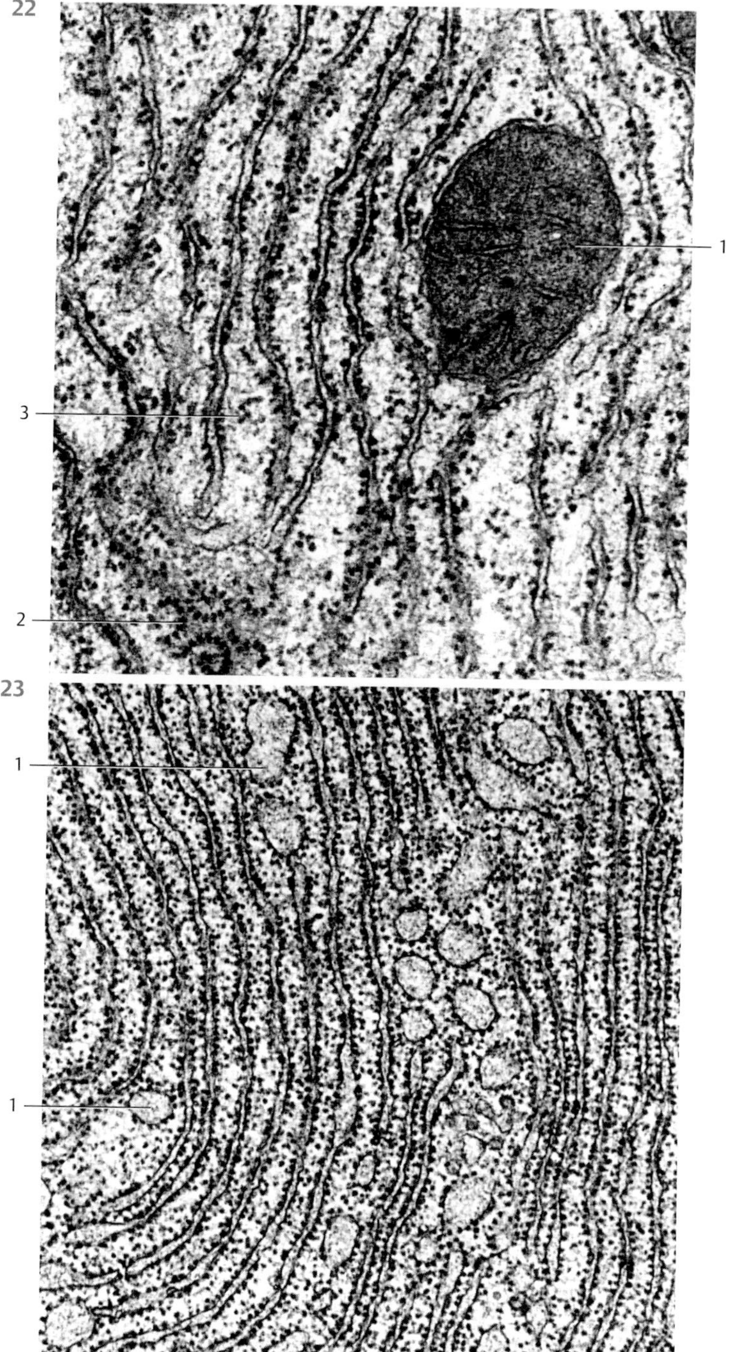
22
1
3
2
23
1
1

24 Granular (Rough) Endoplasmic Reticulum (rER)—Ergastoplasm—Nissl Bodies

The bluish-violet bodies or patches shown in Fig. 20 (*Nissl bodies, Nissl substance*) are ultrastructurally identical to the highly developed ergastoplasm (*rER*) 1, which consists of anastomosing stacked double membranes with bound ribosomes (cf. Figs. 21–23), rER-derived cisternae as well as regions with many free ribosomes 2.
Ribosomes are the smallest cell organelles. With a diameter of about 25 nm, they are clearly visible as *ribonucleoprotein particles* in transmission electron microscopy. Ribosomes are involved in the biosynthesis of proteins, including secretory, lysosomal and membrane-bound proteins. They consist of a large and a small subunit (see cytology or cytobiology textbooks).
Free ribosomes are present in large numbers in the cytoplasmic matrix, either as single ribosomes or in smaller groups (*polysomes*). It depends on the type of neuron whether groups of free polysomes or rER-bound ribosomes predominate.
While G.E. Palade described ribosomes as particles with high affinity to contrast dyes as early as 1955, the name "ribosome" was introduced later by R.B. Roberts in 1958.
This picture shows part of a Purkinje cell from the cerebellum. In the perikaryon are crista-type mitochondria and neurotubules.

1 rER
2 Ribosomes
L Lipofuscin granule (see Figs. 66–68, 256)
Electron microscopy ; magnification: × 14 000

25 Graular (Rough) Endoplasmic Reticulum (rER)—Ergastoplasm

Morphology and expansiveness of the rER can vary widely with cell function. In contrast with the stacked parallel membranes of the rER in Figs. 21–23, in this gland cell, the rough endoplasmic reticulum is distended into large cisternae of different sizes. Inside the cisternae is a very finely dispersed, only slightly osmiophilic material ("*reticuloplasm*") (cf. Fig. 23), which represents mostly secretory protein after its synthesis on membrane-bound ribosomes and segregation into the cisternae.
Lacrimal gland (glandula lacrimalis) from rhesus monkey.

1 rER cisternae
2 Secretory granules
3 Nucleus
4 Expanded intercellular spaces
Electron microscopy; magnification: × 33 000

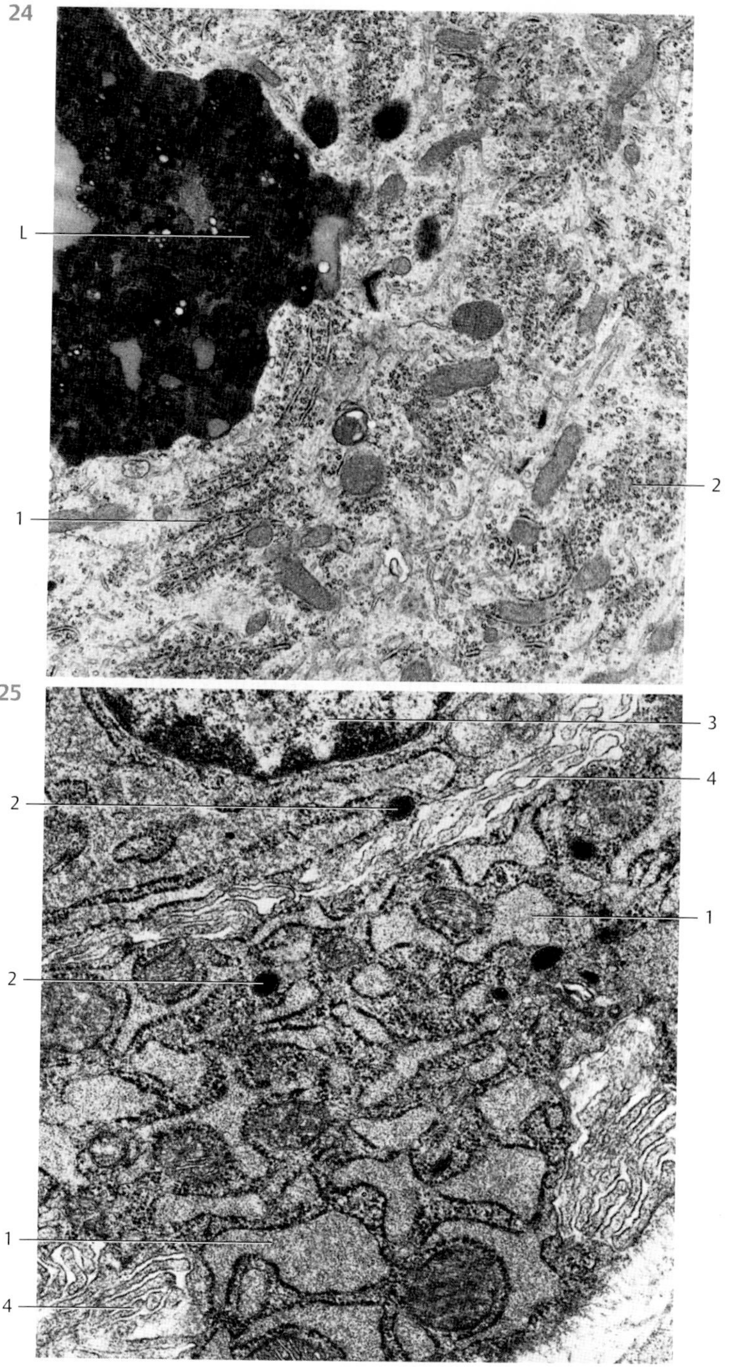
24
L
1
2
25
3
4
2
1
2
1
4

26 Agranular (Smooth) Endoplasmic Reticulum (sER)

The morphological difference between smooth or agranular ER and the granular form of ER is the absence of ribosomes. Rough ER proliferates to smooth ER, where the synthesis of lipid and steroid molecules occurs, cholesterol among others. In addition, *sER* metabolizes many xenobiotic substances, such as pharmaceuticals, pesticides and carcinogens, etc. The *sER* is therefore the most important intracellular detoxification system. It usually takes the form of a tightly woven network of branched tubules of various diameters (30–100 nm). Cisternae are usually absent. As in liver cells, for example, rough and smooth ER are often confluent. There is a pronounced expansion of the agranular ER (*sER*) in steroid hormone-producing cells, particularly in cells of the adrenal cortex, the corpus luteum and in the interstitial cells of the testes. Smooth ER is called sarcoplasmic reticulum in striated skeletal muscle tissue, where it serves to store calcium.
In this picture of an ovarian cell from the corpus luteum, the sER forms many membrane layers around a mitochondrion.

Electron microscopy; magnification: × 60 000

27 Agranular (Smooth) Endoplasmic Reticulum (sER)

Abundant smooth (agranular) ER in an interstitial hormone-producing ovary cell (see Figs. 26, 28–30). This picture shows another *membrane labyrinth*, which consists mostly of coiled tubules. The tubules are rarely cut to show their entire length over a longer distance. The tubules of the sER stream around the mitochondria ①. In the lower left corner ↗ is the section through a desmosome.

Electron microscopy; magnification: × 21 000

28 Agranular (Smooth) Endoplasmic Reticulum (sER)

Freeze-fractured smooth (agranular) ER (freeze-etching). This technique allows a three-dimensional view of the smooth ER membranes. The smooth membranes of the tubules appear interconnected and form a network of branched tubules in the cell. The darts point to the outer surfaces of the smooth tubules, the heads of the darts to the inside of the tubules. These tubules, which point toward the viewer and out of the picture, have been broken off.
Section showing part of the perikaryon of a sensory cell (rat) from the Jacobson organ (organum vomeronasale, VNO) (cf. Figs. 29, 30).

Electron microscopy; magnification: × 33 000

26

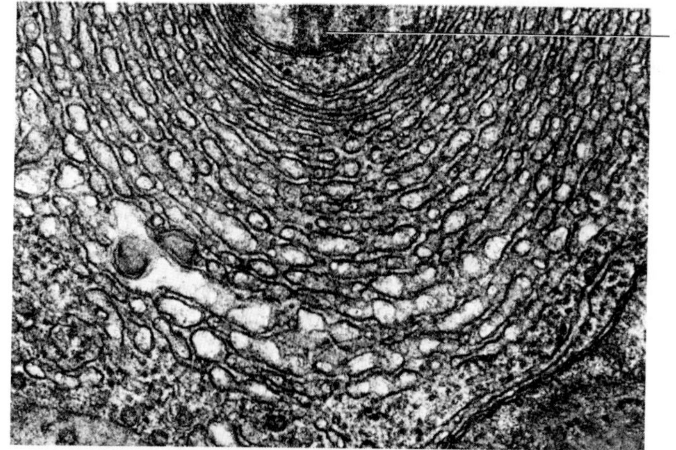

27

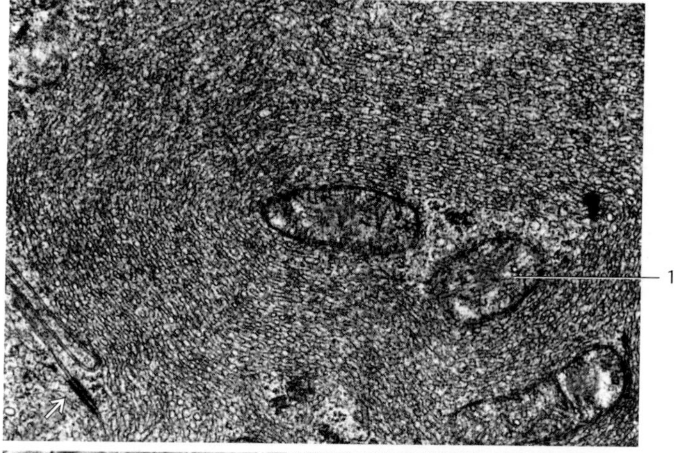

28

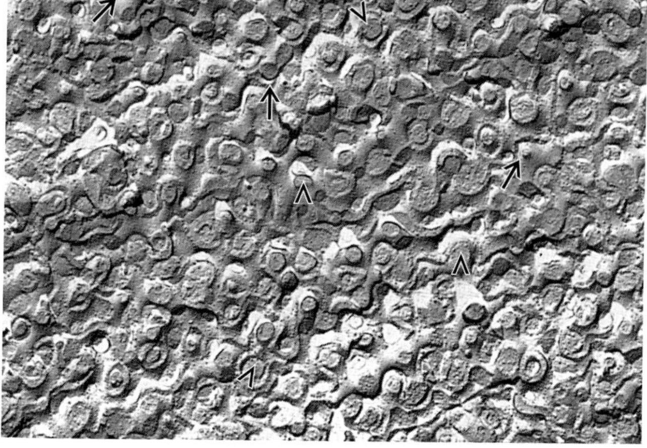

29 Agranular (Smooth) Endoplasmic Reticulum (sER)

Dependent on the cell type, the morphology of smooth (agranular) ER may vary considerably. The fixation technique will obviously influence the preservation and electron-microscopic presentation of the delicate membrane system as well. In this figure, the tubules of the agranular ER are arranged in loops and meandering lines (cf. Fig. 28). Note the only marginally stained cytoplasm between the tubules.

Striated muscle cells are also interspersed with smoothly lined tubules (*T- and L-system*) (see Fig. 232). All tubules combined form the *sarcoplasmic reticulum* of muscle cells or muscle fibers. This highly organized system of tubules exists in a characteristic relationship with the striation pattern of the myofibrils, and both combined will form impressive patterns.

Partial section of the perikaryon of a sensory cell from the rat Jacobson organ (organum vomeronasale, VNO)

Electron microscopy; magnification: × 30 000

30 Agranular (Smooth) Endoplasmic Reticulum (sER)

In some cells, both forms of endoplasmic reticulum coexist. The lower left half of the adjacent figure shows granular ER (*rER*), which is apparently continuous with the looped tubules of the agranular ER (sER) 2. The enzymes for the lipid and glycogen metabolisms are localized in the smooth ER membrane system. Various lipoids, for example, are synthesized in the sER of steroid-producing cells, which biosynthesize steroid hormones from cholesterol.

Partial section of a sensory cell perikaryon from the Jacobson organ of the rat (organum vomeronasale, VNO).

1 Granular ER (rER) membranes
2 Meandering tubules of the smooth ER (sER)
Electron microscopy; magnification: × 30 000

31 Annulate Lamellae

Annulate lamellae are a specialized form of smooth endoplasmic reticulum membrane. They articulate from the nuclear membrane and form concentric layers of lamellae or, as seen here, membrane stacks. The cisternae show *porecomplexes* 1, which are identical to those of the nuclear pore complexes (cf. Fig. 11). Osmiophilic material is more abundant in the pore regions.

Annulate lamellae are prevalent in cells with a high membrane turnover, such as tumor cells, testicular Sertoli cells and gametes. This figure shows details from a human oocyte.

1 Pores with osmiophilic material
2 Mitochondria
3 Granular ER (rER)
Electron microscopy; magnification: × 50 000

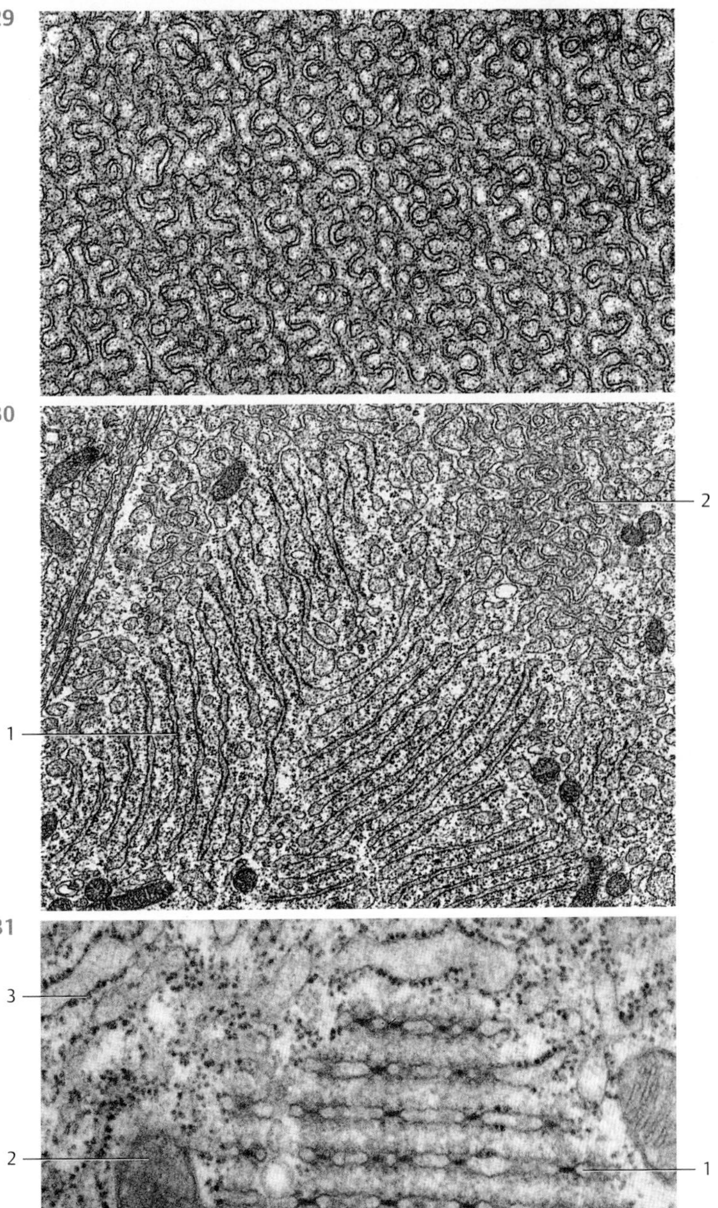
29
30
2
1
31
3
2
1

32 Golgi Apparatus

The Golgi apparatus was named after Camillo Golgi (Nobel Prize 1906), who discovered this cell structure in nerve cells (1898) and assigned it the role of a cell organelle. The Golgi apparatus is ubiquitous in cells. The figure shows spinal ganglion cells with cytoplasmic structures in the form of black rods, hooks or loops 1. In differentiated polar cells from exocrine glands, they are located in the apical third of the cell, frequently in close proximity to secretory granules (see Figs. 33–37). Inspired by its appearance, Golgi named this cell structure the inner reticular apparatus (“*apparato reticolare interno*”). The Golgi apparatus is not stained in routine histological preparations. However, components of the Golgi apparatus can reduce metal ions.

1 Golgi apparatus (apparato reticolare interno)
2 Ganglia nucleus with clearly visible nucleolus
3 Nuclei in satellite cells
Stain: Kopsch-Kolatschew osmium stain; magnification: × 260

33 Golgi Apparatus

The *Golgi apparatus* consists of membranes that are about 6–8 nm thick. The basic unit of the Golgi apparatus is the *dictyosome* or *Golgi field*. In this section, it consists of a stack of 3–8 smooth (i.e., ribosome-free) slightly arcuate stacked membranes in close proximity to each other. The membranes enclose long narrow cisternae, which are slightly wider at both ends. The dictyosome can be compared to a stack of flat membrane sacs with osmiophilic content (*export proteins*). Golgi cisternae are always accompanied by Golgi vesicles 1, which deliver and export material (*transport vesicles*). The Golgi apparatus has therefore two faces, a *convex* (*cis-*), or *forming face* 2 and a *concave* trans-*face*, or *secretory face* 3. Prespermatid from *Eisenia foetida.*

1 Golgi vesicle (transport vesicle)
2 Convex, *cis*-face
3 Concave, *trans*-face
4 Nucleus, partial section
Electron microscopy; magnification: × 33 000

34 Golgi Apparatus

Large *Golgi apparatus* with smooth double membranes and Golgi vacuoles (see Figs. 35–37). Some of the cisternae are distended 1. At the concave side (trans-*face*) of the cisternae, there are very small vesicles (transport vesicles); among them are coated vesicles, but also somewhat larger vacuoles. They contain variable amounts of secretory products. The more or less sharply curved membrane stacks of the Golgi complex feature a *convex* cis-*face* (*uptake side*) and a *concave* trans-*face* (*export side*). These two distinct sides also contain different sets of enzymes.

1 Distended Golgi cisternae
2 Secretory granules
3 Mitochondria
4 Golgi vesicles (transport vesicles)
Electron microscopy; magnification: × 25 000

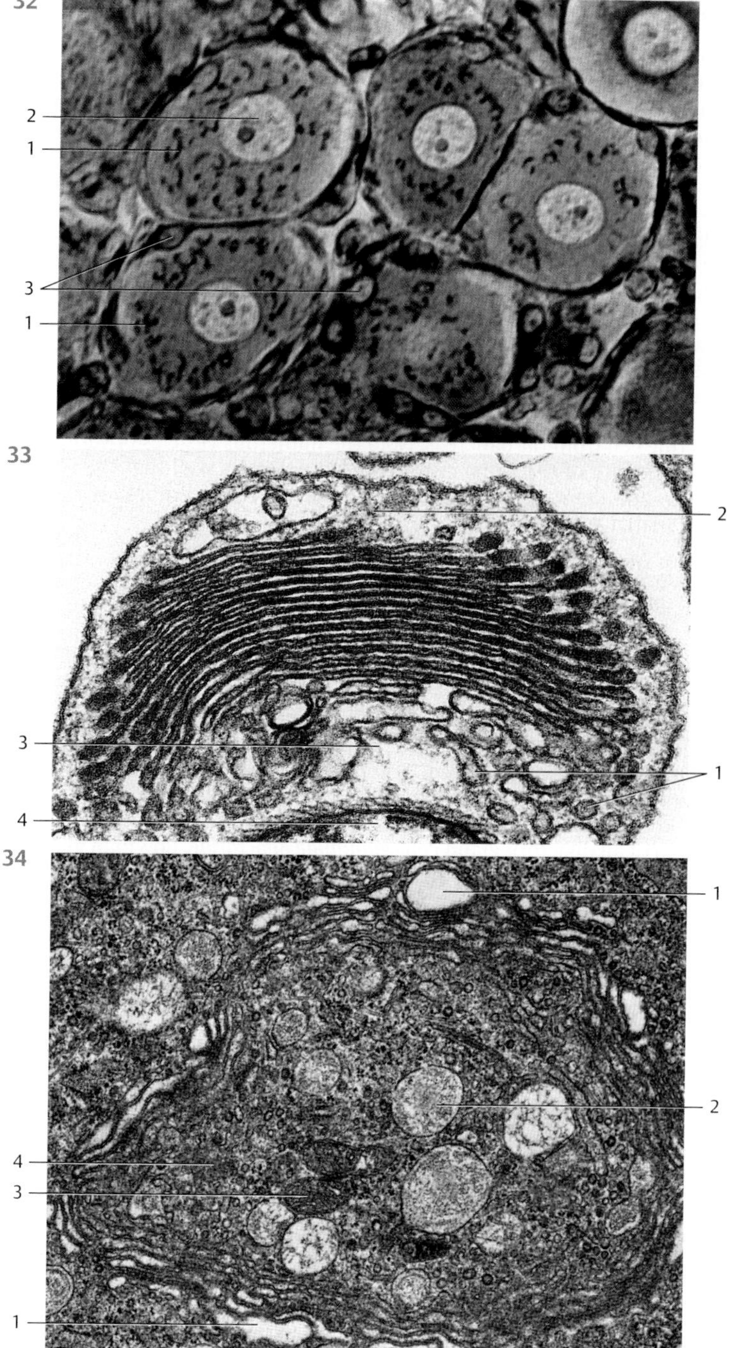
32
2
1
3
1
33
2
3
1
4
34
1
2
4
3
1

35 Golgi Apparatus

The Golgi apparatus often contains several *dictyosomes* (Golgi fields). In cells with a polar structure, dictyosomes are usually localized in the supranuclear region. The basic structural unit of the Golgi apparatus, however, is the Golgi cisterna. It is a flat, 1–2 μm wide membrane sac, which is often dilated and fenestrated at the outer edges. Several of these cisternae form a functional dictyosome. All dictyosomes in a cell combined make up the Golgi apparatus. The ultrastructure of the Golgi apparatus (*Golgi complex*) is distinct in its detail. The electron-microscopic examination of thin sections of cells reveals the Golgi apparatus as a characteristically structured system of smooth double membranes (*sacculi*), which are either arranged in parallel stacks, or are layered around vacuoles. The membranes do not communicate with each other. Often, 6–8 membrane profiles form a stack of flat or arcuate cisternae. Most of them are distended at the ends, like flasks. At those ends are small vesicles (*transport vesicles*) and vacuoles, which have been pinched off from the distended cisternae (*sacculi*) (see Fig. 34, 36, 37).
Exocrine cell from rat pancreas. Note the numerous vesicles of various sizes in the vicinity of the Golgi cisternae, and notice as well that the Golgi apparatus and the rough endoplasmic reticulum (rER) membranes 4 are in a close spatial arrangement.

1 *cis*-Face
2 *trans*-Face
3 Mitochondria
4 Granular ER (rER)
Electron microscopy; magnification: × 30 000

36 Golgi Apparatus

This figure and Fig. 37 show that dictyosomes can have quite different shapes. In contrast to the cisternae depicted in Figs. 33, 34 and 35, the *Golgi cisternae* here are very bloated 1. At the *trans*-face 2 are numerous vesicles, some are covered by a *protein coat* 3. However, this coat is different from the well-known coat of "*coated vesicles*," which is made of *clathrin*.
Section of an olfactory gland cell (*glandulae olfactoriae*, Bowman glands).

1 Golgi cisternae
2 *trans*-Face
3 Golgi vesicles with coat (protein cover)
4 Granular ER (rER) membranes
5 *cis*-Face
Electron microscopy; magnification: × 33 000

37 Golgi Apparatus

This picture displays a mightily developed Golgi apparatus in an exocrine gland cell. It consists of several distended membrane cisternae 1 and shows on its concave side (trans-*face*) 2 numerous Golgi vesicles of various sizes 3 and large, sometimes confluent secretory vacuoles 4. Section from a cell from the tissue of the Harder gland from *Passer domesticus* (sparrow).

1 Golgi cisternae
2 *trans*-Face
3 Golgi vesicles
4 Secretory vacuoles
5 *cis*-Face
Electron microscopy; magnification: × 22 000

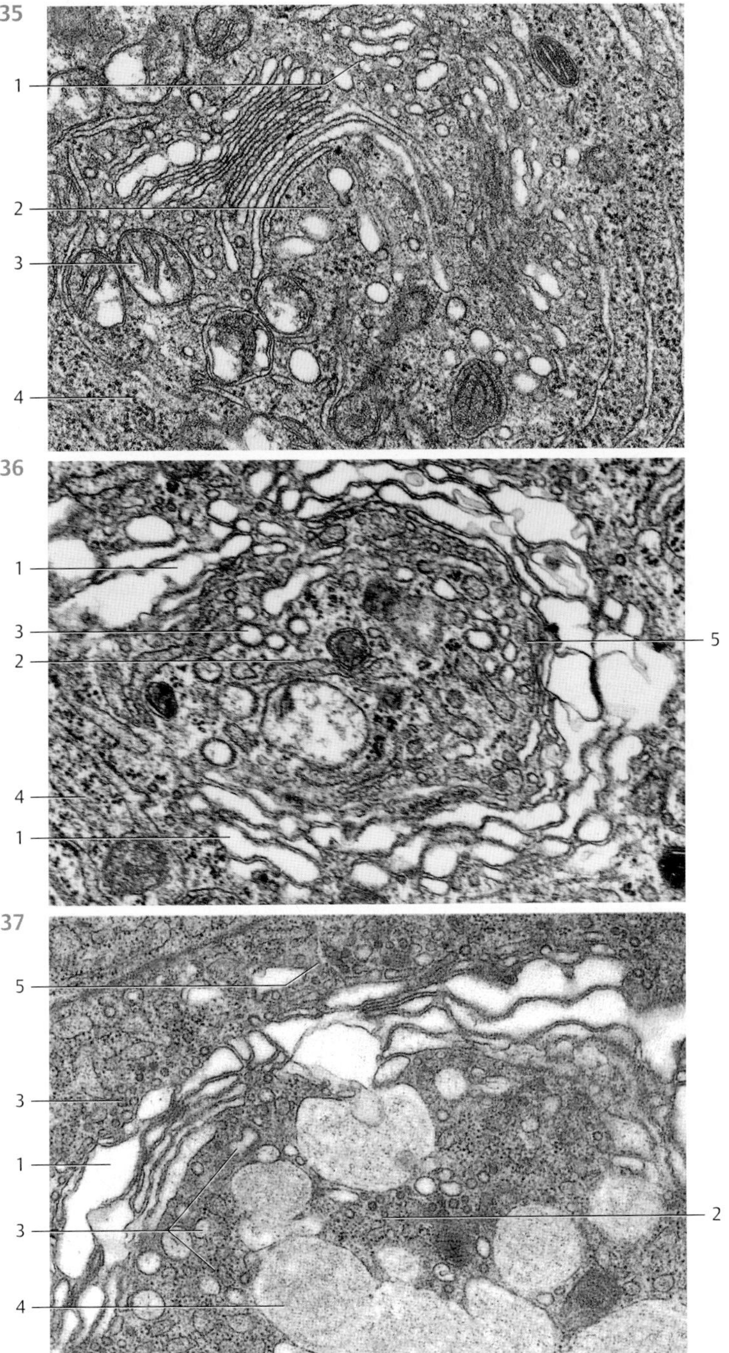
35
1
2
3
4
36
1
3
2
4
1
5
37
5
3
1
3
4
2

38 Mitochondria

Before the turn of the 19th century, Altmann discovered and described mitochondria, the power plant organelle of cells, as granular, rod-like stringy cell components. In 1898, C. Benda introduced the term *mitochondria* for these "*threaded bodies*" (mitos, Greek: thread; chondros, Greek: granulum). Later (1952–1953), electron microscopy made it possible for G.E. Palade and F.S. Sjöstrand to show the characteristic structural details of mitochondria. This figure shows mitochondria [1] in the epithelial cells of renal tubules. The mitochondria stand out as long, black-brown rods, which line up in the basal cytoplasm to almost parallel rows. The cell nuclei [2] are not visible; their positions appear as gaps.

1 Mitochondria in the form of short rods
2 Epithelial cell nuclei
3 Blood vessels
Stain: Heidenhain iron hematoxylin; magnification: × 950

39 Mitochondria

The basic structure follows the same principle layout in all mitochondria. An outer membrane (*outer mitochondrial membrane*) separates the mitochondrion from the cytoplasm. Inside this outer membrane (border) lies the inner membrane. It forms septum-like folds (*cristae mitochondriales*), which extend to various lengths across the organelle (*crista-type mitochondria*). The inner and outer membranes separate two cell compartments. Between the outer and inner membrane, separated by about 8 nm, lies the outer compartment (*outer metabolic compartment, intermembrane space*), which extends into the crevices of the cristae. The inner membrane and its cristae forms the border around the inner compartment (*inner metabolic space*). It contains a homogeneous or granular matrix of variable density (cf. Figs. 40–44). The inner mitochondrial matrix often contains granules, the *granula mitochondrialia* or *matrix granules*, which have a size of 30–50 nm and are rich in Ca^{2+} and other ions.
This picture shows mitochondria from a heart muscle cell.

1 Myofilament bundles of the striated heart muscle cell
Electron microscopy; magnification: × 47 000

40 Mitochondria

Sizes and shapes of mitochondria can be very different. On average, they are 0.25 μm thick and 2–7 μm long. Nevertheless, there are also giant forms (*giant mitochondria*). The number of *cristae mitochondriales* also varies. As a result, the sizes of the inner and outer compartments (cf. Figs. 39, 41–44) are also different. The figure shows mitochondria (crista-type) in a cell from the mucosal stomach lining, which have been cut in different planes. Note the *granula mitochondrialia,* with diameters between 30–50 nm in the matrix (*matrix granules*).

Electron microscopy; magnification: × 28 800

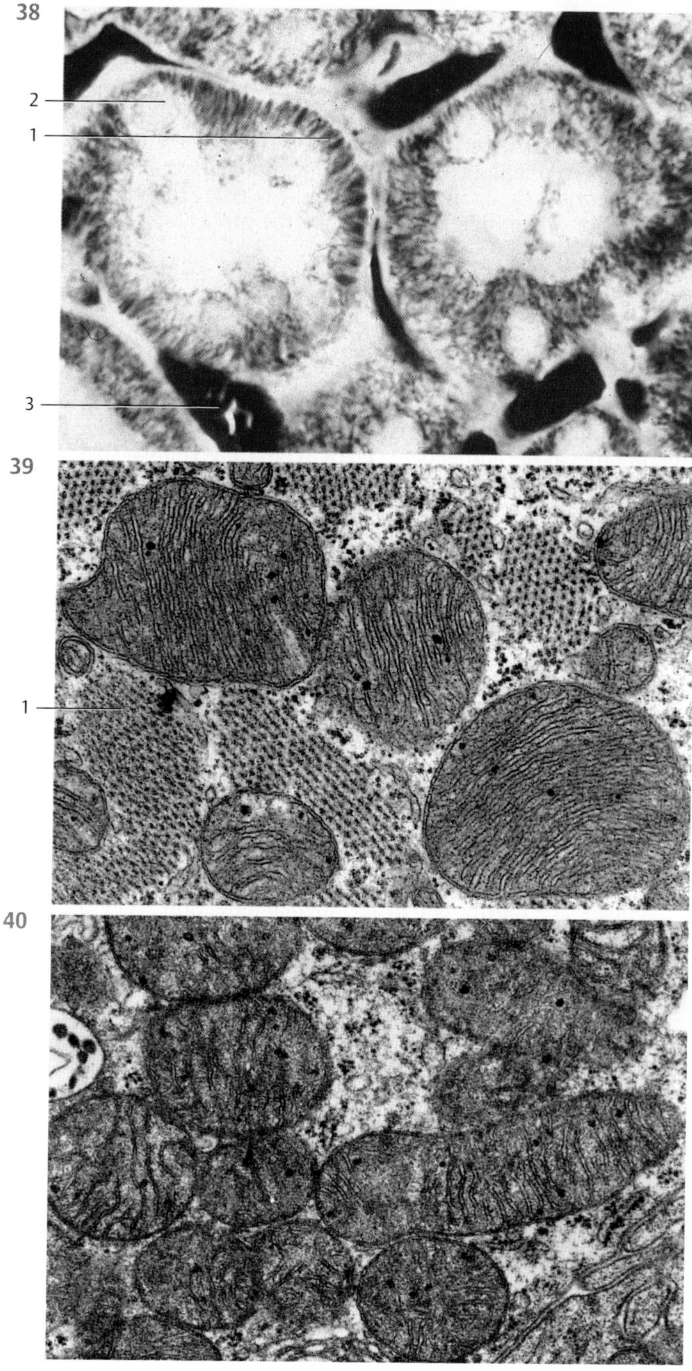
38
2
1
3
39
1
40

41 Mitochondria

Predominantly oval, crista-type mitochondria from an epithelial cell of a proximal kidney tubule. The folds that originate at the inner membranes and extend into the inner centers of the mitochondria—the *cristae mitochondriales*—are different in length and form a series of incomplete transverse septa. Note the osmiophilic *granula mitochondrialia* in the matrix. Some of the mitochondria are cut tangentially, and their cristae therefore appear diffuse, or are not discernible at all. Between the mitochondria are the basal plasmalemma folds.

Electron microscopy; magnification: × 26 000

42 Mitochondria

Oval-shaped, often arcuate, crista-type mitochondria with an electron-dense (osmiophilic) matrix (cf. Figs. 39–41) are lined up alongside the inner cell membranes at the border between two cells (intercellular space) 1. Note the *interdigitations* 1 between neighboring gland cells.
Gland cells with secretory granules 2 from the human lacrimal gland (glandula lacrimalis).

1 Intercellular space with interdigitations
2 Secretory granules
↑ Contact between cells (desmosome)
Electron microscopy; magnification: × 8400

43 Mitochondria

Apart from crista-type mitochondria, there are also mitochondria with inner membranes, which protrude into the mitochondrion like fingers or sacs 1. These are *tubular* or *saccular*-type mitochondria. The processes can also be rod-like or have edges, as they do in prismatic-type mitochondria. Tubular and saccular-type mitochondria occur in steroid hormone-producing cells.
The figure shows oval, slender mitochondria in cells from the adrenal cortex. Their tubules are mostly cut in rectangular direction. They are visually empty. Note the dense mitochondrial matrix and the light space between the outer and inner membranes. Between the mitochondria are smooth ER membranes and ribosomes.

1 Tubuli mitochondriales, cut lengthwise
2 Lipid vacuole
3 Cell nucleus, cut tangentially
Electron microscopy; magnification: × 20 000

44 Mitochondria

Tubular-type mitochondria in an adrenal cortex cell from the *zona fasciculata* (cf. Fig. 43). Winding tubules extend from the inner mitochondrial membrane. They are cut at different angles along their winding paths. The result is a section with a variety of profiles.

Electron microscopy; magnification: × 22 100

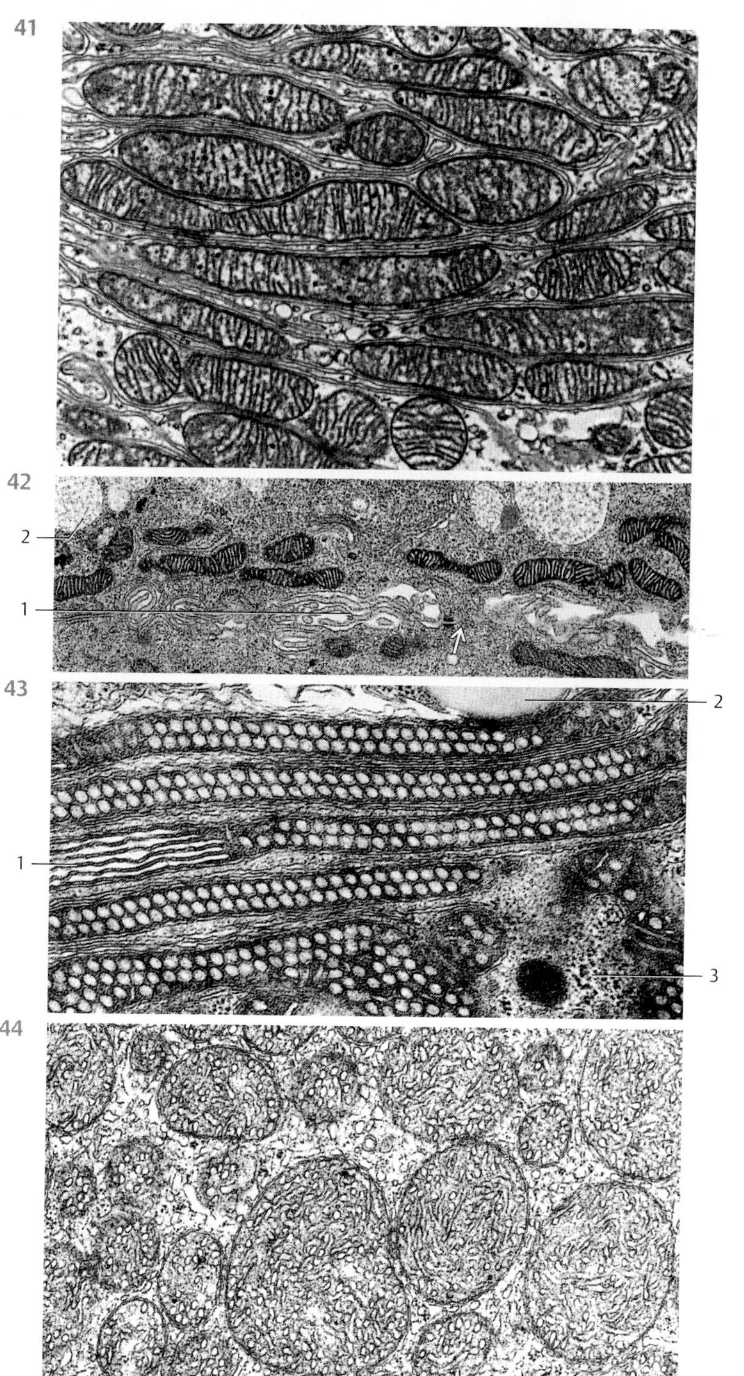
41
42
2
1
43
2
1
3
44

45 Lysosomes

C. de Duve identified *lysosomes* as unique cell organelles relatively late—only in 1955. Their membrane-contained bodies are rich in *acid hydrolases* with pH-optima between 4.5 and 5.0. These enzymes are specific to lysosomes and can be used as marker enzymes. Histochemical identification of these marker enzymes allows it to localize and visualize lysosomes using light microscopy. Due to their acid hydrolase content, lysosomal cell compartments play an important role in the intracellular digestion or *degradation* of endogenous substances (*autophagy*) and phagocytosed substances (*heterophagy*). Lysosomes store insoluble metabolites and participate in the autolysis of cells. This figure shows cells from the adrenal gland (see Figs. 480, 495). Four glomeruli and numerous sections through different parts of the urinary tubules are visible. The epithelial cells from these tubules contain different numbers of red-stained granular bodies. These represent lysosomes, which contain *acid phosphatase*, the marker enzyme for this organelle (cf. Figs. 46, 47, 66–68).

Burstone histochemical acid phosphatase stain; magnification: × 80

46 Lysosomes

In electron microscopy, lysosomes appear as membrane-enclosed bodies of varied geometry. Their sizes are 0.1–1.2 µm. Before lysosomes participate in intracellular digestive functions, they contain only lysosomal enzymes. At that stage, they are called *primary lysosomes* or *lysosomal transport vesicles*. They arise from the *trans*-face of the Golgi apparatus. Primary lysosomes are able to fuse with phagocytotic vacuoles (*phagosomes, autophagosomes,* or *heterophagosomes*, respectively). These vacuoles contain substances, which must be digested. The fusion leads to *cytolysosomes* (*autophagolysosomes* or *heterophagolysosomes*), commonly called *secondary lysosomes*. The figure shows two phagolysosomes with many ingested granules and vacuoles with different content. There is also a primary lysosome ⧄. Lysosomes are also referred to as the lytic (acid) cell compartment. Pericyte from a capillary.

1 Endothelium of a capillary
Electron microscopy; magnification: × 13 000

47 Lysosomes

Telophagolysosome (*residual body*) in a human cell from the submandibular gland, with heteromorphic content. Lipofuscin granules, which are seen in some cell types (see Fig. 66), represent tertiary (permanent) lysosomes (*residual lysosomes, telolysosomes*). In contrast, the rod or disk-shaped granules in neutrophil granulocytes (see Fig. 351) and the discus-shaped granules with crystalloid content in eosinophil granulocytes (see Fig. 143) are primary lysosomes.

1 Secretory granules
2 Granular ER (rER) membranes
Electron microscopy; magnification: × 30 000

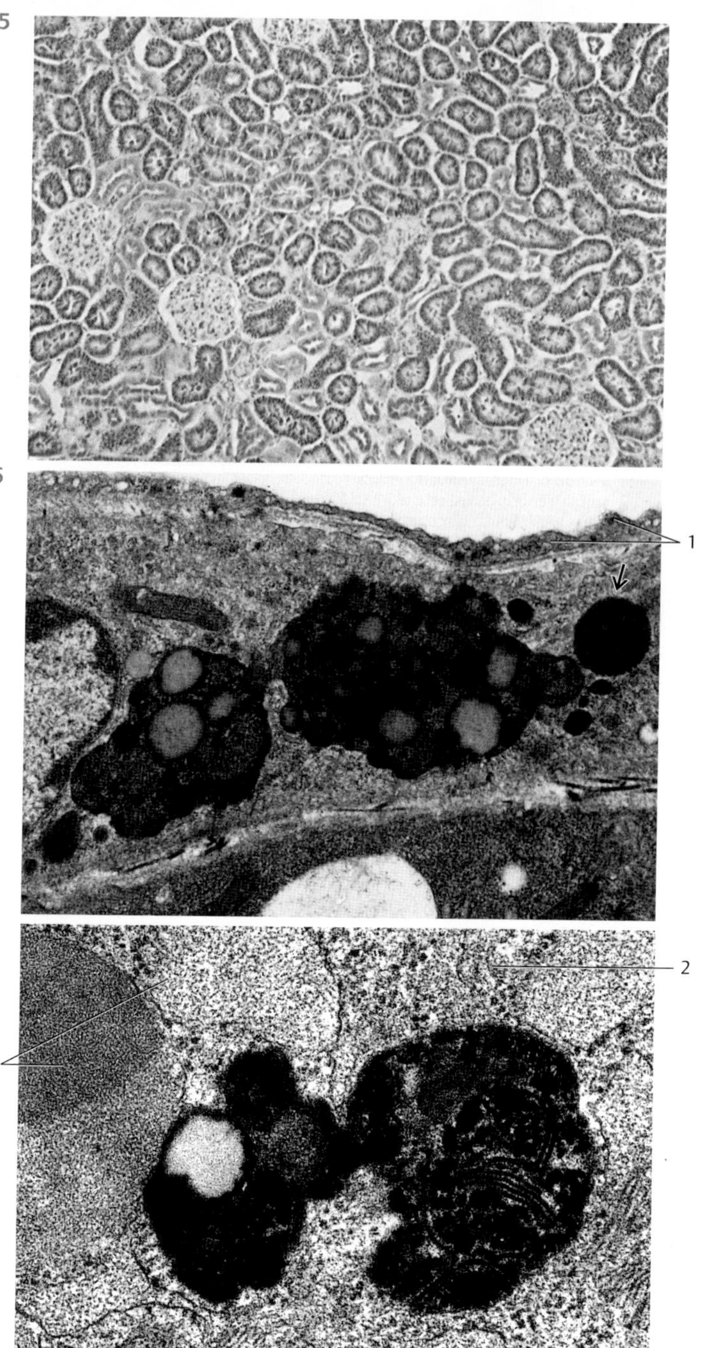
45
46
1
47
2
1

48 Peroxisomes

In 1965, C. de Duve discovered *peroxisomes* in liver cells. J.A. Rhodin had previously described them as "*microbodies.*" They are small, spherical organelles with a diameter of about 0.2–1.5 μmm, which are ubiquitous in cells. Peroxisomes have a single membrane as their outer border. Their finely granular or homogeneous content is electron-dense. Occasionally, peroxisomes enclose paracrystalline materials. Peroxisomes are respiratory organelles. They contain various oxidases, catalase and the enzymes for the β-oxidation of fatty acids. Peroxisomes owe their name to their peroxidative enzyme content. They play an important role in the detoxification of cells. Example: the enzyme catalase will split hydrogen peroxide, a lethal cell poison. Genetic diseases that are based on peroxisomal defects include *Zellweger syndrome*, *Refsum syndrome* and *adrenoleukodystrophy* (see textbooks of pathology and internal medicine).
Section from an epithelial cell (human liver) with two peroxisomes of different sizes.

1 Section through a mitochondrion
2 Smooth endoplasmic reticulum (sER) membranes
3 Areas with cellular glycogen (glycogen removed)
Histochemical catalase staining; magnification: × 60 000

49 Peroxisomes

Section through a mouse epithelial cell from a proximal kidney tubule with several *peroxisomes*, which are rich in *catalase* 1.

1 Peroxisomes
2 Nucleus (partial section)
3 Mitochondria (crista-type)
4 Granular ER (rER) membranes
5 Peritubular connective tissue space
Histochemical catalase staining; magnification: × 10 000

50 Multivesicular Bodies

Multivesicular bodies (*MVBs*) 1 in a canine epithelial cell (liver), which are located in the cytosol, close to the apical cell border. Multivesicular bodies are vacuoles with a surrounding membrane and a variable number of enclosed small vesicles. They are part of the group of secondary lysosomes and contain acid phosphatase, among other components. MVBs probably play a role in *crinophagy*, meaning that they help recapture an excess of secretory products in the cells of endocrine and exocrine glands.

1 Multivesicular bodies
2 Protein-coated vesicles
3 Mitochondrion (section)
4 Gall capillary
5 Glycogen containing areas (glycogen removed)
6 Granular ER (rER) membranes
Electron microscopy; magnification: × 40 000

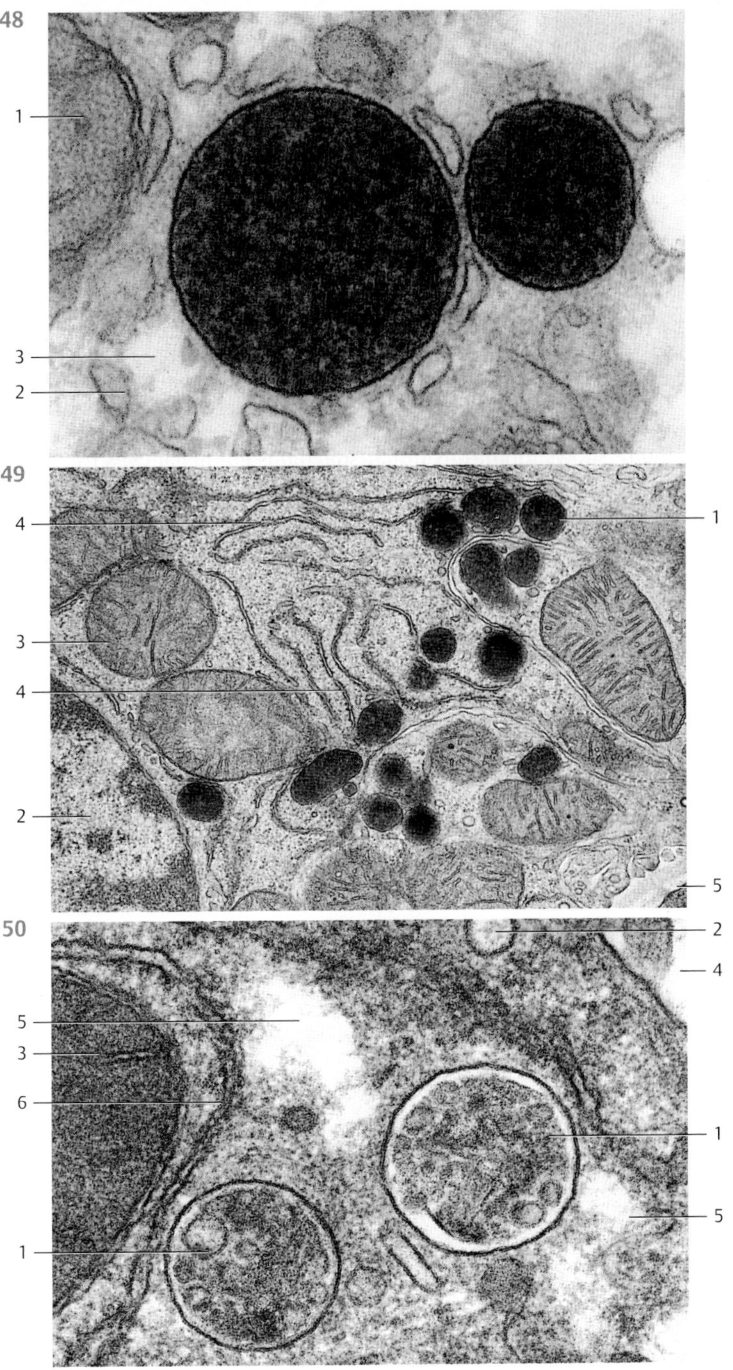
48
1
3
2
49
4
1
3
4
2
5
50
2
4
5
3
6
1
1
5

51 Tonofibrils

Strings of several different filament networks span the cytoplasmic matrix of cells to form the cytoskeleton. These networks are a dynamic system. There are three distinct networks with morphologically different structures: *microfilaments, intermediary filaments* and *microtubules*. Among others, there are *desmin, vimentin* and *spectrin* filaments, also *neurofilaments* in neurons, *glial filaments* in glial cells and *keratin filaments* in epidermal epithelium. Each of these networks is built from specific proteins. As a group, they are sometimes still referred to as "*metaplasmic*" structures—a name that was coined in the era of light microscopy. The tonofibrils (resistance fibrils) often serve as a well-known demonstration example of a fiber network. Tonofibrils are particularly impressive in cells from multilayered squamous epithelium in mechanically resilient tissue. These tonofibrils are dense bundles of *intermediary protein filaments* (*cytokeratin filaments*) of undefined lengths (see Figs. 52, 55) and can be seen using a light microscope. Intermediary filaments have diameters of 8–10 nm.
This figure shows tonofibrils in flat squamous epithelial cells from bovine hoof.

Stain: Heidenhain iron hematoxylin; magnification: × 400

52 Tonofilaments—Cytokeratin Filaments

Using electron microscopy, the light microscopic images of intracellular *tonofibrils* (see Fig. 51) prove to be bundles of very fine filaments. The bundles are either strictly parallel or wavy bundles, which create the image of brush strokes in electron micrographs. Tonofibrils pervade especially the cells in the lower layers of the multilayered squamous epithelium. They line up in the direction of the tensile force. However, filament bundles also extend from the cell center to areas with many desmosomes (see Figs. 55, 95–98).
Tonofilament bundles in the epithelial cell of the vaginal portio uteri.

Electron microscopy; magnification: × 36 000

53 Microtubules

Microtubules exist in all cells and consist of extended noncontractile tubes, which are several micrometers long and have no branches (see Fig. 59). Their outer diameter is 21–24 nm, the inner diameter is 14–16 nm. The tubule wall is about 8 nm thick and densely structured. It is built from globular, helical proteins (*tubulin*), which themselves are composed of 13 lengthwise running protofilaments. Microtubules not only maintain the geometry of cells (*cytoskeleton*), they also participate in the construction of kinocilia, centrioles, kinetosomes and the mitosis spindles. Another of their many functions is the regulated intracellular transport of materials and organelles.
Microtubules ⤢ in an epithelium cell from the endometrium.

Electron microscopy; magnification: × 46 000

51

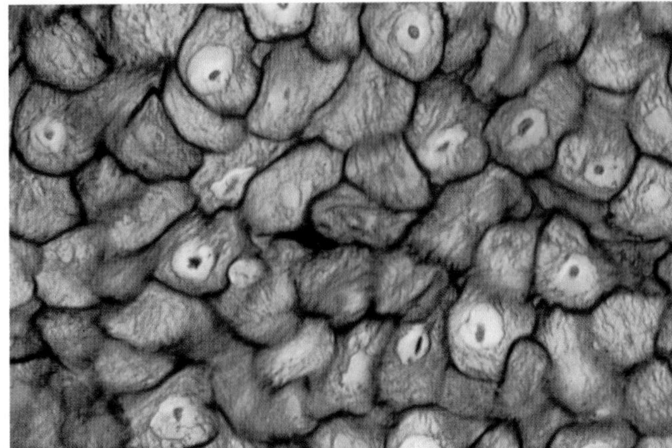

52

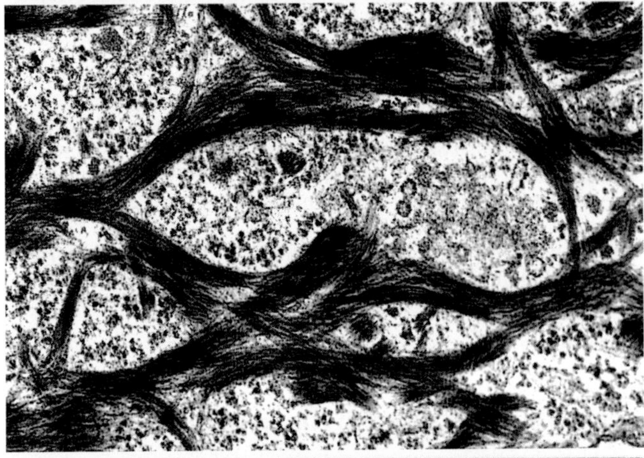

53

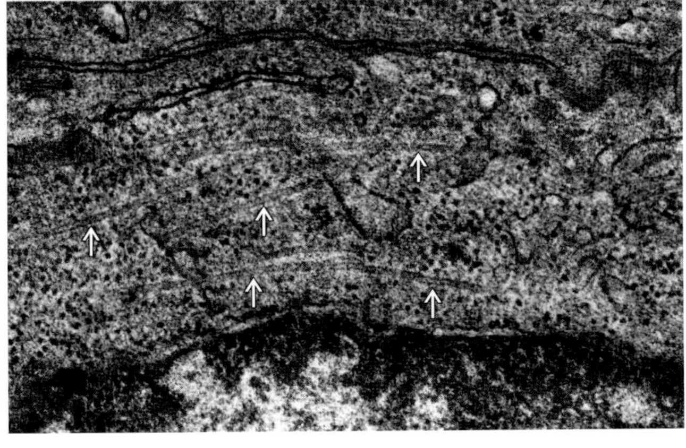

54 Microfilaments—Actin Filament Cytoskeleton

Microfilaments consist of G-actin (actin filaments) and have a diameter of 5–7 nm. They occur as single filaments or as bundles—for example, underneath the cell membrane, in cell processes and in microvilli (see Figs. 56, 75, 77, 78). This figure shows the system of *actin filaments* in endothelial cells from the human umbilical vein, using fluorescence-labeled antibodies against actin. Thick, 100–200 nm wide bundles of actin filaments are characteristic of endothelial cells in culture (shown here) and in situ. These filaments, named stress fibers, improve the adhesion of endothelial cells and protect them from the shearing forces of the bloodstream.

Fluorescence microscopy; magnification: × 690

55 Intermediary Filaments—the Tonofilament System

In addition to actin filaments and microtubules, *intermediary filaments* (*tonofilaments*) are the third system making up the intracellular cytoskeleton of eukaryotic cells. Their diameter is 7–11 nm. This makes them thicker than microfilaments (5–7 nm) and thinner than microtubules (20–25 nm). Currently, five subclasses of intermediary filaments are defined: the *cytokeratin filaments* in epithelial cells (see Figs. 51, 52); *desmin filaments*, the characteristic structures in smooth cells and striated muscle fibers; glia filaments, *glia acidic fibrillary protein* (*GAFP*) in astrocytes; *neurofilaments* in neurons from the central and peripheral nervous system; and *vimentin filaments*, which are characteristic of cells of mesenchymal origin (fibroblasts, chondrocytes, macrophages, endothelial cells, etc.).
This figure shows vimentin-type intermediary filaments (tonofilaments) in human endothelial cells from the umbilical vein. Staining was done using a fluorescence-labeled antibody against vimentin.

Fluorescence microscopy; magnification: × 480

56 Microfilaments—Actin Filament Cytoskeleton

Immunohistochemical reactions are also helpful on the level of electron-microscopic investigations. The figure shows evidence for the presence of actin in human *brush border* epithelium from the small intestine using electron microscopy. For this immunohistochemical preparation, antibodies against actin were adsorbed to colloidal gold. In the section, gold particles will then indicate the location of actin. The microvilli in this image exhibit a supporting skeleton of actin filaments, which continues downward to the apical cytoplasm of the enterocytes (see Figs. 77, 78).

1 Cytoplasm
2 Intercellular space
Electron microscopy; magnification: × 32 000

54

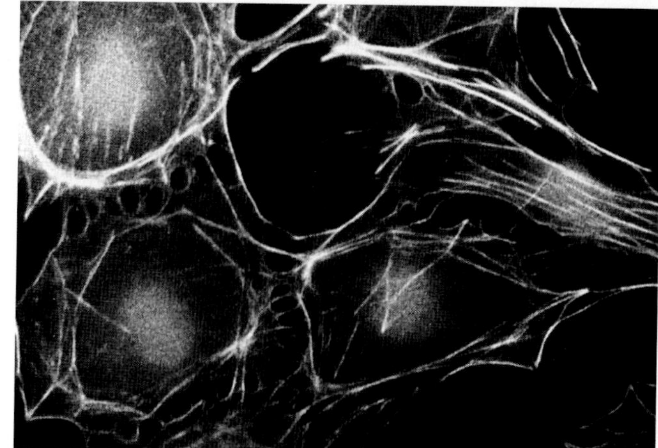

55

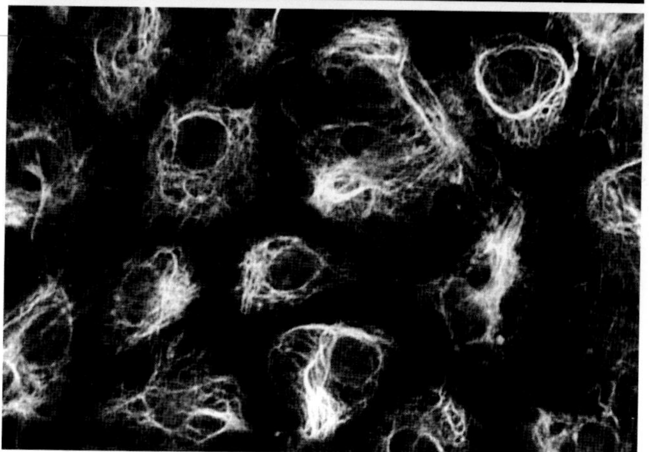

56

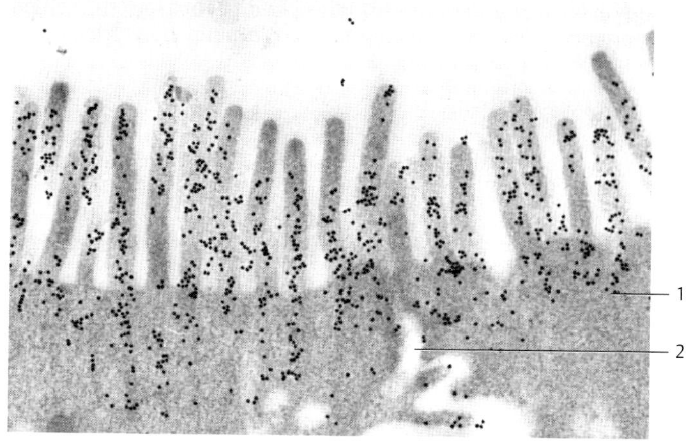

57 Microfilaments—Actin Filament Cytoskeleton

Actin is a polymer protein and the main component of the actin filaments, which are about 7 nm thick. Actin filaments are double filaments (*F-actin*), which contain two rows of globular proteins in helical configuration (*G-actin*). They are usually assembled in slender bundles. In nonmuscle cells, they are called *stress fibers*, because they lend structured support to cells (see Fig. 54). Bundles of actin filaments (*stress fibers*) can be seen using nothing more elaborate than phase-contrast microscopy. However, their identity can be elegantly proven by indirect immunofluorescence using antibodies against actin. The figure on the right shows stretched actin filament bundles (stress fibers) in isolated endothelial cells from bovine aorta. The actin antibody is labeled with the fluorescent dye fluorescein isothiocyanate (FITC) + phalloidin. Phalloidin is the poison in the *Amanita phalloides* mushroom. It binds to F-actin filaments, stabilizes them and by doing so prevents polymerization.

Fluorescence microscopy; magnification: × 700

58 Intermediary Filaments—Vimentin Filaments

Vimentin is the *intermediary filament* protein, which occurs in fibroblasts and endothelial cells as well as in other nonmuscle mesenchymal cells.
This figure shows *vimentin filaments* in cytokeratin-negative endothelial cells in tissue culture after their isolation from bovine aorta. Vimentin in these cells was traced by immunohistochemistry. The vimentin antibody was labeled with the fluorescent dye rhodamine. Bundles of vimentin filaments were shown to envelop part of the cell nuclei.

Fluorescence microscopy; magnification: × 700

59 Microtubules

Microtubules, in conjunction with intermediary and actin filaments, form the *cytoskeleton* (see Fig. 53).
This figure shows *microtubules* in isolated cytokeratin-negative endothelial cells from bovine aorta. The microtubules originate with a location called *microtubule organization center* (*MTOC*) and fan out into the cell periphery. The antibodies against the α-tubulin and β-tubulin dimer from microtubules were labeled with rhodamine.

Fluorescence microscopy; magnification: × 700

57

58

59

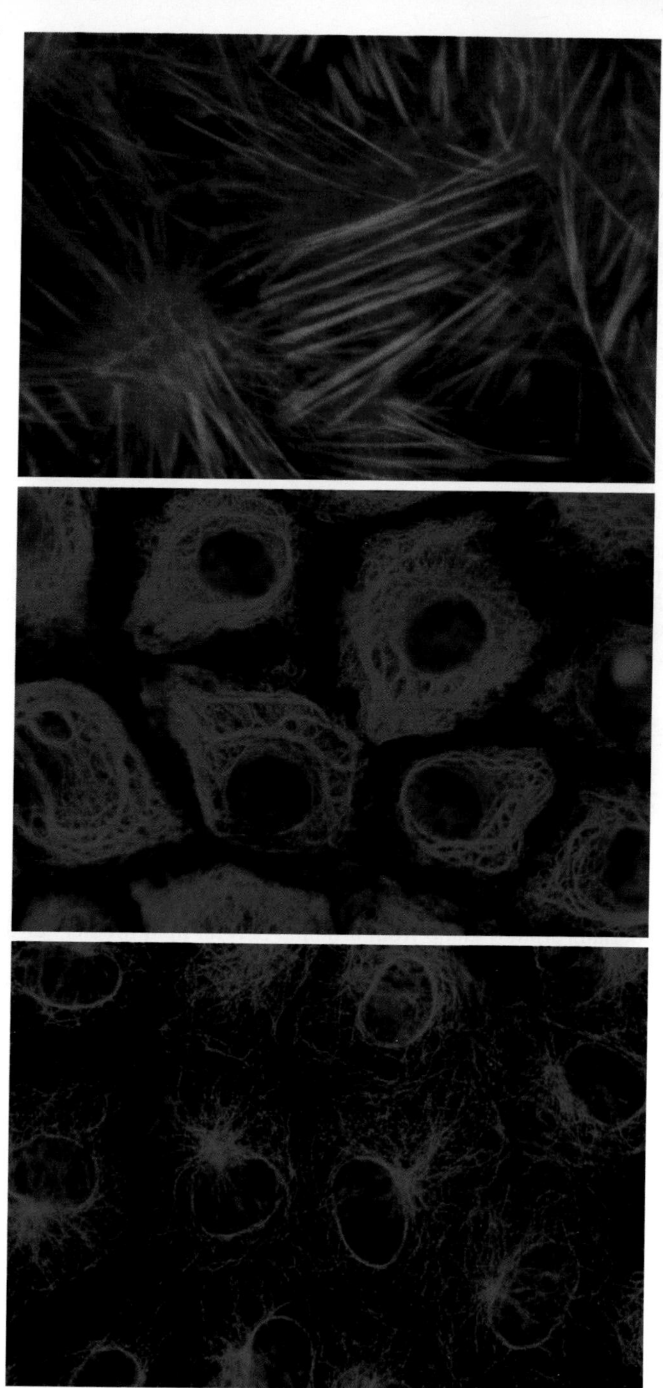

60 Lipid Droplets—Hyaline Cartilage

Paraplasmic substances (*cell inclusions*, stored materials) are either derived from metabolic activities (*storage materials*) or from the enclosure of "dead" substances (*metabolic residue* or *phagocytosed materials*). Carbohydrates, proteins, fat (mostly triglycerides), ferritin (iron storage particles) and pigments are among the most important paraplasmic inclusions.
This figure shows four isogenous cartilage cells (two *chondrons* or *territories*) with fat droplets of different sizes. These fat droplets (stained red) are characteristic of mature *chondrocytes* (see Fig. 61). The cell nuclei are stained blue. There is a narrow border between the cartilage cells, which stands out because of its high refractive index. This is the *cartilage cell capsule* 1, which is part of the *territorial extracellular matrix* (see Figs. 193–198).

1 Territorial extracellular matrix, cartilage cell capsule
2 Interterritorial extracellular matrix
Stain: Sudan red-hemalum; magnification: × 500

61 Lipid Droplets—Hyaline Cartilage

Chondrocytes with stored cytoplasmic fat droplets 1. The finely granulated cytoplasm also contains small oval mitochondria, glycogen particles 2 and filament tufts 3. A cartilage capsule 4 encloses the *territorial extracellular matrix.*
Hyaline cartilage from tracheal cartilage (cartilago trachealis).

1 Fat droplet
2 Glycogen granules
3 Filaments
4 Cartilage cell capsule
5 Chondrocyte nuclei
6 Extracellular interterritorial matrix
Electron microscopy; magnification: × 3900

62 Lipid Droplets—Exocrine Gland Cells

Harderian (orbital) gland from a rabbit. Several lipid droplets of different sizes 1 from an exocrine gland cell (section) after freeze-etching. Freeze-fracture makes it possible to examine cells by electron microscopy without fixation. This special procedure circumvents both the removal of water from the tissue and embedding in synthetic resin. *Freeze-etching* often brings out different structural properties for individual lipid droplets in different fracture planes 2. These structures hold clues to the lipid composition. Lipids are predominantly stored as triglycerides, with cholesterol esters mixed in.
In 1694, Johann Jakob Harder described a large gland in the medial upper quadrant of the orbit in the deer. Today, we know that it exists in many mammals and reptiles. Subsequently, this gland became known as the Harderian gland, although its function is still not completely elucidated.

1 Lipid droplets
2 Freeze-fracture plane of a lipid droplet
Electron microscopy; magnification: × 18 000

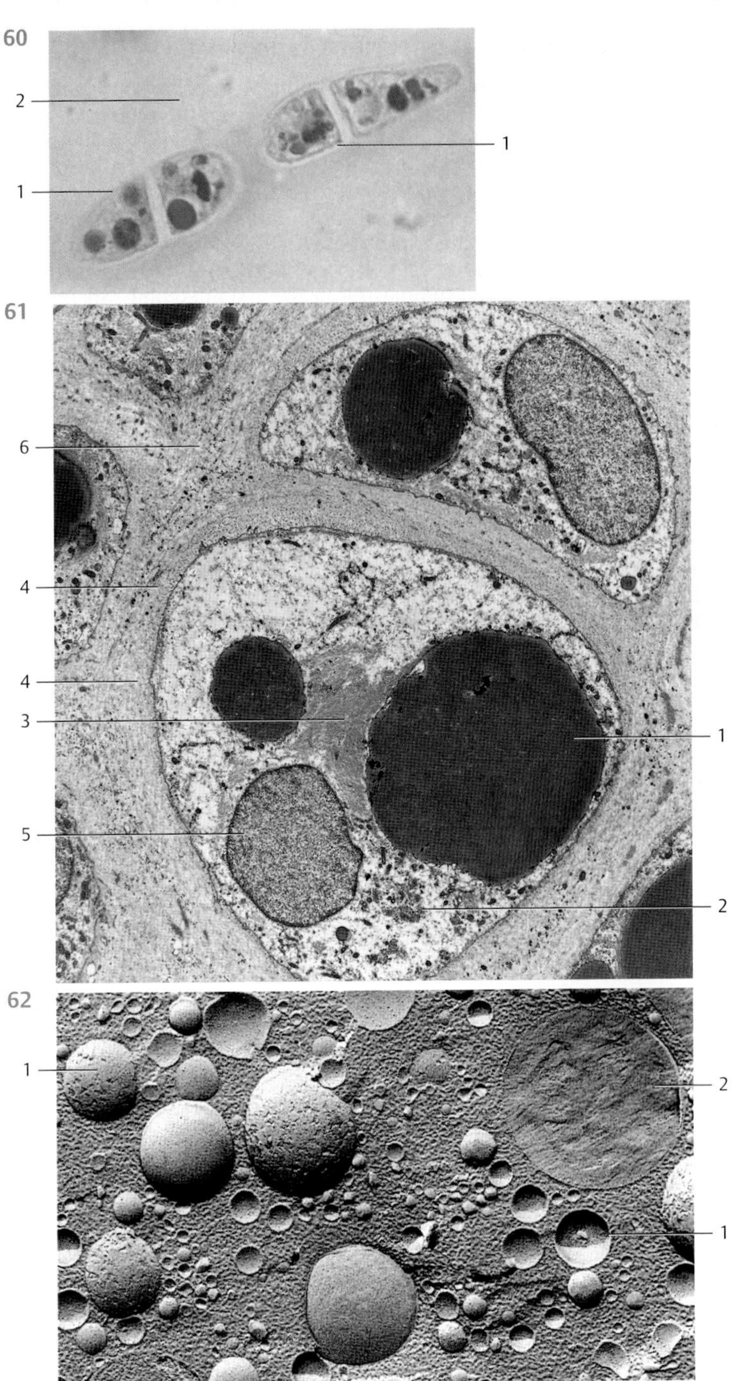
60
2
1
1
61
6
4
4
3
1
5
2
62
1
2
1

63 Lipid Droplets—Endocrine Gland Cells

Small lipid inclusions are particularly abundant in cells from steroid hormone-producing glands. This figure shows cells from the *zona fasciculata* of the adrenal gland. The cells are densely populated with small vacuoles, which correspond to small lipid droplets. With suitable fixation methods, these lipid droplets remain intact, and they can then be stained with lipophilic dyes. At the time of preparation, other fatty substances were removed from the tissue. This accounts for the holes in these large round or polygonal cells and explains the name "*spongiocytes*." Between fat vacuoles, the delicate cytoplasmic septa and cytoplasmic bridges (stained blue) are preserved (see Figs. 351–354). Note the intensely stained cell nuclei (blue) 1, their clearly visible nucleoli, and the abundance of capillaries 2.

1 Cell nuclei
2 Capillaries
Semi-thin section; stain: methylene blue-azure II; magnification: × 400

64 Glycogen—Liver

Glycogen, a large glucose polymer, is a frequently observed paraplasmic inclusion. It can be found in the cytoplasm of many cells in the form of fine or coarse granules.

This figure shows the central region of a liver lobule (see Fig. 438). The center represents a cut through the central vein 1. The red stain in the radially oriented liver cells corresponds to glycogen particles. Between the cells are the liver sinusoids 2. Note the uneven distribution of the *glycogen granules* (see Fig. 65). The liver cell nuclei are not stained. It should also be noted that glycogen particles are not stained in routine histology preparations. With hematoxylin-eosin (HE) staining, they leave small empty spaces in the red-tinged cytoplasm. However, their identification can successfully be accomplished with the Best carmine stain and the periodic acid-Schiff (PAS) reaction.

1 Central vein of a liver lobule
2 Liver sinusoids
Stain: PAS reaction; magnification: × 80

65 Glycogen Granules—Liver

Glycogen is a typical inclusion in liver cells (see Fig. 64). It forms electron-dense, irregularly shaped granules (β-*particles*) 1 with diameters of 20–40 nm. β-Particles aggregate to form α-particles with diameters approaching 200 nm. β-Particles often assemble and form rosette structures with diameters of 0.2–0.4 mm.

This figure shows two liver cells with osmiophilic glycogen granules 1 and numerous mitochondria 2.

1 Glycogen granules
2 Mitochondria
3 Lumen of a liver sinus
4 Endothelial cell with nucleus
5 Disse's space (perisinusoidal space)
6 Hepatocyte microvilli
Electron microscopy; magnification: × 2000

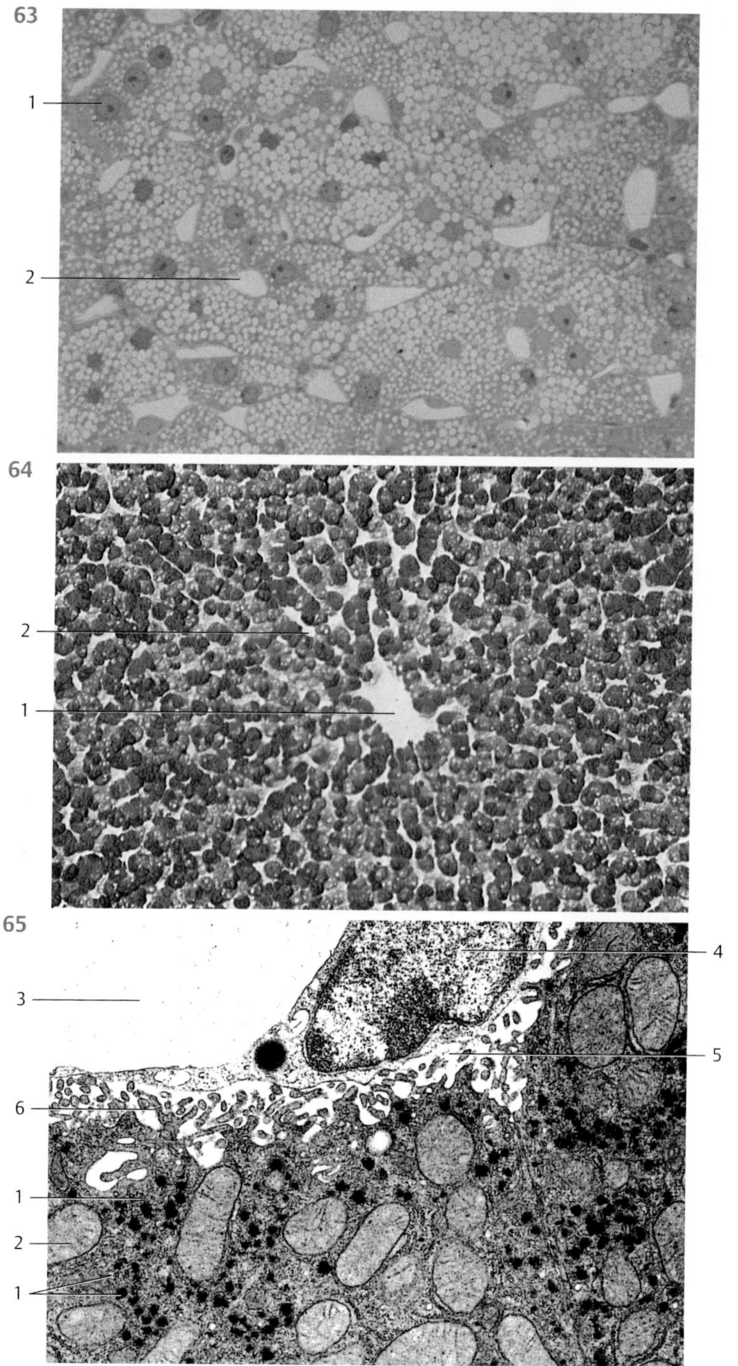
63
1
2
64
2
1
65
4
3
5
6
1
2
1

66 Pigments—Spinal Ganglion Cells

Pigments have their own color attributes, and this makes them visible in tissues without staining. Pigments are either biosynthesized by the cells from unpigmented precursors (*endogenous pigments: porphyrins, iron pigments, melanin, lipofuscin*), or they are exogenous substances that have been engulfed and stored by certain cells (*exogenous pigments: carbon dust, vitamin A, lipochromes*). *Hemoglobin* is the most important endogenous pigment. *Hemosiderin* , its degradation product, is a pigment inclusion in some cells (see Fig. 70a, b).

Both ganglion cells in this figure contain accumulations of yellow-brown small *lipofuscin granules* 2 in the vicinity of their nuclei. Lipofuscin particles are often called age or wear-and-tear pigments (see Fig. 251, 256). As *residual bodies,* they are derived from lysosomes (telolysosomes). See also Fig. 1.

1 Pigments
2 Nucleus from a ganglion cell with nucleolus
3 Nuclei in satellite cells
Stain: molybdenum-hematoxylin; magnification: × 260

67 Pigments—Purkinje Cells

The enzymatic degradation of endocytosed material is often incomplete. Vesicles and vacuoles with such material are called *residual bodies*. Lipofuscin is a membrane-enclosed, indigestible residue that is left over after lysosomal degradation. Lipofuscin-loaded *residual bodies* are called *lipofuscin granules*. In long-lived muscle and nerve cells, lipofuscin granules become more abundant with age. Lipofuscin is therefore known as an aging or "wear-and-tear" pigment.

Lipofuscin granules in Purkinje cells from rat cerebellum. The small lipofuscin granules show an endogenous yellow fluorescence. They appear in small piles at the upper cell pole between nucleus and dendrite. Small granules can occur anywhere in the perikaryon.

Stain: Einarson gallocyanine; fluorescence microscopy (BG-12 excitation filter, 530-nm barrier filter); magnification: × 1000

68 Pigments—Purkinje Cell

This figure shows the ultrastructure of a lipofuscin granule. Note the bizarre shape (*lipofuscin* has an irregular surface), the osmiophilic electron-dense matrix, which consists of numerous very small granules, and the differences in electron densities. In the immediate vicinity of the granule, there are areas with polysomes 1 as well as short ergastoplasmic lamellae 2 (*Nissl bodies*, see Fig. 24).

1 Polysomes
2 Nissl bodies
Electron microscopy; magnification: × 13 000

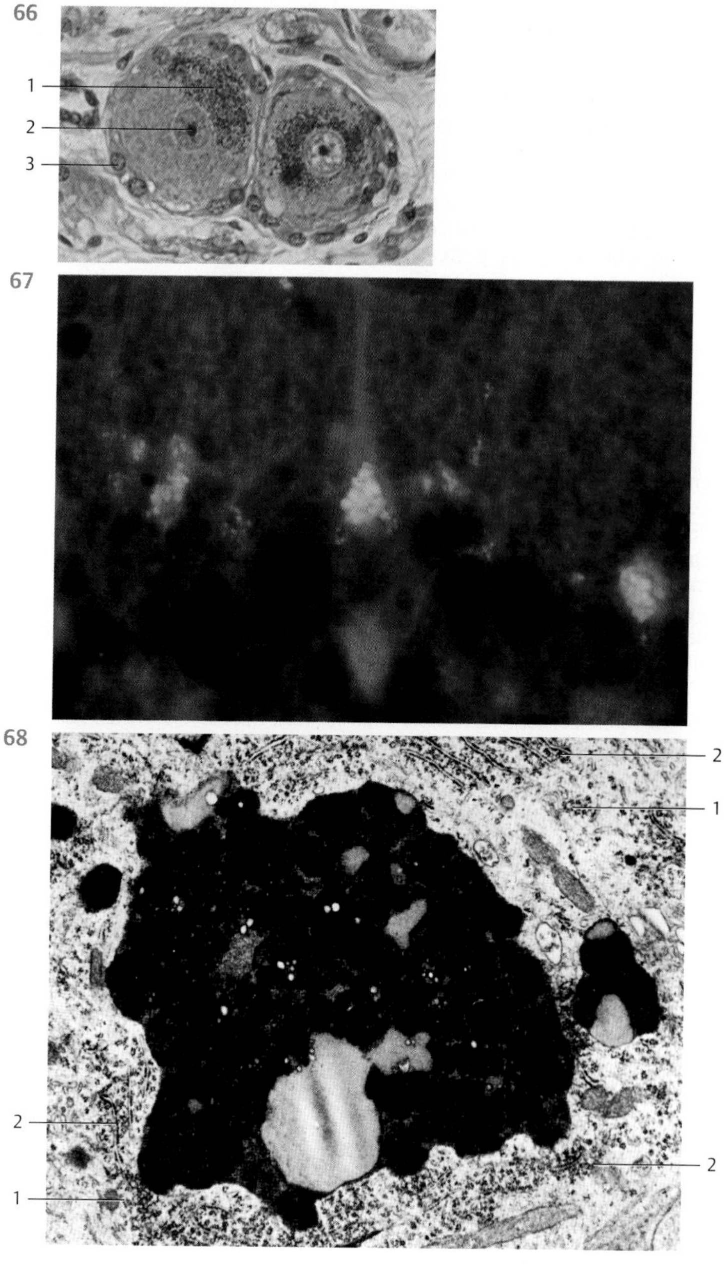
66
1
2
3
67
68
2
1
2
2
1

69 Protein Crystals

Protein accumulations in the form of *protein crystals* exist in several different mammalian cells. In humans, for example, they occur in the intermediary cells of the testes (*Reinke crystals*, see Fig. 522). While these *paracrystalline* bodies can have a multitude of forms, morphologically they are always characterized by a more or less definite geometric organization.
The figure on the right depicts crystalline inclusions of different sizes and structures 1 in an epithelial cell from sheep chorion. Crystalline bodies also exist in mitochondria, peroxisomes and in eosinophil granulocytes (cf. Fig. 143).

1 Paracrystalline bodies
2 Glycogen particles (cf. Fig. 65)
Electron microscopy; magnification: × 50 000

70 Hemosiderin Pigments—Spleen

Hemosiderin is the iron-containing product of hemoglobin degradation. It is the iron-containing pigment of red blood cells (erythrocytes). Hemosiderin is formed in certain cells of the liver, spleen and the bone marrow, following phagocytosis of erythrocytes (lifespan about 120 days). It is stored in form of small yellowish-brown granules.
Figure a shows *hemosiderin pigment* in its natural color in cells of the red splenic pulp. In Figure b, the free iron in hemosiderin is visualized with Turnbull's blue reaction.

a) Pappenheim stain; magnification: × 160
b) Tirmann and Schmelzer variant of Turnbull's blue reaction—the nuclei are stained with lithium carmine; magnification: × 50

71 Exogenous Pigments—Lymph Nodes

Section from a bronchial lymph node. Its reticulum cells have taken up brownish-black particles, probably dust or carbon particles (*anthracotic lymph node*), by phagocytosis. The organism takes up carbon dust with the inhalation of air. Lymph nodes owe their ability to work as filters to the phagocytotic capacity of the reticulum cells. By a similar mechanism, reticulum cells also retain endogenous materials such as lipids, bacteria, cell fragments and carcinoma cells.
Carotene is another exogenous pigment in animal cells. The yellowish-red plant pigment (carrots, tomatoes) is stored almost exclusively in adipose tissue. At the right edge of this figure is a section of adipose tissue 1 (cf. Figs. 320–326).

1 Adipose cells
2 Marginal sinus
3 Lymph-node capsule
4 Lymph-node cortex
5 Medullary sinus
Stain: hematoxylin-eosin; magnification: × 40

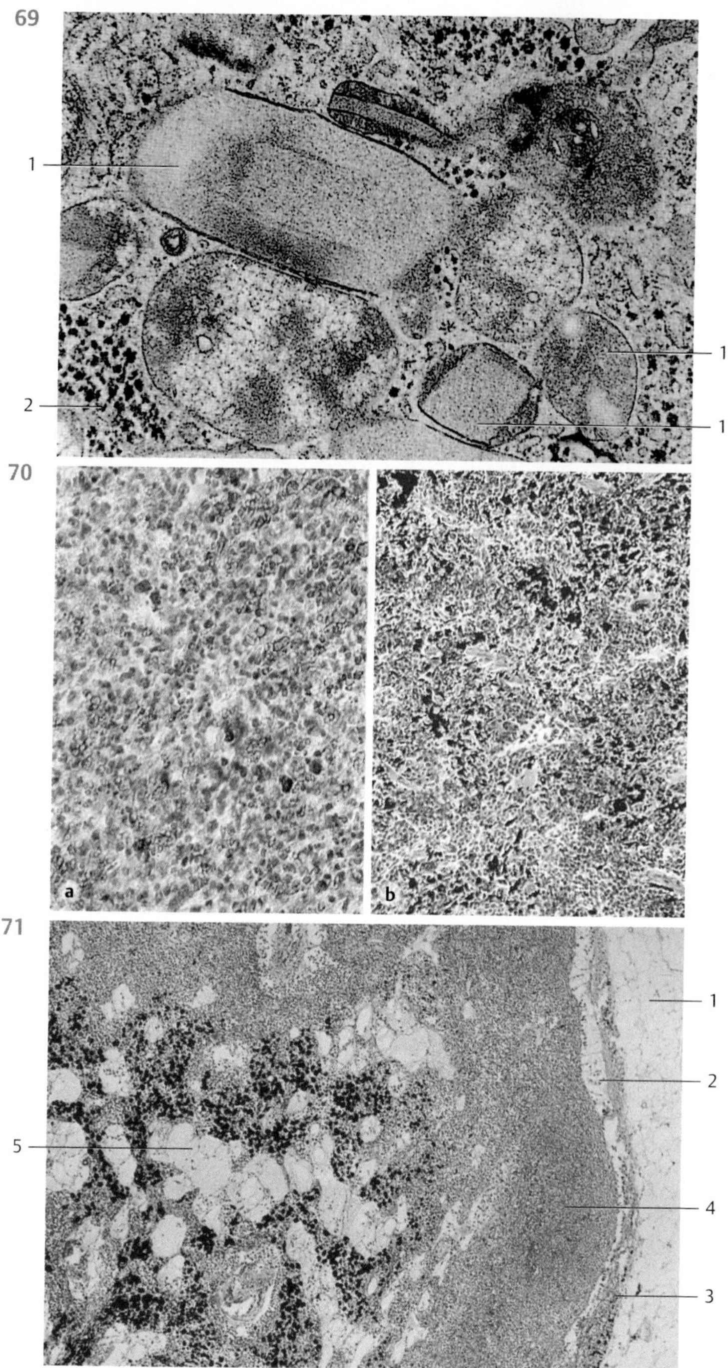
69
1
1
1
2
70
a
b
71
1
2
5
4
3

72 Microvilli—Uterus

Many epithelial cells form processes, named *microvilli*, at their free surfaces. These processes are finger-shaped; they are about 100 nm thick and of various lengths. The structure of microvilli is static and without any particular organization. However, protrusions from the plasmalemma increase the cell surface area. Scanning electron microscopy provides a method of examining the outer elements of the tissue surface in detail.
This figure offers a view of the surface of the uterine cavum epithelium. The cells are either polygonal or round and covered with short stub-like microvilli. The image is that of small patches of lawn. The dark lines between the cells are cell borders. In the lower right part of the figure are two erythrocytes. Compare this figure with Figs. 73–78 and 86–88.

Scanning electron microscopy; magnification: × 3000

73 Microvilli, Brush Border—Duodenum

The cell surfaces of resorptive cells feature a dense cover of microvilli. The microvilli extend upward from the surface and create a pattern, which can be recognized in light microscopy as a light, striped border, the *brush border* 1. It is PAS-positive and contains several marker enzymes, which partake in resorptive cell activities. The figure shows pseudostratified columnar epithelial surface cells from a small intestinal crypt. *Goblet cells* 2, filled with secretory products, exist side by side with the epithelial cells (cf. Figs. 108, 109, 122, 415, 417, 426–429). Compare the slender epithelial cell nuclei with those in Fig. 74.

1 Brush border
2 Goblet cell with secretory product
3 Lamina propria mucosae
4 Intestinal crypt
Stain: azan; magnification: × 160

74 Microvilli, Brush Border—Kidney

Brush borders and the resulting enlargement of the luminal cell membranes are characteristic of resorptive epithelium. Brush borders are highly specialized structures. They are dense with microvilli, which are covered by a *glycocalix* (see Figs. 77–79). This cross-section shows the proximal tubules of a nephron. A high *brush border*, stained light blue with azan, covers the single-layered, medium height epithelium of the proximal tubules. Approximately 6000–7000 microvilli cover each of the epithelial cells from the proximal tubule. The microvilli can be up to 0.2 μm long. The left half of the figure shows a cut through the center part of the distal tubules 2 of the kidney (cf. Figs. 73, 497, 498).

1 Brush border
2 Distal tubule
3 Capillaries
Stain: azan; magnification: × 800

72

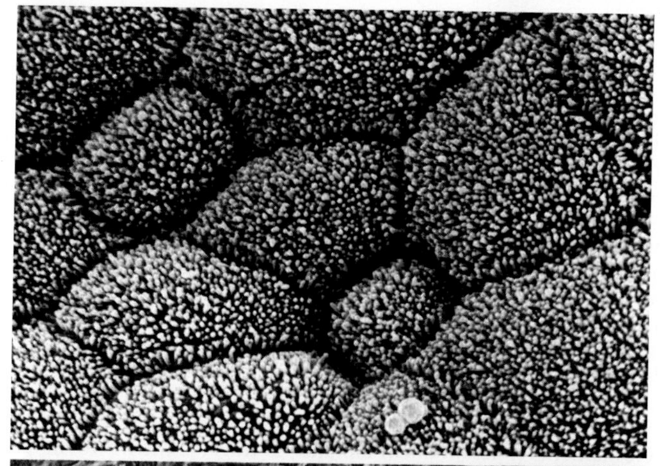

73

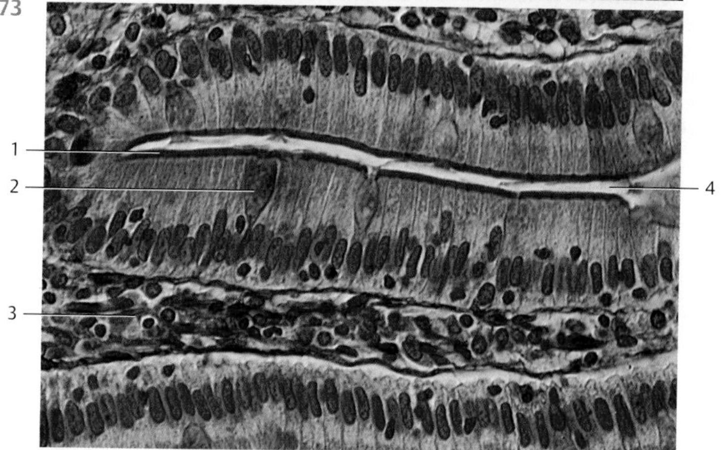

74

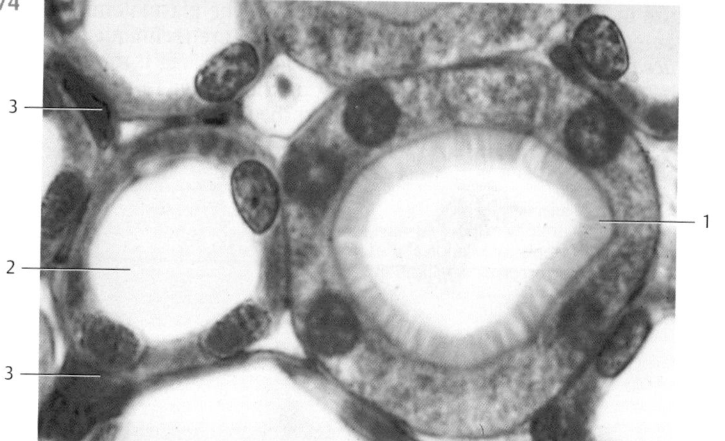

75 Microvilli, Brush Border—Duodenum

Microvilli are finger-like protrusions from the plasmalemma. They are about 50–120 nm thick and up to 3 µmm long. In resorptive epithelium (e.g., in *enterocytes* from the small intestine and *epithelium* from the proximal renal tubules) the microvilli form a dense lawn, which can be recognized as a *brush border* in light microscopy (cf. Figs. 73, 77, 78).
Electron microscopy reveals that the rod-shaped processes (*microvilli*), which extend from the free surface of the epithelial cells, are encased by the plasmalemma (*three-layered structure*). On the microvilli surface is a finely granular, sometimes filament-like material (cf. Figs. 77, 78). This layer is the *glycocalix* (*cell coat*) (cf. Fig. 79). The glycocalix (calyx, Greek: chalice, bud) consists of the polysaccharide chains of glycolipids and glycoproteins. Enlargement will bring out these chains as *antennulae microvillares*. The glycocalix provides the basis for cell specificity. It exposes antigenic determinants, which determine the serological attributes of cells. The glycocalix mediates cell-cell recognition.
Microfilaments (*microfilament bundles*) [1] traverse the microvilli parallel to the long axis. They consist of actin and actin-binding proteins (see Fig. 56) and extend to the *terminal complex* (*terminal web*) [2] in the apical cytoplasm. The terminal web also contains myosin at its border. This apical terminal web area of the epithelial cell is mostly free of organelles.
Duodenal enterocytes.

1 Bundled actin filaments providing mechanical support (skeleton)
2 Terminal web
3 Crista-type mitochondria
Electron microscopy; magnification: × 34 000

76 Microvilli, Brush Border—Jejunum

Freeze-fracture image of microvilli (*brush border*) from the apical portion of an epithelial cell of the small intestine (cf. Figs. 72–74, 77, 78). In the freeze-fracture technique, membranes are split into two membrane complements. This makes it possible to investigate and interpret the structures of the two complementary inner membrane surfaces. It is hardly possible to render a picture of the real outer and inner surfaces of the plasmalemma with the freeze-etching technique alone. The freeze-fracture technique exposes the *extracellular face* (*EF*) and the *protoplasmic face* (*PF*) [2]. EF is the exposed face of the half-membrane that started out as the border to the extracellular space; PF was the half-membrane toward the cytoplasmic side (cf. Figs. 75, 77).
Jejunal enterocytes.

1 Extracellular face (EF)
2 Protoplasmic face (PF)
3 Apical cytoplasm, location of the terminal web (see Fig. 75)
Electron microscopy; magnification: × 35 200

75

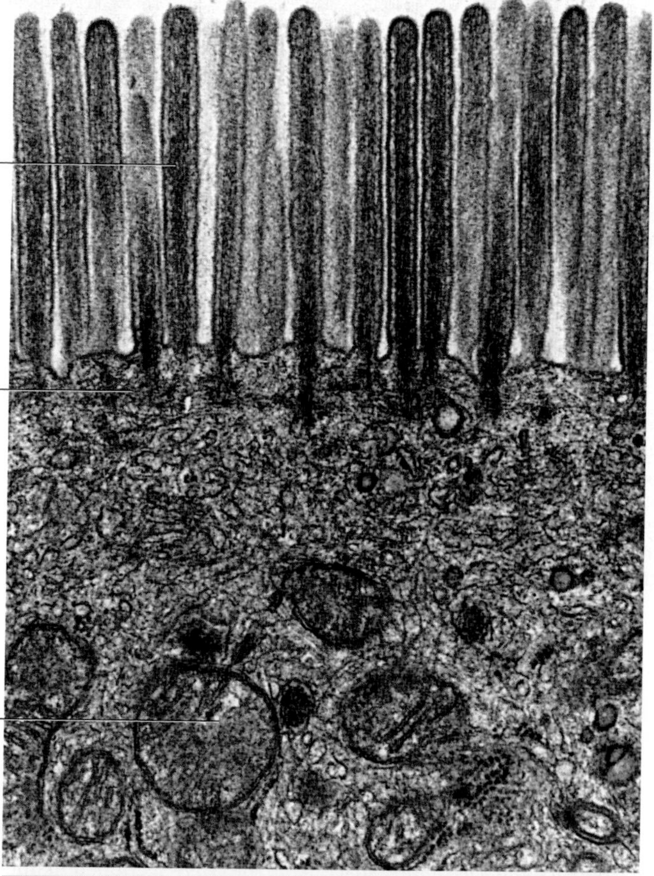

1

2

3

76

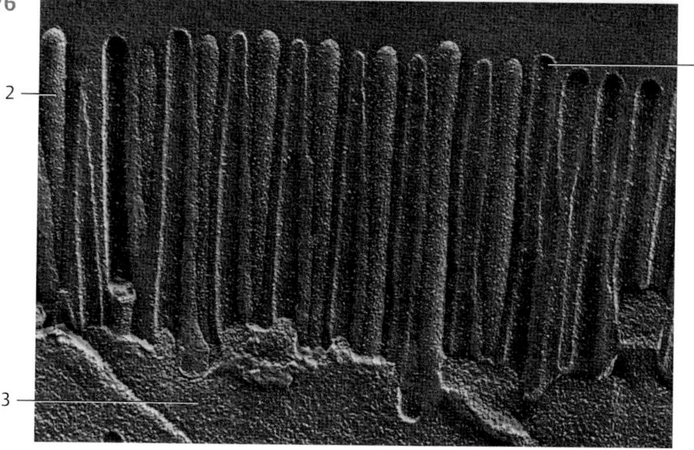

77 Microvilli Brush Border—Duodenum

Microvilli (*brush border*) around a duodenal enterocyte at large magnification (cf. Fig. 72–76, 415, 416). Each of the *microvilli* contains a central *microfilament bundle* (central bundle traversing the length of the villi) 1, which emerges from an apical dense spot 2. Each longitudinal bundle consists of 20–30 *actin filaments*, which fan into the terminal web 3 area. Note the finely granular, sometimes filament-like material on the surfaces of the microvilli. This is the glycocalix (see Figs. 75, 79). The central actin filaments (*inner skeleton*) create a contractile element that can shorten the microvilli and presumably facilitate resorption. The microvilli, in conjunction with the terminal web, form a protein filament system, which achieves parallel movement and cytoskeletal stability. The apical, terminal web area of the epithelium contains few if any organelles. Among other structural proteins, the microvilli contain *villin*, which cross-links the actin filaments. Another component is *calmodulin*. Together with Ca^{2+}, it apparently regulates the function of villin. There are actin filaments in the *terminal web* as well. These run parallel to the cell surface. Other elements of the terminal web are myosin, tropomyosin and 10-nm filaments, which are probably cytokeratin filaments that connect to the zonulae adherentes of the duodenal absorptive cells (cf. Fig. 56). This complex system apparently supports the microvilli, gives them rigidity, and anchors them in the terminal web 3. On the other hand, this system also provides microvilli with a controlled level of motility.
Duodenal enterocytes (absorptive cells).

1 Central microfilament bundle (actin filaments, diameter 7 nm)
2 Apical dense spot
3 Terminal web
Electron microscopy; magnification: × 95 000

78 Microvilli, Brush Border—Duodenum

In this figure, the free tissue surface of a duodenal cell is cut across the brush border. The section shows the plasmalemma around each of the microvilli. It is triple-layered and consists of two osmium tetroxide-stained black lines of equal density and a light interspace. Note the cross-sectioned filaments (central longitudinal bundle) in the centers of the microvilli. Also, note the partly granular, partly filament-like or fuzzy material on the surfaces of the microvilli, the *glycocalix*.
Duodenal absorptive cells (cf. Figs. 73–79, 415, 416).

Electron microscopy; magnification: × 70 000

77

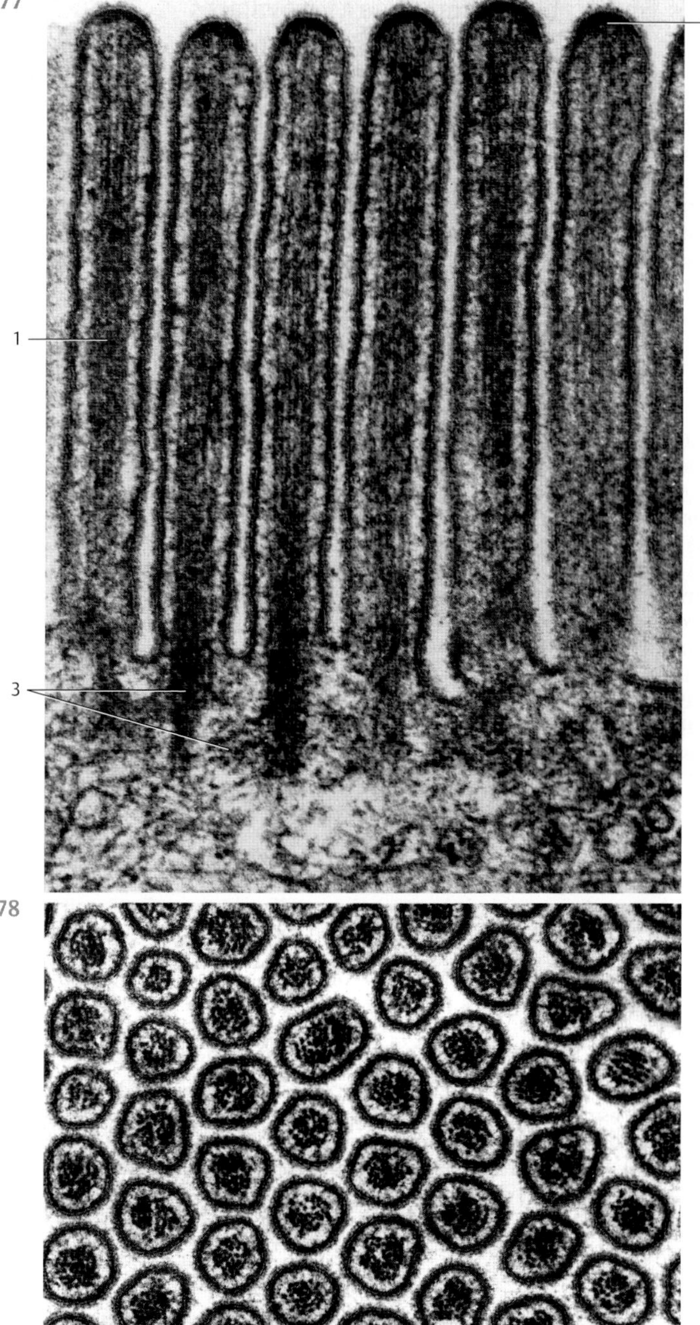

78

79 Glycocalix—Antennulae Microvillares

A dense layer of carbohydrate chains covers the outer plasma membrane. They are part of the *glycolipids* and *glycoproteins* of the cell membrane. The layer of oligosaccharides is called *glycocalix* (cf. Figs. 75, 77, 78). The patterns of *oligosaccharide distribution* show much variation and are characteristic of a particular cell type. The glycocalix determines cell specificity and serves as a cell-specific antigen. The protein-carbohydrate complexes extend outward as tufts of filament-like structures and are called *antennulae microvillares*.
Cross-section through several microvilli around a jejunal absorptive cell with clearly developed antennules. The 7-nm thick actin filaments can be recognized in the centers of the cross-sectioned microvilli.

Electron microscopy; magnification: × 95 000

80 Endocytosis

Phagocytosis, pinocytosis, transcytosis and potocytosis are distinct cellular functions. In phagocytosis, the cell membrane engulfs the material to be taken up. Adjacent parts of the lamellae fuse, and the particle is now enclosed in a vacuole inside the cell, the *phagosome*. During *pinocytosis*, liquids or substances in soluble form in the extracellular space are transported into the cell (*internalization*). Pinocytosis starts with the formation of invaginations or valleys in the plasma membrane (*membrane vesicularization*), with subsequent pinching off as a membrane vesicle from the plasma membrane into the cell. There are two types of pinocytosis—receptor-mediated pinocytosis and nonspecific pinocytosis (*endocytosis*). In *receptor-mediated pinocytosis*, coated vesicles (coated pits) form. At their cytoplasmic face, they are coated with *clathrin*, among other proteins. Clathrin-coated vesicles have a diameter of 200–300 nm.
The figure shows the part of a myofibroblast cell that contains the nucleus. On the cell surface, there are round or oval plasma membrane invaginations with diameters of 60–100 nm. They are lined up at the plasmalemma like pearls on a string. These are *caveolae*, which do not have a clathrin coat but are enveloped by the protein *caveolin*. Caveolae are considered to be static invaginations, because their invaginations will only sporadically pinch off as vesicles. This mechanism of uptake and transport is called *potocytosis*.

Electron microscopy; magnification: × 25 000

81 Potocytosis—Caveolae

Cytoplasmic protrusion from a myofibroblast to illustrate *caveolae* [1]. It was isolated from the perineurium of the median nerve. Caveolae are small round or oval invaginations of the plasma membrane. They are particularly numerous in smooth muscle cells, myofibroblasts, fibroblasts and endothelial cells.

1 Caveolae
2 Myofilaments
3 Collagen fibrils
Electron microscopy; magnification: × 35 000

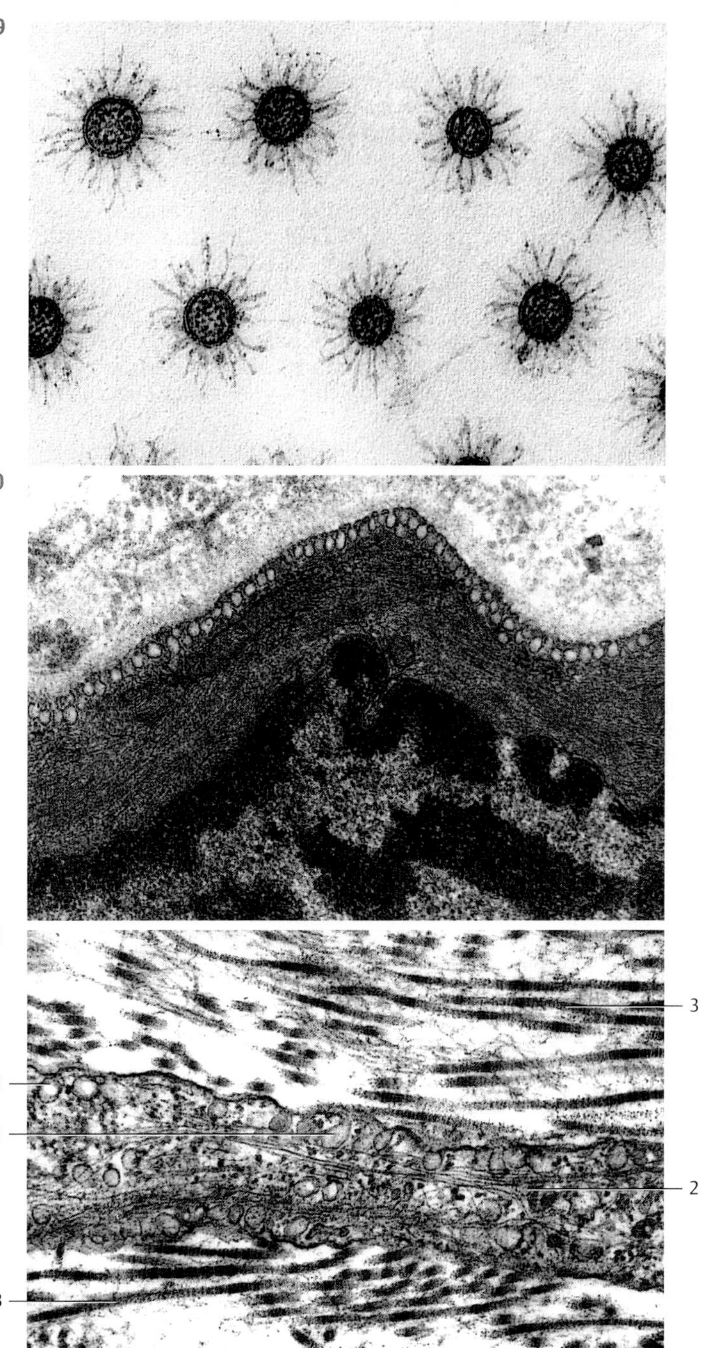
79
80
81
1
1
2
3
3

82 Kinocilia—Uterus

Some eukaryotic cells have *cilia* or *flagellae*. Kinocilia are cylindrical motile processes, which are 0.2 μm thick and about 2–5 μm long. Their central structure consists of microtubule aggregates that are covered by the cell membrane. Kinocilia occur singly or as bushels (*cilia border*). Extremely long kinocilia, such as the tails of spermatozoa, are called *flagellae* (cf. Fig. 524). Cilia and flagellae have a uniformly organized system of microtubules.
Scanning electron microscopy of epithelium reveals a particular clear and impressive image of their surface relief. This figure shows a ciliated cell surrounded by cells from the uterine cavum epithelium. The cilia form a tight bushel (cf. Figs. 84, 85, 469–471, 565). They are slender, sometimes arcuate and slightly thicker at their ends. In this preparation, the surfaces of the neighboring epithelial cavum cells can be smooth or show a more or less dense population of microvilli, which may look like buttons or rods (cf. Fig. 72).
In contrast to *stereocilia*, kinocilia are motile cell processes with a complex internal composition and structure (cf. Figs. 83, 84).

Scanning electron microscopy; magnification: × 3000

83 Kinocilia—Uterine Tube

The detail structure of cilia is particularly impressive in cross-sections: there are two tubules in the center, and nine pairs of tubules (*doublets*) are located around them in the periphery (9 × 2 + 2 pattern). The peripheral twin tubules (*microtubule doublets, axonemes*) are close to each other and share a common central wall. The wall consists of two or three protofilaments that are predominantly composed of the protein *tubulin* (α- *and* β-*tubulin*). This particular arrangement creates two different tubules within the twin tubules (doublet); only one of them, the *A-microtubule*, features a complete ring structure with 13 protofilaments. The *B-tubule* forms an incomplete ring. The B- tubule itself consists of only nine protofilaments. Three or four protofilaments in its structure belong to the A-ring. In contrast to the central microtubule pair, the A-tubules at the periphery have small "arms," which reach to the adjacent pairs of microtubules. This figure shows these arms only vaguely. The arms consist of the protein *dynein* and *ATPase*. They play an important role in the motility of cilia. The two central microtubules are separate, side-by-side units. The peripheral axonemes are clearly connected to each other via the binding protein (*nexin*).
Axial view of the ciliated cells from oviduct (cf. Fig. 84, longitudinal section through cilia).

Electron microscopy; magnification: × 60 000

82

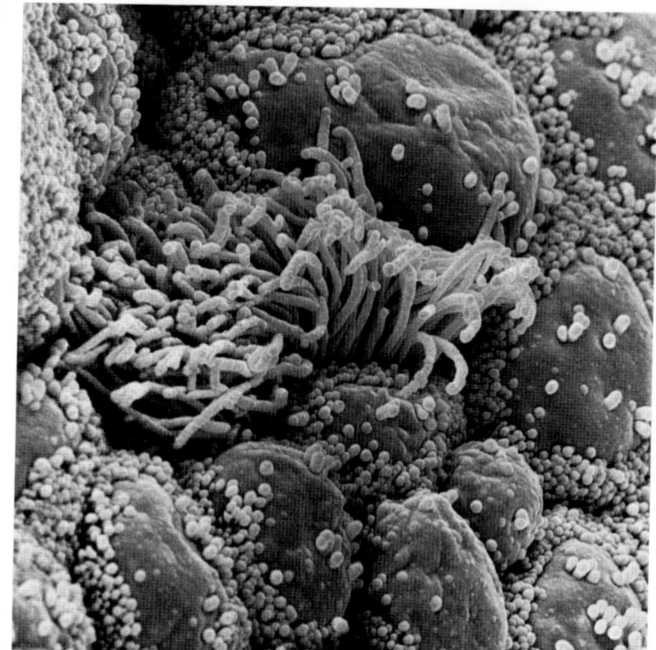

83

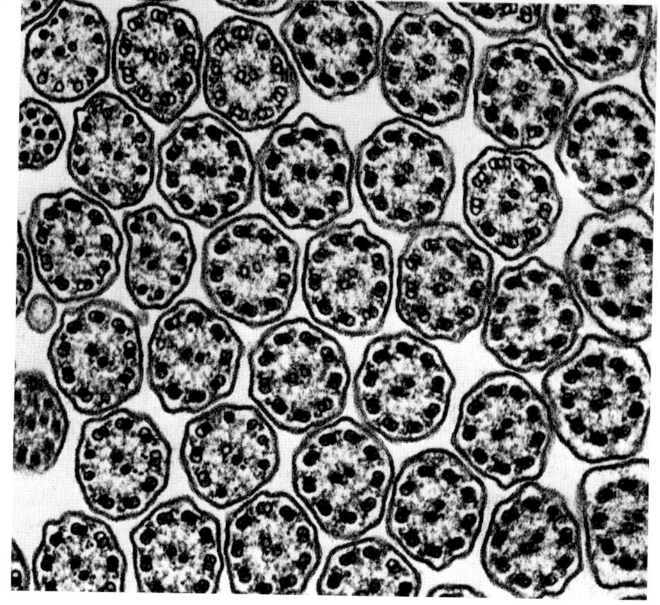

84 Kinocilia—Uterine Tube

Longitudinal section through the kinocilia of a ciliated epithelial cell from oviduct (cf. Figs. 83, 85, 561, 563–565). Between the cilia are several sections through arcuate microvilli in different angles. Inside the cilia, microtubules form the longitudinal axis (*axonemes*), which consist of two central tubules (central tubule pair) and nine peripheral double tubules (*doublets*, each made of *A- and B-tubules*): 9 × 2 + 2 structure (cf. Fig. 83). The nine parallel outer axial tubules are connected to the central two tubules via *spoke proteins*.

The two peripheral double tubules are different: in an axial section, *tubule A* forms a ring. In contrast, *tubule B* looks like an incomplete circle, like the letter C (cf. Fig. 83). The peripheral ciliary microtubules extend into the apical cytoplasm region. There, underneath the cell surface, they form *basal bodies* (*basal nodes, kinetosomes, cilia root*) ↗. *Kinetosomes* form the cytoplasmic anchor places for microtubules. Their structure is that of *centrioles*. At the basal side, there is often a structure called rootstock, which shows a striation pattern. The rootstock contains the protein *centrin*. Kinetosomes are densely packed in richly ciliated epithelium. This accounts for the layer of basal bodies (*basal nodule row*) that is visible in light microscopy (see Fig. 85).

1 Apical cytoplasm in a ciliated cell
Electron microscopy; magnification: × 30 000

85 Kinocilia—Tuba Uterina

Kinocilia are motile, membrane-enclosed cell processes. They emerge from small bodies (*basal bodies* or *kinetosomes*) under the cell membrane (see Fig. 84). Cilia are usually 2–5 µm long and have diameters of about 0.2–0.3 µm. That makes them considerably longer than microvilli and easily discernible using light microscopy. Kinocilia are often abundant (cilia border) and form very dense groups at the cell surface. Such cells are called *cilia cells*.

This figure shows single-layered columnar epithelial cells from the oviduct mucosa, which consists of *cilia cells* and *secretory cells*. As seen in light microscopy, the cilia originate with the row of heavily stained basal bodies (*line of basal bodies*). The secretory cells protrude like domes into the lumen of the duct ↗. They interrupt the rows of basal bodies at the inner plasmalemma (cf. Fig. 84).

1 Loosely organized connective tissue of the mucosa folds
2 Oviduct lumen
3 Horizontal or angular section through oviduct epithelium
Stain: Masson-Goldner trichrome stain; magnification: × 200

84

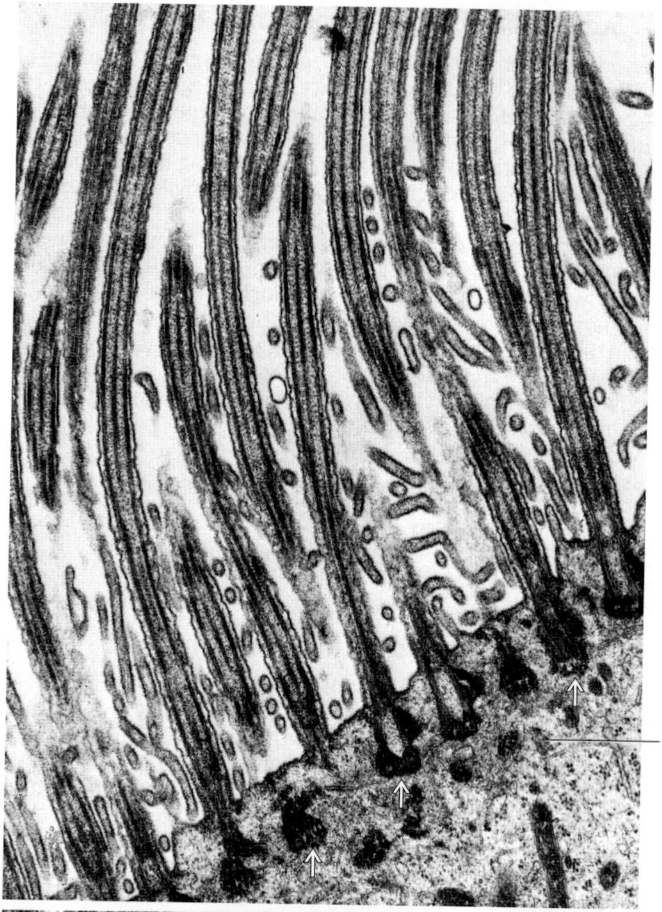

1

85

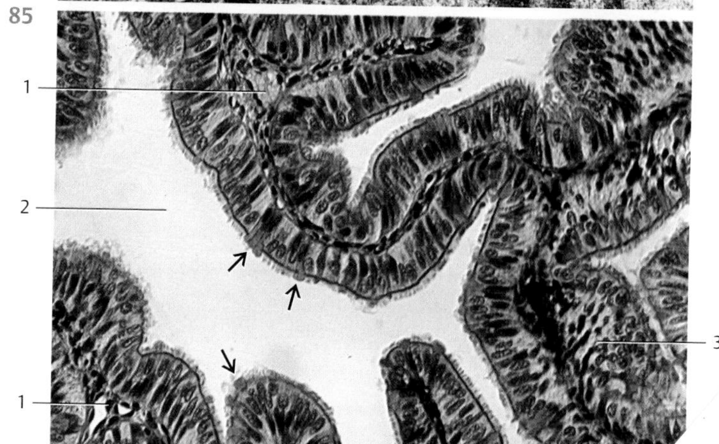

86 Stereocilia—Duct of Epididymis

Stereocilia (stereos, Greek: rigid, hard) are processes on the surface of epithelial cells. They line the epididymal duct and the beginning part of the sperm duct. Stereocilia and kinocilia show different morphologies and have different functions. The sperm-duct stereocilia are not motile, although flexible. In light microscopy, they have the appearance of long hairs, which often stick together in tufts 1. Stereocilia are branched microvilli and therefore do not have kinetosomes (see Fig. 87).

The duct of the epididymis (paratestis) is lined by a double-layered pseudostratified epithelium 2 (see Figs. 110, 527–530). The basal cells are usually round 3 with round nuclei, while the nuclei of pseudostratified cells are oval. The pseudostratified columnar epithelial cells show dot-like expansions in their apicolateral regions. These are the terminal bars (terminal web, junctional complex) (see Fig. 99).

Inflexible stereocilia also exist on the surfaces of the sensory cells (*hair cells*) in the inner ear (*inner ear stereocilia*).

1 Stereocilia tufts
2 Oval nuclei of pseudostratified epithelial cells
3 Nucleus of a basal cell
4 Remaining spermatozoa
5 Delicate subepithelial fibers from the lamina propria
Stain: van Gieson iron hematoxylin-picrofuchsin; magnification: × 400

87 Stereocilia—Head of the Epididymis

Protrusions, sometimes bizarrely shaped, project from the apex of epithelial cells of the epididymal head (*caput epididymidis*). They are the bases for the emerging stereocilia, which are cut lengthwise in this figure (a). The stereocilia of the epididymal head are thin, thread-like cytoplasmic processes. Each contains a densely packed microfilament bundle (*actin filament skeleton*). Some of the microfilaments are connected via thin bridges. Several such thin bridges between cytoplasmic processes (*stereocilia*) are visible in the cross-section (b). Note the terminal bar network in Figure a. Compare this figure with Figs. 72–77 and Fig. 415, which show an even distribution of microvilli.

Electron microscopy; magnifications: a) × 11 300; b) × 17 500

86

87

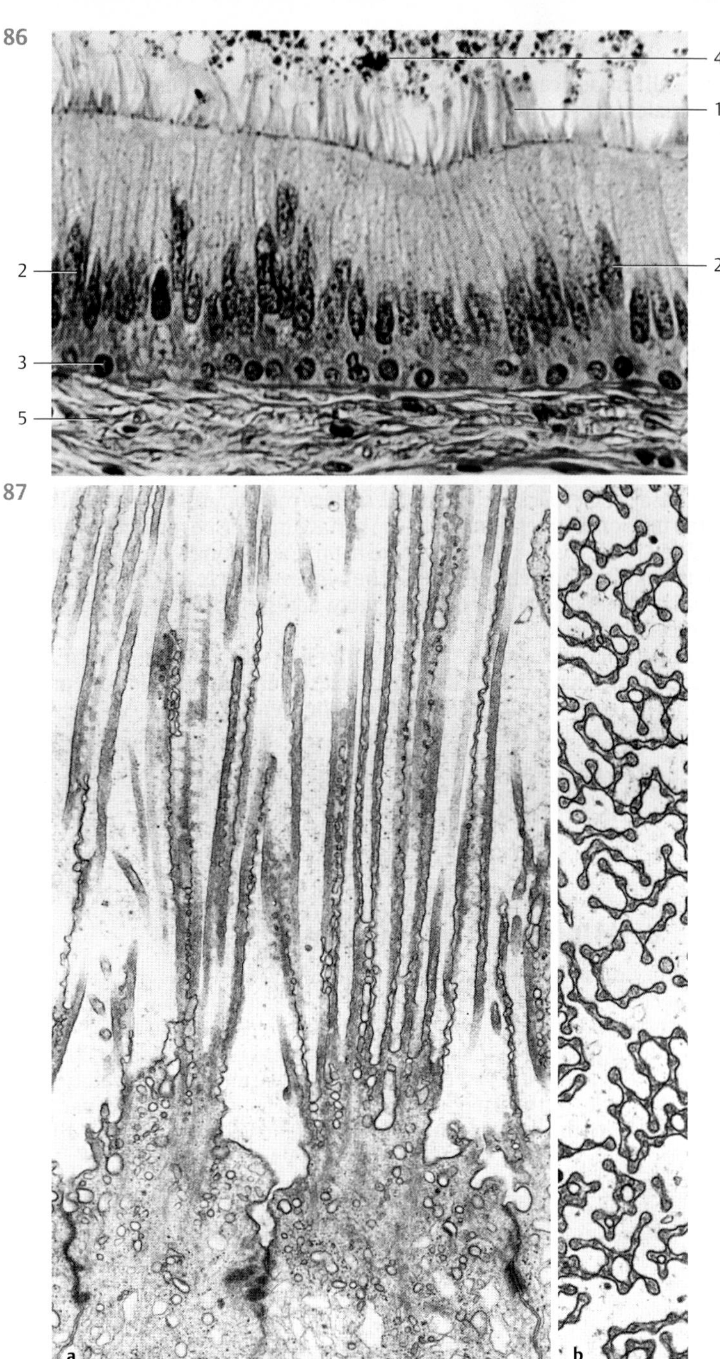

88 Microvilli—Microplicae

The cell surface can also be enlarged by raised, leaf-like formations of the plasmalemma—i.e., by outward extension in the form of folds. The figure shows flat epithelial cells from the canine tongue with a dense pattern of *microplicae*—i.e., raised folds of the plasma membrane. Such microplicae folds are commonly observed in a multitude of patterns. Microplicae also exist at the bottom face of flat epithelial cells, and therefore may play a role in intercellular adhesion. The more pronounced "edges" in this figure correspond to the cell borders. In transmission electron microscopy, vertical cuts show microplicae often as short, stump-shaped microvilli.
Located on top of the epithelial cells are two erythrocytes and a rod-shaped form, which can be categorized as an oral cavity saprophyte.

Scanning electron microscopy; magnification: × 3600

89 Basolateral Interdigitations

The basal, and especially the lateral, surface membranes of epithelial cells are often uneven. Elements at the tissue surface include be microvilli, microfolds and cell processes 1, which partake in an interlocking system of *interdigitations* with the neighboring cells. The processes increase the lateral surface areas of the epithelial cells considerably, and sometimes there are extended intercellular spaces 2.
The adjacent figure displays the view of cells from gallbladder mucous membranes, which have been pulled apart. The columnar epithelial cell processes can form many interdigitations along their entire surface 1. The surfaces show deep crevices (see Figs. 90, 91, 92).

1 Lateral membrane surfaces
2 Intercellular spaces
3 Surface of an epithelial cell
4 Basal membrane
Scanning electron microscopy; magnification: × 780

90 Basal Infolds—Basal Labyrinth

Secretory duct from the submandibular gland with adjacent capillaries 1 and secretory acini 2. The pseudostratified epithelial cells of the secretory duct show a clearly expressed striation pattern rectangular to the basis 3. It is caused by plasmalemma involutions and rows of mitochondria (*basal striation*, "*basal labyrinth*") (see Fig. 91). These plasmalemma involutions relegate the nuclei of the pseudostratified epithelial cells to the upper third of the cells. Note the basal basophilia of the gland cells (see Figs. 18, 19).

1 Capillaries
2 Secretory acini
3 Basal striations
Semi-thin section; stain: methylene blue-azure II; magnification: × 500

88

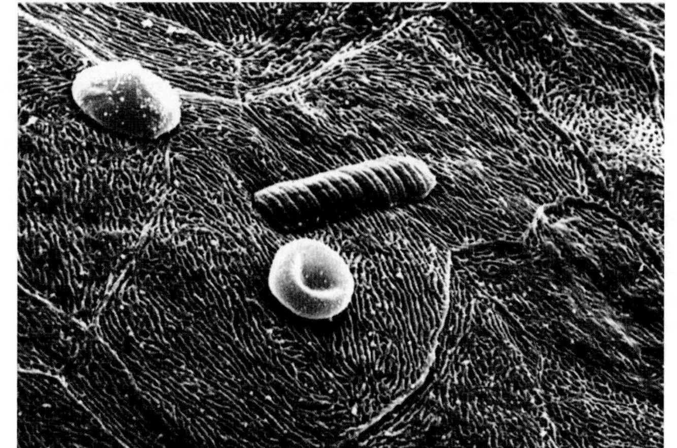

89

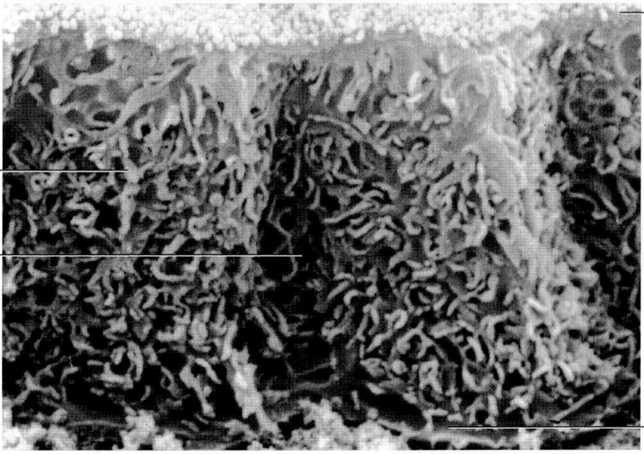

90

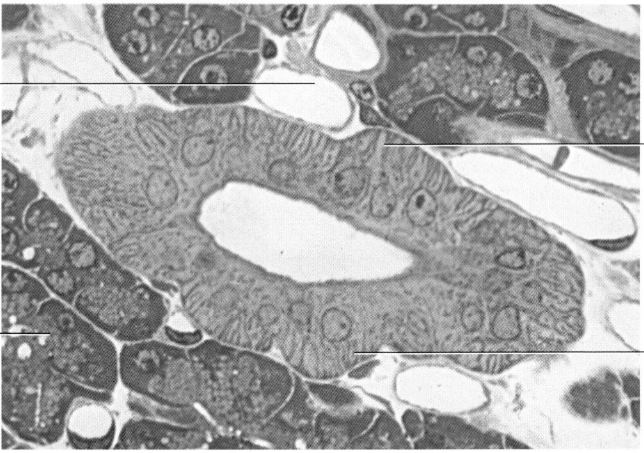

91 Basal Plasmalemma Infolds—Basal Labyrinth—Basolateral Interdigitations

Epithelial cells, which are involved in an extensive transport of ions and liquids, have deep, often complex, vertical involutions of the basal plasmalemma. In earlier descriptions, they were known as the "*basal labyrinth*" [2]. Involutions of the plasmalemma obviously serve to enlarge the basal cell surface area. Involutions exist in different variations. Separating curtains of membrane folds create high, narrow cytoplasmic spaces, which contain large, mostly oval crista-type mitochondria [3]. Constituents of these plasma membrane involutions mediate transport functions. Involutions and the rows of mitochondria between them create the appearance of a *basal striation* in light microscopy (see Figs. 89, 90, 92).

Part of an epithelial cell of the *tubulus proximalis* from a rat nephron.

1 Cell nucleus, pushed up to the apical cell region
2 Basal membrane involutions
3 Mitochondria
4 Basal lamina
5 Lumen of a peritubular capillary
6 Endothelial cell, region with nucleus
7 Fenestrated epithelium
8 Lysosomes
Electron microscopy; magnification: × 10 000

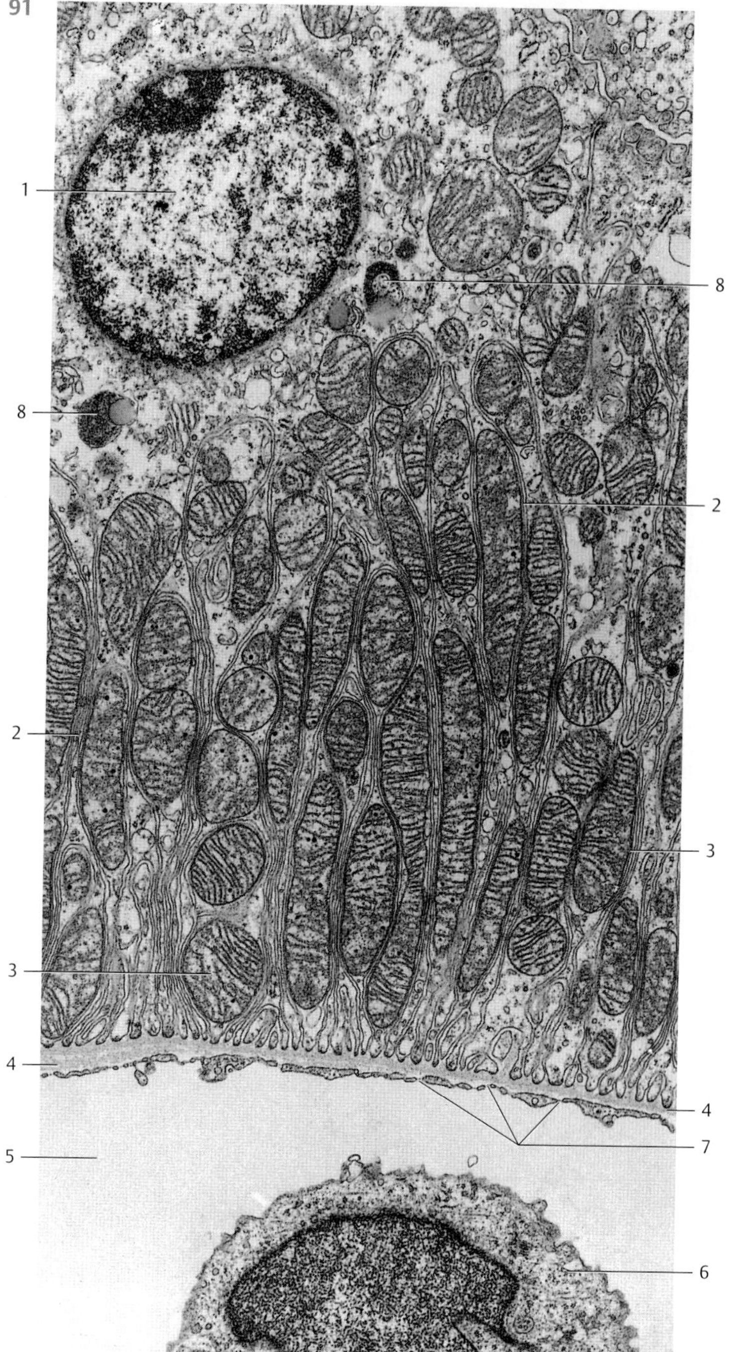
1
8
8
2
2
3
3
4
4
7
5
6

92 Basolateral Interdigitations

Interdigitations ① between cell processes in the epithelium of a *secretory duct* from the parotid gland. The tissue is cut parallel to the cell surface. The interlocking digitations of neighboring plasmalemma are particularly impressive in this picture. They convey the impression of a labyrinth. As in other sections, the processes, which create the interdigitations, contain large mitochondria ②. The shape of the mitochondria adjusts to the spacing within the cell processes.
The cells of the secretory duct of salivary glands have all the structural criteria of a transport epithelium (see Figs. 89, 90, 91, 96).

1 Interdigitizing cell processes
2 Mitochondria
3 Desmosomes
Electron microscopy; magnification: × 4000

93 Dermoepidermal Junction—Rootstocks

The deepest epidermal cell layer is the *stratum basale*. It consists of columnar cells with variably shaped branched cell processes, which form a *rootstock* structure in the basal cell region. The rootstock structures anchor the basal cells in the *stratum papillare* ① of the corium, which consists of reticular fibrils. This enlarges the contact area between basal cells and the vascularized connective tissue. The basal lamina between rootstocks and stratum papillare remains. The rootstocks contain a multiplex of tonofilament bundles ④ (*intermediary filaments, prokeratin*), which radiate into the row of half-desmosomes at the plasmalemma.
In light microscopy, skin sections display the transition from epidermis to dermis (*dermoepidermal junction*) as an irregular, wavy line (see Figs. 595, 599–601, 603).

1 Stratum papillare with collagen fibrils (type III collagen)
2 Desmosomes
3 Stratum spinosum cells
4 Tonofilaments (intermediary filaments)
Electron microscopy; magnification: × 6000

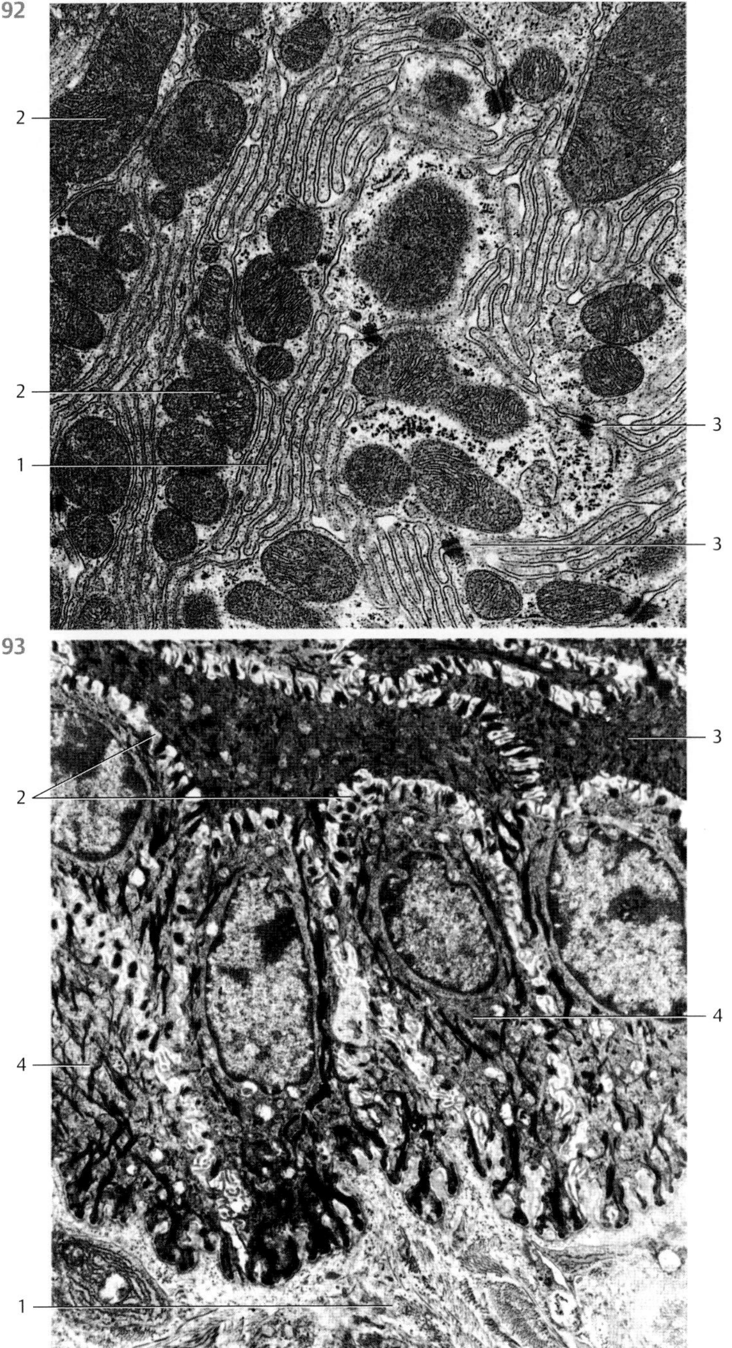
92
2
2
1
3
3
93
3
2
4
4
1

94 Intercellular Junctions

Horizontal section through the *stratum spinosum* of the skin, with polygonal prickle cells (*Malpighian cells, keratinocytes*) and large intercellular spaces. These spaces are spanned by thorn-like cell processes (intercellular junctions) 1. Small, thicker nodules form at the points of contact between the cell processes of adjacent cells. These are the *junction nodules* (*nodes of Bizzozero*), which are complicated attachment structures known as desmosomes (desmos, Greek: connection; soma: body) (see Figs. 93, 95–98).

Stain: hemalum-eosin; magnification: × 675

95 Intercellular Junctions

Cytoplasmic processes from neighboring epithelial cells, some slender processes, some wider ones, protrude into the extended extracellular space 1 (*intercellular junctions*). When they make contact, attachment structures (desmosomes) 2 form. These structures are identical to the *junction nodes* seen in light microscopy (see Fig. 94). Bundles of intermediary filaments (*tonofilaments*) 3 connect to the attachment structures (cf. Figs. 93, 96, 101).

Electron microscopy; magnification: × 23 000

96 Interdigitations

Intercellular contact between two neighboring epithelial cells via interlocking cell processes (*interdigitations*) 1. In this case, the intercellular space is narrow (*cell junction*). The darts point to two *maculae adherentes* (*focal desmosomes, spot desmosomes, type 1 desmosomes*) (cf. Figs. 95, 97, 98).

Electron microscopy; magnification: 23 000

97 Desmosome—Macula Adherens

Desmosomes can take the shape of a button (*punctum adherens, focal desmosome*), of a disk (*macula adherens*), a band (*fascia adherens*) or a belt (*zonula adherens, belt desmosome*). In this figure, two cells have attached to each other via a *macula adherens* in a push-button style. In the 20–40 nm wide intercellular space, microfilaments provide a form of glue (desmoglea), which condenses in a center line (*mesophragma*). Tonofilaments, 10 nm thick, radiate into the condensed, disk-shaped cytoplasmic area (*tonofilament-associated focal desmosome, type I desmosome*) (cf. Fig. 95).

Electron microscopy; magnification: × 46 500

98 Desmosomes—Maculae Adherentes

Typical desmosomes (*maculae adherentes*) between two secretory duct cells from the parotid gland. Note the striation pattern in the intercellular junction (glue). As seen before, tonofilaments radiate into the disk-shaped condensed cytoplasmic area (cf. Figs. 96, 97).

Electron microscopy; magnification: × 58 000

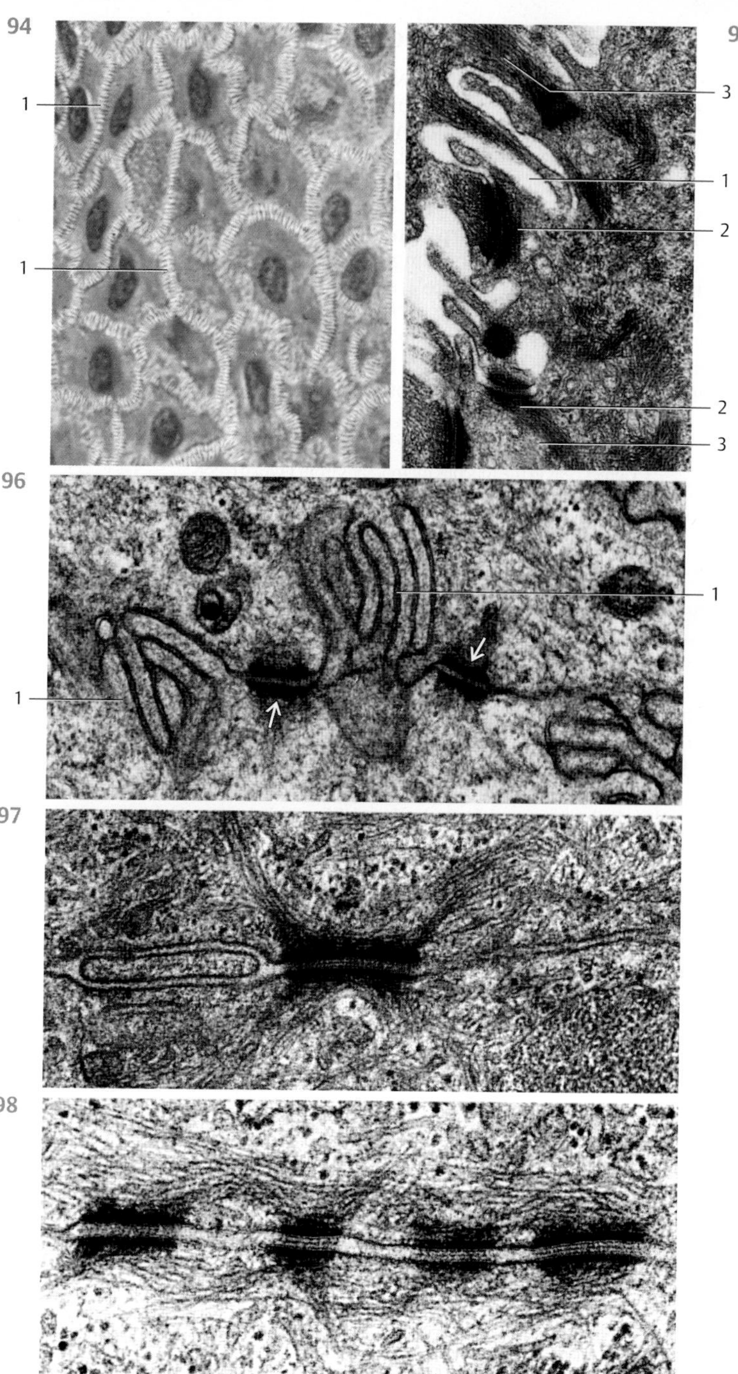
94
1
1
95
3
1
2
2
3
96
1
1
97
98

99 Terminal Bar—Junctional Complex

The terminal bar is defined as a web-like attachment system at the apicolateral zones of the prismatic (cuboidal) epithelium. It surrounds single endothelial cells like a belt. In light microscopy, this terminal network 1 is particularly conspicuous in tangential or horizontal cuts through the apical regions of cells from single or multilayered epithelium. In vertical cuts, only the profiles of these terminal bars can be observed. They appear as clearly defined granules with sharp borders (see Fig. 86). Electron microscopy reveals complex systems of binding components behind the light microscopic images of terminal bars. There are two distinct structures at the apicolateral region of the cells, the *zonula occludens* (*occluding or tight junction*) and the *zonula adherens* (*belt desmosome*). Usually, a macula adherens (focal desmosome) (cf. Figs. 101, 632) follows the zonula adherens in close proximity. Tangential cut through the mucous membrane from a human colon.

1 Terminal web
2 Lamina propria mucosae
3 Goblet cells in the mucous membranes from human colon
Stain: iron hematoxylin-benzopurpurin; magnification: × 125

100 Tight Junction—Zonula Occludens

The two outer lamina of the plasma membrane from two neighboring cells fuse at the zonula occludens and form a bar-like, *occluding junction*. At the point of fusion, the whole connecting membrane is only about 15 nm thick. There are three different types of *tight junction*. In this case, it is a continuous belt-type tight junction at the apicolateral plasma membrane from a jejunal enterocyte. The junction is part of the terminal web (see Figs. 99, 101). In the PF freeze-fracture plane, the zonula occludens usually consists of a web-like lattice system ↗. The intercellular space is occluded and the tight junction completely impermeable to hydrophilic molecules, such as ions, digestive enzymes and carbohydrates.

1 Microvilli
Electron microscopy; magnification: × 36 000

101 Terminal Bars—Junctional Complex

Electron micrograph of neighboring epithelial cell borders from a secretory duct of the submandibular gland. The junctional complex consists of a zonula occludens (ZO) and a zonula adherens (ZA). Desmosomes (D) occur in the more basal part of the junction (cf. Figs. 99, 100). The neighboring cells are cut tangentially through the area of the zonula occludens (ZO). Therefore, the occluding junction is not clearly discernible.

1 Mitochondria
2 Microvilli with glycocalices
Electron microscopy; magnification: × 31 000

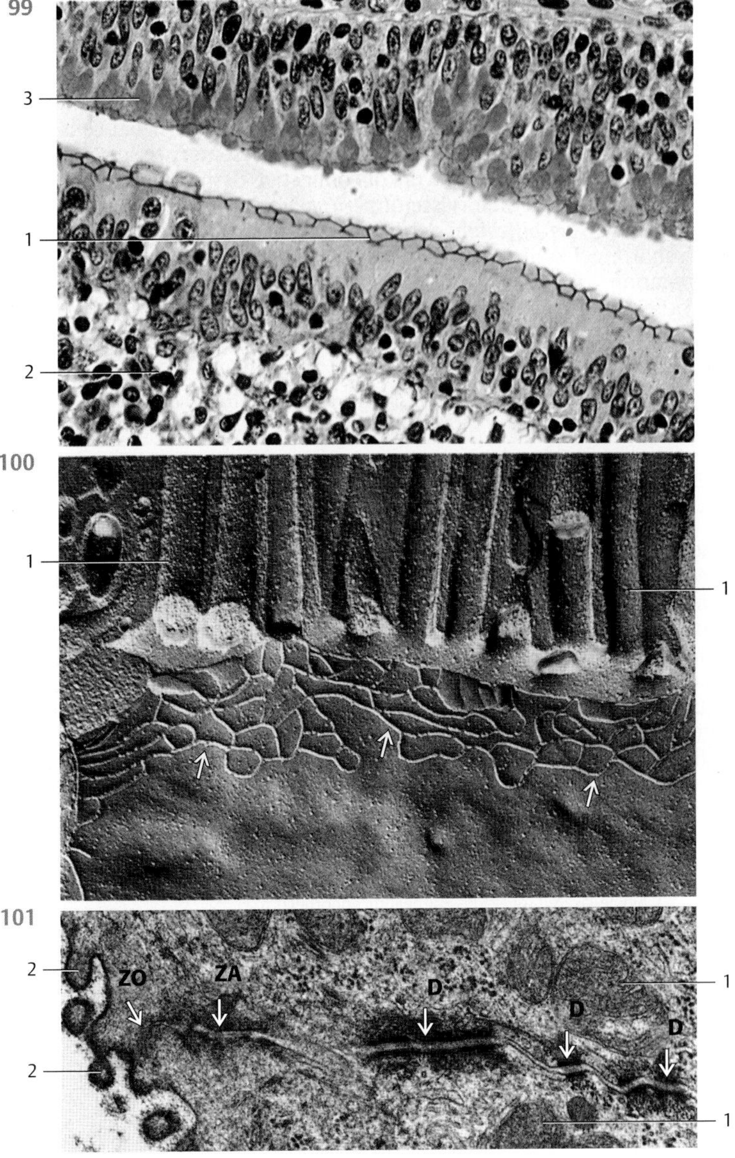
99
3
1
2
100
1
1
101
2
ZO
ZA
D
D
D
1
2
1

102 Single-Layered Squamous Epithelium—Mesentery

Single-layered (simple) squamous epithelium consists of only one layer of cells. Simple squamous epithelium occurs in the lining of the blood and lymph vessels (*endothelium*), of the heart (*endocardium*), the pleura and the peritoneal lumen (*serosa, mesothelium*). Squamous epithelial cells show a polygonal pattern when viewed from the top. Mesentery tissue, as shown in this picture, consists of flat layers of connective tissue and a layer of serous membranes at each side (*visceral peritoneum*). The epithelial cells of the serous tissue (*mesothelium, peritoneal epithelium*) are flat, polygonal cells with short microvilli, which form a single-layered epithelium. In this cuticle preparation, the cells look like pieces on a puzzle board. Silver impregnation has accentuated the cell borders (see also Figs. 103–105, 633, 634, 640). The borders from underlying cells in this cuticle preparation are visible through the top layer as gray, shadowy lines.

Whole-mount preparation; stain: silver nitrate staining; magnification: × 300

103 Single-Layered Squamous Epithelium—Posterior Epithelium of the Cornea

The surface epithelium is a continuous layer of cells without vessels. Separated by a basal membrane, it is located on top of connective tissue. The apical border is either an inside or an outside body surface. The single-layered squamous epithelium 1 of the cornea, the posterior corneal epithelium (*"corneal endothelium"*), covers the surface of the cornea opposite to the anterior chamber of the eye (see Figs. 104, 634, 640). It is a typical single-layered squamous epithelium. A vertical section shows the flat cell profiles. This figure also allows a view of the spindle-shaped nuclei in the flat epithelial cells. Underneath the epithelium is the *lamina limitans posterior, Descemet's membrane* 2. This is the thick basal lamina between the flat epithelium and the *substantia propria corneae*. It is thought to arise from the corneal epithelium. Next to it follows the wide layer of the *substantia propria corneae* 3 (see Figs. 634, 638, 640). The light spaces are technical embedding artifacts.

1 Single-layered squamous epithelium, endothelium
2 Descemet's membrane
3 Proper cornea substance
4 Fibrocytes ("cornea cells")
Stain: hematoxylin-eosin; magnification: × 400

104 Single-Layered Squamous Epithelium—Posterior Epithelium of the Cornea

View of the *posterior epithelium of the cornea* at the border to the anterior chamber (cf. Figs. 103, 634, 640). The cells are arranged evenly in a polygonal pattern. The cell regions containing the nuclei slightly protrude forward. The surfaces of the layer of flat cells are predominantly smooth. There are no microvilli. The ridged lines are the cell borders where the slender processes of neighboring cells tightly connect and are joined via macula adherentes (*desmosomes*).

Scanning electron microscopy; magnification: × 800

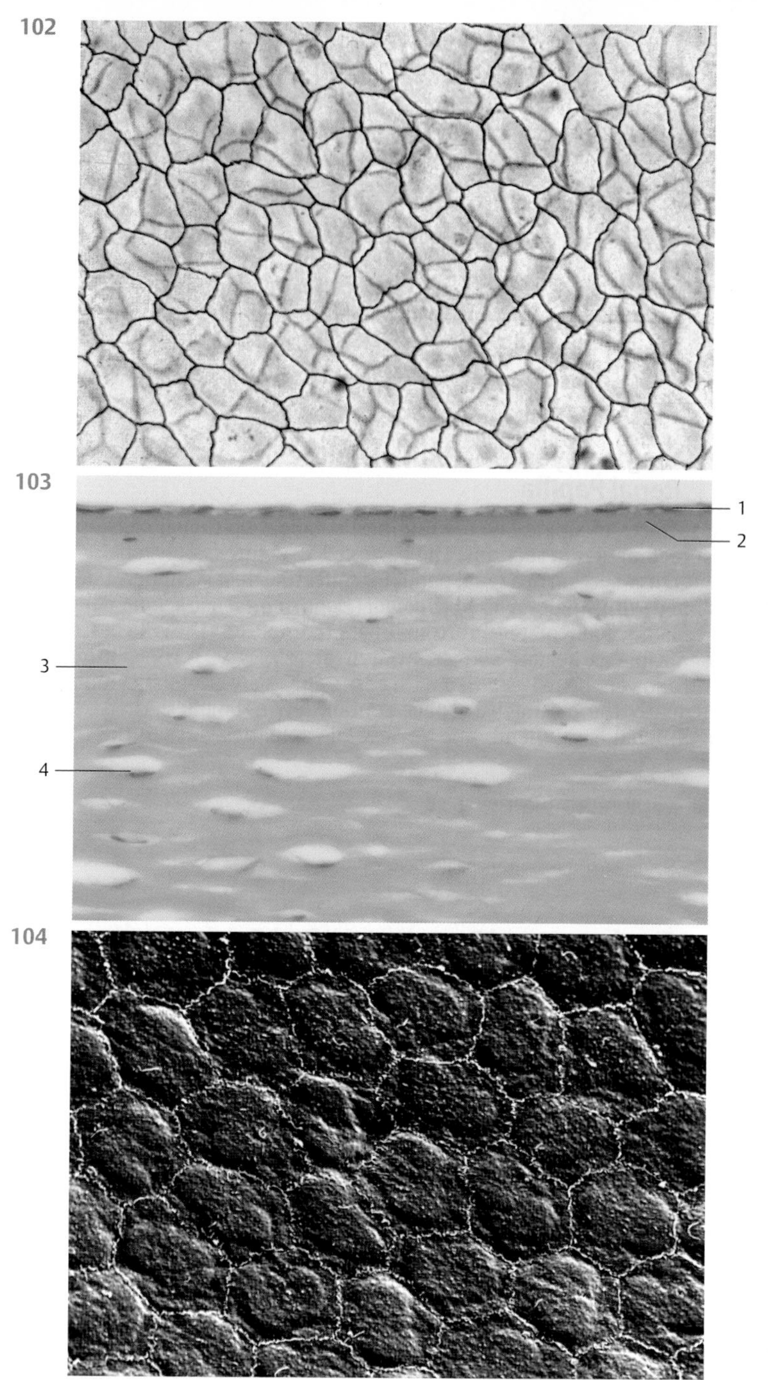
102
103
1
2
3
4
104

105 Single-Layered Squamous Epithelium—Peritoneum—Serosa

The peritoneum, the *serosa* of the peritoneal cavity, consists of a layer of peritoneal single-layered (simple) squamous epithelium and a subepithelial layer of collagenous connective tissue—i.e., the *lamina propria serosae*. The free surface of the flat epithelium (mesothelium, serosa lining) is covered with microvilli.
The cells of the peritoneal epithelium are flat, polygonal cells with serrated cell borders that can be accentuated by silver impregnation (see Fig. 102). The cell borders in the figure are clearly defined and look like short bars. The nuclei have the shape of lentils. Raised plasmalemma domes indicate their location. The surface above the nuclei has fewer microvilli (cf. Fig. 104).

Scanning electron microscopy; magnification: × 1650

106 Single-Layered Cuboidal Epithelium—Renal Papilla

The surfaces of single-layered (simple) cuboidal epithelial cells appear almost rectangular in sections. The basic cell structure is polygonal.
In this cross-section of a renal papilla, a collecting duct is cut perpendicularly. It is lined with single-layered *cuboidal* (*isoprismatic*) *epithelium*. The epithelial cells have apicolateral terminal bars (complexes) 1, which are clearly recognizable as heavily stained focal areas (cf. Fig. 99). The cell nuclei are round and very heavily stained with eosin. The finely granular cytoplasm and particularly the perinuclear space contain few organelles. There is a thick subepithelial basal membrane 2. Several capillaries close to the collecting duct are cut 3.

1 Terminal bars (complexes)
2 Basal membrane
3 Capillaries
Stain: hemalum-eosin; magnification: × 400

107 Single-Layered Pseudostratified Columnar (Cylindrical) Epithelium—Renal Papilla

Cross-section through the kidney papilla at the height of the ductus papillares 1. The ducts are lined with *single-layered pseudostratified epithelium* (*cylindrical epithelium, columnar epithelium*) (cf. Figs. 106, 505). The epithelial nuclei (light red) are located in the basal portion of the cell. The cytoplasm contains few organelles and shows only faint staining. The cell borders are a prominent detail. Between the ductus papillares are blood-filled capillaries 2. The connective tissue components in this renal papilla preparation are stained blue.
The diameter for collecting tubes in the ductus papillares is about 20 µm.

1 Ductus papillaris
2 Capillaries
Stain: azan; magnification: × 200

105

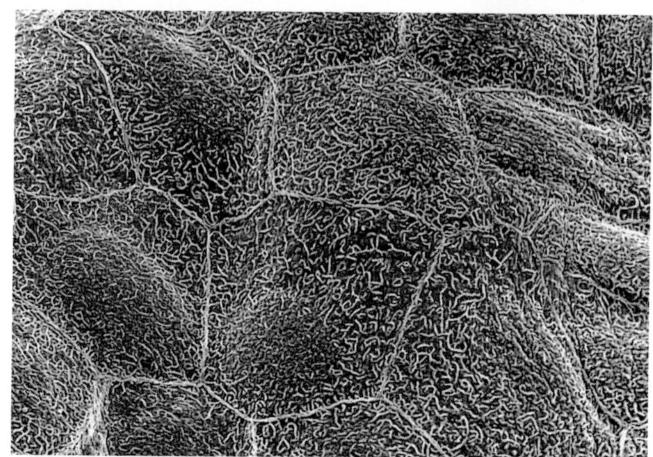

106

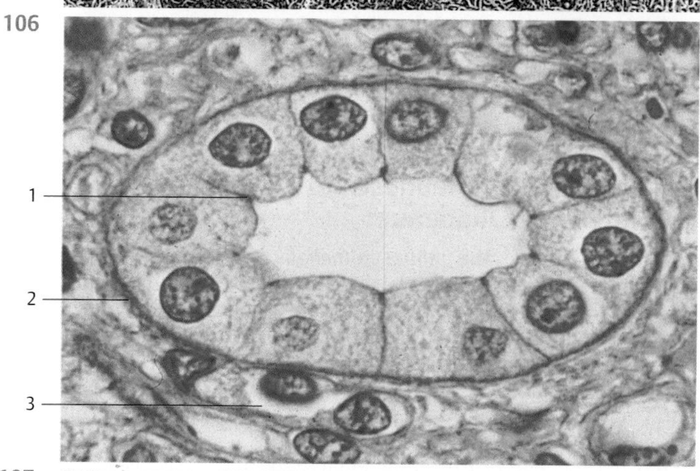

107

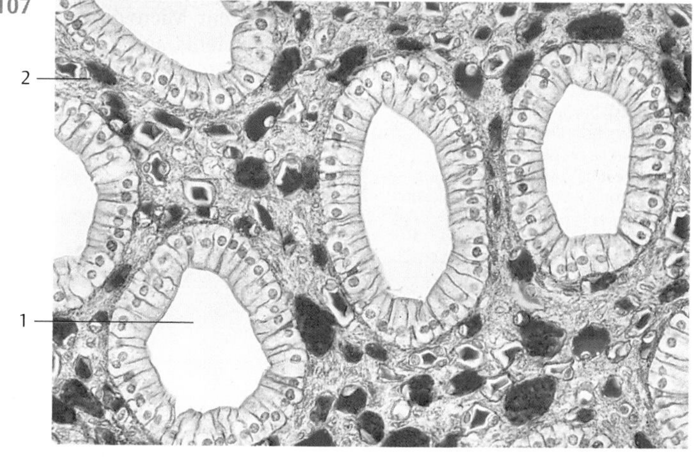

108 Single-Layered Pseudostratified Columnar Epithelium—Duodenum

In single-layered pseudostratified epithelium, the longitudinal axis of the cells is always oriented vertical to the tissue surface. The cells appear polygonal in cross-sections. A row of oval nuclei mostly occupy the basal part of the cell, while most of the cell organelles are located in the supranuclear cell region. The free surfaces of the epithelial (*enterocytes*), cells in this figure have a clearly visible striated border 1 which consists of microvilli (cf. Figs. 73, 75, 76, 415). Sporadically, goblet cells 2 occur interspersed with the epithelial cells of the tissue. The cells of the *lamina propria mucosae* 3 form a connective tissue layer underneath the epithelium, which also contains smooth muscle cells 4, apart from blood and lymph vessels, nerve fibers and myofibroblasts. A thin basal membrane (stained blue in this section) separates the epithelium from the lamina propria mucosae 3. Compare the geometry of the nuclei in Figs. 90 and 91.

1 Brush border
2 Goblet cells
3 Lamina propria mucosae
4 Smooth muscle cells
5 Terminal web
Stain: azan; magnification: × 400

109 Single-Layered Pseudostratified Columnar Epithelium—Duodenum

Vertical section through the *lamina epithelialis mucosae* of the duodenum to describe single-layered pseudostratified columnar epithelium (enterocytes, cf. Fig. 108).

The slender pseudostratified epithelial cells are evenly covered with a brush border 1 (*microvilli*, cf. Figs. 73, 75, 76, 77, 110). The oval nuclei are located in the basal third of the cell. All enterocytes contain a large number of mitochondria, both in the perinuclear (basal) space and in the apical third of the cell 2.

Microvilli, here seen as *brush border*, enlarge the duodenal surface and allow considerably more contact with the intestinal content. Microvilli-associated enzymes are important for the resorption of nutrients and digestion. The lamina propria mucosae 3 is visible in the lower part of the figure.

1 Brush border (microvilli)
2 Mitochondria
3 Lamina propria mucosae
4 Intestinal lumen
Electron microscopy; magnification: × 2000

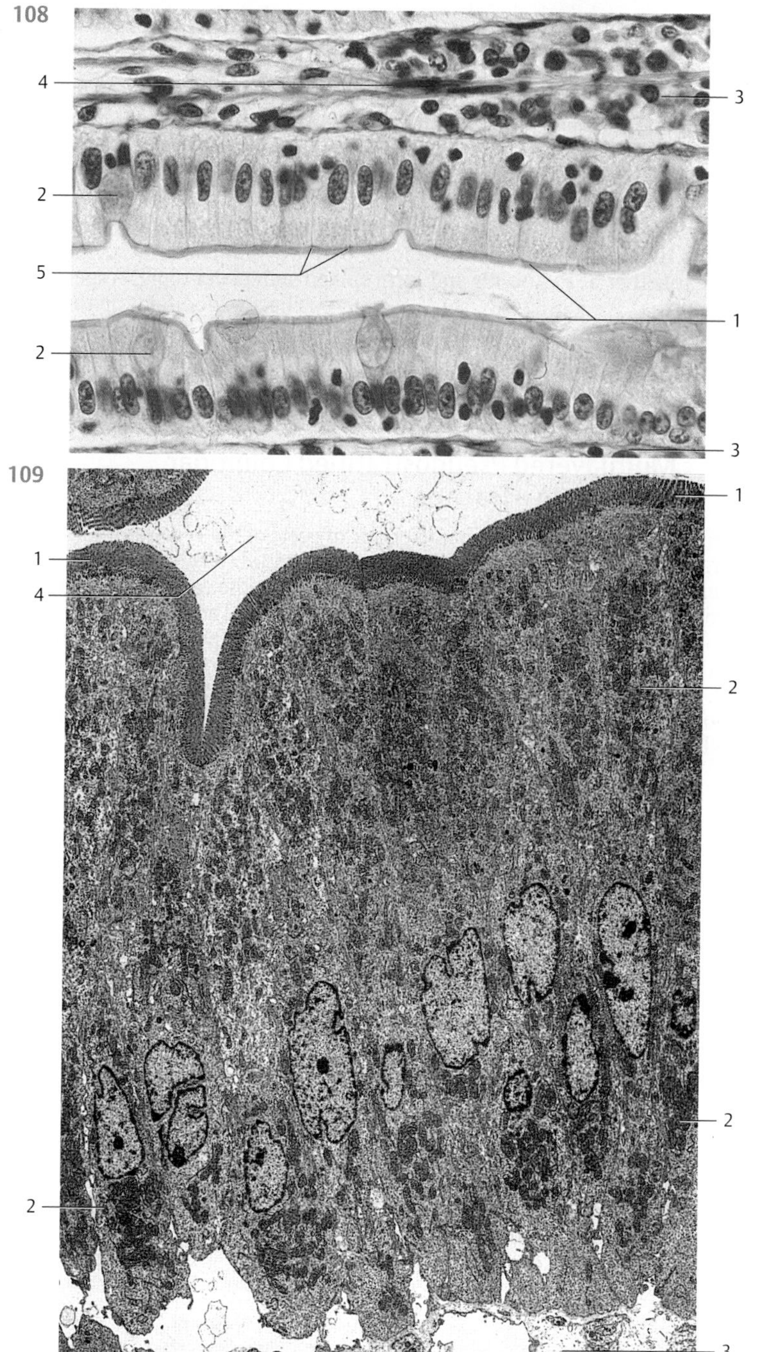
108
4
3
2
5
1
2
3
109
1
1
4
2
2
2
3

110 Two-Layered Pseudostratified Columnar Epithelium—Ductus Epididymis

In a two-layered pseudostratified epithelium, all cells originate at the basal membrane. However, not all epithelial cells extend to the surface; the cells have different heights. In this epithelial cell arrangement, the cell nuclei are located at different heights from the basal membrane. This creates the picture of two bands of nuclei (two-layered epithelium). The dark nuclei of basal cells 1 and the lighter, oval nuclei of high columnar cells 2 can be recognized. High columnar cells have long, partially branched microvilli, which stick together at their ends and form spiked stereocilia tops 3 (sperm duct stereocilia), (cf. Fig. 82, 83, 527–530). Stereocilia are modified microvilli and contain microfilament bundles.

1 Basal cell nuclei
2 Pseudostratified columnar epithelium cells
3 Stereocilia
4 Connective tissue
Stain: iron hematoxylin-eosin; magnification: × 180 .

111 Multilayered Pseudostratified Columnar Epithelium—Trachea

This type of epithelium is characteristic of parts of the respiratory tract (respiratory epithelium). In this form of epithelium, all cells touch the basement membrane but reach different heights. Therefore, the cell nuclei are not only visible in one or two, but at least in three layers. There are small, usually round basal cells 1, intermediary cells in the form of pyramids or spindles 2 and long columnar cells 3. The long columnar cells are ciliated 3 (kinocilia) (cf. Fig. 78–81, 469–471). Heavily stained lines at the apex of cilia cells correspond to rows of basal bodies 4 (cf. Fig. 80, 81). Underneath the epithelial cells is a thick lamina propria mucosae.

1 Basal cells
2 Surface cells
3 Kinocilia
4 Basal bodies
5 Goblet-cell nucleus
6 Lamina propria mucosae
7 Vessel
Stain: azan; magnification: × 400

112 Multilayered Pseudostratified Columnar Epithelium—Larynx

This section through cells from the *plica vestibularis* more strikingly presents the *multilayered structure* (banding) of the pseudostratified columnar epithelium (*cylindrical epithelium*) than the section in Fig. 111. Intermingled with cells that extend through the entire thickness of the cylindrical epithelium are smaller basal replacement cells 1 and higher *intermediary cells* 2, (cf. Fig. 110, 111). The mostly round nuclei of basal cells 1, the oval nuclei of intermediary cells 2, which do not yet reach the surface, as well as the stretched, long nuclei of fully differentiated pseudostratified epithelial cells 3, appear to occupy different layers. Therefore, there are bands with rows of cell nuclei when the epithelium is cut in a right angle to the surface. While all epithelial cells touch the basement membrane, not all of them reach all the way to the surface. Note the row of basal bodies at the apical surface of the tall ciliated cells (cf. Fig. 111). Sporadic goblet cells 6 are present amid the epithelial cells.

1 Basal cells
2 Intermediary cells
3 Tall columnar cells
4 Basement membrane
5 Basal bodies
6 Goblet cells
7 Cilia
8 Lamina propria
Stain: azan; magnification: × 400

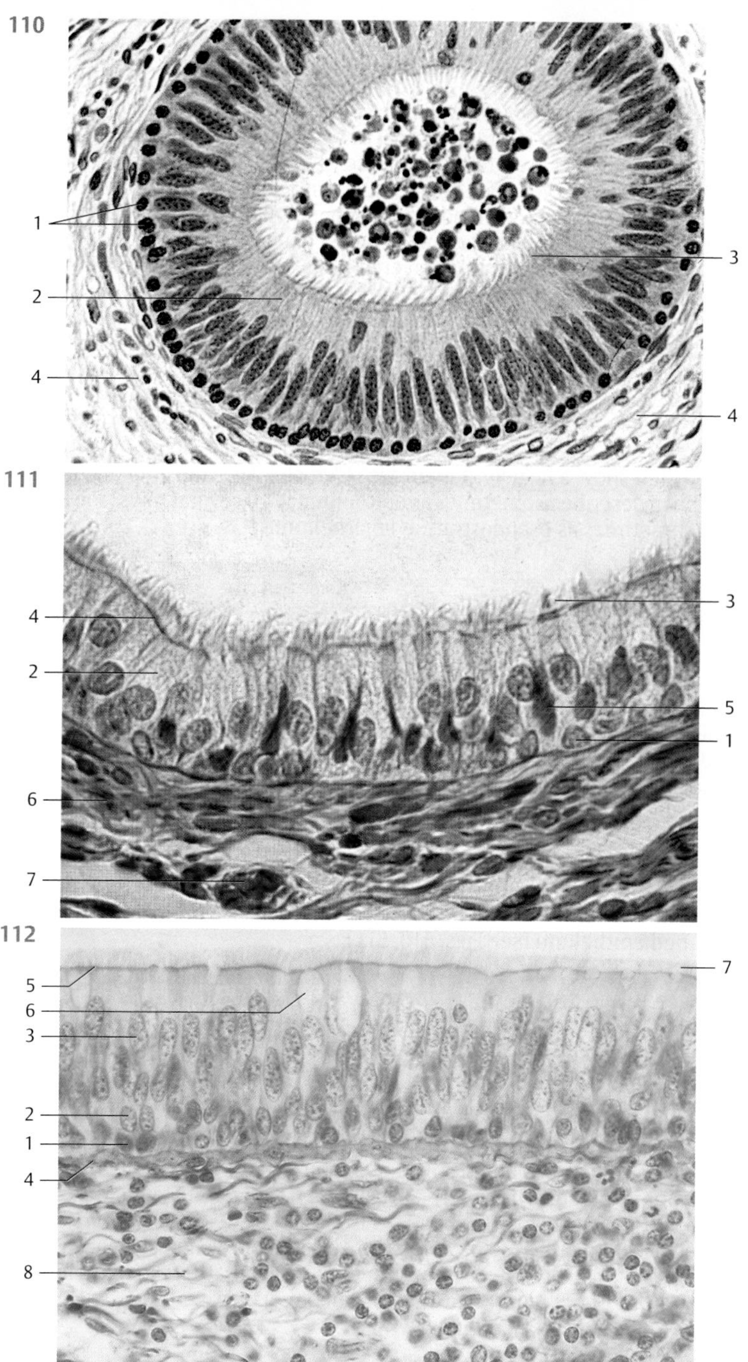
110
1
2
3
4
4
111
3
4
2
5
1
6
7
112
5
7
6
3
2
1
4
8

113 Transitional Epithelium—Urothelium—Urinary Bladder

Transitional epithelium (urothelium) forms a superficial layer, which is specific for the ureters – i.e., for the renal pelvis, ureters, urinary bladder and the initial part of the urethra. The unique characteristic of urothelium is its ability to adapt to volume changes and respond to the tensile forces in the lumen of the urothelium-lined organ. Dependent on the relaxed or distended state of the urinary bladder, urothelium changes its configuration, undergoing a transition from a multilayered type to a type with ostensibly fewer layers (= *transitional epithelium)*. In most instances, at least three layers are present. The layers are identified as the basal layer [1], followed by the intermediary layer [2] and, spanning the intermediary cells like an umbrella, the *superficial cells*. The cells in the intermediate layer [2], in particular, show irregular shapes, and they are separated by wide intercellular spaces. Polyploid nuclei are characteristic of the superficial cells. There are also superficial cells with two nuclei. Underneath their apical plasmalemma, superficial cells often show a heavily stained area (*"crust"*). The transitional epithelium has been described sometimes as epithelium with several rows (see Fig. 114), and sometimes as pseudostratified epithelium.

1 Basal cells
2 Intermediary cells
3 Superficial cell (cells of the superficial layer)
4 Lamina propria

Stain: hematoxylin-eosin; magnification: × 400

114 Transitional Epithelium—Urothelium—Ureter

This figure illustrates the basis for the controversy about the configuration of the urothelium. Seemingly, all cells are anchored on the basal membrane. Since they are of different heights, their nuclei appear at different heights from the basal membrane—*"multilayered pseudostratified epithelium."* There are basal [1], intermediary [2] and superficial cells [3]. Large cells in the superficial layer often have two nuclei. They bulge into the lumen, each one covering several intermediary cells—*superficial cells*. By definition, the superficial cells must be anchored at the basal layer, if seen as a multilayered pseudostratified epithelium (see Figs. 510, 511).

1 Basal cells
2 Intermediary cells
3 Cells of the superficial layer
4 Capillaries of the lamina propria

Semi-thin section; stain: methylene blue; magnification: × 350

115 Transitional Epithelium—Urothelium—Ureter

Cross-section through a moderately distended ureter (detail magnification). The transitional epithelium appears as multilayered squamous epithelium. It contains no glands. The superficial cells are flattened (distended, cf. Figs. 113, 508, 509). As the bladder expands, the cells of the deeper layers are also flattened. Now, the microfolds at the cell surfaces between epithelial cell junctions (see Fig. 114) are less prominent. Underneath the epithelium, the *lamina propria* extends as a thick layer of connective tissue with a tight-meshed network of capillaries.

Stain: azan; magnification: × 200

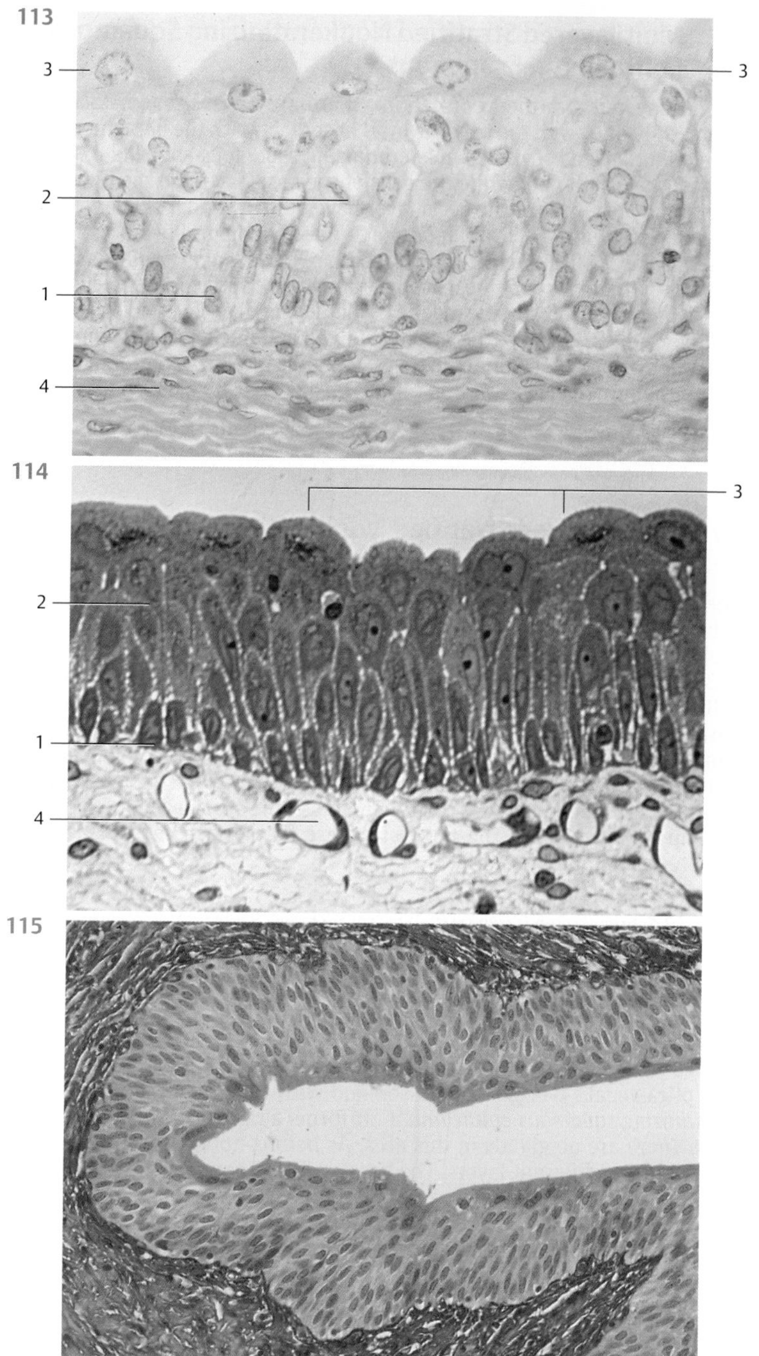
113
3
3
2
1
4
114
3
2
1
4
115

116 Multilayered Stratified Nonkeratinizing Squamous Epithelium—Esophagus

In multilayered stratified epithelium, there are always many stacked cell layers. Only one layer, the basal layer, is in contact with the basal membrane. In the *multilayered stratified nonkeratinizing squamous epithelium*, the surface cells are flattened, while the cells of the basal layer are seemingly prismatic. In reality, cells of the basal layer have quite irregular shapes. The cells in layers following the *stratum basale* 1 have polyhedral geometry and are generally larger. In successive layers, cells are more and more flattened, until the largest diameters are measured parallel to the surface. The nuclei are intact even in the top surface layer 2. The dense, dark layer of basal cells is clearly visible because of the heavily stained cell nuclei. The *lamina propria mucosae* with its high connective tissue papilla 3, 4 is layered underneath the epithelium (cf. Figs. 371 399–401, 583, 627, 628, 633, 635, 636).

1 Basal layer
2 Superficial layer
3 Connective tissue papilla, across
4 Connective tissue papilla
Stain: hemalum-eosin; magnification: × 50

117 Multilayered Stratified Nonkeratinizing Squamous Epithelium—Cornea

Vertical section through the human cornea with *Bowman membrane* 1 and *substantia propria corneae* 2. The anterior corneal epithelium is a typical multilayered stratified nonkeratinizing squamous epithelium 3 (cf. Figs. 633–636). It consists of only a few epithelial cell layers. Several epithelial cells are densely layered one over the other. The resulting layers contain basal cells, intermediary cells or superficial cells, respectively. The basal layer consists of prismatic cells; only these are in contact with the Bowman membrane 1. From the basal membrane toward the free surface, the cells are increasingly flattened and are extremely flat at the surface, about 5 µm thick and up to 50 µm long. The nuclei in these flat surface cells are long and oriented parallel to the surface.

1 Bowman membrane
2 Substantia propria corneae (the crevices are technical artifacts)
3 Multilayered stratified nonkeratinizing squamous epithelium
Stain: hematoxylin-eosin; magnification: × 400

118 Multilayered Stratified Nonkeratinizing Squamous Epithelium—Plica Vocalis

The plica vocalis (vocal fold) is also lined with a *multilayered stratified nonkeratinizing squamous epithelium* 1. It forms a rigid attachment to its support. There are no glands in this area. As before, notice the changes in cell shapes in the different layers. The basal cells are between isoprismatic and columnar and border on the basal membrane 2. In the following layers, the cells have polyhedral shapes. Closer toward the free surface, they are more and more flattened until their longest diameter is parallel to the surface. The two uppermost layers stain intensely (cf. Figs. 117, 468).

1 Multilayered stratified nonkeratinizing squamous epithelium
2 Basal membrane
3 Lamina propria
Stain: azan; magnification: × 400

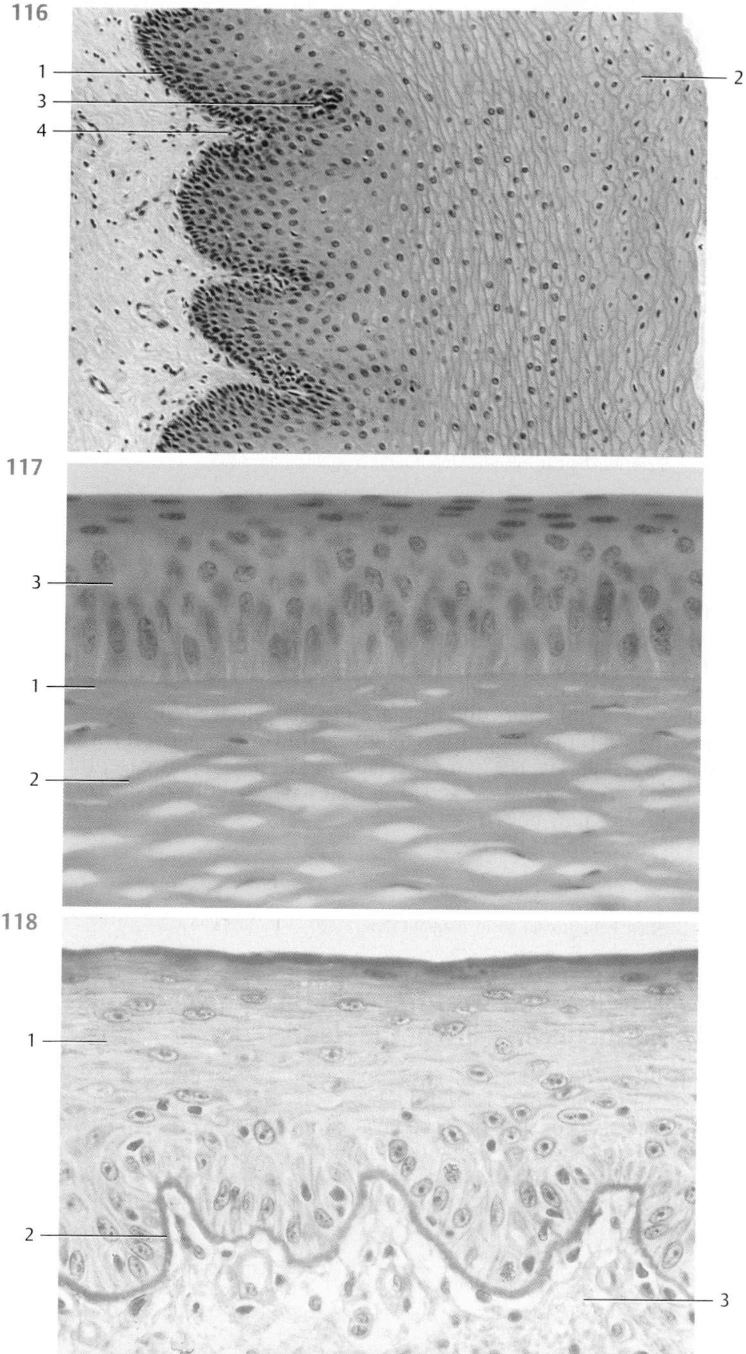
116
1
3
4
2
117
3
1
2
118
1
2
3

119 Multilayered Stratified Keratinizing Squamous Epithelium—Vestibulum Nasi

In this form of epithelium, the surface layers go through the process of keratinization. This turns the *keratinocytes* into a layer of small "dead" keratin scales, the *stratum corneum* 1. The stratum corneum is only slightly expressed in the vestibulum nasi (in contrast, see Figs. 597, 599–601, 603, 604). In this figure, it is stained light green. Nuclei can no longer be recognized. Underneath the stratum corneum is a layer of cells with dark cytoplasmic granula. It is termed *stratum granulosum*. Underlying this layer, follow several layers of prickle cells, the *stratum spinosum* (see Fig. 94). Again, only the cells of the basal layer have contact with the basal membrane. Stratum basale and stratum spinosum combined form the germinative layer, the *stratum germinativum*. Under the epithelium is the *lamina propria*, with bundles of collagen fibers and many vessels 2 (see Figs. 120, 121, 597–601, 603, 604).

1 Stratum corneum
2 Vessels of the lamina propria
Stain: iron hematoxylin-benzopurpurin; magnification: × 135

120 Multilayered Stratified Keratinizing Squamous Epithelium—Axillary Skin

Skin thickness varies for different parts of the body. For example, the epidermis of the palm and the soles is thick. However, the thin skin of the back, for example, has a strikingly thick corium (dermis). Skin is thinner and less cornified if not stressed very much. The epidermis in this figure consists of only a few cell layers and furthermore, the surface relief reveals reserve folds. The stratum corneum 1 is relatively thin by comparison with the equivalent layers in Fig. 119 and especially in Fig. 121. In this case, the keratin layers are already loosened and form scales, which will scuff off. Up to 16 g of keratin scales may be scuffed off daily.
Skin in the armpit.

1 Stratum corneum
2 Dermis (corium)
Stain: hematoxylin-eosin; magnification: × 130

121 Multilayered Stratified Keratinizing Squamous Epithelium—Palm of the Hand

The palm of the hand is subject to considerable wear and tear. Because of this stress, the epidermis is tightly attached to the dermis (corium). The epidermis also consists of more layers and is more cornified than the thin epidermis (cf. Figs. 597, 599–601, 603, 604). Note the thick *stratum corneum* 1, the abundant epidermal processes 2 and the configuration of the *corium papillae* 3. Intact cells with nuclei do not exist in the stratum corneum (keratin layer).

1 Stratum corneum
2 Epidermal projections
3 Corium papillae
4 Dermal stratum papillare
Stain: Masson-Ladewig trichrome staining; magnification: × 80

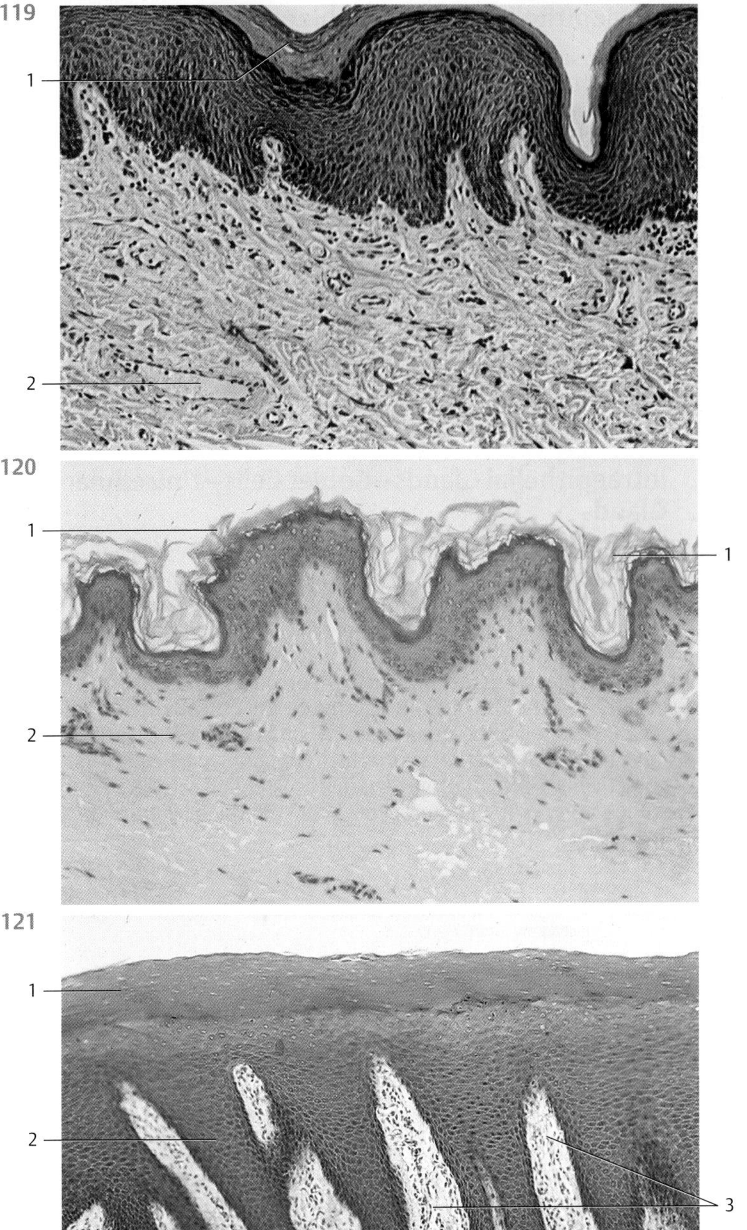
119
1
2
120
1
1
2
121
1
2
3
4

122 Intraepithelial Glands—Goblet Cells

Goblet cells are unicellular intraepithelial gland cells (see Figs. 79, 99, 108, 111, 112, 415–417, 420, 426–429). They release their secretory products by merocrine extrusion (*exocytosis*) to the free tissue surface.
This figure shows several goblet cells interspersed with ciliated epithelium. The apical part of the goblet cells show slightly stained blue secretory plugs, some extending beyond the free apical tissue surface. Around the goblet cells, the ciliated border is interrupted. The ovoid, sometimes wedge-shaped goblet cell nuclei 1 are located in the *goblet stem*. Goblet cells often form distended drum-like bodies or they expand like a chalice. Their bellies narrow at the apical membrane. Toward the basal membrane, their circumferences are also progressively reduced ("*goblet stem*"). With their secretory products released, goblet cells turn into small, spike-shaped cells ("spike cells"). Under the layer of epithelium are bundles of collagen fibers 2 and vessels 3.
Pharyngeal roof (frog).

Stain: azan; magnification: × 400

123 Intraepithelial Glands—Goblet Cells—Unicellular Glands

Goblet cells are found in many epithelial tissues. As *intraepithelial* gland cells, they have become the prototype for mucin-producing gland cells. Goblet cells occur in large numbers in the prismatic epithelium of the small and large intestines and the respiratory tract. They produce mucous materials (*mucins*). A larger luminal surface is necessary for the discharge of mucins. In the colon, this is accomplished with the development of tube-like crypts, which are rich in goblet cells (cf. Figs. 426–429). In this figure, the mucous membranes of the colon are cut parallel to the tissue surface (surface cut). This cut exposes the deeply invaginated part of the crypt, which contains a particularly large number of goblet cells. Here, they are strikingly distended into large bulbs. They relegate the scanty crop of enterocytes almost to the background.

1 Goblet cells
2 Goblet-cell nuclei
3 Slender enterocytes
4 Lumen of a crypt
5 Lamina propria mucosae

Surface cut through the mucous membranes of a human colon.
Stain: azan; magnification: × 400

124 Mucous Gland Acinus

Dependent on the morphology of the acini and the type of secretory materials from exocrine glands, there are *serous glands* (see Figs. 127, 129, 379–381, 630–632), *mucous glands* (see Figs. 128, 130, 378) and *mixed glands* (see Figs. 131, 132, 382–387). Mucous end pieces are tubules with relative wide lumina. Their nuclei 1 are flattened. They are located at the cell border or in the basal space. In contrast to serous acini, the cell borders of mucous acini can be stained and made clearly visible. The cytoplasm has a honeycomb structure. Mucous gland cells possess terminal bars 2. There are no *intercellular secretory canaliculi.*
This figure displays a typical mucous end piece from the mixed glands of the uvula of the soft palate.

1 Flattened nucleus
2 Terminal bar (complex)
3 Connective tissue of the uvula

Stain: azan; magnification: × 400

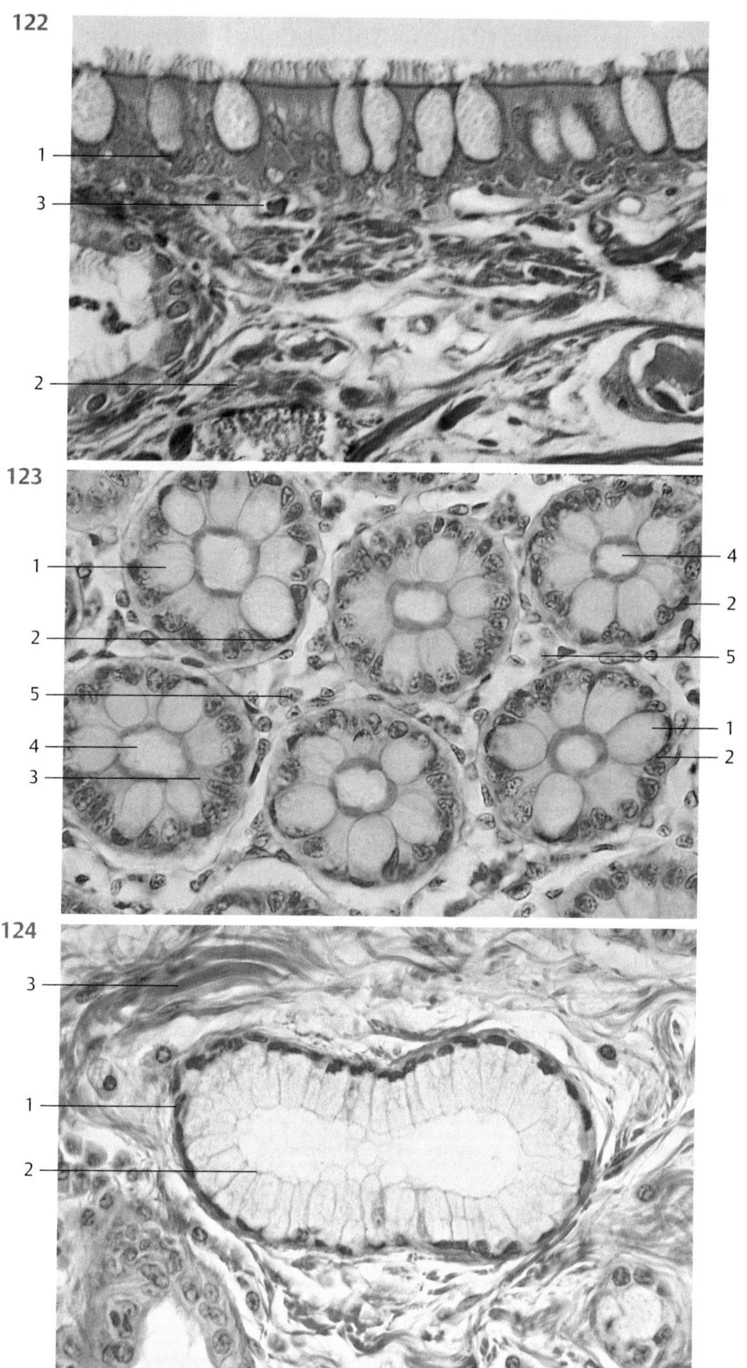

Exocrine Glandular Epithelium

125 Intraepithelial Glands—Goblet Cells—Unicellular Glands

Two goblet cells in the epithelium from the mucous membrane of the colon are filled to capacity with secretory granules. The *mucus droplets* (*secretory granules*) 2 are tightly packed. They are separated only by thin cytoplasmic partitions. The left goblet is cut tangentially. In its apical region are several secretory granules. In the absence of cytoplasmic septa, they have coalesced into a secretory lake. The stack of secretory products has reduced the cytoplasm to small peripheral bands. In the right goblet cell, lamellae of the basal ergastoplasm 3 and the nucleus 4 have been cut (see Figs. 108, 111, 112, 415–417, 420, 426–429). First, the protein components of the *mucins* are biosynthesized in the granular endoplasmic reticulum. The carbohydrate components are added in the Golgi apparatus, and the two components are then coupled.
The lifespan of a goblet cell is approximately 3 days.

1 Lumen of the colon crypt
2 Mucus droplet
3 Ergastoplasm
4 Cell nuclei
5 Enterocyte
Electron microscopy; magnification: × 6500

126 Multicellular Intraepithelial Glands

Several secretory cells can combine to small groups in the surface epithelium. This creates *multicellular intraepithelial glands* 1, which can be found in the multilayered stratified columnar epithelium of the nasal cavities as well as in the epithelium of the urethra and the conjunctiva of the eye (*goblet-cell groups*).
This vertical section through the ciliated, multilayered stratified columnar epithelium of the nasal cavity shows goblet cells 2 and a multicellular intraepithelial gland. The cytoplasm of the secretory cells is only faintly stained.
Note also the loosely organized connective tissue of the *lamina propria* 3.

1 Multicellular interepithelial gland
2 Goblet cells
3 Lamina propria
Stain: alum hematoxylin; magnification: × 400

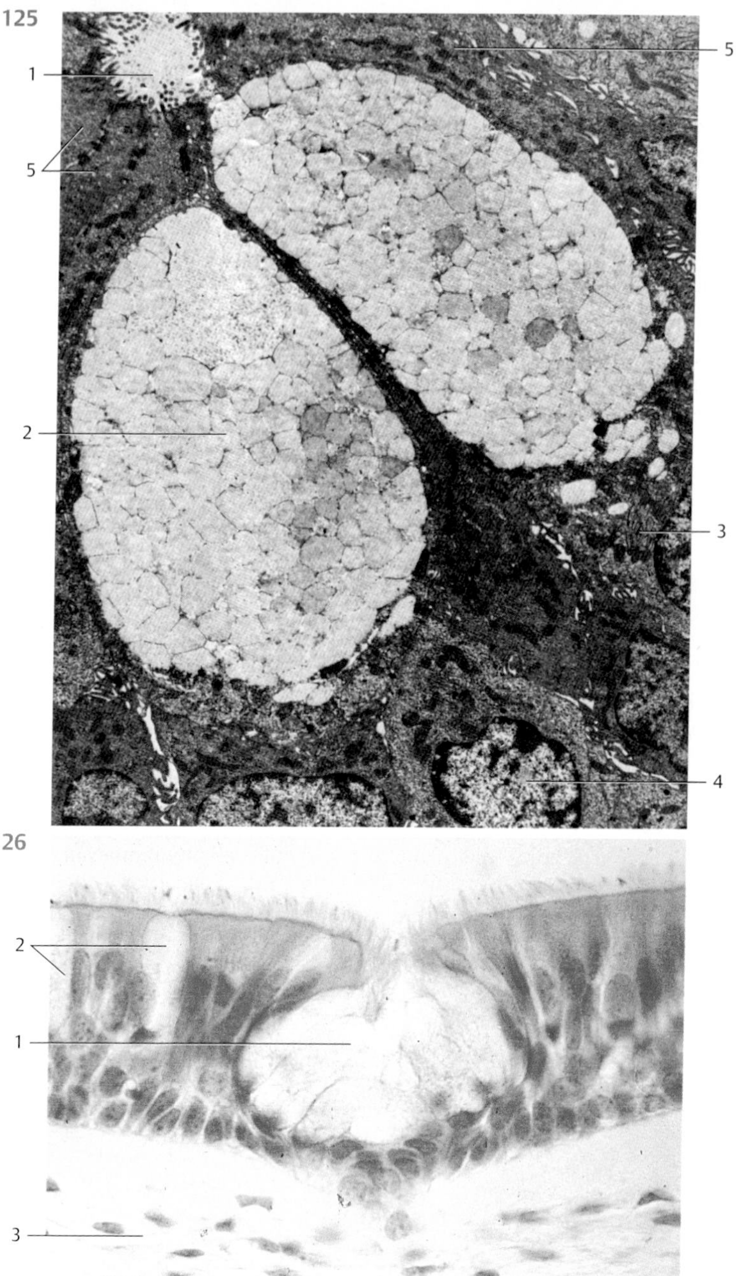
125
1
5
5
2
5
3
4
126
2
1
3

127 Extraepithelial Glands—Serous Glands

The secretory cells of active glands accumulate visible supplies of secretory products. This leads to enrichment in secretory materials and their precursors. In the process, the number of conspicuous secretory granules or secretory droplets increases. The acinar cells of the parotid gland show the typical attributes of serous glands. Their many secretory granules are distributed over the entire cell. In electron microscopy, they appear as osmiophilic spheres. The electron densities of granular membrane and contents are the same. The granular membrane is therefore hardly visible, even at high magnification. The secretory granules are generally released into the lumen 1 as single granules (exocytosis). However, occasionally the secretory granules in serous gland cells may fuse before they are extruded.
This figure shows an acinus of the parotid gland (cf. Figs. 129, 379–381, 455–459, 630–632) with osmiophilic secretory granules. On average, the gland cells are cone-shaped. There are secretory canaliculi 2 between gland cells. The nuclei 3 are located in the basal space.

1 Acinar lumen
2 Intercellular secretory canaliculi
3 Cell nuclei
4 Connective tissue cells
5 Capillary
Electron microscopy; magnification: × 1800

128 Extraepithelial Glands—Mucous Glands

In light microscopy, the cytoplasm of mucous gland cells appears light. Frequently it is structured like a honeycomb. The flattened nuclei are located in the basal cell space (see Figs. 130, 378). As in serous glands, cells from mucous glands produce many secretory granules, which will finally occupy the entire cell body (see Fig. 125). Electron microscopy shows different patterns of density for the mucus droplets. These droplets will fuse with each other, especially in the apical cell region, and lose their cell membranes in the process. The mucous droplets are so densely packed that they will supplant other cell organelles and inclusions. Only small cytosol septa are left between the secretory granules. At the cell periphery is a narrow layer of cytoplasm, which contains the mitochondria, other cell organelles and, in the basal cell region, the flattened nucleus. This figure shows mucus droplets in submandibular gland cells. Neighboring cells interconnect via cell processes. The basal region contains myoepithelial 2 cells.
Mucins can be selectively stained using special staining procedures, e.g., Alcian blue staining or the PAS reaction (mucin staining; see Fig. 428b).

1 Secretory granules
2 Myoepithelial cell
3 Gland lumen
4 Intercellular space, can be recognized as cell border using light microscopy
Electron microscopy; magnification: × 7800

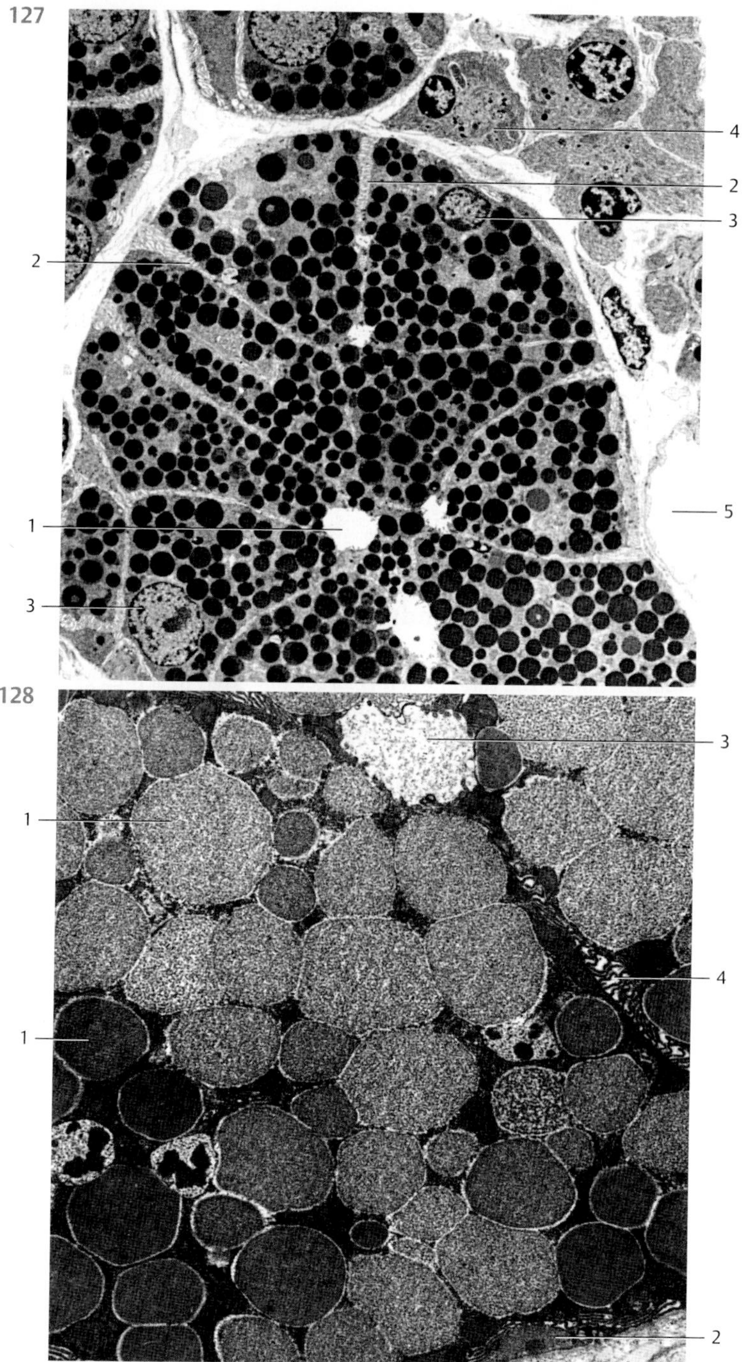
127
4
2
3
2
1
5
3
128
3
1
4
1
2

129 Extraepithelial Glands—Serous Glands

Extraepithelial glands consist of many epithelial cells in an organized group with the attributes of an organ. They originate with the surface epithelium. During their development, they become part of the underlying connective tissue. However, they maintain open connections to the surface epithelium via secretory ducts (*ductus excretorii*). The terminal portion of a serous gland duct has the form of an acinus (cf. Figs. 132, 379–381, 455–459). The mostly cone-shaped serous gland cells show polar differentiation. They display round nuclei and an elaborate ergastoplasm (basal basophilia, cf. Figs. 18, 19). Staining clearly reveals secretory granules in the supranuclear cell space. The cytoplasm is therefore granulated (cf. Figs. 379–381, 455, 457). The acinar lumina are narrow. Between glandular cells are intercellular secretory ductules (see Figs. 127). Staining will only marginally bring out the cell borders. Serous gland cells secrete an easy flowing solution of proteins and enzymes. The serous gland in this preparation is from parotid gland, which is an exclusively serous gland. There are fat cells 1 between the acini. This figure shows two acini, one (on the left) was cut across the axis, and another connecting duct (in the right upper corner) was cut lengthwise (cf. Figs. 379–381).

1 Fat cells
2 Acinus
Stain: hematoxylin-eosin; magnification: × 200

130 Extraepithelial Glands—Mucous Glands

Most terminal portions of mucous glands are tubular (*glands with tubular terminal portions*). The total lumen is larger than that in serous gland acini. The lumina are relatively wide, the nuclei are flattened and distorted and look like sickles or spindles. Nuclei are always located in the basal cell region. Basal basophilia does not exist, or is barely detectable after staining. The cell bodies of mucous gland cells display large, only lightly stained secretory granules, which occupy most of the cellular space. These stacked granules cause the cytoplasmic honeycomb structure (cf. Figs. 124, 378, 401). The cell borders are clearly visible. In the apical regions are terminal bars (see Figs. 99, 128). There are no *intercellular secretory canaliculi*.
Human sublingual gland.

1 Terminal portion of the mucous gland
2 Serous acinus
Stain: hematoxylin-eosin; magnification: × 200

131 Extraepithelial Glands—Mixed (Seromucous) Glands

This figure displays a mucous terminal portion (*tubulus*) 1. It is flanked by several serous acini 2. The nuclei of serous acinar cells are round 3 while the nuclei of mucous tubule are more flattened 4. The cytoplasm of serous gland cells is stained red, that of mucous gland cells is light. Note the wide lumen 5 of the mucous tubule (cf. Figs. 132, 382–387).

1 Mucous tubule
2 Serous acini
3 Nuclei of serous gland cells
4 Nuclei of mucous gland cells
5 Lumen of a mucous tubule
Mixed glands from the mucous membrane of the uvula.
Stain: azan; magnification: × 400

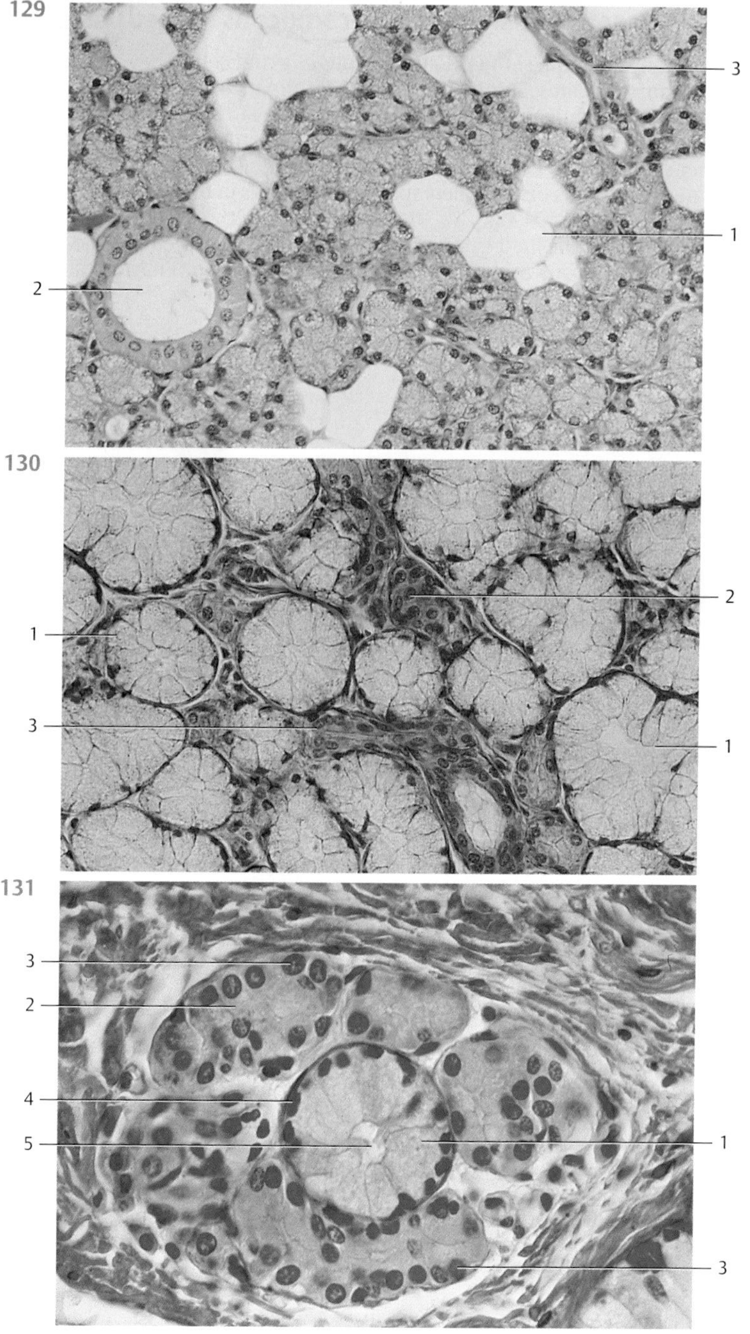
129
3
1
2
130
2
1
3
1
131
3
2
4
5
1
3

132 Extraepithelial Glands—Seromucous (Mixed) Glands

Some glands contain serous 1 and mucous 2 gland cells. They are therefore termed *mixed glands*. Serous and mucous terminal portions can exist side by side. However, mucous tubules 2 often feature at their ends serous gland cells, which form a cap-like structure, termed serous cap or demilunes 3 (*Ebner's or Giannuzzi's crescents, semiluna serosa*). Note that both serous and mucous gland cells display their specific characters in terms of structure and staining (cf. Figs. 387–387). The flattened nuclei in the basal cell region, the cell borders and the light cytoplasm of the mucous gland cells are clearly discernible. The serous acini are smaller, their lumina more narrow and their nuclei are round.

1 Serous acini
2 Mucous tubule
3 Serous demilune
Stain: azan; magnification: × 400

133 Extraepithelial Glands—Apocrine Sweat Glands

The apocrine sweat glands (*aroma glands*) are long, unbranched epithelial tubules with wide lumina, which end at the follicle. The coiled secretory tubules of the sweat glands are lined with single-layered epithelium. Its height depends on the functional state. It is characteristic of these gland cells to form raised domes on the cell surface. These domes are filled with secretory material and will finally separate as vesicles from the cell body 1 by constriction and membrane fusion: *apocrine extrusion, apocytosis*. In the process, part of the cytoplasm may be extruded as well. After secretion, the glandular tubules are lined by a flattened epithelium. The small dark spots 2 at the basis of the gland cells represent myoepithelial cells (cf. Figs. 609–611). Apocrine sweat gland from the human axilla (armpit).

1 Cytoplasmic dome with secretory material
2 Myoepithelial cell
Stain: van Gieson iron hematoxylin-picrofuchsin; magnification: × 240

134 Extraepithelial Glands—Holocrine Sebaceous Glands

Sebaceous glands consist of bulbous multilayered *epithelium cones*, termed *sebaceous bulbs* or sacs, which lack a luminal space (cf. Figs. 612, 613). The neck of the main bulb opens to the hair shaft. The cells inside the bulb grow larger, produce sebum and consequently, change into sebum cells 2. Their nuclei then die (*apoptosis*). In the usual preparations used for teaching purposes, the fat droplets are removed. This leads to more and more vacuoles in the cells at the center. While producing the *secretory product*, the cells die and are extruded together with the secretory material (*sebum*): holocrine extrusion, holocytosis, (cell lysis). New cells arrive from a supply line, which start at the peripheral cell layer (substitute cells, basal cells) 3.

1 Sebum in the neck of the gland
2 Sebaceous gland cells
3 Peripheral cells (substitute cells, basal cells)
4 Dense regular connective tissue
Stain: azan; magnification: × 65

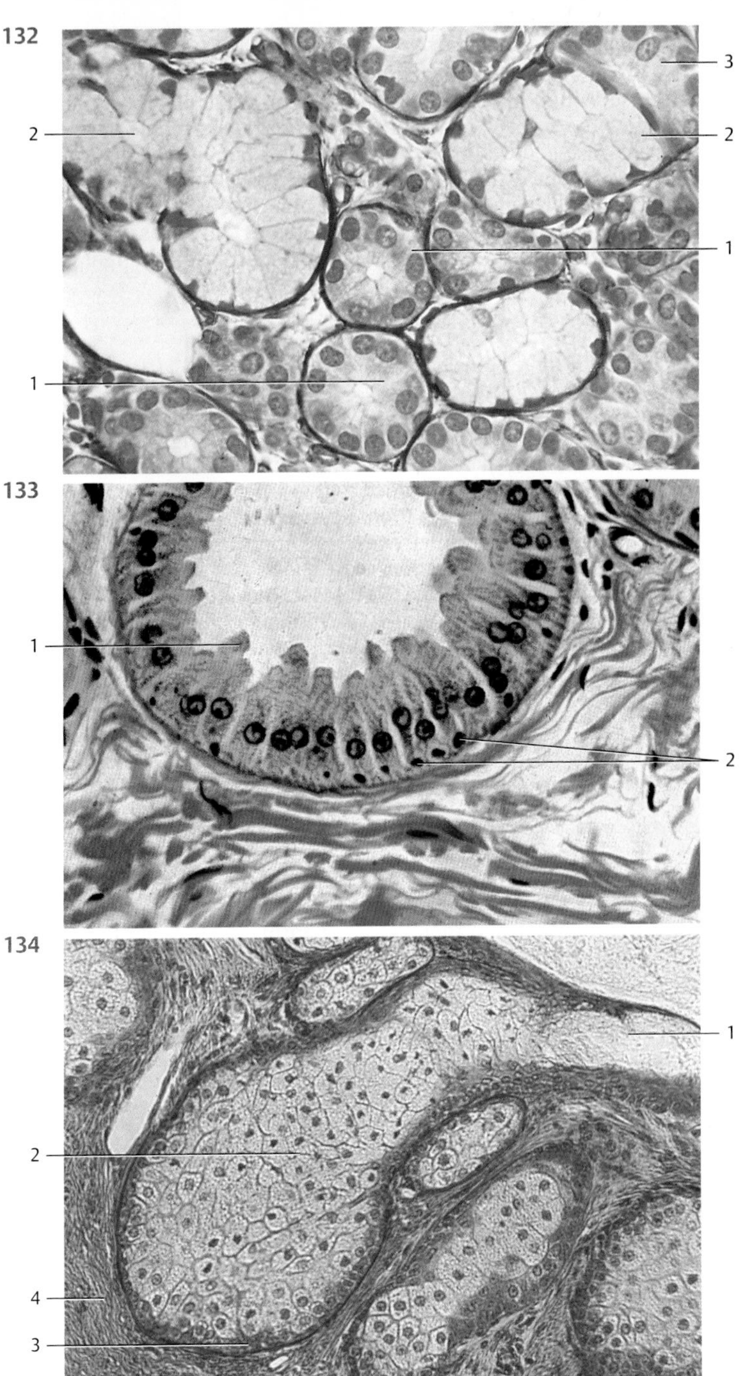
132
2
3
2
1
1
133
1
2
134
1
2
4
3

135 Mesenchymal Cells

Mesenchymal cells are specific cells of the embryonic connective tissue. They will give rise to the adult connective and supporting tissue. The mesenchyme itself originates with the mesoderm early in the embryonic development. Mesenchymal cells have little cytoplasm; their large (euchromatin) nuclei show weak basophilia and contain one or more nucleoli. Mesenchymal cells show many cytoplasmic processes: thin, branched cell processes connect with each other and form a loose, spongy network that spans an intercellular substance (*extracellular matrix*) that is not specifically differentiated.
Mesenchymal cells from a 10-day old mouse embryo.

Stain: Heidenhain iron hematoxylin; magnification: × 200

136 Fibroblasts—Fibrocytes

Fibrocytes are local (fixed) connective tissue cells (cf. Fig. 4). They are branched and connect to each other via cytoplasmic processes of different sizes. Otherwise, the appearances of fibrocytes differ, dependent on the type of the connective tissue and their function. In the usual sections, they attach so tightly to the surrounding connective tissue fibers that it often renders their cytoplasm invisible. The name *fibroblast* shows that the connective tissue cell has a specific functional role. Fibroblasts play an important role in the synthesis of extracellular substances (*extracellular matrix*), as in *fibrillogenesis*. This figure shows strongly basophilic fibroblasts in the connective tissue of a fetal jawbone.

Stain: hemalum-eosin; magnification: × 500

137 Fibroblasts—Fibrocytes

Fibroblasts from the edge fog of a cell culture (*cover-glass culture*). After seeding a cell culture, the propagating cells will spread. Their spreading in a sparse, thin layer to the underside of the cover glass allows a microscopic examination. Fibroblasts are stretched, flattened cells. Their cytoplasmic processes may look like a membrane, or form spikes. They feature large, usually oval nuclei with prominent nucleoli and display a very delicate chromatin structure. The cytoplasm appears vitreous and is only lightly stained. Occasionally, it contains small fat droplets and vacuoles. Note the cells in mitosis 1.

Stain: methylene blue; magnification: × 400

138 Fibroblasts—Fibrocytes

Fibrocytes from the connective tissue of a human amnion. Some of the oval or spindle-shaped fibrocytes have long processes, which will make contact with processes from other fibroblasts.

Whole-mount preparation. Stain: Heidenhain iron hematoxylin; magnification: × 50

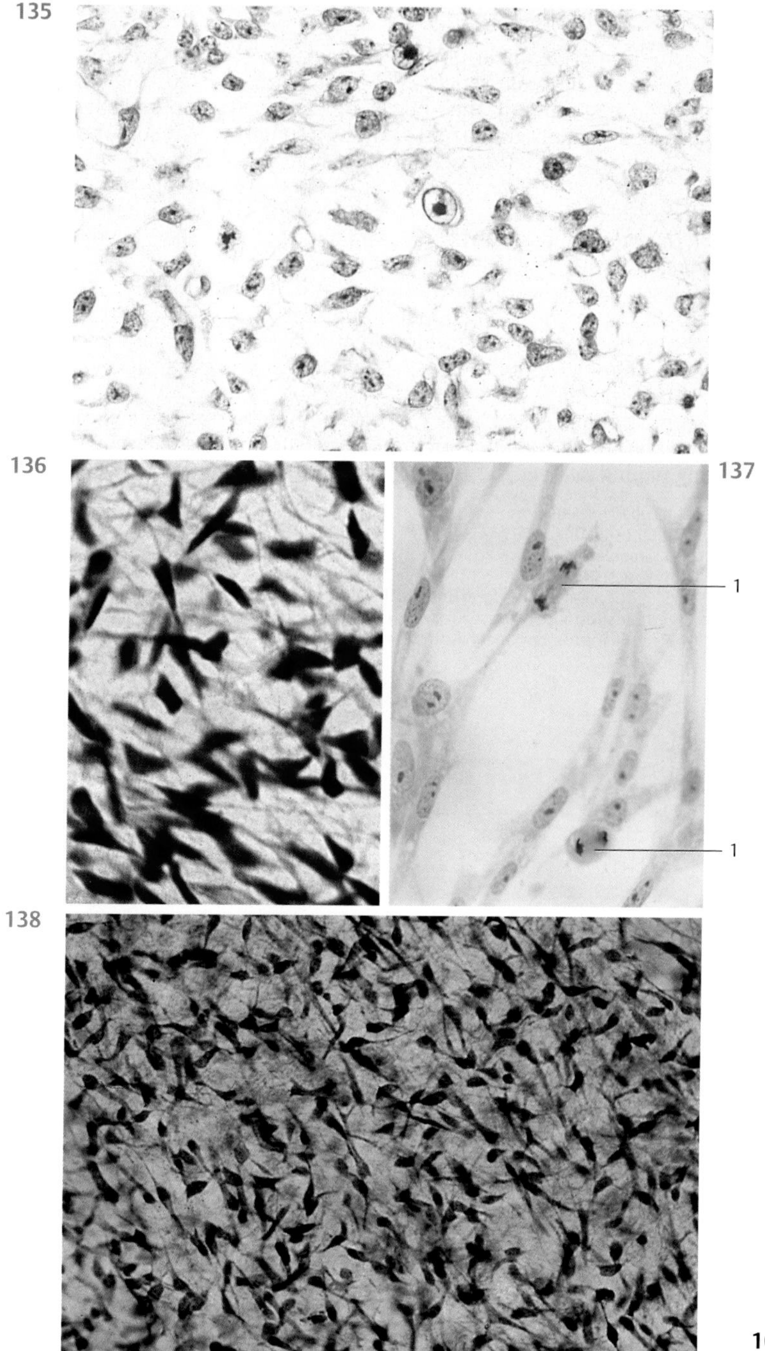
135
136
137
1
1
138

139 Fibroblasts—Fibrocytes

Fibrocyte from the epineurium of the median nerve with arcuate, slender processes 5 of different lengths. Fibrocytes tend to have the shape of a spindle and consequently, their nuclei are elongated and often lobed 1. The electron-dense, finely granulated cytoplasm contains many small mitochondria 2 with an electron-dense, osmiophilic matrix (cf. Fig. 40) and close to the surface, vacuoles of various sizes 4. The granular endoplasmic reticulum 3 and the Golgi apparatus are only poorly developed. Close to the fibrocytes—i.e., in the extracellular matrix of the connective tissue—there are multitudes of collagen fibrils 6, which are all cut vertical to their axis.

Fibroblasts and fibrocytes are always present in connective tissue. They are important for the formation of fibers and the synthesis of nonstructural intercellular substances (*glycosaminoglycans*). The cells discharge procollagen molecules into the extracellular space, which assemble to tropocollagen and finally to microfibrils.

Different stimuli convert fibrocytes back to fibroblasts. They will then synthesize structural and nonstructural extracellular substances, for example during wound healing.

1 Lobed nucleus
2 Mitochondria
3 Granular ER
4 Vesicles
5 Cell processes in the form of tentacles and microvilli
6 Basic substance (extracellular matrix) with collagen fibrils
Electron microscopy; magnification: × 7000

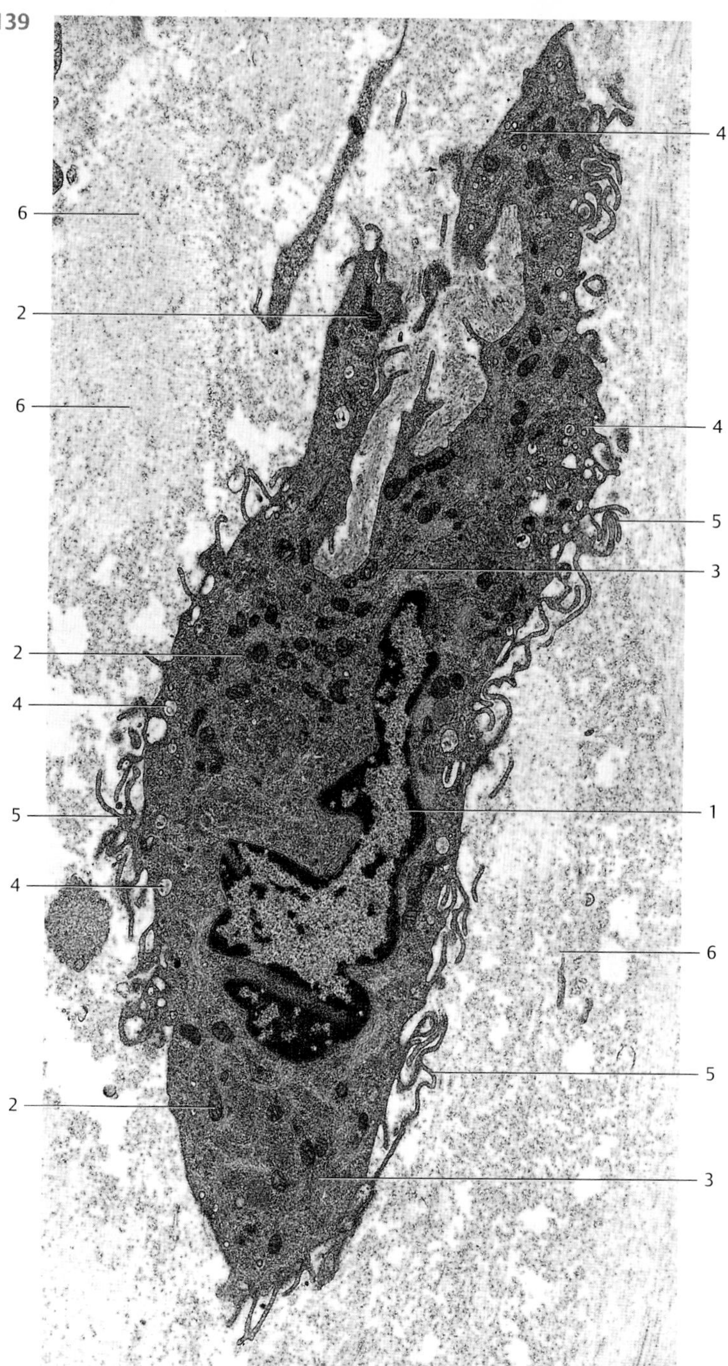
4
6
2
6
4
5
3
2
4
5
4
1
6
5
2
3

140 Free Connective Tissue Cells—Macrophages

Connective tissue macrophages are also called *histiocytes, sessile macrophages* or *resting migratory cells*. They are part of the mononuclear phagocyte system (MPS; reticuloendothelial system, RES). The precursor cells of connective tissue macrophages are monocytes, which are derived from bone marrow. Their characteristic attribute is their ability to phagocytose and store substances (*scavenger cells*). Phagocytes have irregular shapes, they are flattened and often show pseudopodia-like processes. Their eccentrically located nuclei are smaller and more densely structured than fibroblast nuclei. The cytoplasmic organization is particularly striking in electron micrographs. Apart from the usual cell organelles, there are small vesicles, vacuoles, filaments and osmiophilic inclusions. These may be primary lysosomes, secondary lysosomes 1 or often also *inclusions*, which have become part of *phagolysosomes* or *residual bodies*. Therefore, light microscopy often reveals a "granular cytoplasm" in macrophages. *In-vivo* injection of a vital dye (trypan blue, lithium carmine, Indian ink) will selectively stain macrophages, because macrophages opsonize these substances and store them in their cytoplasm in the form of granules. The granules and the phagocytosed substances can be recognized in light microscopy.
Macrophage from human subcutaneous connective tissue.

1 Lysosomes
2 Collagen fibrils cut vertical to their axis
Electron microscopy; magnification: × 15 000

141 Free Connective Tissue Cells—Macrophages

This electron-microscopic image shows the characteristic attributes of human macrophages. During periods of very active phagocytosis, macrophages ("large scavenger cells") show a diameter of about 20 µm and are indeed voluminous. Their cytoplasmic processes may look like the tentacles of pseudopodia or like hooks. In the vicinity of their kidney-shaped nuclei 1 are crista-type mitochondria 2. The granular endoplasmic reticulum (rER) is poorly developed. In contrast, note the elaborately developed Golgi apparatus 3 as well as the osmiophilic granules, which can be identified either as lysosomes or as phagosomes. Note the cross-section of a centriole ↗.
Macrophages are able to move around in the connective tissue like ameba. Therefore, they are also called wandering (mobile) phagocytes.

1 Nucleus
2 Mitochondria
3 Golgi apparatus
Electron microscopy; magnification: × 12 000

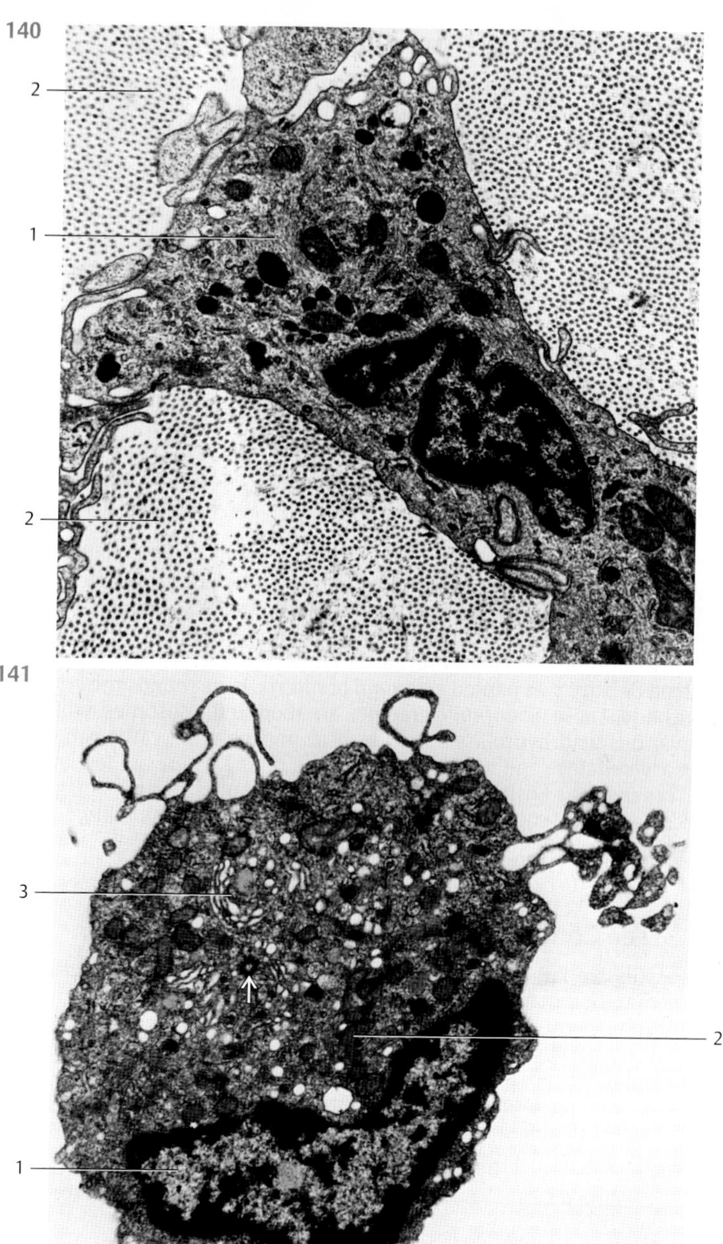
140
2
1
2
141
3
2
1

142 Free Connective Tissue Cells—Macrophages

Human macrophages can be isolated from subcutaneous connective tissue and grown in cell culture like the macrophage seen here. The flat, sprawling cell shows a characteristic surface relief. In the central region, it forms a dome over the cell nucleus. In this central area, the cytoplasmic processes appear relatively cloudy. However, the raised, partially branched microfolds (*microplicae*) in the periphery create a veil-like edge. The microfolds can be of different lengths.

Scanning electron microscopy; magnification: × 4300

143 Free Connective Tissue Cells—Eosinophilic Granulocyte

Eosinophilic granulocytes occur not only in blood (1–4% of the leukocytes) but also in connective tissue. Eosinophilic granulocytes measure about 12 µm in diameter. That makes them slightly larger than neutrophil cells. They have a bilobed nucleus (spectacle form). In the figure, the connection between the two lobes is not visible (see Fig. 308f).
The characteristic marker for eosinophils are eosin-stained acidophilic or eosinophilic granules (see Figs. 308e, f). In electron microscopy, these show a remarkably regular and characteristic structure. The oval, discus-shaped granules contain a central, oblong crystalloid body, termed *internum*. At higher magnification, the internum reveals a lamellar structure. A layer of lesser electron density was named *externum* or *matrix*. It surrounds the crystalloid inner body. These acidophilic granules are modified lysosomes, which contain various acid hydrolases, such as acid phosphatase, cathepsin, peroxidase, arylsulfatase and ribonuclease, among others. There are few cytoplasmic organelles. Eosinophilic granulocytes recognize and phagocytose antigen-antibody complexes, and they show ameba-like mobility.

Electron microscopy; magnification: × 16 400

144 Free Connective Tissue Cells—Monocytes

Monocytes are large blood cells that are rich in cytoplasm. Blood analysis shows that their diameters can reach 16–20 µm (see Fig. 308m). The nuclei of monocytes are rounded but mostly kidney-shaped or lobed. The cytoplasm contains numerous mitochondria, ribosomes and small granules. The granular endoplasmic reticulum membranes (rER) are only sparse. As in this figure, the Golgi apparatus is usually located in a perinuclear cove. Monocytes can also assume the functions of macrophages. Along with an erythrocyte [1], this monocyte occupies a capillary. Monocytes develop in the bone marrow.

1 Erythrocyte
2 Endothelium
Electron microscopy; magnification: × 4000

142

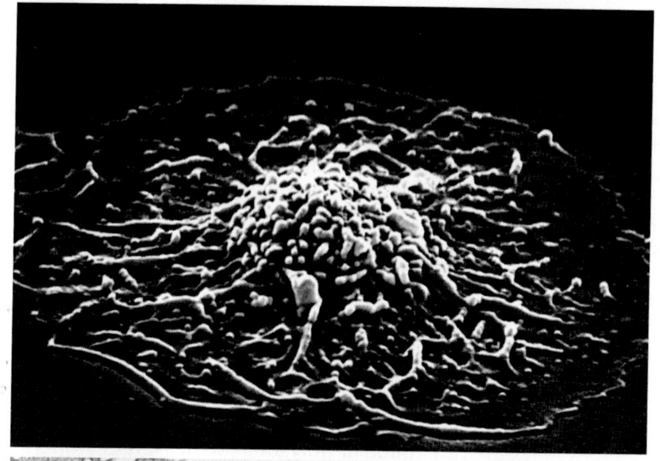

143

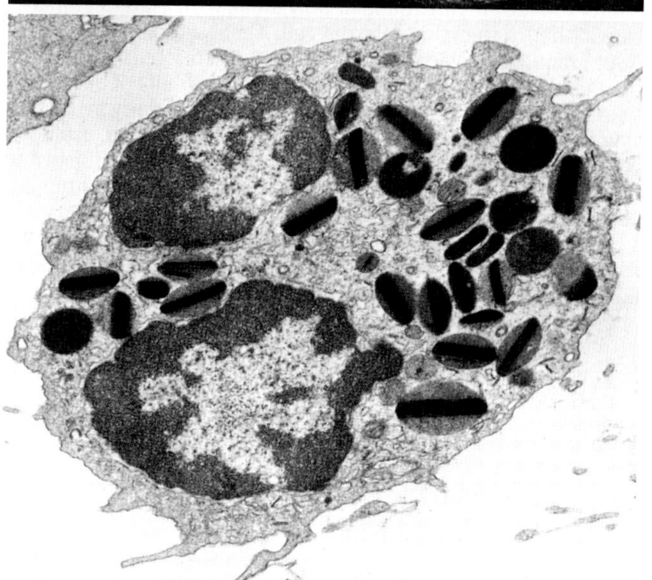

144

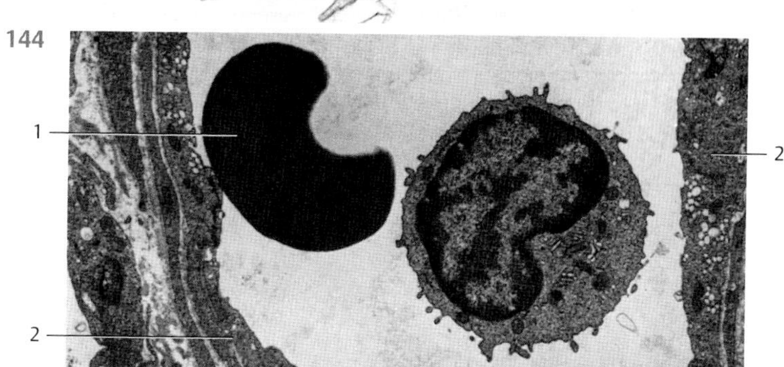

145 Free Connective Tissue Cells—Mast Cells and Plasma Cells

Figure a shows two oval, basophilic granulated mast cells from connective tissue of the greater omentum. As single cells, but more frequently in small groups, mast cells occur particularly often in the vicinity of small vessels (see Fig. 148). Mast cells (diameter 6–12 µm) contain a rounded nucleus. Their cytoplasm is loaded with basophilic, metachromatic granules. Paul Ehrlich (1877) interpreted these as alimentary storage granules (Ehrlich's mast cells). Mast cells synthesize, store and extrude the acid and sulfatized glycosaminoglycan *heparin*, the biogenic amines *serotonin* (only rat and mouse) and *histamine*, also two additional factors, which play a role in anaphylactic reactions. Histamine is released in large amounts during allergic reactions. It causes a widening of the capillaries.
Figure b depicts plasma cells in the lamina propria from pyloric mucous membranes. Like mast cells, they are free cells and occur in loosely organized or in reticular connective tissue, usually in small groups. Plasma cells (diameters 10–20 µm) are round or polygonal, with a large cytoplasmic compartment—hence the name plasma cell. Their cytoplasm is basophilic and without granules. In electron micrographs, plasma cells are rich in ergastoplasm and free ribosomes. This explains the basophilia of plasma cells. They participate in the synthesis of serum proteins, particularly in the synthesis of *gamma globulins*. One of their characteristics is the round, usually eccentric nucleus and its nuclear membrane. Chromatin bodies are attached to the nuclear membrane in a regular pattern. Often, there is a radial chromatin organization pattern (*wheel-spoke nucleus*) (cf. Fig. 146–150). Plasma cells represent the final stage in the series of B-lymphocytes. They arise from B-lymphocytes after contact with an antigen. The B-lymphocytes migrate from blood to the connective tissue.

1 Lymphocyte
2 Fibrocyte
3 Histiocyte
a) Stain: toluidine blue-paracarmine; magnification: × 510
b) Periodic acid-Schiff (PAS) leucofuchsin stain-hematoxylin; magnification: × 410

146 Free Connective Tissue—Mast Cells

This mast cell was isolated from lung tissue. It shows long cell processes, some of which are branched. The cells establish contact with each other via these processes (in contrast, see Fig. 147). This creates the image of a three-dimensional, more or less elaborate, peripheral network. In the cell center is an arcuate, notched nucleus with heterochromatin at its periphery. The cytoplasm displays a dense, finely granular matrix. Apart from this specific granulation, there are few organelles. The cell-specific, membrane-enclosed granules have diameters of about 0.5–1.5 µm. They are amorphous, both in form and structure. There are two distinct mast cell types—*mucosa mast cells* in the connective tissue of mucous membranes and *tissue mast cells* in the connective tissue of the skin.

Electron microscopy; magnification: × 13 600

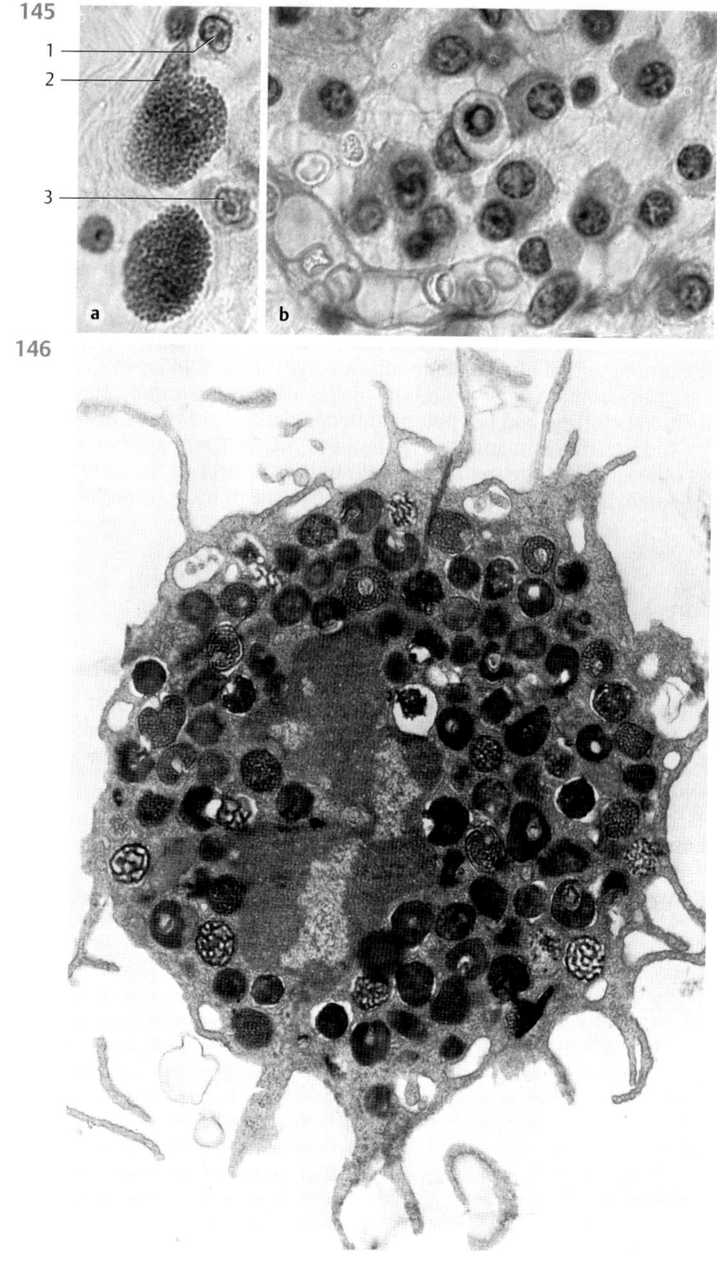
145
1
2
3
a
b
146

147 Free Connective Tissue Cells—Mast Cells

This transmission electron microscopic image displays the typical ultrastructure of a *tissue mast cell* from a rat. On the surface are sporadic short plasma membrane processes. The central nucleus is relatively small and shows peripheral heterochromatin. The nucleus is dented in several places because of the close vicinity to cell-specific granules. The cytoplasm contains the specific round or oval granules, which have diameters of about 0.5–1.5 µm. The granules are always enclosed by a membrane and separated from other granules by cytoplasmic septa, which contain crista-type mitochondria, Golgi complexes and, sporadically, filaments. The matrix of each granule is homogeneous and electron-dense (cf. Fig. 146).

Based on their sulfated glycosaminoglycan content, mast cells show a metachromatic reaction—i.e., their granules appear between blue-violet and red after staining with a blue alkaline thiazine dye (cf. Figs. 145a, 148).

The granules contain *heparin* and the biogenic amine *histamine*. Heparin inhibits blood clotting and is a potent anticoagulant. Histamine causes the arteries and arterioles in connective tissue to dilate. There are two different types of mast cells—the *tissue mast cells* in the connective tissue of the skin and the *mucosa mast cells* in the connective tissue of mucous membranes.

Electron microscopy; magnification: × 11 400

148 Free Connective Tissue Cells—Mast Cells

Several mast cells are lined up along a dividing arteriole. They are about 10–12 µm long and contain blue-violet (*metachromatic*) granules (cf. Fig. 145a). The cell nuclei in the center are often obscured because granules cover them. The release of mast cell granules into the extracellular space (*exocytosis*) is triggered either by nonspecific stimuli or by antigen-antibody reactions. In this preparation, there are also many metachromatic granules present in the free connective tissue space.

This whole-mount preparation (not a section) is from the peritoneal lining of a rat diaphragm. The arteriole contains blood cells.

Stain: toluidine blue; magnification: × 400

147

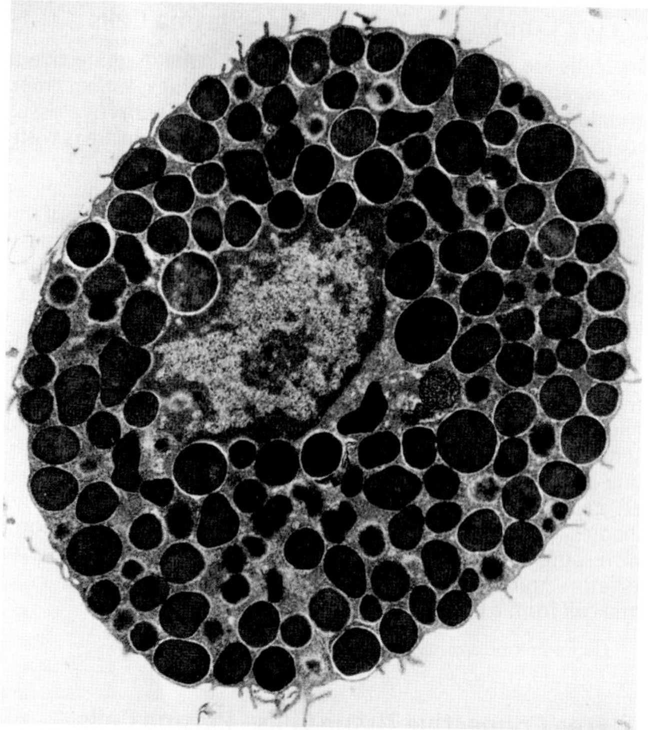

148

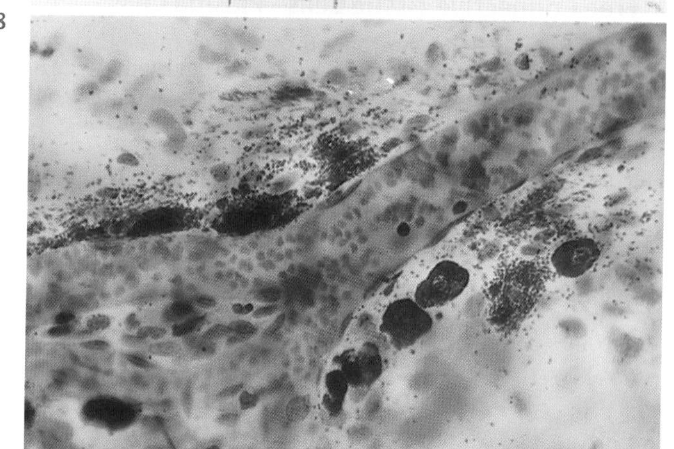

149 Free Connective Tissue Cells—Plasma Cells

Plasma cells are most frequently found in the cellular connective tissue of various organs (*lymph nodes, spleen, bone marrow, lung, lamina propria of the intestinal mucosa*). They are sporadically found in connective tissue everywhere in the body, except in blood. They are abundant in areas with chronic inflammation.

Plasma cells are round or polyhedral with rounded or oval nuclei, usually in an eccentric location. The chromatin structure is characteristic of these cells. Starting at the nucleolus, it extends to the inner nuclear membrane in a star-like fashion. Chromatin accumulates at the inner nuclear membrane. This creates the *wheel-spoke nucleus*, as seen in light microscopy (cf. Fig. 145b).

Plasma cells are remarkably rich in intracellular granular membrane systems (*ergastoplasm*), which account for the basophilia (cf. Figs. 18–23). The membranes of the rough (granular) endoplasmic reticulum (rER) organize in a circular pattern and form cisternae in some locations. Rough ER membranes are absent from the Golgi region in the cell center. Crista-type mitochondria are present in the cytoplasm as well.

Plasma cells are the final stage in the B-lymphocyte series. They are local (fixed) cells and do not divide; their lifespan is 10–30 days. They synthesize antibodies (proteins), and their function therefore serves the humoral immune response. Antibodies are released (*by extrusion*) without the formation of secretory granules.

Plasma cell from a lung (cat).

Electron microscopy; magnification: × 17 000

150 Free Connective Tissue Cells—Plasma Cells

Plasma cells from the loosely organized connective tissue from the orbital gland of a sparrow. The cells are close together and form a small group. Plasma cells, the final cells in the B-lymphocyte series, are large, either oval or round (see Fig. 149) and usually have round nuclei with dense coarse heterochromatin. Their characteristic is the abundance of granular (rough) endoplasmic reticulum (rER) as a location for immunoglobulin synthesis. It explains the conspicuous basophilia in light microscopy (cf. Fig. 145b, also Figs. 18–25). In the plasma cell in the top right part of the figure, the rER cisternae are distended. All cells contain mitochondria of different sizes.

Electron microscopy; magnification: × 9000

149

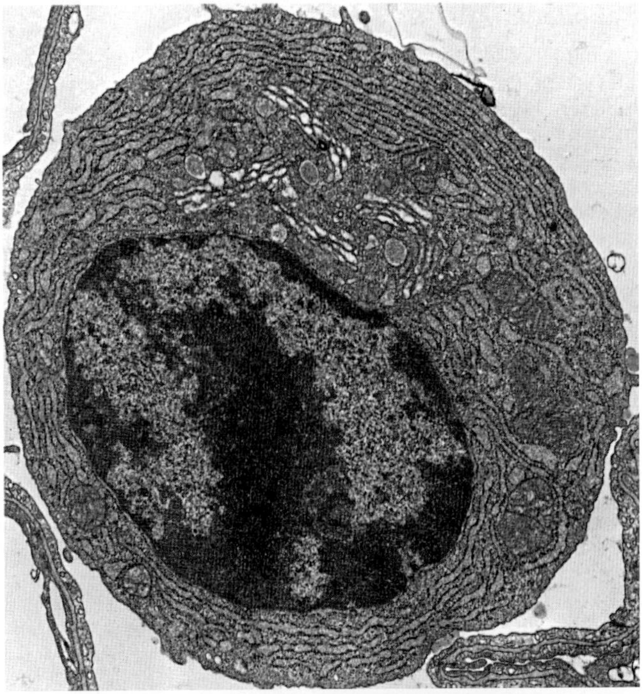

150

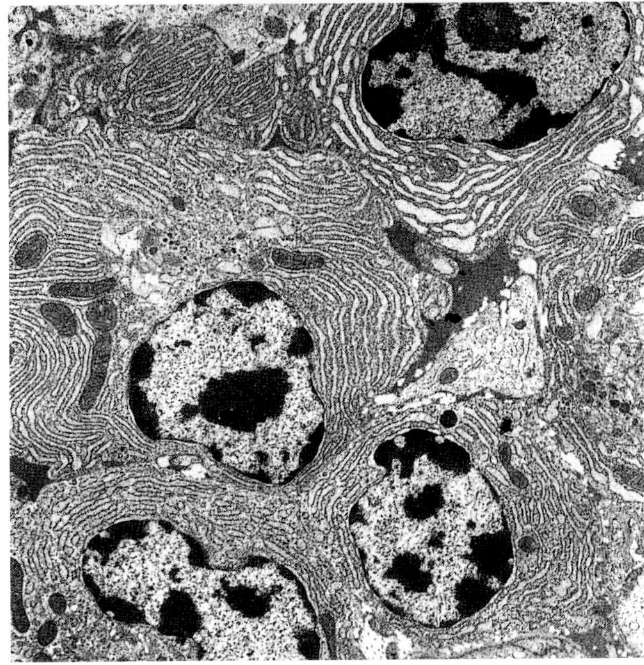

151 Collagen Fibers

Collagen fibers exist almost everywhere in the body; they are the most prevalent type of fiber in connective tissue (*collagen type I*). They can be clearly identified in histological sections by staining with various acidic dyes. Collagen fibers are unbranched. They consist of collagen fibrils. Most of the fibrils have diameters of 30–70 nm (see Figs. 152–155). Collagen fibers with diameters of 2–10 µm often form wavy fibers, like undulating locks of hair. This figure shows wavy collagen fibers (blue) in connective tissue from the corium (*stratum reticulare of the corium*). The connective tissue cells between them are stained red. Collagen (colla, Greek: glue, bone glue) is the prevalent fiber protein in the extracellular matrix.

Stain: azan; magnification: × 200

152 Collagen Fibrils

In electron micrographs, the collagen fibrils, which are approximately 30–70 nm thick, show a striation pattern of lighter and darker bands (termed *cross-striation*) with a periodicity of about 64 nm and range limits of 50 and 70 nm, respectively. This typical cross-striation is brought about by the arrangement of the 280 nm long *tropocollagen*, which consists of three polypeptide chains (α-triple helix). The tropocollagen molecules are lined up one after another, forming gaps after each molecule. They are also packed one over another in a staggered way. In the process, the protocollagen molecules are shifted by a quarter of their length (*parallel aggregation*). This causes the cross-striation seen in microfibrils.

Electron microscopy; magnification: × 52 800

153 Collagen Fibrils

Collagen fibrils with cross-striation as an example of a highly organized biological system.
Tail tendon from a rat (cf. Figs. 152, 154, 155).

Electron microscopy; magnification: × 18 000

154 Collagen Fibers—Collagen Fibrils

Collagen fibrils organize in the organism to collagen fibers. Their organization and distribution vary and adjust to changing tensile forces. The width of the fibril bundles varies too. In this figure, a fibril bundle (fiber) is cut vertical to its axis. A fibroblast is also cut and shows a nucleus, which is surrounded by a small plasma seam ①. Notice the fine intracellular filaments. In the finely granulated intercellular substance adjacent to the fibrocyte are collagen fibrils, either singly or in small groups. They are mostly cut across their axis. Some fibrils in the lower third of the figure are cut tangentially.
Section through the mitral valve of a human heart (cf. Fig. 155).

Electron microscopy; magnification: × 18 000

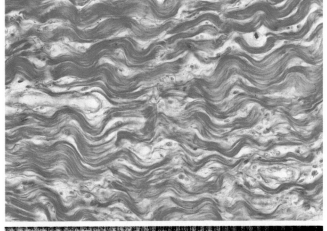

151

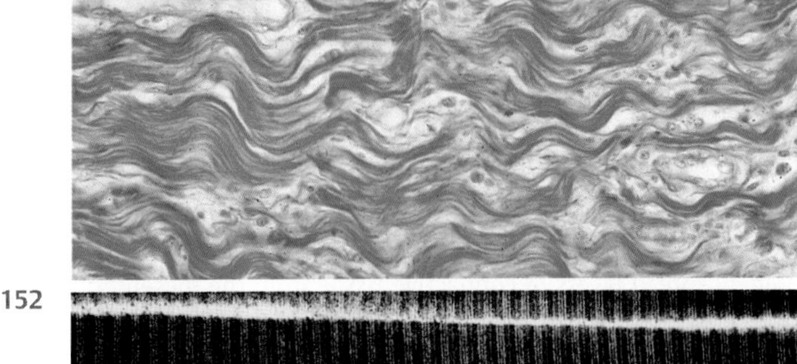

152

153

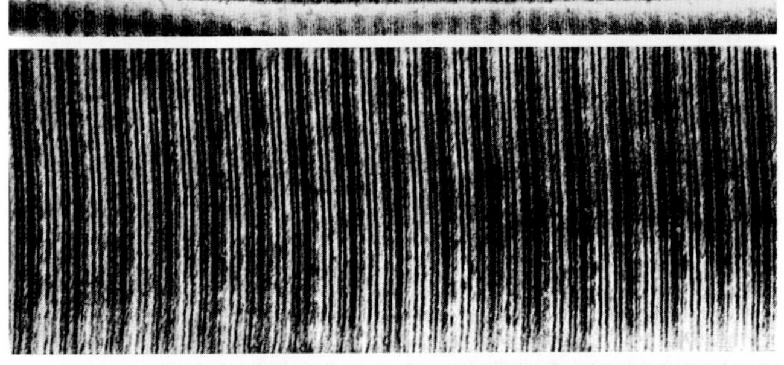

154

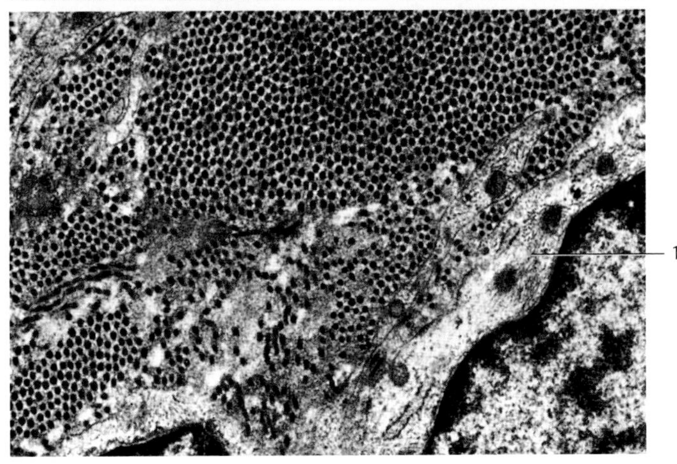

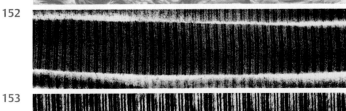

155 Collagen Fibers—Collagen Fibrils

Collagen fibers are the main portion of the structural intercellular elements. While fresh, the fibers are shiny white. In light microscopic images, the fibers look like strands of hair curling in spirals (see Fig. 151). In thin sections for electron-microscopic examination, they are inevitably cut in different planes and directions. In this figure, the *fibril bundles* are cut either across or longitudinally, but mostly tangentially. Lengthwise-cut fibrils faintly show periodic cross-striation (cf. Figs. 152, 153). There are also elastic fiber elements ↗. Collagen is the most widely found protein; by weight it represents about 25% of the protein in the human body.
Bundles of collagen fibrils from the *stratum papillare* of the corium.

Electron microscopy; magnification: × 10 000

156 Collagen and Elastic Fibers—Mesentery

The widely spread layers of connective tissue from the mesentery contain strong undulating bundles of collagen fibrils (stained red), which are interspersed with thin elastic fibers (stained blue-violet) and argyrophilic fibers. Built into these extended fiber networks are blood and lymph vessels, fat cells and nerves (not shown). Fibrocytes and a large number of different free cells are found in the fiber mesh.

Stain: van Gieson iron hematoxylin-picric acid-fuchsin; magnification: × 200

157 Reticular Fibers—Larynx

The *PAS* reaction (because *fibronectin* is present) or the *silver salt impregnation* technique brings out the fine, about 0.2–1 μm thick reticular fibers in sections from reticular connective tissue, adipose tissue and from the borders between different tissues. The reticular fibers are therefore also called *argyrophilic* fibers or *silver fibers*. Reticular fibers are similar to collagen fibers. However, they consist of type III collagen. In contrast to the unbranched collagen fibers, they form extended tight-meshed networks and grids (*matrix fibers*). Reticular fibers are, for example, part of the lamina propria of the epithelium. They exist in many organs, where they build a supportive structure (see Figs. 159–161).
Reticular fibers from the infraglottic fibroelastic membrane of the larynx. The elastic fibers are not visible.

Stain: Gomori silver impregnation; magnification: × 400

158 Reticular Fibers—Amnion

Reticular fibers in the amnion of a young chicken. They form a dense meshwork. The amnion epithelium and the cellular elements of the amnion connective tissue are not visible.

Stain: Gomori silver impregnation; magnification: × 400

155

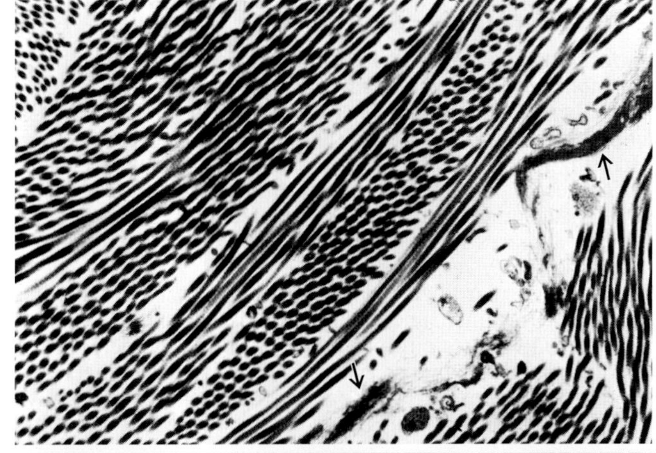

156

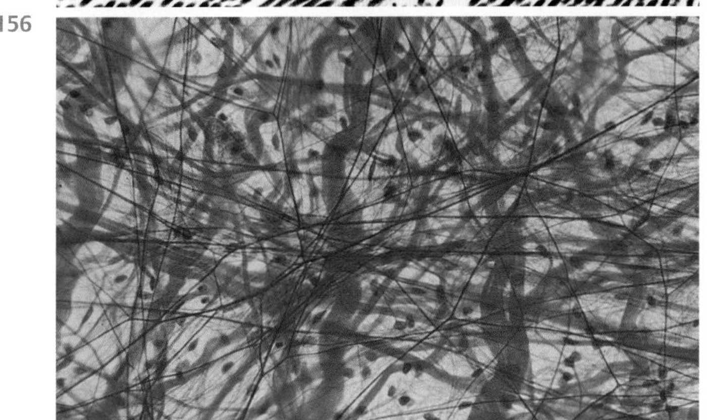

157

158

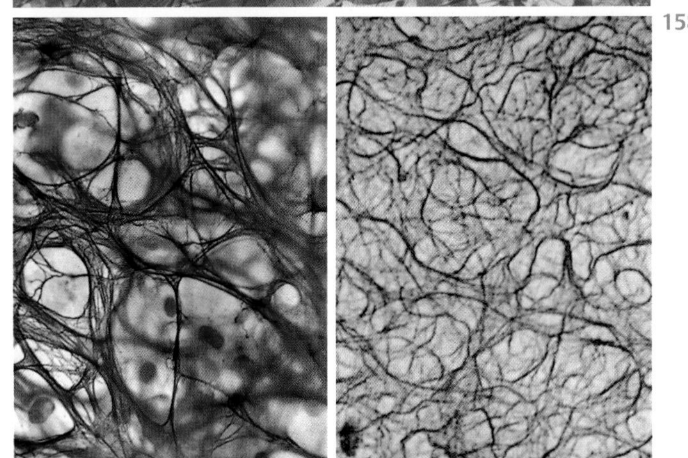

159 Reticular Fibers—Kidney

In contrast with the strong unbranched collagen fibers, the reticular fibers (*predominantly collagen type III*) are delicate and only about 0.5–2.0 µm thick. Reticular fibers often form branched networks. They are therefore called *reticular (matrix) fibers* or *argyrophilic fibers* (*silver fibers*), because they can be stained using silver salt impregnation. Reticular fibers build delicate supportive structures for parenchymal cells in almost all organs (see Fig. 444).
The fine reticular fibers form a dense layer of reticular fibers—for example, in the interstitial spaces between kidney tubules, which contain the collecting ducts and the kidney vessels.
Very delicate reticular fibers weave a net around parallel renal tubules (in this figure lightly stained, undulating, band-like structures). The epithelium is not visible with this staining procedure. The reticular fibers are also a component of the *basal membranes*. Like other fibers, reticular fibers consist of fibrils with a typical cross-striation pattern. With a diameter of 20–45 nm, reticular fibers (type III collagen) are smaller than type I collagen fibrils.

Stain: Gomori silver staining; magnification: × 2500

160 Reticular Fibers—Thyroid Gland

Interstitial connective tissue from the thyroid gland. The round glandular follicles (see Figs. 358–363) appear to bulge forward. A densely woven network of reticular fibers surrounds them. In the connective tissue between the follicles, there are also collagen fibers, some of them thick ropes of intertwined fibers. Connective tissue cells are not visible in this preparation.

Scanning electron microscopy; magnification: × 2500

161 Reticular Fibers—Amnion

The amnion (Greek: sheep skin, membrane covering the embryo) is a transparent, shiny *embryo sac*. The outer amnion layer consists of the amnion connective tissue, which attaches to the chorion connective tissue (see textbooks of embryology). The inner surface is smooth and lined by the single-layered *amnion epithelium*. The *amnion connective tissue* has several distinct layers. Immediately underneath the epithelium are reticular fibers, which run in different directions and cross over each other, forming a matrix (cf. Fig. 158). Sporadically, thicker bundles of collagen fibers are found between the woven strings of these delicate reticular fibers.
Human amnion, subepithelial weaves of reticular fibers. The procedures in this preparation do not support the demonstration of the epithelium or the cellular elements of the connective tissue in the fibrous mesh.

Scanning electron microscopy; magnification: × 5000

159

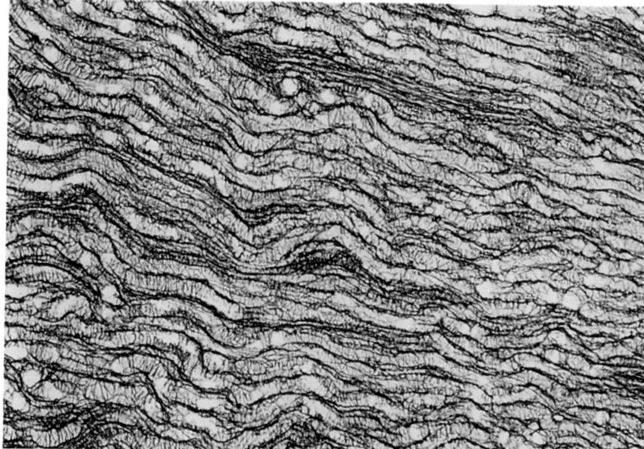

160

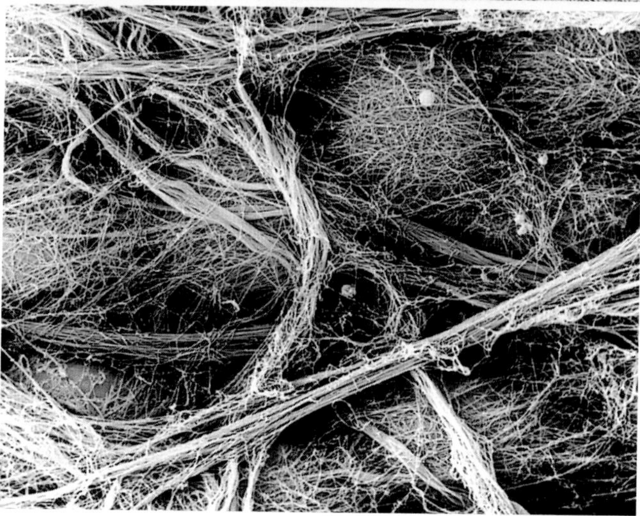

161

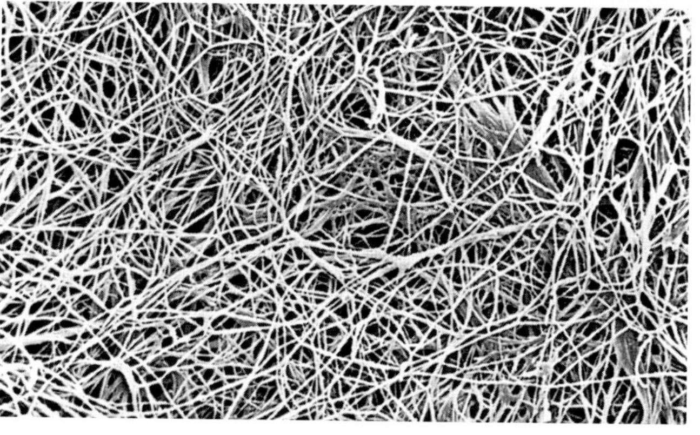

162 Elastic Fibers—Corium

The attributes of elastic fibers (elastin fibers) are different from those of collagen or reticular fibers. One of these differences rests with their affinities to stain. Elastic fibers can be specifically stained using elastin-specific dyes, such as resorcin-fuchsin, aldehyde-fuchsin, or orcein. Elastic fibers are heavily branched and form irregular, often dense fiber networks or fenestrated membranes, due to webbed extensions at their nodal points, reminiscent of the webbed feet of waterfowl (see Fig. 279). The fibers show diameters between 0.5 μm and 5 μm. This wide range covers thin fibers and very thick ones, such as the fibers of the elastic neck band (see Figs. 190–192).
Elastic fibers in vivo are slightly yellow (yellow fibers). Tissue elasticity depends to a large degree on the number of elastic fibers and their arrangement. Elastic fibers are particularly abundant in the connective tissue of the lung, in elastic cartilage (see Fig. 163), in the skin, in organ capsules and in the walls of vessels.
This figure shows a dense elastic fiber network in the *stratum reticulare* of the corium. Cellular elements are not stained (cf. Fig. 156).

Stain: orcein; magnification: × 300

163 Elastic Fibers—Auricle (Ear Flap)

The components of elastic fibers, microfibrils (diameter about 12 nm) and amorphous elastin are ubiquitous in connective tissue.
In this figure, staining emphasizes the elastic fibers in human skin from the earflap (concha of auricle). There are long, thin, slightly undulating fibers, thick fibers and short fragments of elastic fibers. The light pink stained structures are robust collagen fibers. The nuclei are not stained.

Stain: resorcin-fuchsin; magnification: × 200

164 Elastic Fibers—Aorta

This figure shows a vertical section through the media of the thoracic aorta. In contrast to Figs. 162 and 163, the elastic fibers run in the wavy pattern of corrugated sheets. Between the black-violet elastic fibers are yellow-stained smooth muscle cells. Compare this figure with Figs. 156, 162, 165, 166 and with Figs. 274–280.
In arteries of the elastic type, elastic structures can be seen as fibers only in vertical sections through the vessel wall. In fact, these structures are *elastic membranes or lamellae* (see Fig. 279). The regular staining methods, as used in histology courses, rarely show elastic fibers. The fibers do not display an organized structural scheme. There is no cross-striation (see Figs. 166, 167).

Stain: van Gieson resorcin-fuchsin-picric acid; magnification: × 200

162

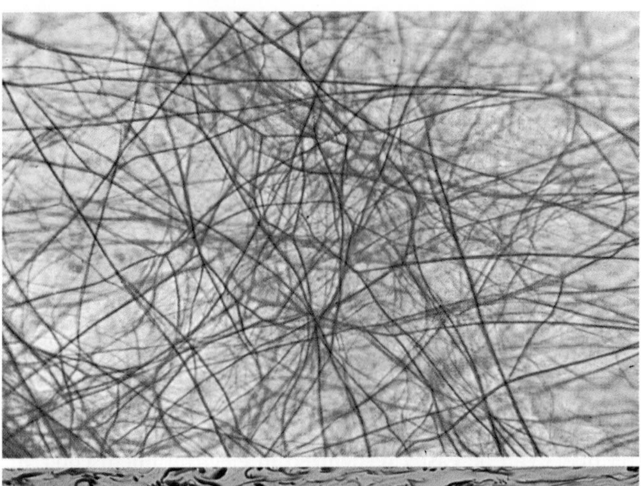

163

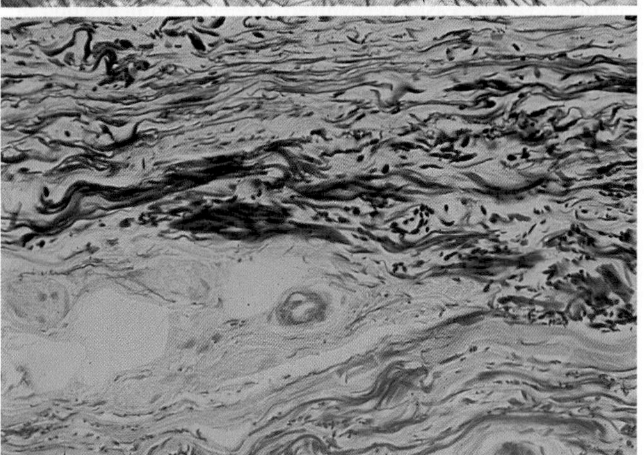

164

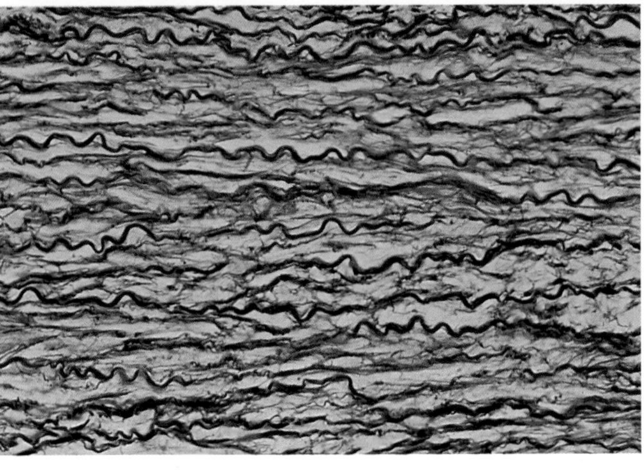

165 Elastic Fibers—Aorta

This section from an aorta wall shows elastic fibers, which dominate the picture in the form of undulating or stretched elements (stained deep blue) (cf. Figs. 164, 275–280). Smooth muscle cells (stained light blue) are present between elastic fibers (cf. Fig. 164).

Only a vertical section of this artery close to the heart will display the elastin as more or less wavy fibers. However, parallel sections show that these are in fact *elastic membranes* (see Fig. 279). Elastic fibers withstand degradation using trypsin, heat (cooking) or hydrolysis with dilute acid or alkali. However, *elastase*, a pancreatic enzyme, will hydrolyze elastin.

Tunica media of the human thoracic aorta.

Semi-thin section; stain: methylene blue-azure II; magnification: × 320

166 Elastic Fibers—Aorta

Elastic fibers can be easily recognized in electron microscopic images by their mostly homogeneous central structure with low electron density, called amorphous component or *amorphous center*. Nevertheless, with appropriate contrasting and higher resolution of a small sector in an edge zone, it is possible to display the fibrils. The fibers show no periodic cross-striation. The small edge zone is called *fibrillar component* and consists of 15–20 nm thick fibrils.

This preparation is from the tunica media of the aorta. The snake-like undulating, remarkably light elastic fibers 1 clearly stand out against the smooth muscle cells 3 (cf. Fig. 167).

Elastin, the scleroprotein of elastic fibers, is rich in lysine and alanine. The presence of *desmosine* and *isodesmosine peptides* is also characteristic of elastic fibers. Different from collagen, elastin contains little hydroxyproline and no hydroxylysine.

1 Elastic fibers
2 Collagen fibrils
3 Smooth muscle cells
Electron microscopy; magnification: × 4500

167 Elastic Fibers—Corium

Electron micrographs show elastic fiber material also in the form of spot-like, weakly osmiophilic patches of different sizes. However, with suitable contrasting procedures, elastic fibers can also be rendered heavily blackened. Elastic fibers do not show the cross-striation pattern that is characteristic of collagen fibers. Two elements can be distinguished, an amorphous *center* of even density, which contains elastin, and a small outer zone (edge) with about 10 nm thick microfilaments and 15–20 nm thick microfibrils (*fibrillar component*).

Cross-sections and tangential sections through elastic fibers from the corium of human skin with accumulations of osmiophilic material near the outer borders. The dimensions of the elastic fibers differ.

Electron microscopy; magnification: × 28 600

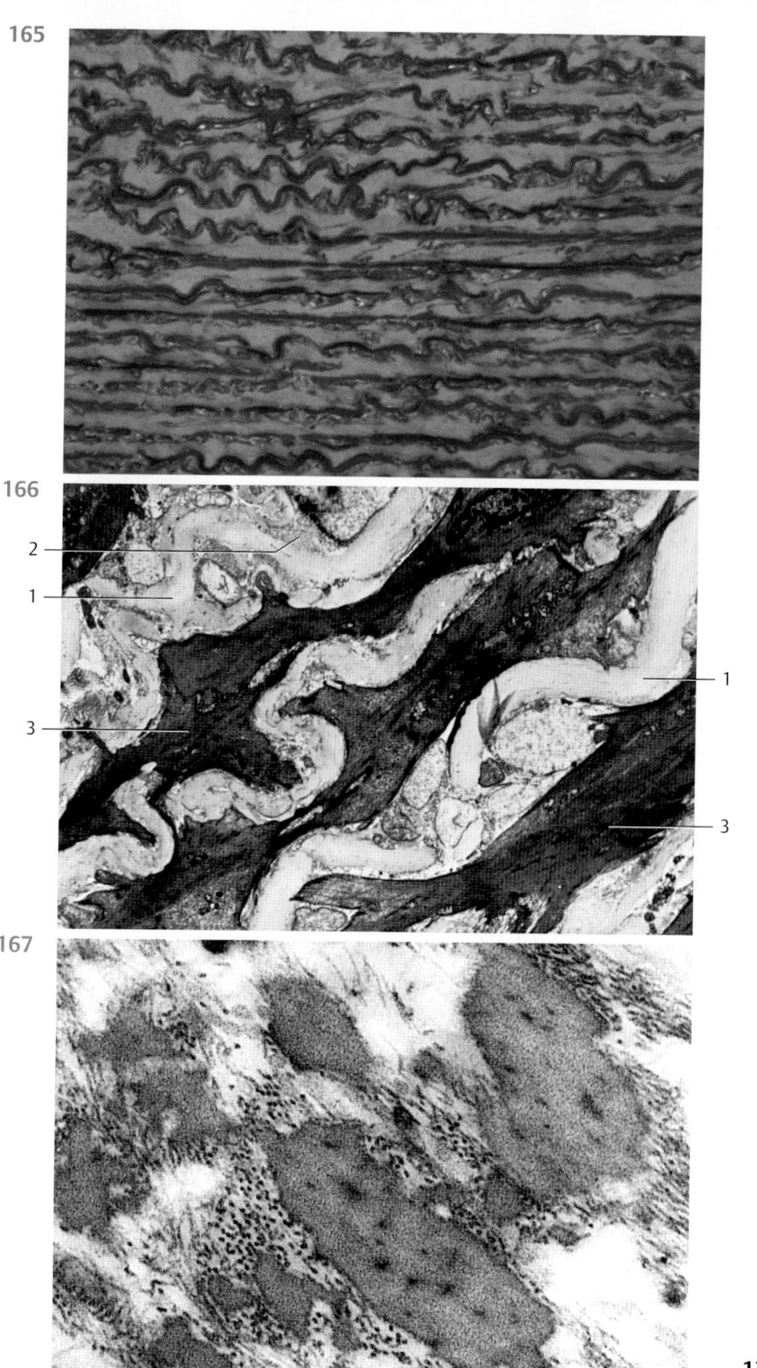
165
166
2
1
3
1
3
167

168 Embryonal Connective Tissue—Mesenchyme

The cells of the mesenchymal connective tissue contain little cytoplasm. Their partially thin, partially spread out, always branched cell processes interconnect the cells. This creates a loosely structured three-dimensional spongy network, which is filled with a viscous intercellular substance (*amorphous gel-like ground substance, extracellular matrix*). The ground substance contains the glycosaminoglycan hyaluronic acid. Intracellular structural components, such as fibers, are not yet or scarcely present. Light microscopy does not reveal cell borders inside the spongy network. All of the connective and supportive tissues, as well as most smooth muscle cells, arise from the mesenchyme. Mesenchyme cells are pluripotent (cf. Fig. 135).
Mesenchyme from a mouse embryo.

Stain: iron hematoxylin-acid fuchsin; magnification: × 400

169 Embryonal Connective Tissue—Gelatinous or Mucous Tissue

This complete section across a mature human umbilical cord reveals at its surface a covering with a single-layered amnion epithelium. Inside, the umbilical cord is filled with a gelatinous or mucous connective tissue, named *Wharton's jelly* (see Figs. 170, 171). Embedded in this gelatinous tissue are the *umbilical vein* (right) and the two *umbilical arteries* (left). A section through the remnant of the *allantoid canal* is seen in the center. The vessels in the umbilical cord are always strongly contracted after birth. The specific gelatinous connective tissue consists of a wide-meshed network of long, stretched fibrocytes with many interconnecting cell processes (see Figs. 170, 171).

Stain: azan; magnification: × 12

170 Embryonal Connective Tissue—Gelatinous or Mucous Tissue

Gelatinous connective tissue exists in the skin of embryos and, particularly well defined, as Wharton's jelly in the umbilical cord. The cells of the gelatinous tissue are flattened fibroblasts and fibrocytes with branched cell processes, which interconnect and form a wide-meshed network. Light microscopy shows that the interstices are filled with a homogeneous gelatinous ground substance with embedded densely interwoven bundles of reticular and collagen fibers. When boiled, these fibers yield glue. The nuclei are stained red (cf. Figs. 168, 171).
The ground substance mostly consists of nonsulfatized glycosaminoglycans. Note the increase in the number of fibers at the time of birth (Fig. 170b).

a) Umbilical cord of a 5-month-old fetus
b) Umbilical cord of a newborn
Stain: picro-Sirius red-lithium carmine; magnification: × 100

168

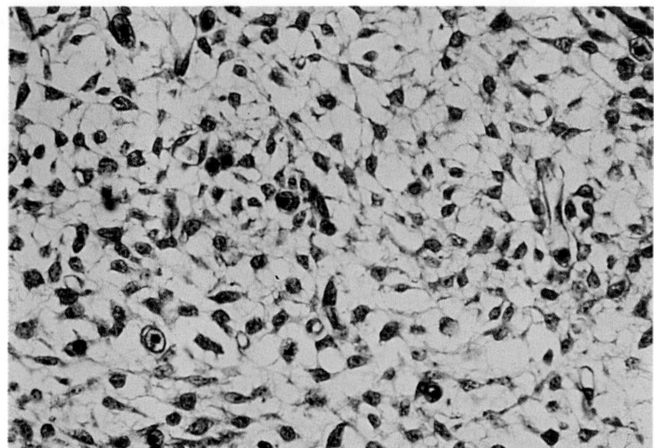

169

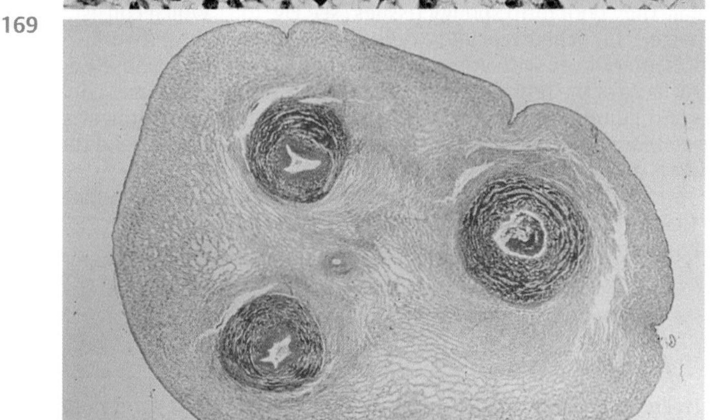

170

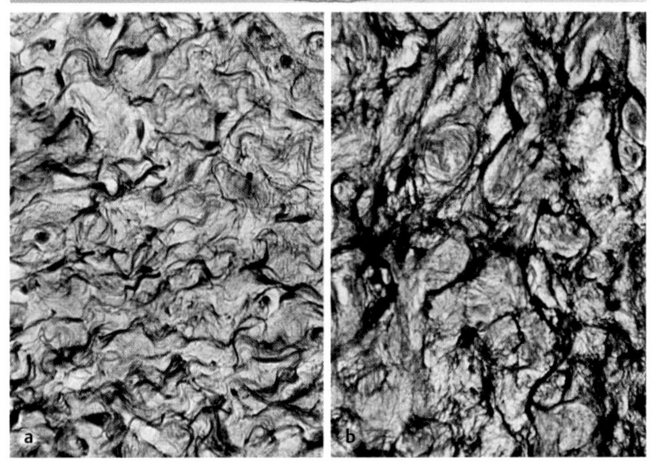

171 Embryonal Connective Tissue—Gelatinous or Mucous Tissue

The embryonal connective tissue (*gelatinous tissue, Wharton's jelly*) from a mature human umbilical cord contains connective tissue cells (fibroblasts, fibrocytes) and a homogeneous gelatinous or gel-like ground substance, which holds the collagen fibers. The fibers run in all directions in this space and consequently, they are cut in all planes, across, lengthwise or tangentially (cf. Figs 168–170a, b). The prevailing ground substances in the gelatinous tissue are amorphous ground substances, which are predominantly *nonsulfatized glycosaminoglycans.*

Stain: azan; magnification: × 400

172 Reticular Connective Tissue—Spleen

Reticular connective tissue and embryonic support tissue (*mesenchyme*) are similar. They both form spongy tissues (see Fig. 168), which consist of interconnected, branched *reticulum cells* in a wide-meshed network. This network is interwoven with argyrophilic (reticular) fibers that closely adhere to the surfaces of the reticulum cells. The large intercellular spaces contain free cells and liquid. The figure shows a spleen perfused with Ringer solution. Free cells are no longer present. The nuclei appear deep blue, and the reticular fibers are stained light blue.
The reticular connective tissue is a special form of connective tissue, with few fibers. It provides the support structure for the spleen, the lymph nodes, the lymph follicles and the bone marrow (cf. Figs. 320–331).

Stain: methylene blue-eosin; magnification: × 200

173 Adipose Tissue

There are two types of adipose tissue: *unilocular* (white) and *multilocular* (brown) adipose tissue. Adipose tissue arises from the pluripotent mesenchymal cells and later from cells of the reticular connective tissue, which can produce grape like fatty tissue lobes also. The reticulum cells store fat droplets that will finally coalesce to one large drop. In the process, the cells become rounder. This often creates remarkably large, about 100 µm wide, vacuole cells. Their nuclei and cytoplasm are squeezed to the cell periphery (*signet-ring form*). In the usual histological routine preparations (paraffin sections), alcohol and xylene have dissolved the fat and removed it from the tissue. This creates empty spaces without stain, which are usually defined as fat vacuoles. In this figure, numerous unilocular fat cells (*adipocytes, lipocytes*) 1 pervade the interstitial space of the connective tissue of the striated musculature 2; at the top left is a section through an artery 3 (see Fig. 174). Unilocular adipose tissue is richly vascularized and contains nerves.
Unilocular fat cells (adipocytes, lipocytes); fatty tissue lobe in the interstitial connective tissue of the musculature 2.

1 Adipocytes
2 Striated muscle fibers
3 Artery

Stain: hemalum-eosin; magnification: × 300

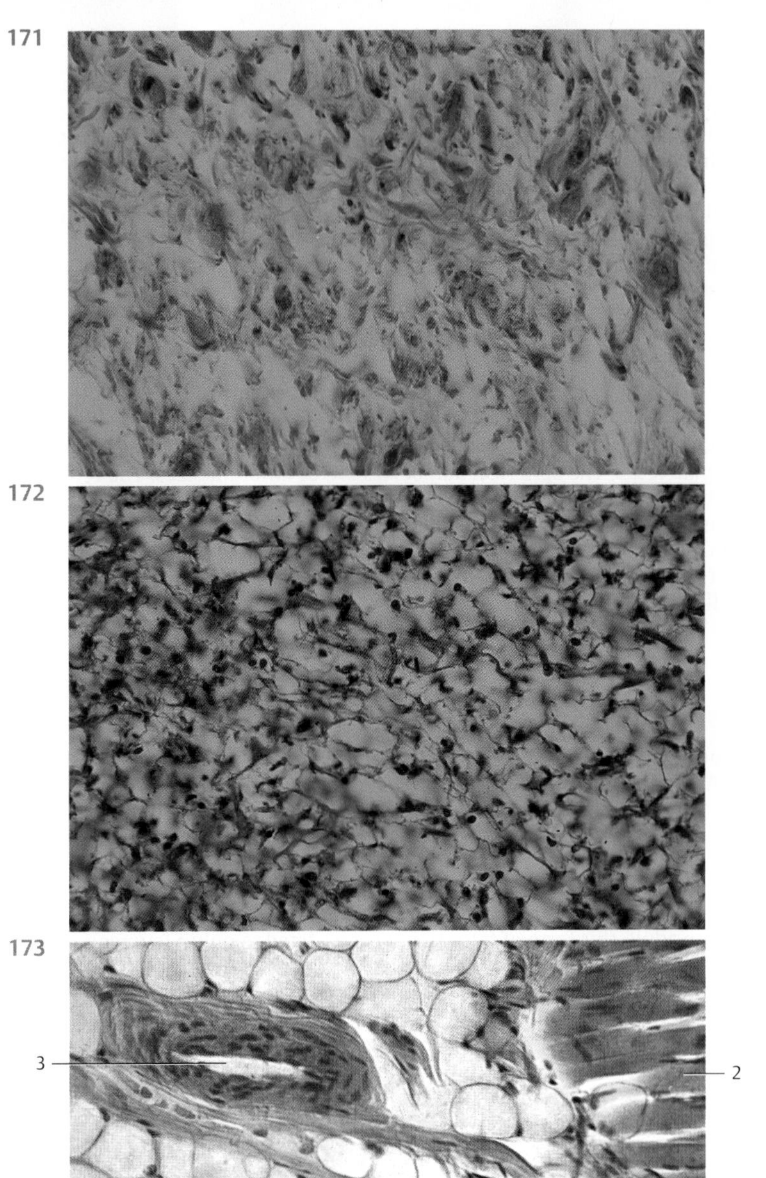
171
172
173
3
2
1
1

174 White Adipose Tissue

Several large, spherical fat cells (*adipocytes*) close to the blood vessels, which run through the human greater omentum. The dense piles of cells are the milk spots, which consist of lymphocytes, reticulum cells and macrophages. In freshly isolated tissue, they appear as opaque milky patches. The histological determination of fat requires fresh tissue or formalin-fixed tissue. Intracellular fatty substances can then be more or less intensely stained using lipophilic (fat-soluble) dyes, such as *Sudan III* or *scarlet red.*
Unilocular fatty tissue (cf. Fig. 173); whole-mount preparation, not a tissue section.

Stain: hematoxylin-eosin-scarlet red; magnification: × 80

175 White Adipose Tissue

Small, lobe-shaped aggregate of adipocytes in the subcutaneous skin of a human fetus. The spherical *adipocytes* are of different sizes. The removal of fatty substances during tissue preparation has created fat vacuoles. The cytoplasm in these *unilocular* fat cells has been pushed to the cell periphery. The nuclei in some of the adipocytes are cut. Note that several adipocytes in the periphery of this lobe still are multilocular. The darker-stained cells are blood cells.

Semi-thin section; stain: methylene blue-azure II; magnification: × 80

176 Brown Adipose Tissue

Plurilocular or multilocular adipose tissue from the brown adipose tissue (BAT) in the vicinity of the thoracic aorta (rat).
Instead of one large fat vacuole, *plurilocular adipocytes* 1 contain many small fat droplets, which are enveloped by an elementary membrane. This gives the cell body a foamy appearance. The intracellular fat droplets are of various sizes, and they stain only slightly. Note the blood vessels 2 in the brown adipose tissue and compare with Fig. 175.
In the adult, this form of fatty tissue is restricted to only a few regions of the body, such as armpits, neck, mediastinum, the skin on the back, etc. The multilocular adipose tissue contains *cytochrome C*, and therefore displays a brownish-yellow color (brown adipose tissue). It plays a large role in thermoregulation in hibernating animals ("*hibernation gland*" of rodents).
Adipocytes contain many mitochondria. There are many sympathetic nerve fibers between the adipocytes in connective tissue.

1 Multilocular adipocytes
2 Capillaries
Semi-thin section; stain: methylene blue-azure II; magnification: × 380

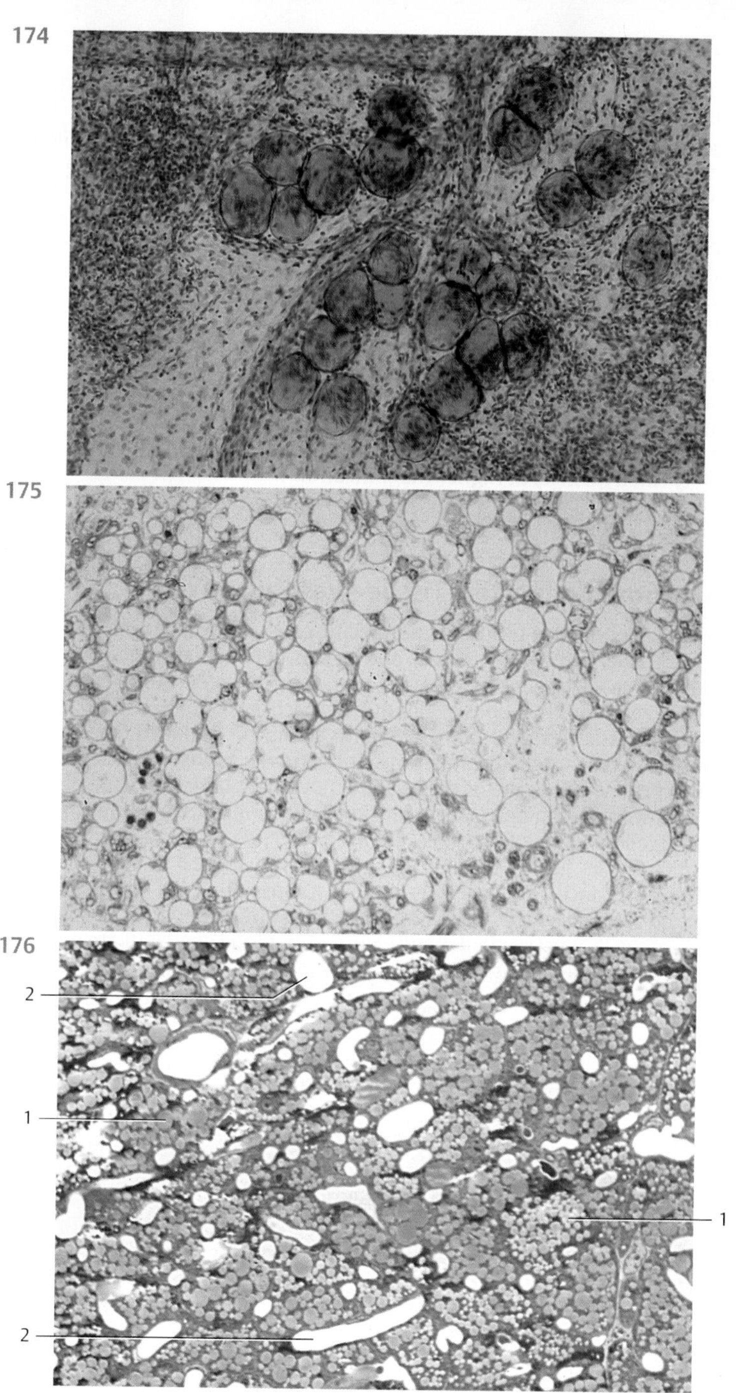
174
175
176
2
1
1
2

177 White Fatty Tissue

In a narrow sense, adipose tissue consists of many adipocytes, which form small aggregates in the connective tissue of organs (cf. Figs. 173, 174). The cell aggregates often form small lobules, sometimes also called *fat lobules.* Among other tasks, they serve a mechanical purpose. White fatty tissue forms cushions in the palms or on the soles, for example, which will dampen an impact (*structural fat, fat cushion*). Fat lobules are also an energy store, such as *storage fat*, which occurs under the skin, in the colon, the omentum and many other locations. These fat lobules are usually encased by a connective tissue like capsule. Connective tissue septa extend into the inside of the capsule and subdivide it into several smaller lobes. At the heel cushion, structural fat accumulates in small compartments with rather tough walls.
The adjacent figure shows a part of a fat lobule from the subcutaneous tissue of a fetus. Note the closely packed round or polygonal fat cells. In this preparation, the sparse connective tissue and the few fibers between the adipocytes have been removed enzymatically. Figure 177b shows round, completely filled fat cells at higher magnification.

Scanning electron microscopy; magnifications: a) × 200; b) × 800

178 Loose Connective Tissue—Vestibular Fold

The loose connective tissue has no specific constant form. As *interstitial connective tissue*, it fills the crevices and spaces between specific components (*parenchyme*) of an organ, occupies the gaps between bundles of muscle fibers or separates the lobes of glands from each other, for example. The loose connective tissue can therefore be seen as a filling material. At the same time, it fulfills diverse metabolic functions. It provides a service reservoir of water and ascertains elasticity for the relative movement of tissues. One of its very important roles is in tissue regeneration. Loose connective tissue consists of local (fixed) cells, the fibrocytes, collagen fibers, elastic and reticular fibers. Reticular fibers go in all directions and fill the spaces. In the amorphous ground substance are numerous free cells, especially cells that mediate the immune response. This preparation is from the subepithelial connective tissue of the larynx (*vestibular fold*). Numerous blood vessels 1 are present in connective tissue (cf. Fig. 179–183).

Stain: azan; magnification: × 200

179 Loose Connective Tissue—Lip

Loose connective tissue from the center part of a human lip. Collagen fibers span the tissue in different directions, some of the fibers are quite strong. In the upper part of the figure, the fibers are more loosely arranged. There are also clearly more connective tissue cells in that area. Vascularized loose connective tissue shows plasticity, and it is soft and pliable. In cases of inflammation or some systemic diseases, it is capable of storing large volumes of water (edema, "swollen cheek"). Loose connective tissue is particularly abundant as subcutaneous layer (cf. Fig. 151).

Stain: azan; magnification: × 200

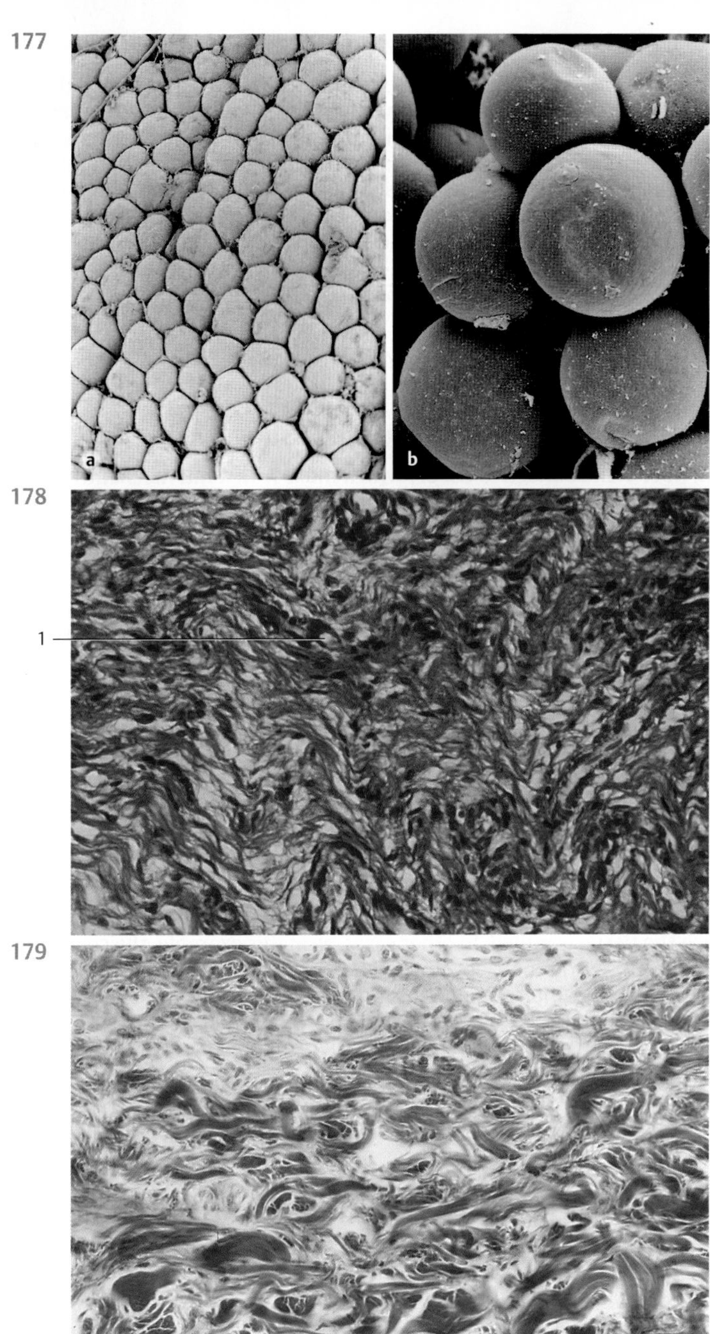
177
a
b
178
1
179

180 Cellular Connective Tissue—Ovary

Tissue from the ovarian cortex, the *stroma ovarii*, is suitable for the demonstration of this type of cellular connective tissue. Apart from a few reticular fibers, the cortex of the ovary contains densely packed, spindle-shaped connective tissue cells, their arrangement often resembling that of a school of fish (*cellular connective tissue*). These cells are still able to differentiate. The collagen fibers are a minor component. The cellular connective tissue of the ovary and the uterus is often considered a special variation of the loose connective tissue. In the endometrium, it partakes in the cyclical changes of the mucous membrane (see Figs. 542–547, 571–574).
Human ovary.

Stain: hematoxylin-eosin; magnification: × 80

181 Dense Irregular Connective Tissue—Eyelid

Taut, fiber-rich connective tissue, which must withstand mechanical stress, is characterized by the arrangement of intercellular supportive structures. This figure shows a planar cut through the lid plate (*tarsus, collagen fiber plate*) of the upper lid. There are densely intertwined bundles of fibers that run in every direction (*woven connective tissue*). This fiber arrangement ascertains a reliable tensile strength in all directions. Sporadically, vessels are cut (cf. Figs. 180, 182). Cells are sparse, and fibers dominate the structure. This braid-like connective tissue (taut, dense connective tissue) is also found in the capsules of many organs (see Fig. 182), the corium (*stratum reticulare of the corium*), the *dura mater* and the *sclera*.
Human upper eyelid.

Stain: azan; magnification: × 70

182 Dense Irregular Connective Tissue—Renal Capsule

In some organ capsules, the taut, fiber-rich connective tissue shows a woven structure. The fibers are densely packed in layers, running in the direction, in which the tissue is pulled. In other cases, as in this example, the coarse fiber bundles are tightly interwoven, which explains the name *matted* or *felted connective tissue*. Intermingled with the coarse bundles of collagen fibers, there are also delicate reticular fibers (cf. Figs. 161, 180, 181, 183).
This preparation does not show the cellular components.
Human renal capsule.

Scanning electron microscopy; magnification: × 5000

180

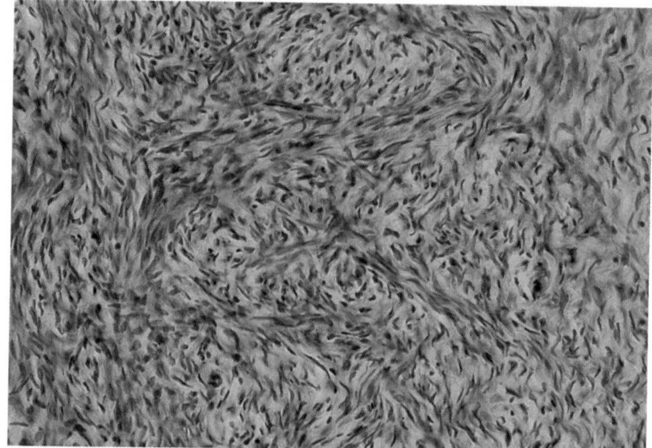

181

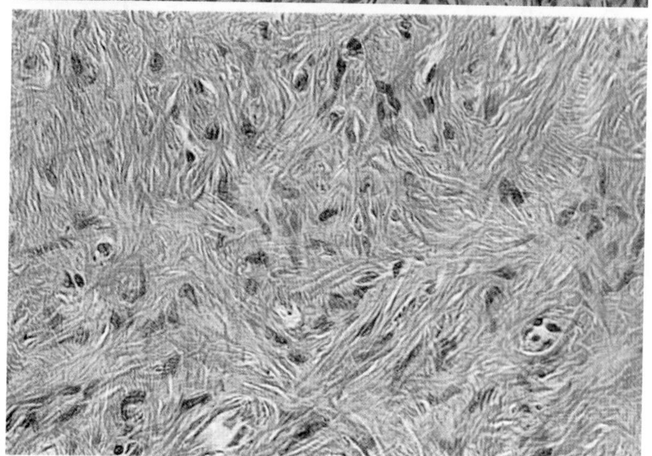

182

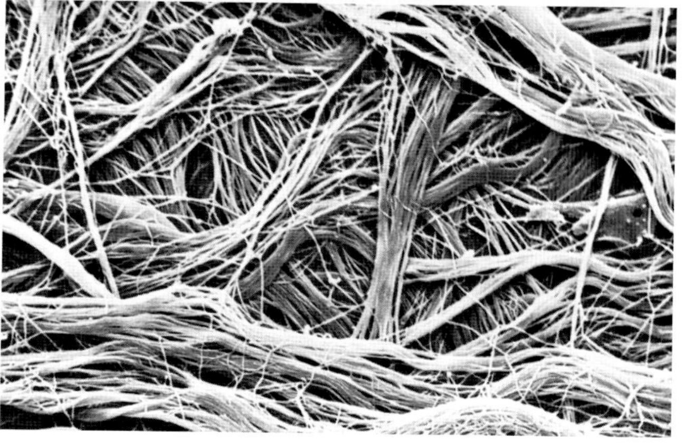

183 Dense Regular Connective Tissue—Tendon

The taut, dense regular connective tissue with parallel fibers is the prototype of tendons (*strand-like form*), aponeuroses (*flat, planar form*) and *ligaments*. This figure shows part of a longitudinal section through a finger tendon. The structural components of tendons are strong, stress-absorbing collagen fibers that are commensurate with their mechanical tasks. The collagen fibers (stained red) assemble in a parallel arrangement (*primary collagen bundles*). Relaxed fibers undulate slightly. Fibroblasts and their row of nuclei line up between fiber bundles. These cells are also called tendon cells (*tenocytes*).

The tenocytes are in part captured in planar view and in part seen as profiles (cf. Figs. 184–189). The geometry of tendon cells adapts to the spatial conditions inside the tendon structure.

Stain: alum hematoxylin-eosin; magnification: × 240

184 Dense Regular Connective Tissue—Tendon

Cross-section through a tendon. Each of the fiber bundles in the tendon are encased by loose, fibrous, vascularized connective tissue (*peritendineum internum*) 1, which subdivides the tendon into secondary bundles. The tendon cells (*winged cells*) extend thin, wing-like cytoplasmic processes in all directions. The cell processes adhere closely to the collagen fibers. The light crevices are technical artifacts (shrinkage due to fixation) (cf. Figs. 183, 185–189).

The tendon surface is covered by the *peritendineum externum* (*epitendineum*), which is a braided web of connective tissue. The epitendineum itself is covered at the outside with loose connective tissue called *peritendineum* .

1 Peritendineum internum

Stain: alum hematoxylin-eosin; magnification: × 130

185 Dense Regular Connective Tissue—Tendon

Cross-section through the tendon (*primary collagen bundle*) of the long finger flexor from a mouse. Several bundles of differently sized collagen fibrils 1 are cut. In light microscopy, every bundle of fibrils corresponds to a fiber (cf. Figs. 183, 184, 186, 187). Between the bundles of fibrils are tendon cells 2 – i.e., modified fibrocytes (*tenocytes*). Their slender cytoplasmic processes extend wing-like into the narrow spaces between fibril bundles ("winged *cells*") 3. These cytoplasmic processes interconnect with each other. Tendon cells contain plenty of granular endoplasmic reticulum (rER) 4, mitochondria and lysosomes 5.

1 Fibril bundles
2 Nuclei of tendon cells
3 Cytoplasmic processes of tendon cells
4 Cytoplasm of tendon cells with rER
5 Lysosomes
Electron microscopy; magnification: × 8300

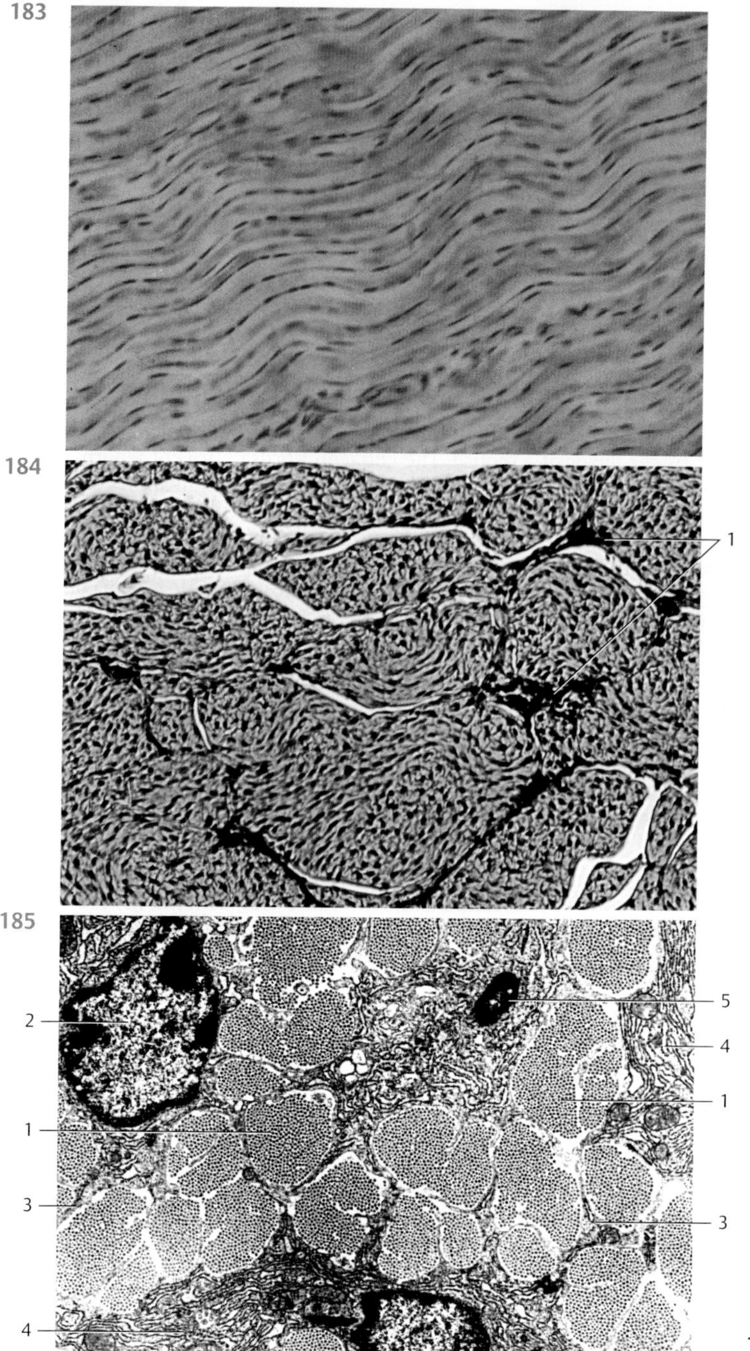
183
184
1
185
5
2
4
1
1
3
3
4

186 Dense Regular Connective Tissue—Tendon

This cross-section through the tendon of the human long finger flexor outlines the wide range for the diameters of collagen fibrils ①. There is also a section through part of a tendon cell (*fibrocyte, tenocyte*) with its nucleus ② and long, extended, slender processes (wings) ③, which adhere snugly to the fibrils. Tendon cells usually have long, extended nuclei (cf. Fig. 183) and little cytoplasm. Note the narrow perinuclear band of cytoplasm ④.

1 Collagen fibrils, cut vertical to their axis
2 Nucleus of a tendon cell
3 Cytoplasmic processes (wing)
4 Small cytoplasmic band (seam)
Electron microscopy; magnification: × 20 000

187 Dense Regular Connective Tissue—Tendon

Longitudinal section through the tendon (*primary collagen bundle*) from the long finger flexor of a mouse. The collagen fibrils ① are cut lengthwise and show the typical cross-striation (cf. Fig. 183). The section shows the perikaryon of a tendon cell (*fibrocyte, tenocyte*) between fibril bundles. The cytoplasm contains rER lamella ② and in some sections, small rER cisternae ③. It also contains mitochondria ④ and Golgi complexes ⑤.
Aponeuroses are planar tendons. Their structures resemble that of collagen ligaments (cf. Figs. 188, 189).

1 Collagen fibrils
2 Granular endoplasmic reticulum, rER
3 Rough ER cisternae
4 Mitochondria
5 Golgi apparatus
Electron microscopy; magnification: × 6500

188 Stretch-Resistant Collagen Band—Ligament

Stretch-resistant bands (*ligaments*) are made up of collagen fibrils in basically the same way as tendons. In the same way as tendons, the collagen fibers of ligaments are assembled in parallel fiber bundles. They can be easily discerned in this figure. The collagen fibers run in characteristic wavy lines. The connective tissue cells are rows of fibrocytes, which have adapted their shapes to their specific localization between collagen fibers. Like tendon cells, the fibrocytes have a long, stretched geometry. Their spindle-shaped nuclei have a wavy geometry as well (cf. Figs. 183, 184). The long light crevices are technical artifacts.
Longitudinal section through a wrist ligament (Lip. collaterale fibulare).

Stain: hematoxylin-eosin; magnification: × 80

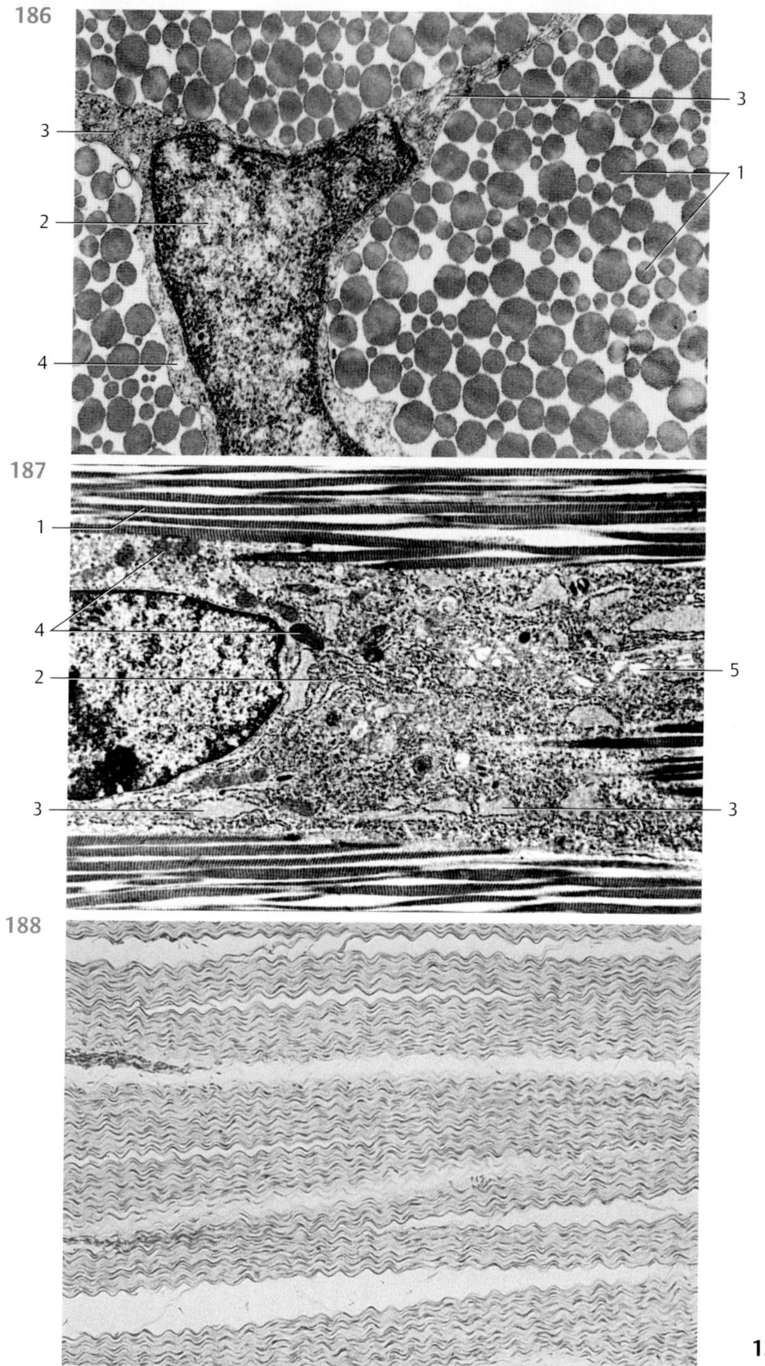
186
3
3
1
2
4
187
1
4
2
5
3
3
188

189 Collagen Band—Ligament

The same preparation has been used for this figure and Fig. 188. The section clearly brings out the wavy pattern of the collagen fibers, and it shows the fibrocytes (dark red) between the fibers. The fibrocytes reflect the arrangement of the collagen fibers in their shape and positioning (cf. Fig. 183). Longitudinal section of a wrist ligament (*fibular collateral ligament*).

Stain: hematoxylin-eosin; differential interference contrast (DIC) image; magnification: × 200

190 Elastic Ligament—Ligamentum Flavum

Elastic ligaments are mostly bundles of thick, parallel elastic fibers. They are branched and connected with each other (see Fig. 191). Because of their yellow color, elastic bands are also called *yellow bands—ligamenta flava*. In humans, they are found at the spine. The neck ligament in hoofed animals, *ligamentum nuchae*, consists of elastic fibers (see Fig. 192).
This cross-section through the ligamentum flavum of the spine demonstrates the characteristic field pattern (patches). The elastic fibers are arranged parallel to each other in bundles of different dimensions and run in the direction of the tensile force (pull). The collagen and reticular fibers (red) are wrapped around the width of the elastic fibers (vertical to the elastic fiber axis). The connective tissue cells are not visible with this staining procedure (in contrast, see Fig. 191).

Stain: van Gieson picric acid-fuchsin; magnification: × 360

191 Elastic Ligament—Ligamentum Flavum

This longitudinal section shows the *network character* of the elastic fibers. The fibers permanently connect with each other in acute angles. Note the cellular connective tissue between the elastic fibers (stained blue), which corresponds to the red-stained fibers in Fig. 190.

Stain: methylene blue-eosin; magnification: × 130

192 Elastic Ligament—Ligamentum Nuchae (Nuchal Ligament)

The elastic ligaments are considered *dense regular connective tissue* (*stretch-resistant parallel fibers*). Their interconnecting bundles of elastic fibers vary in thickness (cf. Fig. 191). In this preparation, the elastic fibers are stained bright red (cf. Fig. 190). The network of collagen fibers and reticular fibers (stained green-blue) contains fibrocytes and small blood vessels.
The smooth muscles, which can raise the neck hair (*arrector muscles of the hair*), have elastic end-tendons.
Bovine neck band, ligamentum nuchae.

Stain: Jerusalem trichrome staining, modified; magnification: × 200

189

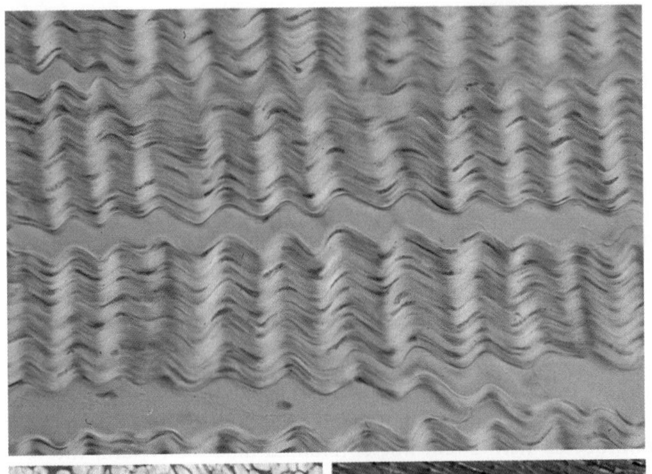

190

191

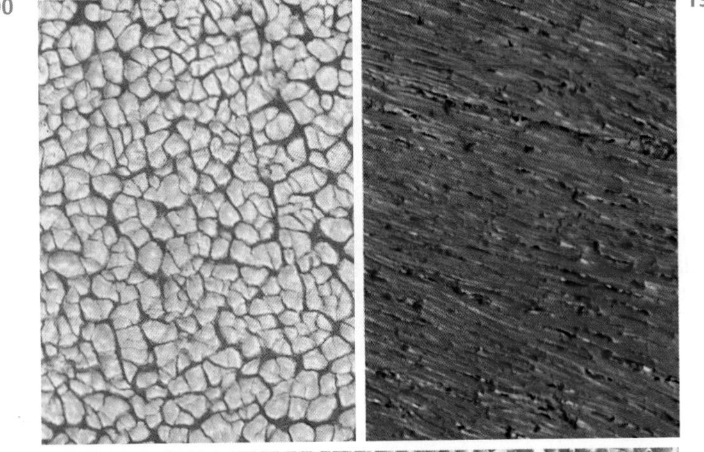

192

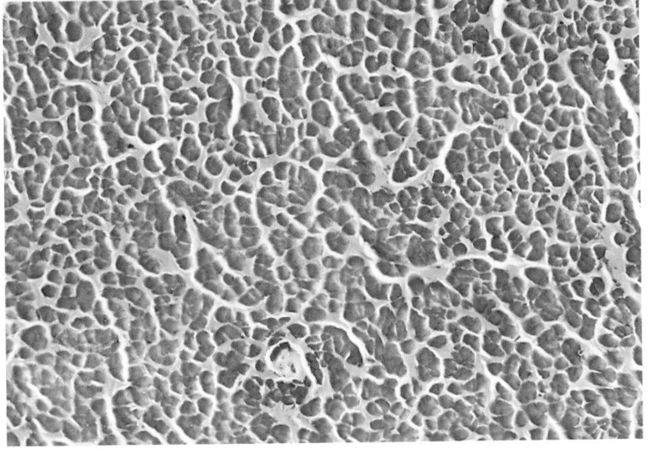

193 Embryonic Hyaline Cartilage

Hyaline cartilage develops from mesenchymal blastema. Mesenchyme cel differentiate into cartilage-forming cells, the *chondroblasts*, and in tur these differentiate into cartilage cells, the *chondrocytes*. Chondroblasts syn thesize the cartilage ground substance (*cartilage matrix*), which consists o water, glycosaminoglycans and collagen fibrils (*type II collagen*). The collage fibrils are masked by components of the ground substance—i.e., by materia in the extracellular matrix. Chondroblasts release their products in all direc tions and consequently wall themselves in. In the process, they turn int chondrocytes, which rest in the smooth-walled caverns of the cartilage ma trix (*cartilage caverns, lacunae*). Even while they are enclosed, chondrocyte will still divide, thus forming isogenous groups of cartilage cells (*interstitia or intussusceptional growth*). The figure shows large round chondrocyte singly or as groups: *chondrons* or *territories*. The space between them is fille with cartilage ground substance: *interterritorial extracellular matrix*.
Iliac tissue from a human fetus, 5th gestational month. Note the spherica chondrocytes with small nuclei (stained blue-violet) and the remarkabl light cytoplasm.

Stain: Masson-Goldner trichrome staining; magnification: × 400

194 Hyaline Cartilage—Costal Cartilage

Mature hyaline cartilage tissue contains cartilage cells amid intercellula substances with different staining attributes—i.e., *the interterritorial extrac ellular matrix*. The cartilage cells occur as single cells or as groups, calle *chondrons* or *territories*. The spotted staining of the interterritorial extracel lular matrix (*interterritories*) is due to different stacking densities of the col lagen fibers (see Fig. 198) and pronounced differences in glycosaminoglyca concentrations in the cartilage matrix. Glycosaminoglycans are considere responsible for the masking of collagen fibrils. At the upper edge of the figure is a thick layer of connective tissue, the *perichondrium*. Starting at the peri-chondrium, cartilage grows by apposition.

Stain: hematoxylin; magnification: × 100

195 Hyaline Cartilage—Costal Cartilage

This figure shows a detail from Fig. 194 at higher magnification. There is a clear organization into *territories and interterritories*. A particularly baso-philic layer surrounds the chondrocytes or the isogenous groups—i.e., cells that have all arisen from one mother cell. This basophilic layer represents the cartilage capsule. It contains only few collagen fibrils, however, it is rich in *chondroitin-4-sulfate*, *chondroitin-6-sulfate* and *keratan sulfate* . These pro-teoglycans are responsible for the strong basophilia. The basophilia extends to the immediate vicinity of the cartilage capsule or cell, thus creating small coronas around the cell groups, sometimes called cartilage coronas or *terri-torial matrix*. The interterritories—i.e., the interterritorial matrix show much less intense staining.

Stain: hematoxylin; magnification × 200

193

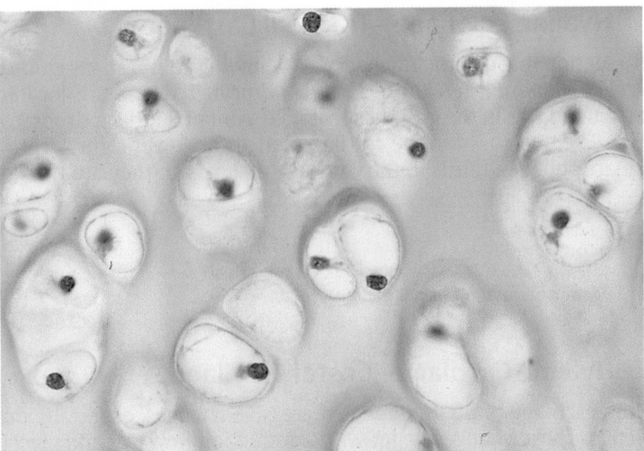

194

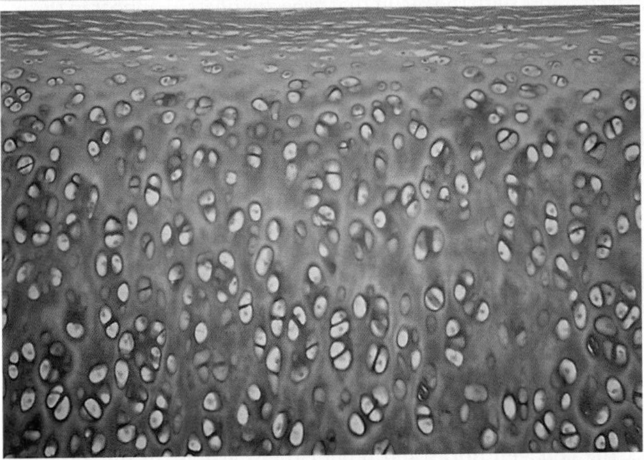

195

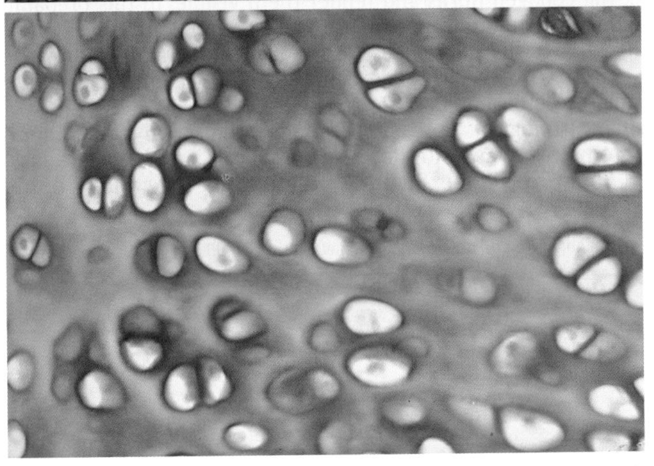

196 Hyaline Cartilage—Tracheal Cartilage

Cross-section through the tracheal yoke showing an *isogenous group of cartilage cells* (*chondron, territory*). The *chondrocytes*, which are located in the cavernous spaces in the ground substance, contain large fat drops 2 (cf. Figs. 60, 61). The nucleus 1 in the cartilage cell at the lower right is cut.
There are collagen fibrils in the cartilage matrix, but they are masked.

1 Cell nucleus
2 Fat droplet
3 Cartilage capsule
4 Territorial matrix
Electron microscopy; magnification: × 1000

197 Hyaline Cartilage—Costal Cartilage

Hyaline cartilage often undergoes regressive changes, especially during senescence. These changes begin with a reduction in water and glycosaminoglycan contents with the result that *asbestos fibers* 1 appear in the intercellular substance. These are collagen fiber aggregates, rendered visible after demasking. Vessels may finally invade these areas, or calcification may occur.
The cartilage cells in the figure appear mostly as part of isogenous groups 2. A corona of cartilage 3 (territorial extracellular matrix) with increased proteoglycan content surrounds the chondrocytes. The lower half of the figure shows demasked collagen fibers, dubbed asbestos fibers, in the interterritorial extracellular matrix 1.

1 Asbestos fibers
2 Isogenous cartilage cells
3 Cartilage corona, territorial extracellular matrix
4 Interterritorial extracellular matrix
Stain: hematoxylin-eosin; magnification: × 400

198 Hyaline Cartilage—Joint Cartilage

Enzymatic digestion of the ground substances in the cartilage matrix can unmask the collagen fibrils and render them visible. In this preparation, the shoulder acetabulum from a mouse, the tangential fiber layer, was exposed by digestion with *hyaluronidase* . The collagen fibers run in one main direction and cross over each other in acute angles. Cell elements are not visible in this microtechnical preparation.
Familiar histological course preparations often reveal striated areas, which are interpreted as asbestos fibers and a typical sign of aging. Demasked collagen *fibrils* explain this finding. In these cases, the ground substance was missing as well.

Scanning electron microscopy; magnification: × 8000

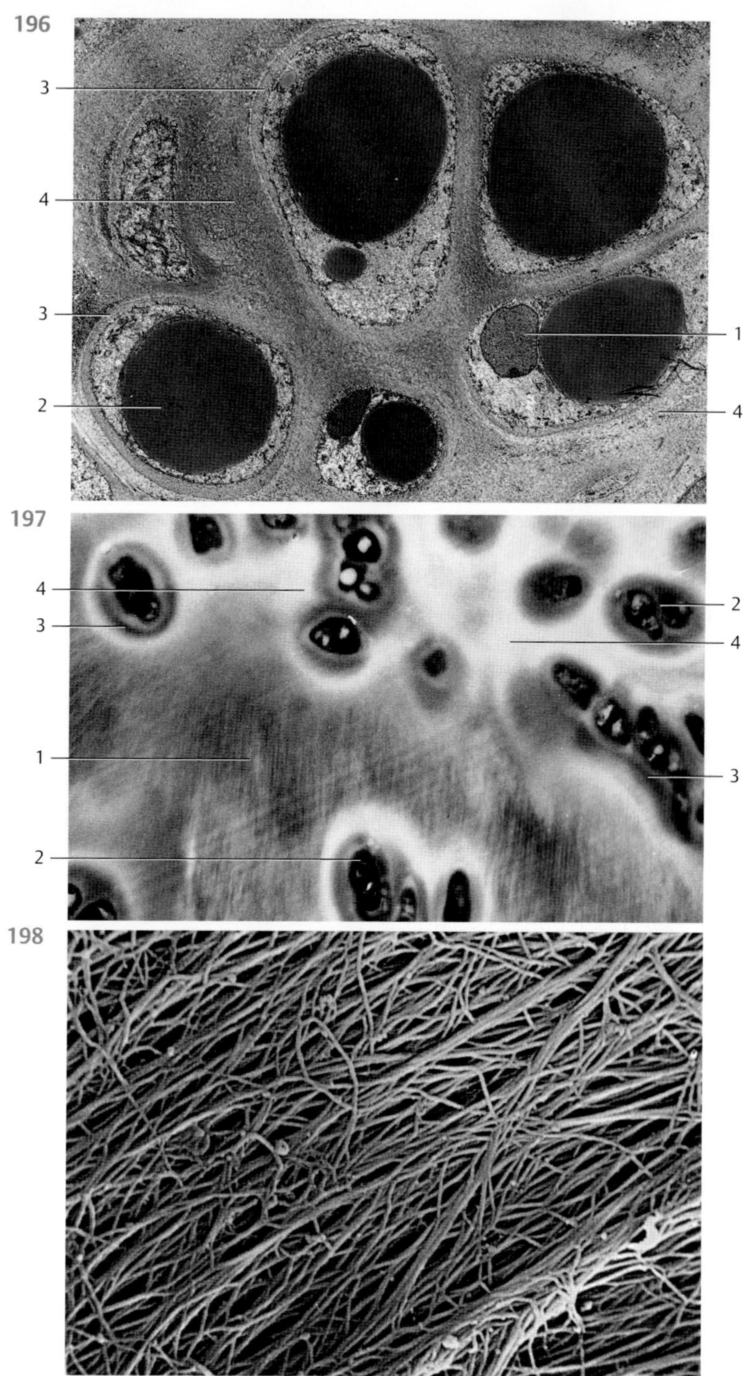
196
3
4
3
2
1
4
197
4
3
1
2
2
4
3
198

199 Fibrocartilage—Intervertebral Disks

Fibrocartilage (*connective tissue cartilage*) expresses the structures and attributes of two types of tissue, dense regular connective tissue and hyaline cartilage. The extracellular matrix consists mostly of collagen fibers (*type I and type II collagen*), which are not masked and therefore visible after staining (*collagen fiber cartilage*). Bundles of collagen fibrils run in the direction, which is determined by the mechanical stress vector. Between the unmasked collagen fibers 2 are single cartilage cells 1 or small groups of chondrocytes. The ovoid to spherical chondrocytes occur singly or often one after the other in a row. However, the overall cell density is low with local differences. As in hyaline cartilage, fibrocartilage features basophilic cartilage capsules and cartilage coronas.
In humans, fibrocartilage is restricted to intervertebral disks, pubic symphysis as well as parts of the joint disks and the menisci.

1 Chondron
2 Collagen fiber bundle
a) Stain: hematoxylin-eosin; magnification: × 240 ;
b) Stain: hematoxylin-eosin; differential interference contrast (DIC) image; magnification: × 200

200 Elastic Cartilage—Epiglottic Cartilage

In its interterritorial matrix, elastic cartilage contains nonmasked elastic fiber networks 1, which can be stained with the dye orcein, among others. At the nodal points, the fibers widen. In principle, the rest of the elastic cartilage structure is like that of hyaline cartilage. Like hyaline cartilage, it contains masked collagen fibers. The round or oval spaces contain the cartilage cells 2, which are only slightly stained. At the left edge of the figure is the *perichondrium* 3, with its fine elastic fibers parallel to the surface.
Elastic cartilage occurs in the auricular cartilage, the epiglottis, in the vocal processes of the arytenoid cartilage (processus vocalis cartilaginis arytaenoideae) and in the cartilage portion of the small bronchi.

1 Elastic fibers
2 Cartilage cells (chondrocytes)
3 Perichondrium
Stain: hemalum-orcein; magnification: × 50

201 Chorda Tissue—Embryonic Spinal Column

The chorda dorsalis (*notochord*) consists of large star-shaped *chorda cells*, which form cell-to-cell contacts with each other. Chorda cells have a high water content, contain microfilaments and synthesize type II collagen. From the chorda dorsalis derives the *nucleus pulposus* of the intervertebral disks.
The figure shows a detail section from the still mesenchymal spine of an embryo with a crown-rump length of 12 mm. The sagittal section is turned by 90°, ventral is up.

1 Chorda dorsalis in slightly ventral position
2 Dense early intervertebral disks
3 Precartilage stage of vertebral bodies with few cells
4 Intersegmental vessels
5 Embryonic mesenchyme
Stain: hematoxylin-eosin; magnification: × 80

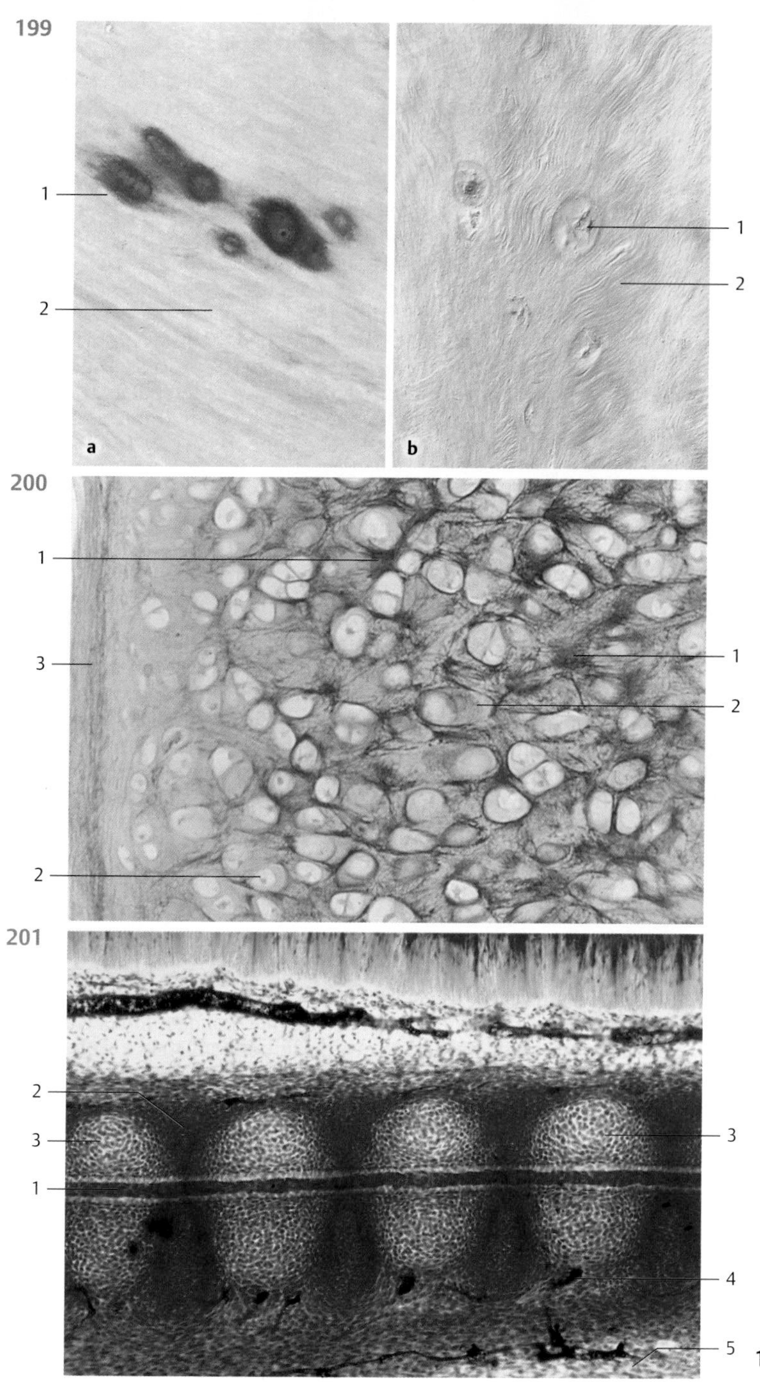
199
1
2
a
1
2
b
200
1
3
2
1
2
201
2
3
1
3
4
5

202 Membranous Osteogenesis—Parietal Bone

Membranous osteogenesis (*intramembranous ossification*) creates connective tissue bones (*direct osteogenesis*). During direct osteogenesis, mesenchyme cells in the embryonic connective tissue differentiate into osteoblasts (initiation of ossification). Osteoblasts are rich in ergastoplasm and secrete an amorphous ground substance, which contains glycoproteins and proteoglycans as well as the precursors of collagen fibrils. Membranous osteogenesis is therefore always accompanied by the appearance of a matted network of very delicate fibrils. Osteoblasts form a soft bone precursor material, which is termed *osteoid* bone. This figure shows red-stained *osteoid lamella* 1. Large osteoblasts line up at their surface. The osteoid lamellae grow by apposition. The cells inside the osteoid lamellae have entrapped themselves during osteogenesis and have differentiated into osteocytes in the process. The connective tissue between the lamellae 2 is rich in cells. In the left half of the figure, there are osteoid lamellae in the immediate vicinity of multinucleated giant cells. These are *osteoclasts* 3, which degrade bone tissue (see Fig. 204).

1 Osteoid lamellae with osteocytes
2 Embryonic connective tissue
3 Osteocytes
Stain: hematoxylin-eosin; magnification: × 90

203 Membranous Osteogenesis—Parietal Bone

Genesis of connective tissue-derived bone in the area of the parietal bone of a human fetus. The osteoid lamella is surrounded by many *osteoblasts* 1. They form prebone tissue, the osteoid 2 (here stained blue) and contain osteocytes 3. A fibrous structure is still discernible (*cartilage bone, fibrous bone*). The richly vascularized mesenchymal tissue between the primary bony lamellae (spongy bone trabeculae) is called primary bone marrow 4. Later, secondary bone marrow, which forms the blood cells, will arise from it.

1 Osteoblasts
2 Osteoid with fibers
3 Osteocytes
4 Primary bone marrow
Stain: azan; magnification: × 400

204 Membranous Osteogenesis—Parietal Bone

Multinucleated giant cells, *osteoclasts*, soon appear on the scenes of osteogenesis. They are part of the *hematopoietic macrophage-monocyte system* and are able to systematically degrade the basic bone substance (*bone resorption*) and phagocytose the products of this degradation. Osteoblasts have irregular shapes. They are branched and may contain as many as 50 or more nuclei. Osteoblasts are located close to the newly formed osteoid lamellae. When they degrade osteoid material, they create small bays, termed *Howship lacunae* or *arrosion bays* (lacunar resorption).
Only a few nuclei are visible in the figure. However, it provides an image of the lacy projections of the osteoclasts. In the lower part of the figure is an osteoid lamella. The area right and left of the osteoclast represents primary bone marrow.

Stain: hematoxylin-eosin; magnification: × 400

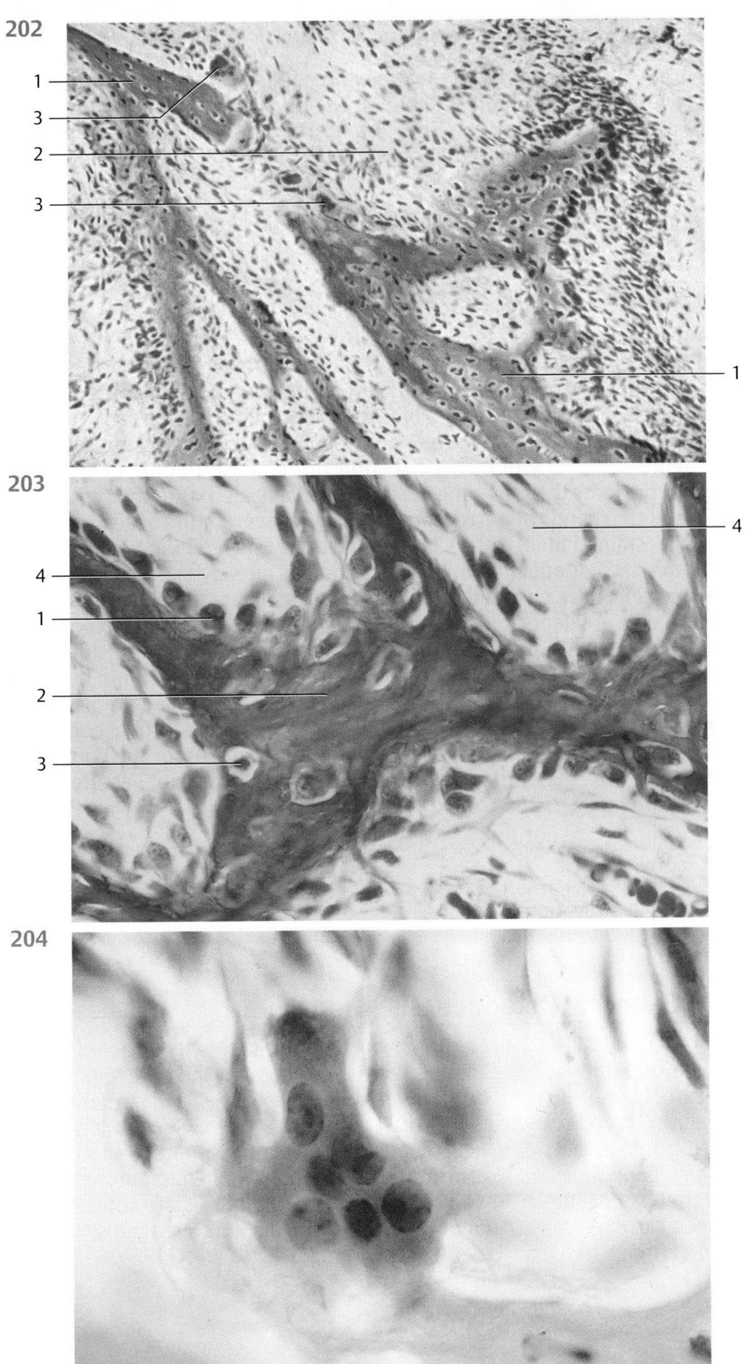
202
1
3
2
3
1
203
4
4
1
2
3
204

205 Chondral Osteogenesis—Finger

Longitudinal section through the index finger of a 6-month-old human embryo, with the base, middle and end of the limb to illustrate chondral osteogenesis (chondral, endochondral ossification), which begins in the *diaphysis*. Note the hyaline cartilage epiphyses (cf. Figs. 206–213). Chondral ossification is also referred to as indirect osteogenesis.

Stain: hematoxylin-eosin; magnification: × 18

206 Chondral Osteogenesis—Finger

In contrast to the membranous, direct osteogenesis (*ossification*), the chondral osteogenesis requires an existing scaffold of hyaline cartilage lamellae (*cartilage model of ossification*). While the cartilage is degraded, it is replaced by bone tissue (substitute bone; *indirect osteogenesis*). Dependent on the location of their synthesis, there are perichondral and endochondral bones. The figure shows a longitudinal section through the middle phalanx of a finger. It presents the following details: the diaphysis 1 is in the center. Both the distal (left) and the proximal (right) *epiphyses* 2 still consist of hyaline cartilage (stained blue-violet). In the light zone between the two epiphyses, the *diaphysis* 1, endochondral ossification has already started. The hyaline cartilage cells have changed into large spherical cells, and at the same time, calcium salts are deposited in the intercellular space. These areas can be recognized as small, branched, gray-blue lamellae. Osteoblasts reside in the connective tissue layer called perichondrium. They have built by membranous osteogenesis a sleeve of perichondral bone in the area of the diaphysis (here stained bright red) 3. The perichondrium is a form of connective tissue. The perichondral bone is a protective encasement for the bony structures in the area of the diaphysis. The two epiphyses are not yet affected by ossification (cf. Figs. 205, 207–213).

1 Diaphysis
2 Epiphysis
3 Perichondral bone
4 Forming muscle cells
Stain: hematoxylin-eosin; magnification: × 15

207 Chondral Osteogenesis—Finger

The perichondral bony sleeve 1 has become thicker by *appositional growth*. At the same time, it has expanded in the direction of the two epiphyses 2. The cartilage cells in the diaphysis 3 have died, and the cartilage has disintegrated. In its place there is now vascular connective tissue, which has invaded from the outside. The tissue is mesenchymal in nature and is called *primary bone marrow*. Concurrently, small bony lamellae are created by chondral osteogenesis. In the direction of the epiphysis are rows of voluminous cartilage cells (*column cartilage*), which stand out against the dormant cartilage tissue at the end of the joint (cf. Figs. 205, 206, 208–213).

1 Perichondral bone
2 Epiphyseal cartilage
3 Diaphysis
4 Periosteum
Stain: hematoxylin-eosin; magnification: × 12

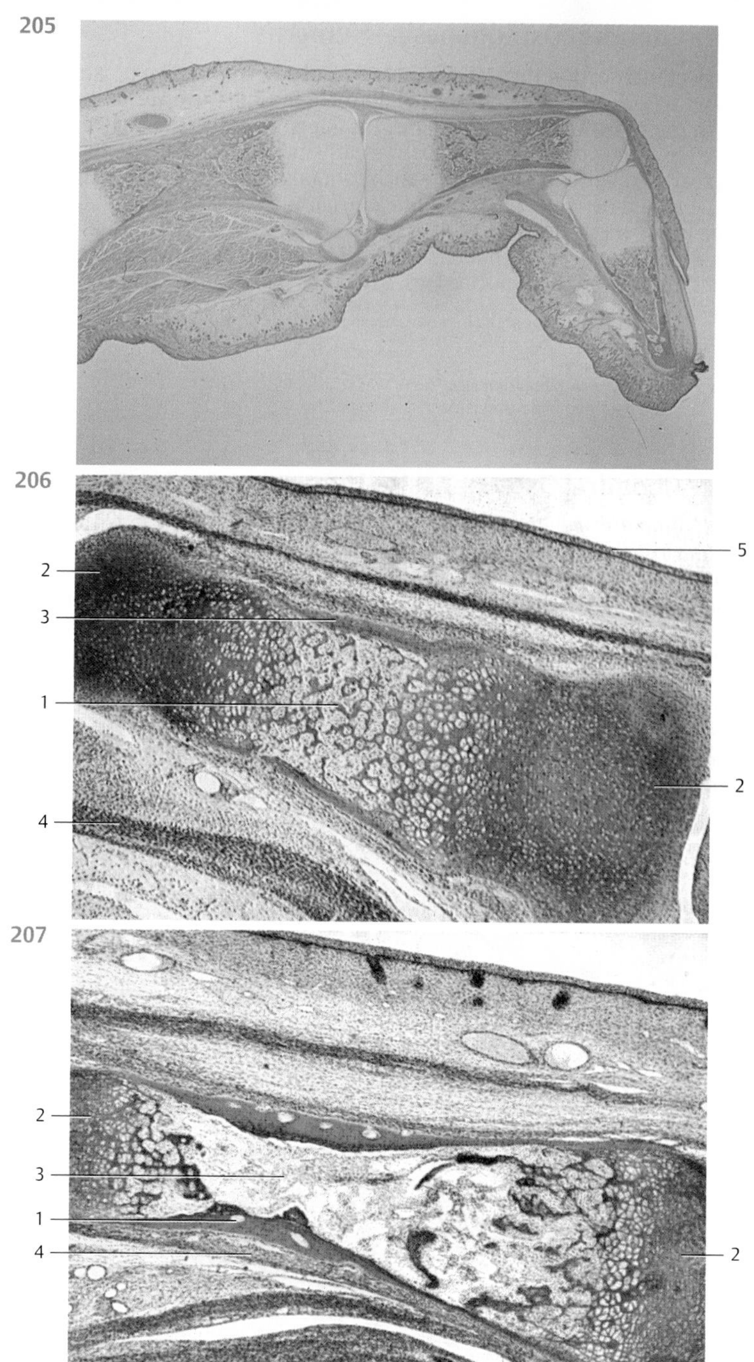
205
206
2
3
1
4
5
2
207
2
3
1
4
2

208 Chondral Osteogenesis—Humerus

Longitudinal section through the humerus of a newborn. The proximal epiphysis 1 (*humerus head*) consists of dormant hyaline cartilage. In the figure, at the top right, an ossification core 2 is already visible. The arched growth plate (*growth gap, epiphyseal gap*) 3 clearly marks the border between epiphyseal cartilage and diaphysis, which contains bone lamellae (stained light red). Located between the *spongiosa lamellae* 4 is blood-forming secondary bone marrow (cf. Fig. 209).
The different stages of endochondral osteogenesis correspond to different zones at the growth plate (see Figs. 211–213).

1 Proximal epiphysis of the humerus, hyaline cartilage
2 Bone core
3 Growth plate
4 Diaphysis with bony lamellae
Stain: Bock hemalum-eosin; magnification: × 2.8

209 Chondral Osteogenesis—Humerus

Enlargement of a detail from Fig. 208. At the top of the image is *epiphyseal cartilage* 1 (red-violet). The following layer represents the growth plate 2 (*epiphyseal plate, metaphysis, growth zone*), identifiable by its darker red stain. In the part of the growth plate that faces the epiphysis, new cartilage is generated by interstitial growth. Endochondral osteogenesis occurs in the metaphyseal part of the epiphysis gap. This entails the mineralization of the cartilage matrix, vascularization and the *resorption of cartilage tissue*. Bone lamellae 3 are generated by primary osteogenesis. They are located close to the diaphysis. The space between the spongiosa lamellae contains blood-forming secondary bone marrow 4. Note: the proximal humeral epiphysis is already vascularized.

1 Proximal epiphysis, hyaline cartilage
2 Growth plate, epiphysial plate
3 Diaphysis with bone lamellae
4 Bone marrow
Stain: Bock hemalum-eosin; magnification: × 13

210 Chondral Osteogenesis—Humerus

Cross-section through the humeral diaphysis of a newborn. Bone lamellae (*spongiosa trabeculae*) 1 have formed by intramembranous osteogenesis. Rows of *osteoblasts* 2 are lined up at their surfaces. The red, heavily stained zones represent endochondral bone, the *osteoid*. The light areas with irregular borders correspond to the calcified ground substance of the cartilage tissue. Note how the osteocytes 3 are walled into their self-generated caverns. Between the spongiosa trabeculae, there is blood-forming secondary bone marrow 4. At this stage, the bone marrow cavity is known as the *secondary medullary cavity*.

1 Spongiosa trabeculae
2 Osteoblasts
3 Osteocytes
4 Blood-forming bone marrow
Stain: azan; magnification: × 200

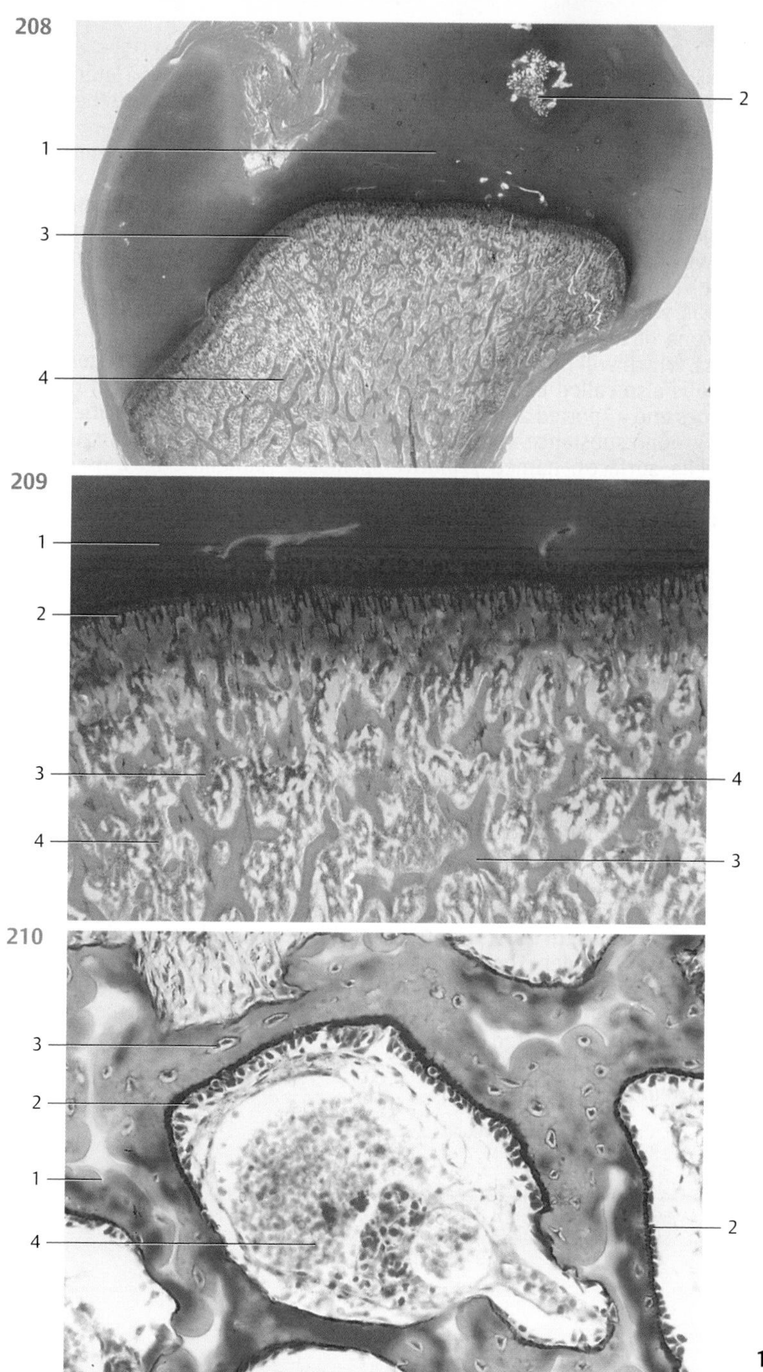
208
2
1
3
4
209
1
2
3
4
4
3
210
3
2
1
2
4

211 Chondral Osteogenesis—Tibia

This longitudinal section from a tibia tissue preparation shows a later stage in osteogenesis (*endochondral ossification*). From the top, there are the following zones:

1 Hyaline cartilage of the epiphysis in the dormant state (*reserve zone*), zone of dormant hyaline cartilage (cf. Figs. 206–209).

2 The cartilage cells in the subsequent zone are arranged like columns (*cartilage column zone, column cartilage*). These cartilage cells ascertain the growth in length by their high proliferation rates (*proliferation or growth zone*). Note the size increase for cartilage cells the closer they are to the diaphysis, while the volume of the intercellular substances decreases.

3 Zone of macerated, voluminous cartilage cells (*hypertrophied cartilage cells*), which will finally be degraded by chondroclasts (*resorptive zone*). This zone is also called *initiation* zone. Next, there are lamellae with different shapes and a spotted appearance. These are remnants of the calcified cartilage ground substance. Osteoblasts deposit newly formed bone tissue at the lamella surfaces, named *primitive spongiosa* (lamella edges, ossification zones). Between the lamellae 4 of the primitive spongiosa, there is the cell rich material of the primary bone marrow 5.

1 Epiphyseal cartilage
2 Column cartilage
3 Distended hypertrophied cartilage cells
4 Primary spongiosa lamellae
5 Medullary cavity, bone marrow
Stain: hemalum-benzopurpurin; magnification: × 30

212 Chondral Osteogenesis—Finger

Proximal phalanx from the finger of a fetus. Section from the zone of cartilage degradation and endochondral osteogenesis.

In the right upper corner, the figure shows the largest cells of the column *cartilage*. The cells in the subsequent layer are the large voluminous *cartilage* cells of the *initiation zone*. The center image shows calcified cartilage ground substance 1, which contains islands of primary bone marrow. Young bone tissue (stained light red) is layered onto this perforated layer (*primitive spongiosa*) like a border. The primary bone marrow 2 contains osteoblasts 3, which are polynucleated cells with all kinds of geometries. The bright red layer in the left corner of the figure is the bony sleeve 4 of the diaphysis, which has been created by membranous osteogenesis. It is covered by a string of osteoblasts. Toward the outside follows the cell-rich layer of the *periosteum* 5.

1 Calcifying cartilage, ground substance
2 Bone marrow
3 Osteoclasts
4 Perichondral bone, bone sleeve
5 Periosteum
Stain: hematoxylin-eosin; magnification: × 65

211

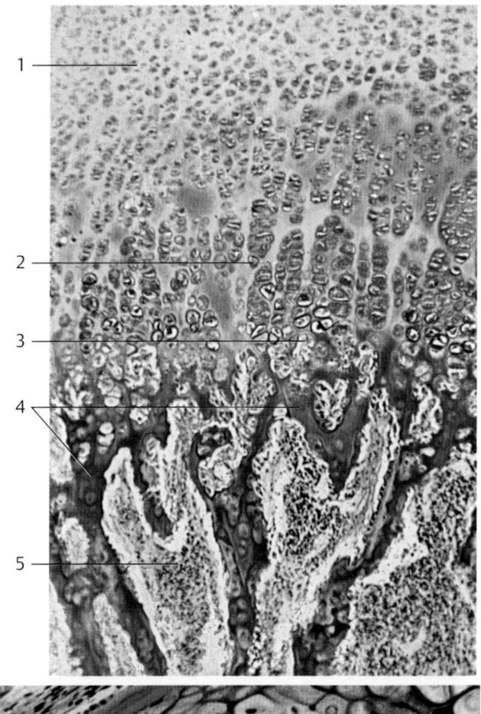

212

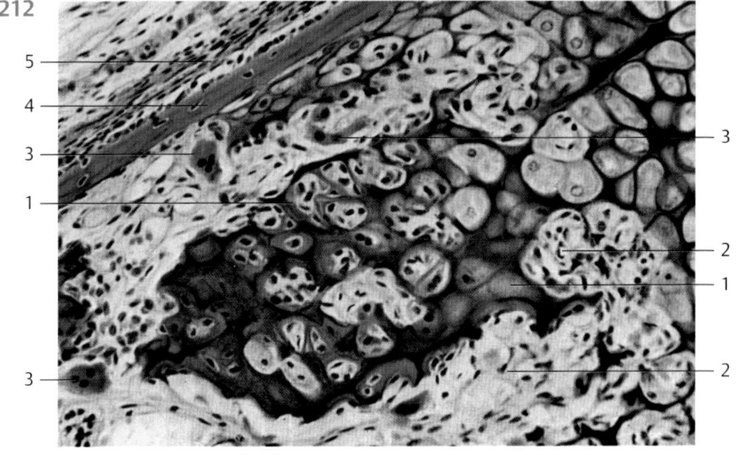

213 Chondral Osteogenesis—Finger

The same ossification processes that operate in the diaphysis also take place in the postnatal period in the epiphyses. In this figure, the epiphysis is located at the left. It is now interspersed with coarse bone lamellae generated by chondral osteogenesis. The subsequent zone (stained red) is *young cartilage*, followed by the wide zone of the column cartilage [2]. The two layers combined form the epiphyseal space or *growth plate*, which remains until the end of growth. The interstitial growth of these cartilage cells ascertains an increase in bone length. In the right part of the figure, the bone marrow of the diaphysis can be seen between the newly formed bone lamellae [3] (cf. 208, 209, 211).

1 Bone lamellae of the epiphysis
2 Column cartilage
3 Bone lamellae of the diaphysis
4 Large voluminous cartilage cells
5 Bone marrow of the epiphysis and the diaphysis
Stain: alum hematoxylin; magnification: × 20

214 Bone Tissue—Compact Bone

In the first years of human life, the primitive fiber-based soft bone (*fibrous bone*) is degraded and replaced by *lamellar bone*. Its structure can be studied in cross-sections through the compact substance (*cortical substance*) of a long bone (as represented by the tibia). The concentric layers of compact substance (*special lamellae*) have central canals (*Haversian canals* or *longitudinal canals, canales centrales*) and blood vessels (*Haversian vessels*) [1]. Bone tubules about 1 cm long (possibly several centimeters long) called *osteons* [2] are created. Their diameters measure about 250–350 µm. The transverse canals, called *Volkmann canals* (*canales perforantes*), break through the Haversian lamellar system and interconnect the vessels in the Haversian canals with those of the *periosteum*. Between osteons are remnants of older, largely degraded bone tubules. They are called *interstitial lamellae* [3]. The fully differentiated *osteocytes* (bone cells) are located between the lamellae in the cavities of the ground substance. They have cemented themselves into their extracellular matrix. The light crevices in this preparation are technical artifacts.

1 Haversian canals, vessels
2 Haversian systems, osteons
3 Interstitial lamellae
Stain: Schmorl thionine-picric acid; magnification: × 70

215 Bone Tissue—Compact Bone

Transverse section of an osteon with its Haversian canal [1]. It is enveloped by lamellae in the ground substance, which may be more or less impregnated with Silver nitrate. The collagen fibers in the more heavily stained lamellae are arranged in a circular fashion; in the lightly stained areas, their orientation follows the longitudinal axis of the osteons. The black spindle-shaped structures with numerous fine black threads extending from their surfaces are osteocytes [2] and their cellular projections. The osteocytes reside in *bone cavities*, and their projections reach into the *bone canals*.

1 Haversian canal
2 Osteocytes
Stain: silver nitrate impregnation; magnification: × 250

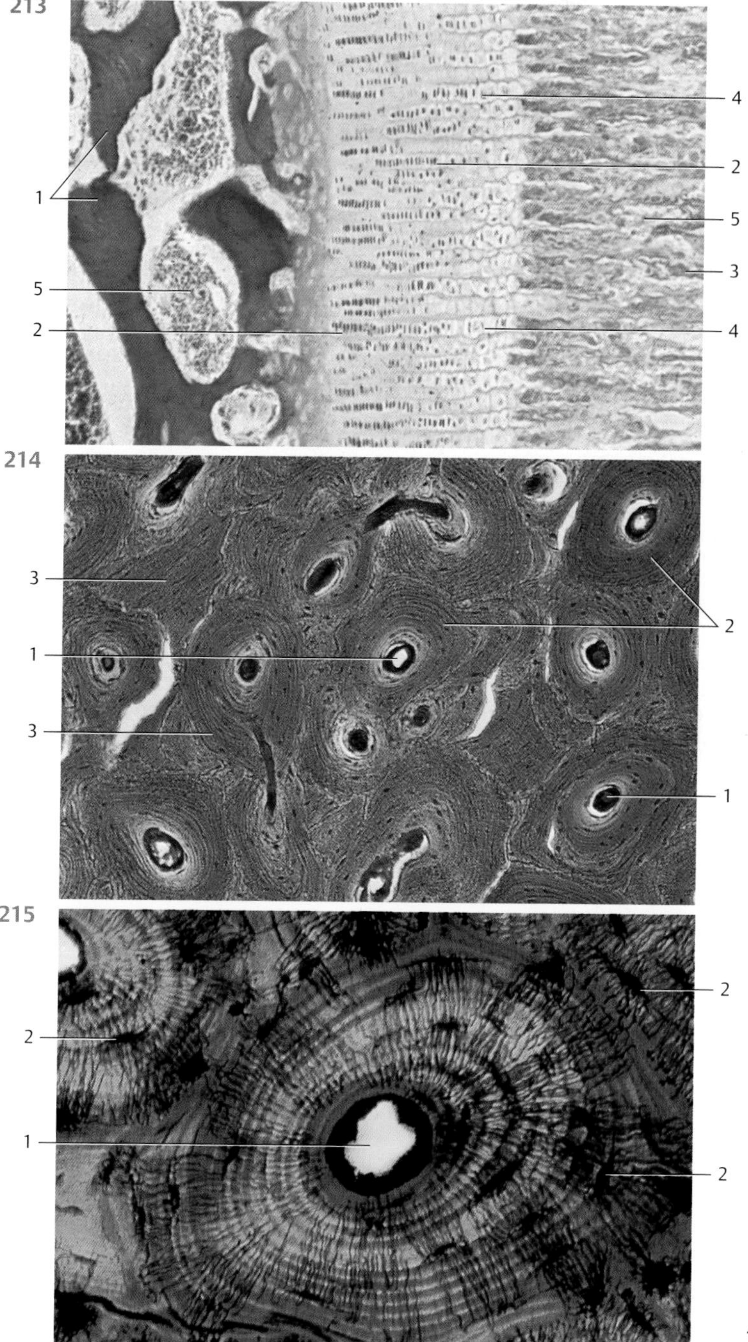
213
1
5
2
4
2
5
3
4
214
3
1
3
2
1
215
2
1
2
2

216 Bone Tissue—Compact Bone

All osteons [1] with their *special lamellae* and the *interstitial lamella systems* [3] are encased by the outer and inner *general lamellae* [4]. Figure 216b shows the outer general lamella [4]. The oblong narrow space represents a vascularized *Volkmann canal* (*transverse canal*) [5]. These transverse canals break through the lamella systems. Different lamella systems are separated by cement lines. These consist of ground substance with a few fibrils, and they stain heavily with hematoxylin.

1 Osteon
2 Haversian canal
3 Interstitial lamella
4 Outer general lamella
5 Volkmann canal
Stain: hematoxylin-eosin; magnifications: a) × 120, b) × 10

217 Bone Tissue—Compact Bone

Cross-section (a) and transverse section (b) through an osteon, demonstrating the lacunae (bone cavities, *lacunae osseae*) and the bone channels (*canaliculi ossei*).
The bone canaliculi cannot be seen in the usual histological preparations. Canaliculi are about 1.0–1.5 μm wide and are devoid of extracellular matrix. They contain many branched, filopodia-like osteoplast projections. Bone canaliculi of neighboring bone cavities interconnect.
The system of canals serves for the exchange of materials between osteocytes and extracellular space.
Osteocytes are spindle-shaped cells with long, slender, interconnecting cell projections.

Stain: Schmorl thionine-picric acid; magnification: × 400

218 Bone Tissue—Compact Bone

Decalcified bone tissue can be processed like any other tissue. It can be cut using a microtome and stained. The cytoplastic processes of osteoplasts occupy bone canals in the extracellular space and connect with each other via nexuses. The exchange of materials probably proceeds via these cytoplasmic processes.
Osteocytes and their cytoplasmic processes (projections) are clearly visible in thin sections of compact bone substance from the femur after decalcification and Schmorl staining.

Stain: Schmorl thionine-picric acid; magnification: × 500

216

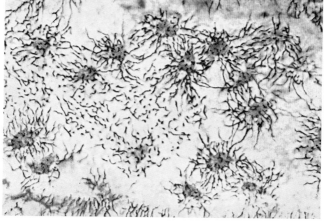

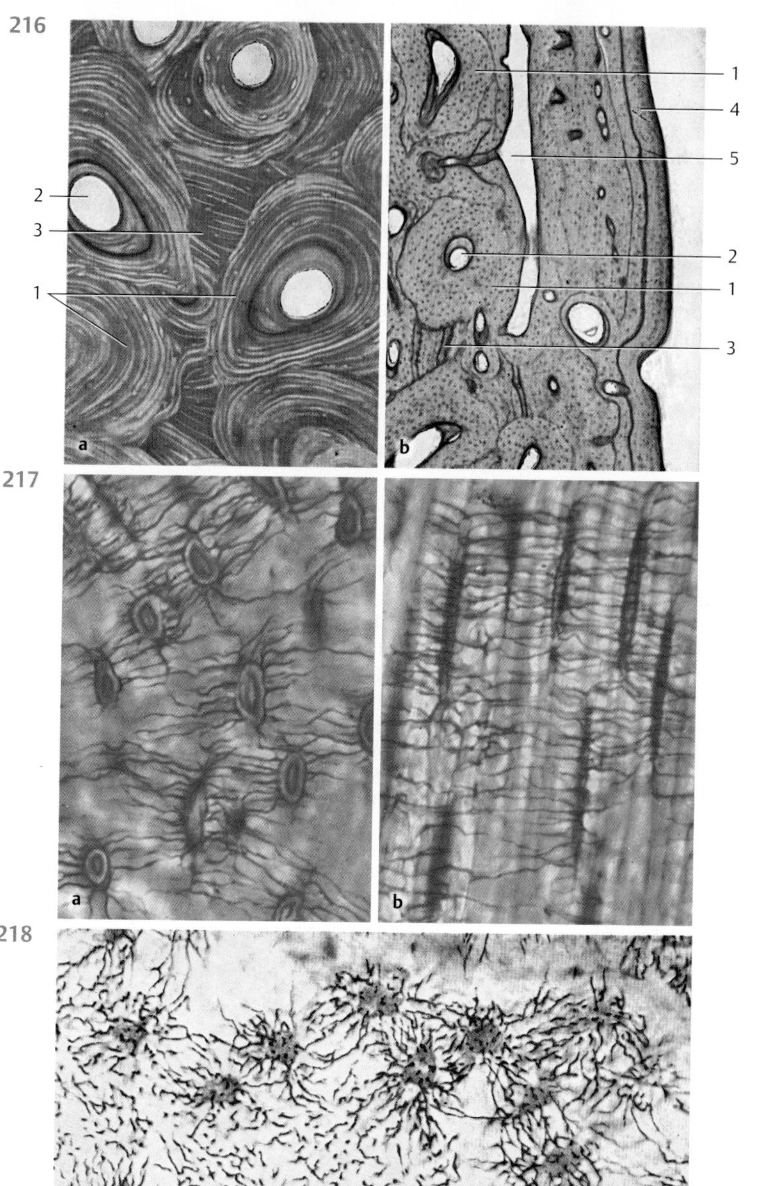

219 Smooth Muscle—Urinary Bladder

The structural units of the smooth muscle consist of spindle-shaped "smooth" cells of different lengths. "Smooth" means that the cells do not show striation. Basis for their contractility is the presence of *myofibrils* in the cytoplasmic matrix (*sarcoplasm*) (cf. Figs. 222, 223). It is difficult to show the cross-striation of these myofibrils in light microscopic images. If visible at all, the cross-striation is rendered barely visible as faint pattern in transverse cuts (see Fig. 220) or as small dots in cross-sections (see Fig. 221). The delicately structured rod-shaped nucleus is always in a central position. This figure shows the spindle-shaped smooth muscle cells in the wall of a urinary bladder from a frog. Outside the focal plane, a vessel shows Y-like branching. Whole-mount preparation.

Stain: hematoxylin-eosin; magnification: × 200

220 Smooth Muscle—Jejunum

Smooth muscle tissue consists of spindle-shaped cells, which are about 5–200 µm long and 3–10 µm thick. Their nuclei reside in the centers of the cells (cf. Figs. 3, 219, 221). Short, compact muscle cells often have an undulating surface. Light microscopy and the usual staining procedures do not bring out any particular structures in the cytoplasm or the embedded myofibrils. Smooth muscle cells converge to bundles of different sizes. Among other tissues, they build the muscular coat of hollow organs. This figure shows the *inner ring layer* 1 and the *outer longitudinal layer* 2 of the jejunal muscular coat. At the upper edge of the image, the submucous coat has been captured. Between the two layers of muscle cells are the ganglion cells of the *myenteric plexus* 3 (*Auerbach plexus*, cf. Figs. 432–434, 437). There is an abundance of blood vessels 5 and loose connective tissue in the outer longitudinal layer of muscle cells 1. They are covered by the *tunica serosa* (peritoneal epithelium) 4.

1 Smooth muscle cells, longitudinal section
2 Smooth muscle cells, cross-section
3 Myenteric plexus
4 Serosa epithelium
5 Capillaries

Semi-thin section; stain: methylene blue-azure II; magnification: × 400

221 Smooth Muscle—Myometrium

Cross-section through a bundle of smooth muscle cells 1, which are interspersed with strong collagen fibers 2. There are capillaries 3 embedded inside these fiber bundles. The nuclei are located in the center of the cell body. Note that not all cells are cut in planes where there are nuclei. This explains the apparent differences in sizes. The differences in the staining intensity of smooth muscle cells should also be noted: there are cells with a light or dark appearance in cross-sections (cf. Figs. 220, 223, 581, 582). During pregnancy, the uterine smooth muscles become hypertrophied. At that stage, their lengths are 800–1000 µm.

1 Smooth muscle cells, cross-section
2 Collagenous connective tissue
3 Capillary

Semi-thin section; stain: methylene blue-azure II; magnification: × 400

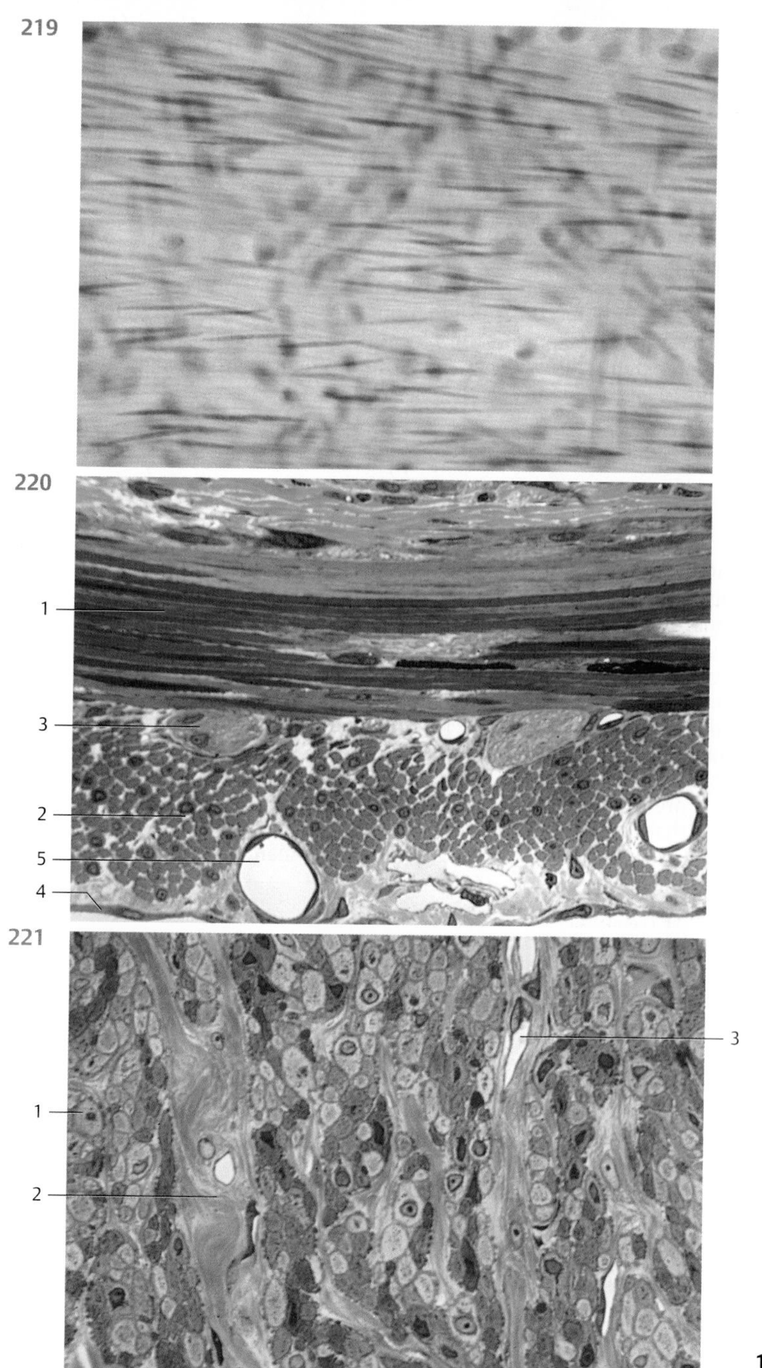
219
220
1
3
2
5
4
221
3
1
2

222 Smooth Muscle—Duodenum

Smooth muscle cells from the *tunica muscularis* of the duodenum with interspersed actin, myosin and intermediary filaments, predominantly actin filaments. There are many small, irregularly distributed denser areas (dense spots) in the cytoplasm. In conjunction with intermediary filaments, they mediate myofilaments attachment. Note the long oval nuclei in the cell centers. The nuclei of contracted muscle cells are often compressed in the form of a spring. Long, oval, strongly osmiophilic mitochondria [1], along with microtubules and sparse granular endoplasmic reticulum membranes are found between the filament bundles, mostly in the pole regions. The cell surface exhibits numerous invaginations. These are *caveolae*, which are considered the equivalents of the T-system in striated muscle fibers. They look similar to *pinocytotic vesicles*. Compare this figure with the light microscopic image in Fig. 220.

1 Mitochondria
Electron microscopy; magnification: × 2500

223 Smooth Muscle—Artery

This figure shows a cross-section through the smooth muscle cells of the tunica media (vascular coat) of the parotid gland. The cell at the top center underneath the endothelium [1] contains a nucleus [2]. In addition, there are small groups of ribosomes, a few crista-type mitochondria and groups or rows of vesicles, called *caveolae*, and predominantly located along the sarcolemma, small dense areas (*dense spots*) [↗], which serve as focal adhesion points for contractile fibers. The myofilaments in this figure are cut across their long axis, and therefore appear as small spots in the cytoplasm. Nexuses (contacts) are present in a few places between neighboring muscle cells [Λ]. They are loci with low electrical resistance and serve as excitation conduits. Note that a basal membrane (see Fig. 222) envelops the muscle cells. The extracellular collagen fibrils have been predominantly cut across their axis (cf. Figs. 220, 221).

1 Endothelium
2 Nucleus
3 Extracellular connective tissue space with collagen fibrils
4 Fibrocyte
Electron microscopy; magnification: × 9500

222

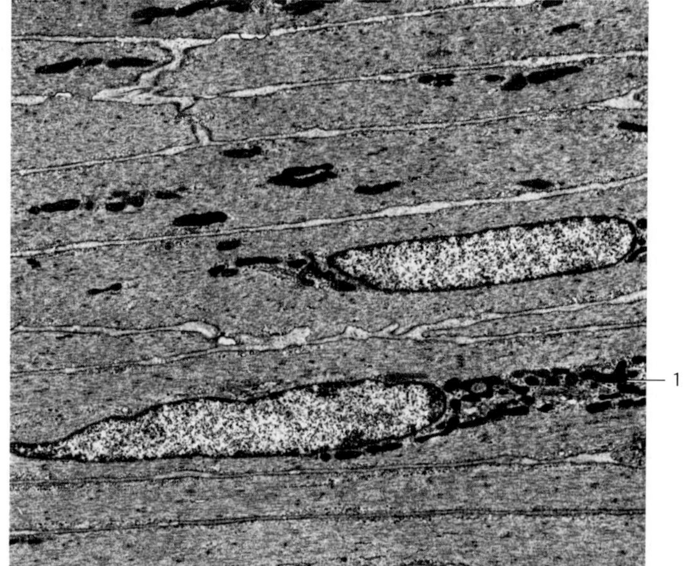

223

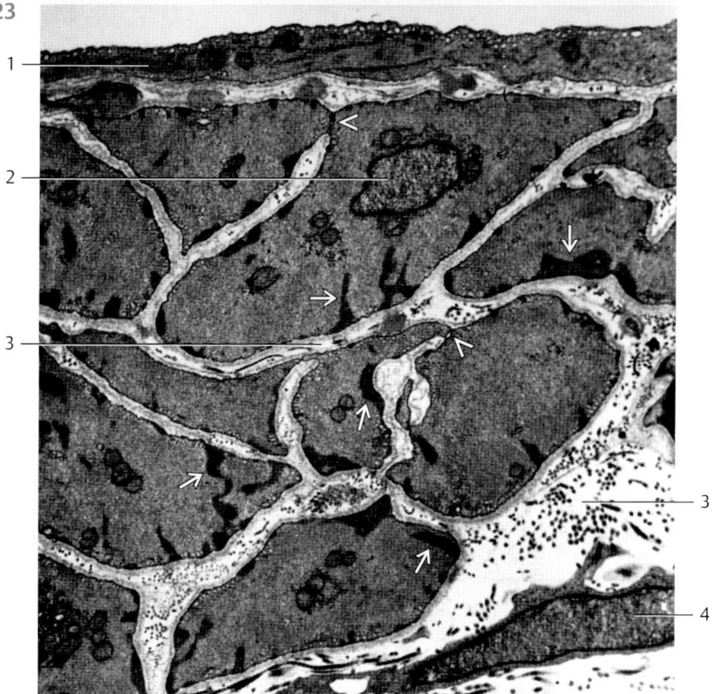

1

2

3

3

4

224 Striated Muscle—Myoblasts

Myotubes from the mylohyoid muscle of an 11-week old fetus. They have arisen from mesodermal tissue aggregates known as somites. The development of skeletal muscle can be traced to a tissue in the somite, the myotome. Expression of the MyoD gene leads to the formation of very actively dividing *muscle progenitor cells*, which will then differentiate and form *myoblasts*. Myoblasts do not divide. They fuse with each other and form syncytes with sometimes thousands of nuclei. The number of fusion cycles determines the size of the fully developed muscle. Myoblasts synthesize muscle-specific proteins and myofibrils. The fusion and assembly of myoblasts to cylinder-shaped myotubes occurs concomitantly in a coordinated process. The myofibrils cause the longitudinal myotube striation. However, there is no cross-striation yet. The nuclei still reside in the cell center (cf. Fig. 225).
The number of muscle fibers does not change in vertebrae after birth. The study of the intricate regulation of their number and size during development may also shed light on the etiology of degenerative muscle diseases.

1 Myotubes
2 Mesenchymal connective tissue
Stain: hemalum-eosin; magnification: × 500

225 Striated Muscle—Tongue

Longitudinal section 1 and cross-section 2 of striated muscle fibers from the tongue of a human embryo in the 22nd week of pregnancy. Compare it with Fig. 224 and note that the striation of the muscle fibers has already become evident. The nuclei are now located at the surface of the muscle fibers (cf. Figs. 226–230).

1 Muscle fibers, longitudinal section
2 Muscle fibers, cross-section
Stain: azan; magnification: × 400

226 Striated Muscle—Psoas Muscle

Longitudinal sections through muscle fibers clearly depict the characteristic striation, i.e., the regular pattern of alternating light and dark cross-bands. The length of striated skeletal muscle fibers ranges from a few millimeters to about 25 cm. Dependent on location and function, they are between 10 and 100 μm thick. The tube-like sarcolemma covers each muscle fiber. The constituents of the *sarcolemma* are the plasmalemma, the basal lamina and a tight covering of delicate reticular fibers. The outer border of this very delicate fibril network and the connective tissue of the *endomysium* 1 interconnect. Every muscle fiber contains numerous rod-shaped or oval nuclei in the cell periphery, close to the sarcolemma.
Note on nomenclature: in descriptions of electron microscopic images, only the plasmalemma of muscle fibers is termed "sarcolemma."

1 Endomysium
Stain: azan; magnification: × 500

224

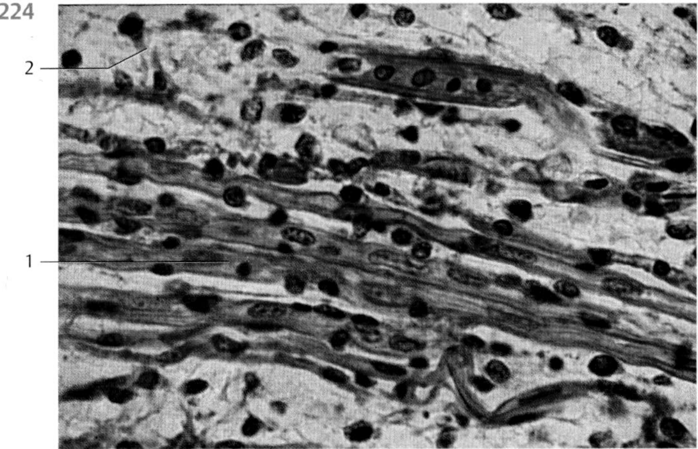

225

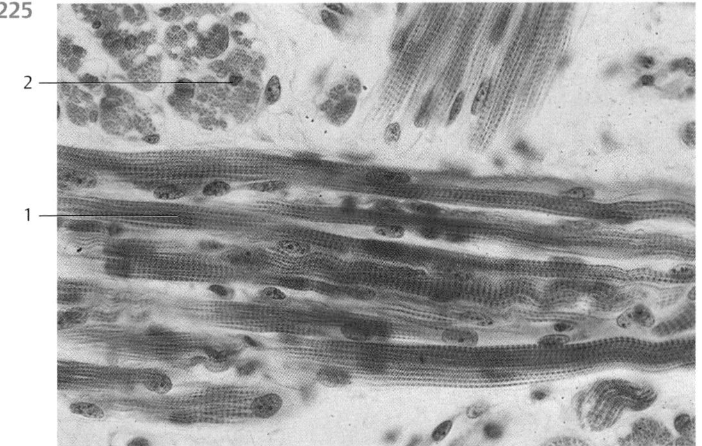

226

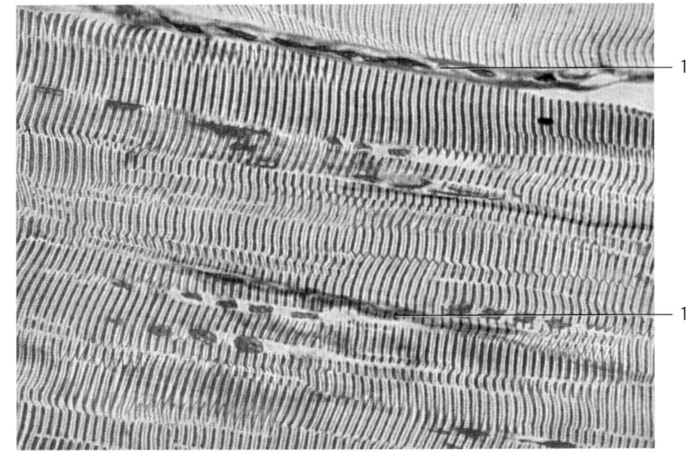

227 Striated Muscle—Thyrohyoid Muscle

The characteristic striation is based on the structure and arrangement of the myofibrils, which traverse the sarcoplasm lengthwise. This longitudinal section of the thyrohyoid muscle shows the parallel orientation of the myofibrils and the resulting fine longitudinal striation. There are alternating light and dark bands, with the dark bands being wider than the light ones. The dark cross-striations appear strongly birefringent in polarized light (*anisotropic, A-bands*). The light bands are refringent (*isotropic, I-bands*). Inside the I-bands are very narrow anisotropic bands with a larger refractive index (Z-bands or intermediary layer). In suitable preparations, a very thin M-band (center membrane) is discernible inside the A-bands. The layers between consecutive Z-bands are called *sarcomeres*. These are the functional units of myofibrils. It should be noted that the nuclei are located at the cell periphery 1. The (blue-stained) endomysium 2 (cf. Fig. 226), which contains capillaries and nerve fibers, should also be noted.

1 Nucleus of a skeletal muscle fiber
2 Endomysium
Stain: azan; magnification: × 1125

228 Striated Muscle—Psoas Muscle

Cross-section of skeletal muscle fibers with evenly distributed myofibrils that are not bundled (*simple fibril pattern*). Note the long, oval nuclei close to the cell surface 1 (cf. Fig. 229) in the muscle fiber. The two darker-stained nuclei in the connective tissue belong to fibrocytes 2.

1 Nucleus in a muscle fiber
2 Fibrocyte
3 Collagenous (dense) connective tissue
Stain: Heidenhain iron hematoxylin; magnification: × 1125

229 Striated Muscle—Psoas Muscle

This cross-section shows striated muscle fibers about 10–100 μm thick. Size and morphology depend on muscle function and workload. The nuclei 1 are clearly located in the periphery of the cells. The plasmalemma envelops the cytoplasm (*sarcoplasm*). The crevices between the muscle fibers contain the loose connective tissue of the *endomysium*, which consists mostly of reticular fibers. The even, dense and only softly stained dots in this cross-section reflect the even distribution of myofibrils (cf. Fig. 228). Occasionally, dependent on the fixation, the fibrils show a grouping pattern (*Cohnheim's fields, groups*). The plasmalemma is often called sarcolemma. This terminology was coined in light microscopy. In fact, the *sarcolemma* consists of the plasmalemma, the basal lamina and a network of delicate reticular fibers. These are not distinct components in light microscopic evaluations.

1 Nucleus of a skeletal muscle fiber
2 Capillary
3 Nucleus of a connective tissue cell
Semi-thin section; stain: methylene blue-azure II; magnification: × 800

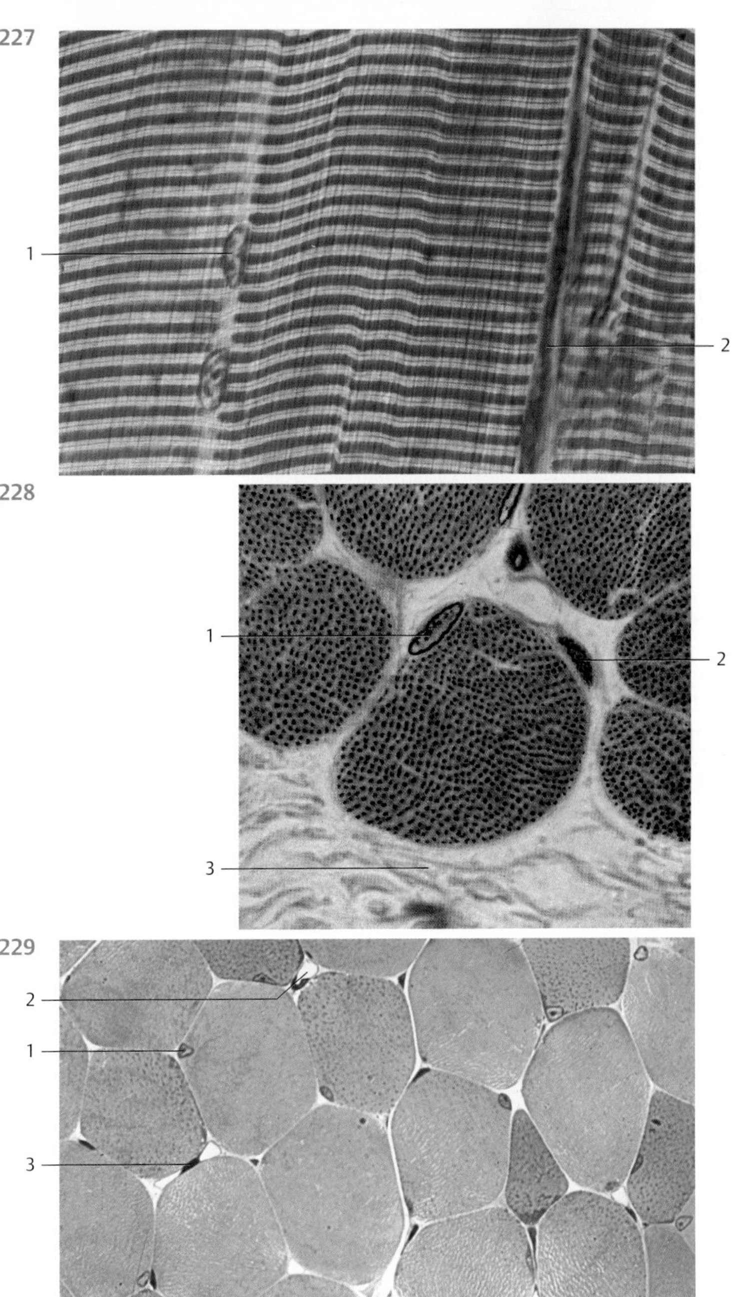

227
1
2
228
1
2
3
229
2
1
3

230 Striated Muscle—Psoas Muscle

Longitudinal section through striated myofibrils with conspicuous sarcomere organization. A sarcomere extends from one Z-band 1 to the next 1. In Z-bands, the actin filaments of two successive sarcomeres twist together and are cross-linked. Actin filaments in the form of I-bands (*isotropic bands*) flank both sides of the Z-band 2. The thicker myosin filaments form the A-band (*anisotropic band*) 3 of the myofibril. Actin and myosin filaments form a twisted helix and leave only the H-band 4 (light zone) in the middle of the A-band. The H-band consists only of myosin filaments, the I-bands only of actin filaments. The dark centerline in the H-zone is the *centermembrane.* Cross-linking of the myosin filaments creates this line. Note the peripheral nucleus 6 close to the fiber surface under the *sarcolemma* (plasmalemma) (see Figs. 226, 227).

1 Z-band
2 I-bands (isotropic)
3 A-bands (anisotropic)
4 H-band (H-zone; Hensen's bands) with M-band (M-line)
5 Mitochondria
6 Nucleus of the muscle fiber
7 Extracellular matrix with collagen fibrils
Electron microscopy; magnification: × 6000

231 Striated Muscle—Psoas Muscle

Longitudinal section through several sarcomeres in a skeletal muscle fibril (cf. Fig. 230). The space between two adjacent Z-bands 1 is called sarcomere. By this definition, a sarcomere consists of an A-band and the two halves of the adjacent I-band 2 on each side.
The Z-band 1 is electron-dense. It runs through the center of the I-band 2. The somewhat lighter stained H-band goes through the middle of the A-band 3. In the center of the H-band is the M-band or M-line (center membrane) (cf. Fig. 230). Between neighboring A-bands are cuts through smooth ER membranes (sarcoplasmic reticulum = L-system). Crista-type mitochondria occur at the level of the I-bands.

1 Z-bands or Z-disk
2 I-bands (isotropic)
3 A-bands (anisotropic)
Electron microscopy; magnification: × 25 000

230

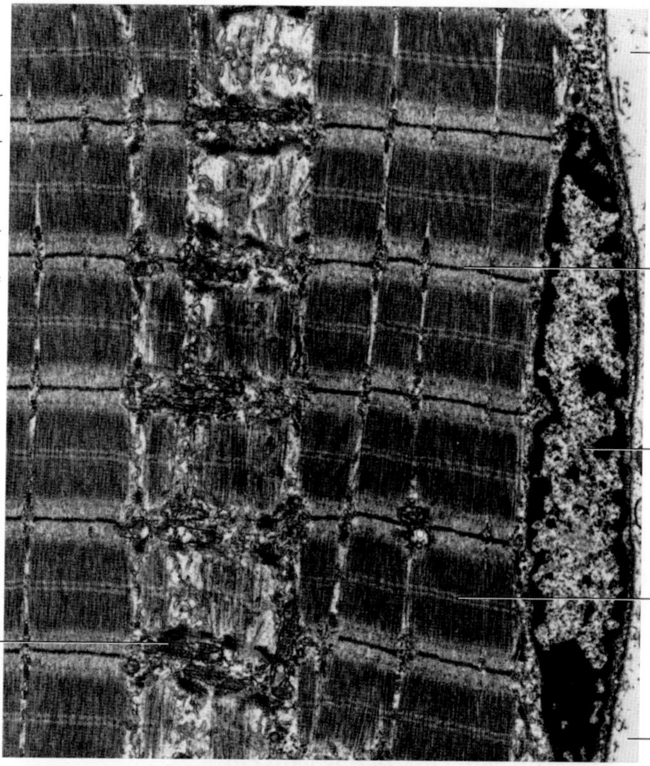

7
2
2
1
3
3
6
2
4
5
7

231

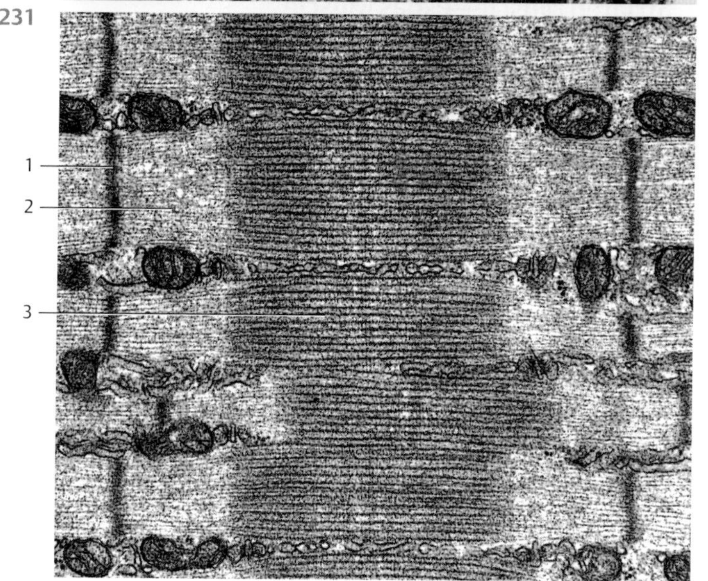

232 Striated Muscle—Psoas Muscle

Cross-section through bundles of myofibrils at the level of an A-band and the T-tubules [1] that cover the myofibril borders. The smooth endoplasmic reticulum, here called sarcoplasmic reticulum (*sarcotubular system*), forms a network around every myofibril as *longitudinal system* (*L-system*) and *transverse system* (*T-tubules, T-system*). Note the hexagonal organization of the thick myosin filaments and the fine spot-like structures, which correspond to cross-sectioned thin actin filaments. There are actin and myosin filaments. Actin filaments are thin (7 nm), about 1 μm in length, and consist of actin, tropomyosin and troponin. Myosin filaments are built from light and heavy *meromyosin* (about 1.5 μm long).

1 T-tubules (transverse system)
Electron microscopy; magnification: × 46 000

233 Striated Muscle—Tongue

The tongue is a *body of muscles*, which is covered by the oral mucous membrane (cf. Figs. 372, 373). The striated muscle fibers form a three-dimensional network. This figure shows a vertical cut (frontal section) through a human tongue. The muscle fibers are arranged almost vertical to each other. This creates a fishbone pattern in the muscle tissue. Strands of muscle fibers go in many directions. The path of the blood vessels follows this pattern. After injection with Indian ink, they are clearly visible here.

Stain: van Gieson iron hematoxylin-picric acid-acid fuchsin, Indian ink injection; magnification: × 40

234 Striated Muscle—Psoas Muscle

The sarcoplasm of striated muscle fibers contains mitochondria (*sarcosomes*) (see Figs. 230, 231). They can be made visible by marker enzyme histochemistry.

The enzyme succinate dehydrogenase is a marker enzyme for mitochondria. Its localization is shown in this freeze-fracture preparation. The products of the histochemical reaction accumulate in the locations of mitochondria. In cross-sections, sarcosome-rich fibers (*aerobic fibers*) appear dark and densely granulated, the sarcosome-poor fibers (*anaerobic fibers*) appear light.

The nuclei are not visible with this marker enzyme mediated visualization. A staining method for the nuclei was not added after the histochemical procedure.

Histochemical reaction of the marker enzyme succinate dehydrogenase (SDH); magnification: × 130

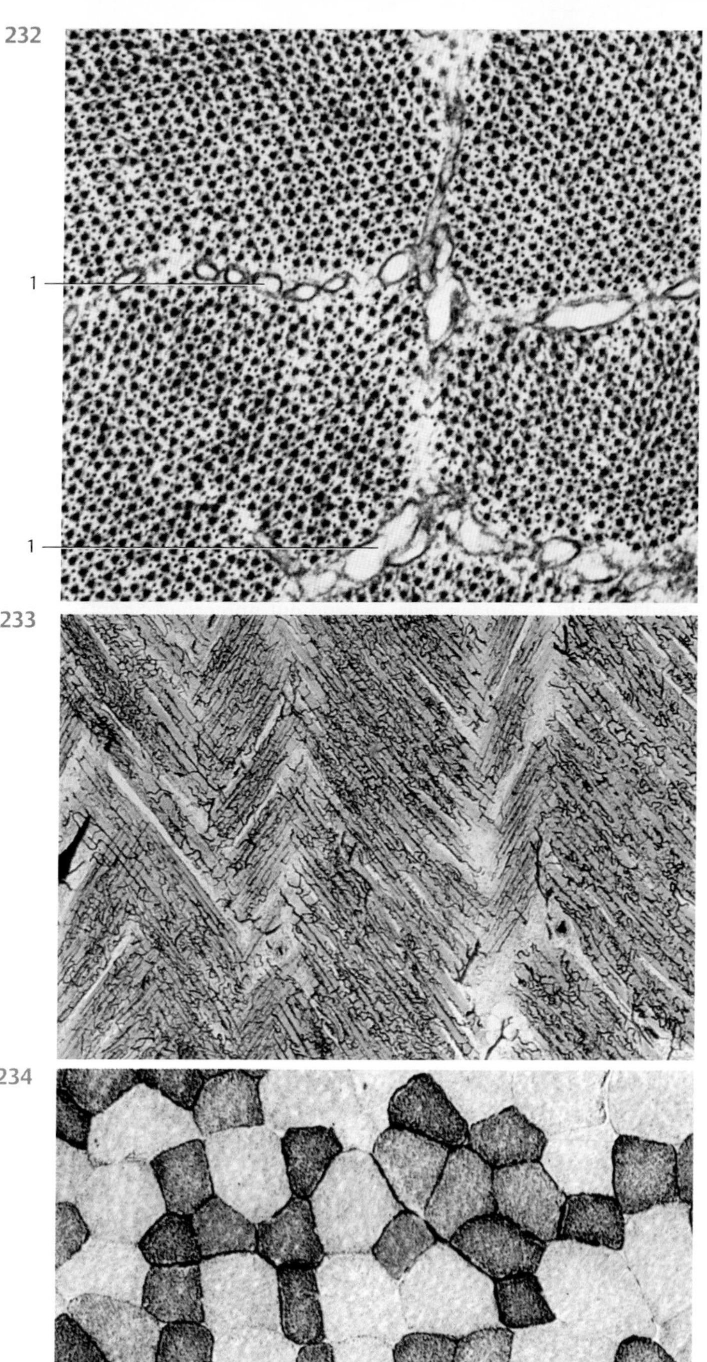
232
1
1
233
234

235 Skeletal Muscle-Tendon Linkage

This figure provides a light microscopic image of the linkage between skeletal muscle fibers 1 and tendon fibers 2. The muscle fibers only appear to continue in the collagen fiber bundles of tendons and aponeuroses. In reality, the connection is made between the fine fiber matrix around the sarcolemma and the loose connective tissue in the immediate vicinity of the muscle fibers. There is no true continuity between contractile myofibrils and collagen fibrils (see Fig. 236). Individual tendon fibers finally merge in an acute angle to form tendons and aponeuroses.

1 Striated muscle fibers
2 Collagen fibers of the tendon
3 Collagenous connective tissue
Stain: azan; magnification: × 500

236 Skeletal Muscle-Tendon Linkage

Finger-like processes of the muscle fibers fan out and establish the link between skeletal muscle and tendon (see Fig. 235). The myofibrils extend into the spaces between these processes, slide over the elongated actin filaments up to the blind ends of the processes and end at the inner plasmalemma. This part of the plasmalemma is condensed to half-desmosomes. Fibrocytes in the tendon tissue (= *tendon cells*) 2 send out numerous cytoplasmic processes. These attach to the ends of the muscle fibers, which stretch toward them like a *fingered glove* 1. The sarcolemma is the center of the liaison between muscle fibers and tendon tissue. The collagen fibrils 3 also pervade the spaces between the finger-like plasmalemma processes of the muscle fiber ends. They are anchored in the outer sarcolemma. A capillary in the immediate vicinity 4 is a regular part of the skeletal muscle-tendon linkage (myotendinal connection).

1 Muscle fiber end with myofibrils
2 Fibrocytes (tenocytes)
3 Collagen fibrils of the tendon
4 Capillary with erythrocytes
Electron microscopy; magnification: × 4250

237 Striated Muscle—Circumferential Myofibrils

Striated muscle fibers may in some places be encircled by thin *spiral muscle fibers*. These peculiar structures are called circumferential myofibrils (*Ringbinden*). They are thought to be signs of degradation. Note that the typical striation has become diffuse in these regions. The number of nuclei is often increased.

The figure shows several circumferential myofibrils in the human uvula. In the lower part of the picture is a regular muscle fiber with well-defined striation. The preparation has been treated with azocarmine as a secondary stain.

Stain: azan; magnification: × 500

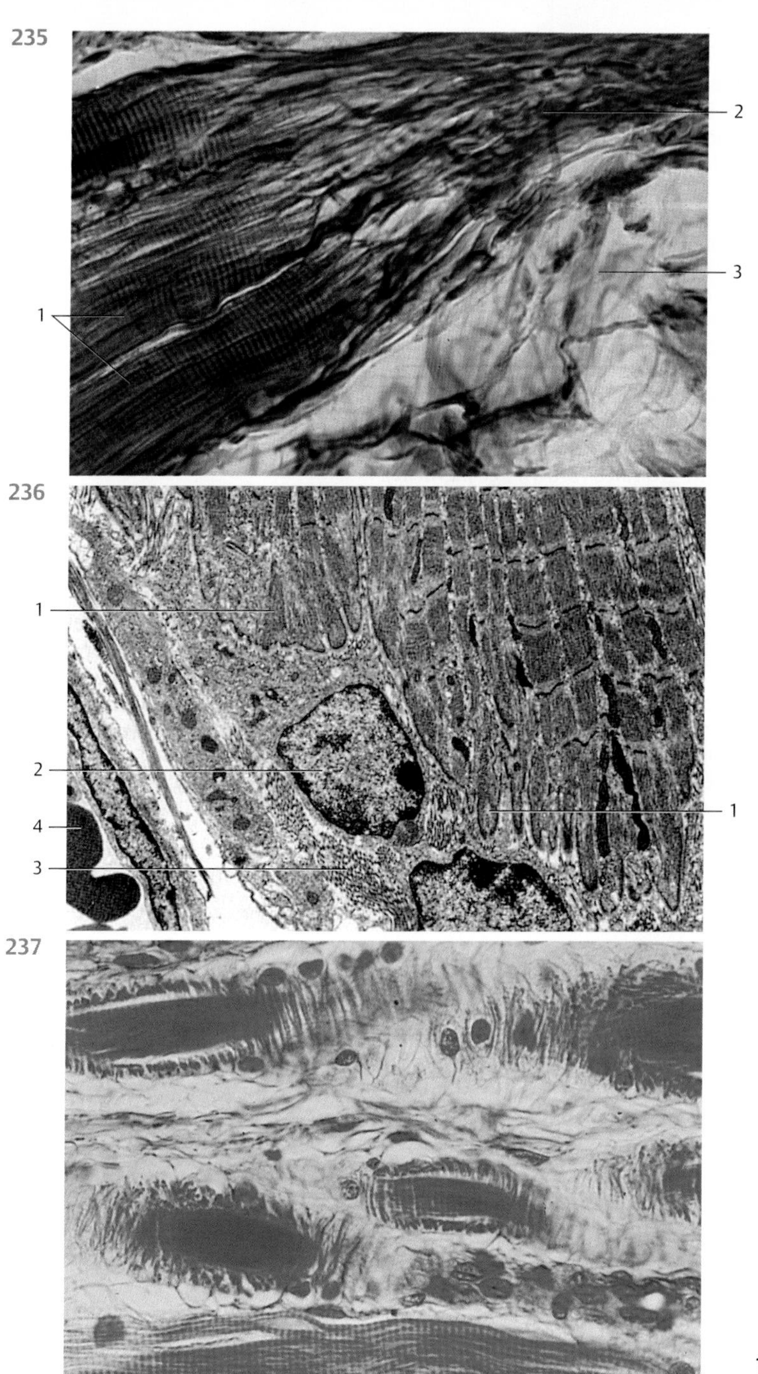
235
1
2
3
236
1
2
4
3
1
237

238 Cardiac Muscle—Myocardium—Left Ventricle

Like the skeletal musculature, the heart muscle tissue is striated. In contrast to skeletal muscles, *cardiac muscle fibers* are branched and anastomose with each other, thus creating a network. The slit-shaped spaces in this web are filled with richly vascularized connective tissue. Cardiac muscle fibers are thinner than skeletal muscle fibers but thicker than smooth muscle cells. This figure clearly shows the capillaries 3 in the web spacing. The heavily stained nuclei are part of fibrocytes 1. Heart muscle cells (*cardiomyocytes*) have only one nucleus. Characteristic of cardiomyocytes are struts (*disci intercalares*), which are dense, heavily stained bands across the muscle fibers. They are regularly spaced and cover the entire width of the fiber (see. Fig. 240). Electron microscopic investigations have shown that struts are co-localized with part of the cell borders (see Figs. 240, 244, 245). The faintly stained nuclei 2 occupy the center of the cardiac muscle cells. There are no fibrils in the perinuclear space. Instead, a rich layer of sarcoplasm surrounds the nuclei. In the sarcoplasmic cones are often fat droplets, glycogen and pigment granules (*brown age pigment*).

1 Fibrocyte
2 Nucleus of a heart muscle cell
3 Capillary
Semi-thin section; stain: methylene blue-azure II; magnification: × 200

239 Cardiac Muscle—Myocardium—Left Ventricle

Cross-sections through cardiac muscle cells show the faintly stained central nuclei 2 and the *Cohnheim fields or groups*. The latter are based on the formation of fibril bundles from myofibrils (*myofibril fields*). The spaces between them contain sarcoplasm. Numerous capillaries 1, which often still contain erythrocytes (cf. Fig. 241), are found in the loose connective tissue between muscle cells.

1 Capillaries
2 Nucleus of a cardiac muscle cell
Semi-thin section; stain: methylene blue-azure II; magnification: × 400

240 Cardiac Muscle—Myocardium—Left Ventricle

Longitudinal section through the myocardium of the left ventricle. Note the branching of the *cardiomyocytes*. The in part terrace-like arranged struts 4 (*disci intercalares*) are very noticeable because they stain heavily. Fibril-free sarcoplasm surrounds the nuclei like a cap 1.

1 Perinuclear space
2 Branching of the cardiomyocytes
3 Vein with erythrocytes
4 Intercalated discs (disci intercalares)
5 Network lamella of the cardiac muscle cell
6 Interstitial connective tissue
7 Cardiac muscle cell with nucleus
8 Capillary
9 Endothelial nucleus
10 Nucleus of a fibrocyte
Stain: brilliant black-toluidine blue-safranin; magnification: × 200

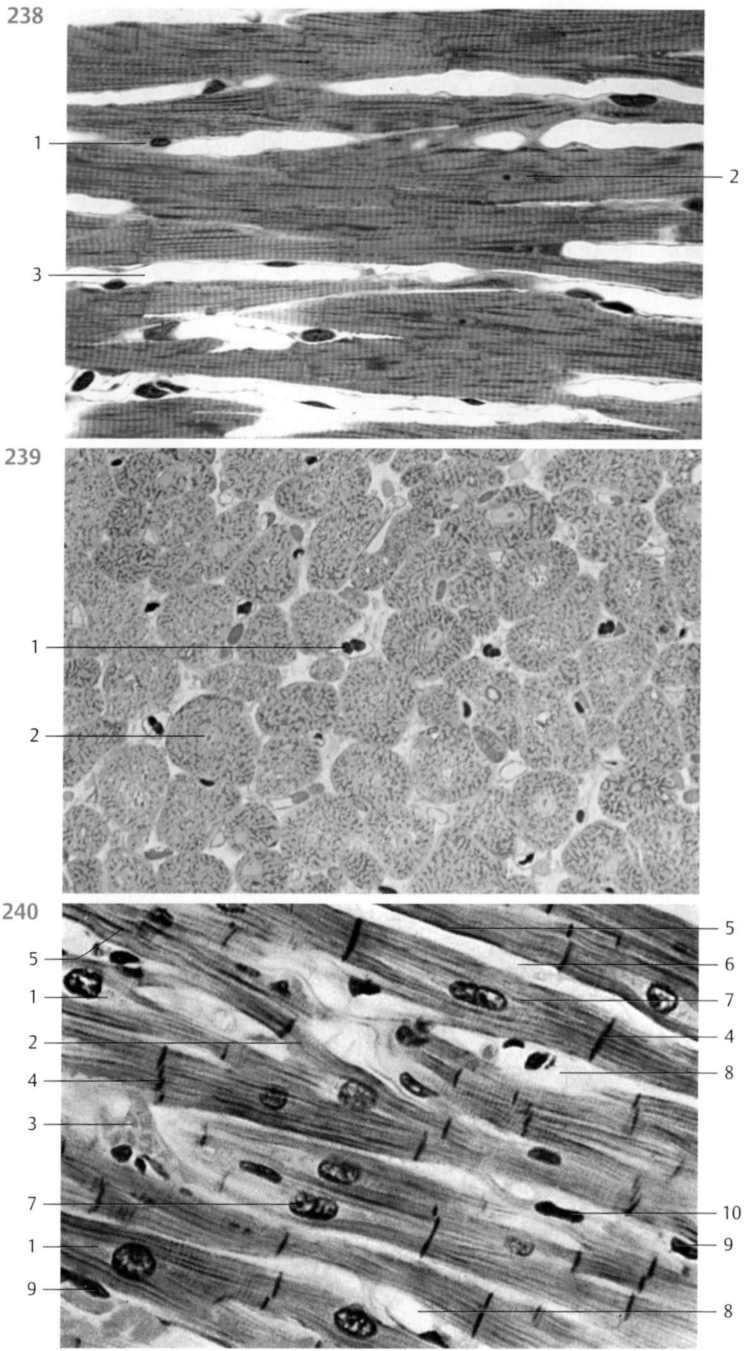
238
1
2
3
239
1
2
240
5
1
2
4
3
7
1
9
5
6
7
4
8
10
9
8

241 Cardiac Muscle—Myocardium—Left Ventricle

This is another cross-section through the cardiac muscle tissue, which gives a clear picture of the *Cohnheim grouping*. Here, myofibrils have aggregated to lamella in a radial formation. The sarcoplasm-rich spaces are free of fibrils and appear light. The size differences among nuclei should be noted [2]. In the sparse connective tissue between heart muscle cells are fibrocytes and capillaries. It should also be noted that the apparent variations in the diameters of the cardiac muscle fibers (*cardiomyocytes*) depend on the presence or absence of their cell nuclei in the section (cf. Fig. 239).

1 Nucleus of a connective tissue cell
2 Nucleus of a cardiac muscle cell
3 Capillary
Stain: alum hematoxylin; magnification: × 600

242 Cardiac Muscle—Myocardium—Left Ventricle

Section from a longitudinally cut cardiac muscle cell with central nucleus [1] (cf. Fig. 238, 240). The sarcomeres of the "*cardiac muscle fibers*" have in principle the same striation pattern as the striated skeletal muscle fibers (cf. Figs. 226, 227, 230, 231). However, in cardiac muscle sarcomeres are not arranged strictly parallel in separate columns, but form a branched three-dimensional web (cf. Figs. 238, 240). Note the mitochondria [2], which are arranged in columns between the microfilament bundles. In the nuclear cones are the sarcoplasm, mitochondria and, in numbers that increase with age, granules with the wear-and-tear pigment *lipofuscin*. In the lower right is a capillary [3].

1 Nucleus of cardiomyocyte
2 Mitochondria
3 Capillary
Electron microscopy; magnification: × 2500

243 Cardiac Muscle—Purkinje Fibers

Apart from the labor musculature, the myocardium also contains specific muscle fibers for the excitation and conduction of excitatory states; among these are the cells of the atrioventricular system, *the Purkinje fibers*. They stand out because they are usually much thicker than the fibers of the labor musculature. These specific myocytes have significantly more sarcoplasm and fewer fibrils. They are also rich in glycogen. The sparse myofibrils of Purkinje fibers are predominantly located close to the cell surface.
This figure (bovine heart) shows numerous subendocardial Purkinje fibers (cardiac conducting cells) with loose connective tissue (here stained green) between them.

Stain: Masson-Goldner trichrome staining; magnification: × 200

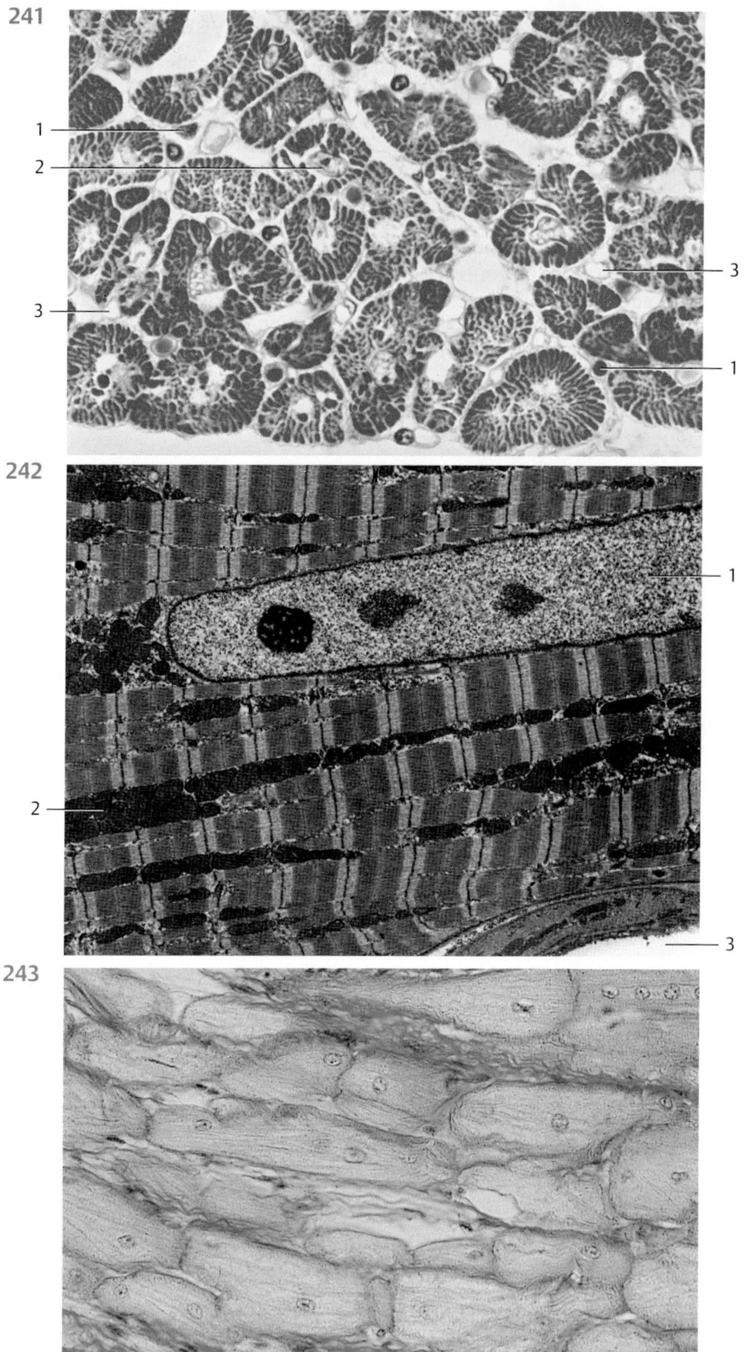
241
1
2
3
3
1
242
1
2
3
243

244 Cardiac Muscle—Myocardium—Left Ventricle

Section from several longitudinally cut cardiac muscle cells (*cardiomyocytes*) after *intravital staining* by injection of ruthenium red. This dye clearly stains the intercellular space, the intercalated discs 1, and the pinocytotic vesicles of the endothelium. The struts follow an irregular, often terrace-like arrangement (cf. Figs. 240, 245), which leads to a tight interlocking of the cells. Located at the inner surface of the cell membrane are electron-dense cadherins that allow actin filaments to attach and anchor themselves to this membrane. Therefore, the filaments do not bridge the intercellular space in the interlocking areas. On the contrary, there is a formation of desmosomes (*maculae adherentes*) as well as focal adhesion centers, which are similar to the *zonulae adherentes* and are named *fasciae adherentes*. The mechanical transfer of the contraction forces between heart muscle cells takes place in these locations.
Note the numerous crista-type mitochondria, which are lined up in rows 3 (cf. Fig. 242, 245).

1 Intercalated discs
2 Capillaris
3 Crista-type mitochondria
Electron microscopy; magnification: × 2800

245 Cardiac Muscle—Myocardium—Left Ventricle

Data about the ultrastructure of heart muscle cells (*cardiomyocytes*) indicate that the struts are arranged in a terrace-like manner. This makes it possible to distinguish between transverse and longitudinal sectors. Inside the struts occur three different types of cell contacts: *fascia adherentes* 1, *maculae adherentes* (desmosomes) 2 and *nexus* 3. The *fascia adherens* exists as contact plate in the transverse sectors. There can be single local desmosomes (maculae adherentes) as part of the fascia adherens or, as in this figure, in the longitudinal sectors of the struts. Gap junctions (*nexus*) occur usually in the longitudinal sectors. They serve for electrical coupling between cardiac muscle cells and consist of the heart-specific nexus protein *connexin 43*.
Note the row of mitochondria with a large number of cristae 4 (cf. Fig. 244).
Note: in contrast with skeletal musculature, the myocardium consists of separate single cells. The heart muscle tissue does not regenerate.

1 Fasciae adherentes
2 Macula adherens
3 Gap junction
4 Mitochondria
5 Plasmalemma with pinocytotic vesicles
6 Basal lamina
7 Axons without myelin sheath
Electron microscopy; magnification: × 30 000

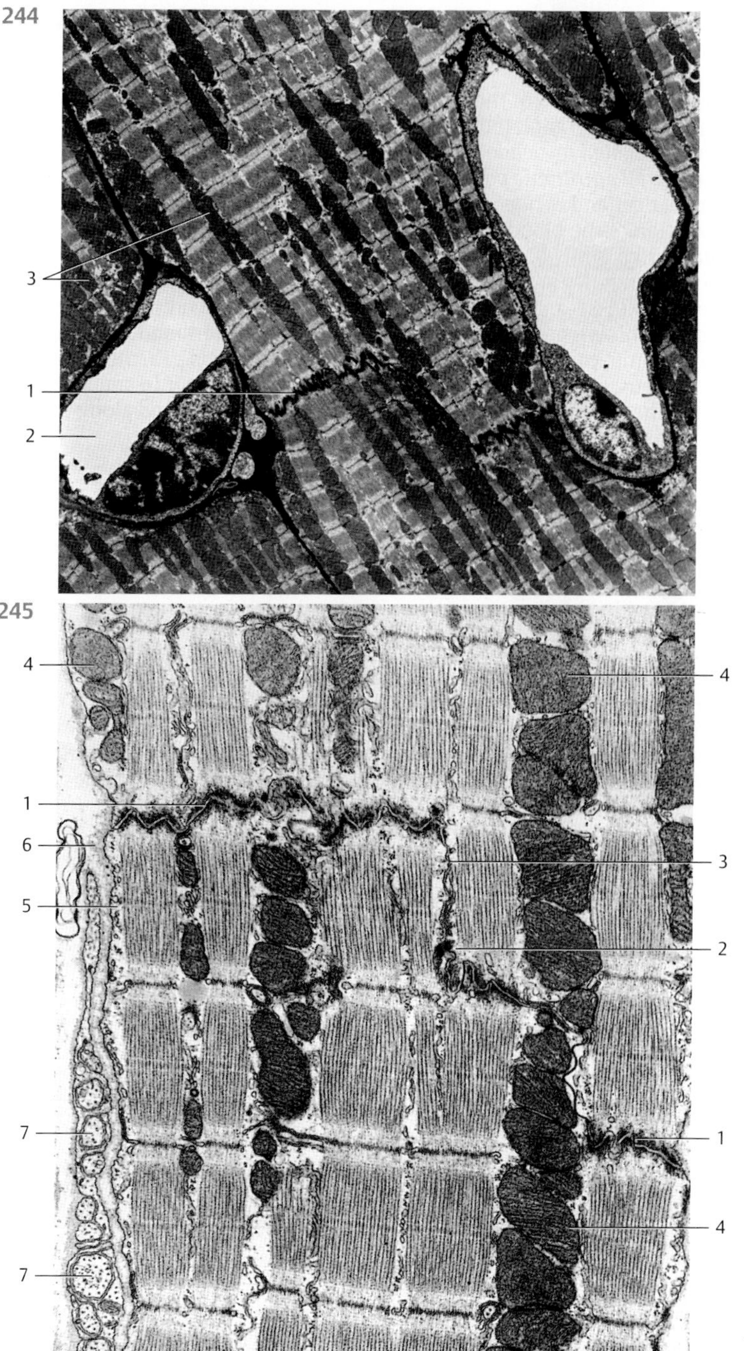
244
3
1
2
245
4
4
1
6
3
5
2
7
1
4
7

246 Cardiac Muscle—Myocardium—Myoendocrine Cells from the Right Atrium

The cardiomyocytes of the atrium contain *osmiophilic granules* (cf. Fig. 247). These specific granulated atrial cells execute endocrine functions and are therefore called *myoendocrine cells*. They secrete the heart polypeptide hormone *atrial natriuretic polypeptide (ANP)* (also known as *cardiodilatin (CDD), cardionatrin* and *atriopeptin*). The hormone plays an important role in the regulation of the blood pressure and the water-electrolyte balance (*diuresis natriuresis*).

This figure shows myoendocrine cells from the atrium dextrum of a pig heart after peroxidase-antiperoxidase staining using an antibody against cardiodilatin. The brown products of these reactions are predominantly found in the sarcoplasmic cones of the cells (*perinuclear localization*). Farther away from the nucleus, staining is weaker. Myoendocrine cells occur in small numbers also in the ventricular myocardium. There, they are detected along the excitatory tissue in the septum.

Preparation; magnification: × 380

247 Cardiac Muscle—Myocardium—Myoendocrine Cells from the Right Atrium

Myoendocrine cells have a typical morphology. The endocrine secretory apparatus, for example, exists only in the Golgi region in or close to the sarcoplasmic cones 1, which is rich in sarcoplasm and poor in myofibrils. Golgi complexes 2 can be located either close to or further away from the nucleus. Secretory granules 3 occur mainly in the Golgi regions, but sporadically there are also secretory granules in the rest of the cytoplasm. They often form lines of vesicles in the space between fibrils. The secretory granules contain antigens, which react with antibody to cardiodilatin.

Note the crista-type mitochondria 4. Left and right in the figure are typical striated myofibrils.

1 Nucleus of a myoendocrine cell
2 Golgi complex (Golgi apparatus)
3 Secretory granules
4 Mitochondria
Electron microscopy; magnification: × 11 000

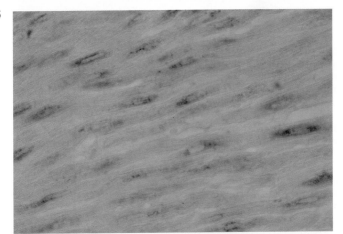

246

247

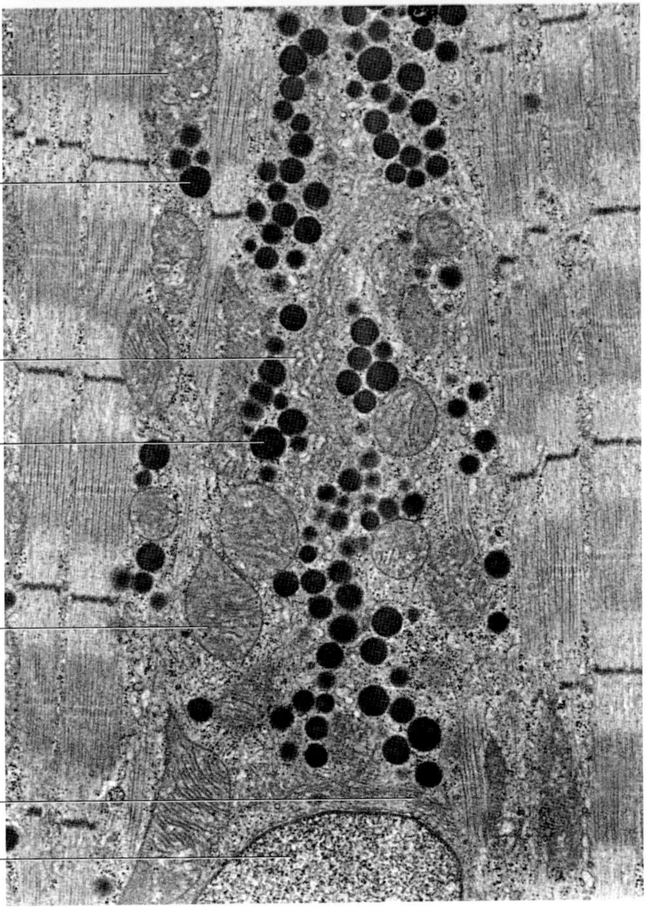

4
3
2
3
4
2
1

248 Multipolar Nerve Cells—Spinal Cord

Nerve cells are remarkably diverse by form and size. This applies to the cell body (*cell soma, perikaryon*) as well as the cell processes and here in particular the processes, which extend from the perikaryon, the dendrites and the axon (neurite). Therefore, it has become customary to classify nerve cells according to the number of processes and their mode of branching. A nerve cell with all its processes is called a *neuron*. By far the most common cell type in the human nervous system is the *multipolar nerve cell*. Its receptor zone is generally localized at the surface of the cell soma and the dendrites. The axons provide the transmission system (*neurite* or *axon cylinder*).
The adjacent figure is a cut through the columna anterior of the spinal cord. There are several deep-red stained cells with processes of different lengths. This staining procedure does not allow it to distinguish between dendrite and axon. The other structures in this figure are small nerve cells, glia cells and nerve cell processes (cf. Fig. 2).

Stain: Weigert carmine; magnification: × 80

249 Multipolar Nerve Cells—Spinal Cord

This figure also shows multipolar motor nerve cells from the *columna anterior* of the spinal cord (*anterior horn motor neurons*). They are considered the prototype of *multipolar cells*. Because of their shape, they are frequently called *pyramidal cells*. Different from Fig. 248, this image at higher magnification shows the large nuclei with clearly defined nucleoli. The dendrites have a wide base at their origin in the perikaryon. A short distance away from the cell body, they form a more or less dense, multibranched open network of processes, which looks like small trees. Axons cannot be identified using the applied staining method.

Stain: Weigert carmine; magnification: × 200

250 Multipolar Nerve Cells—Spinal Cord

In the cytoplasm (*perikaryon*) of nerve cells and in the dendrites, basic dyes bring out fine or coarse granules, which are called *Nissl bodies* (chromophilic or Nissl substance) after their discoverer (cf. Fig. 20). Nissl bodies are portions of the rough endoplasmic reticulum (rER) (cf. Fig. 24). The base of the axon, the *axon hillock*, is free of Nissl bodies and so is the axoplasm. The left process from this multipolar nerve cell from the columna anterior of the spinal cord is in all likelihood an axon (neurite). The other processes are dendrites. Note the large cell nucleus with its clearly outlined nucleolus. The nerve cell is surrounded by a *neuropil*. Neuropils are the structures that fill the spaces between perikarya. The neurophil elements consist of glial cells with their processes, the processes of nerve cells and capillaries.

1 Glial cells
Stain: Nissl cresyl violet; magnification: × 400

248

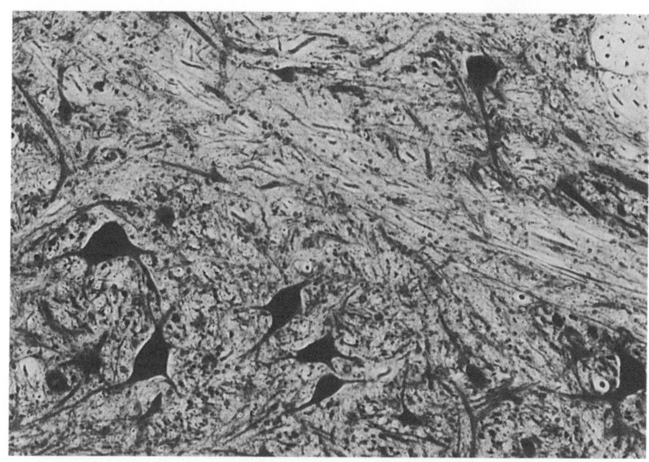

249

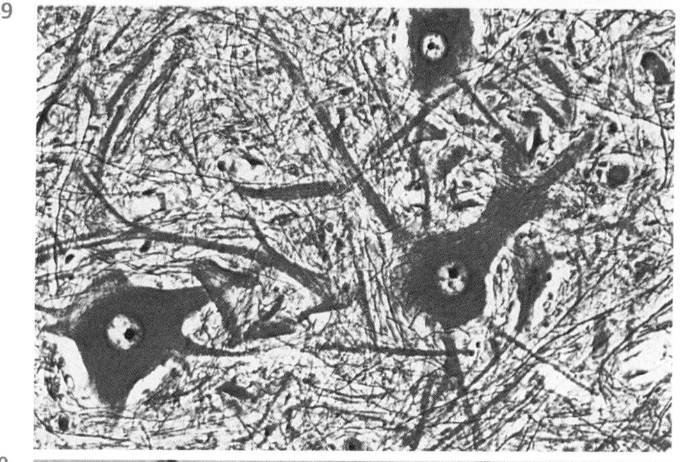

250

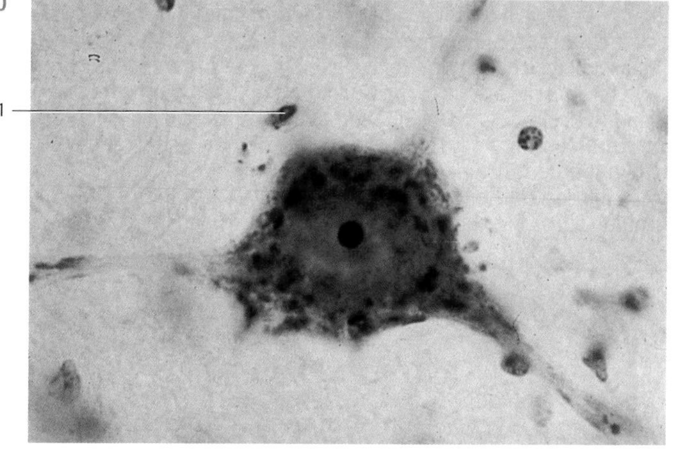

251 Multipolar Nerve Cells—Spinal Cord

The cytoplasm (*perikaryon*) of anterior horn motor cells contains numerous coarse, irregularly shaped particles, the *Nissl bodies*, which frequently impart a spotty, in some areas striped appearance to the cells (*tigroid, tiger skin*) (cf. Figs. 20, 250). Nissl bodies also occur in dendrite sections close to the soma, however, not in axons. The *axon hillock*, the initial section of the axon, is always free of Nissl bodies.

The images of the dendrites in this figure are only faintly visible. Areas free of Nissl bodies, such as the axon hillock, the origin of the axon near the perikaryon, is shown. Note the large, round and only lightly stained nuclei with their dot-like nucleoli in these nerve cells as well as the green-yellow *lipofuscin* inclusions (cf. Figs. 66, 67, 256). The blue stained nuclei 2 of different glial cells are visible in the neuropil between multipolar nerve cells.

1 Dendrite
2 Nuclei of glial cells
Stain: Nissl toluidine blue; magnification: × 300

252 Multipolar Nerve Cells—Spinal Cord

The use of silver impregnation methods makes fine stringy structures in the cell body and the cell processes of nerve cells visible. These are *neurofibrils*, which form a dense web through the perikaryon, some of them as bundles of parallel thin fibers. In nerve cell processes, they always run parallel to the long cell axis and can be traced over longer distances. The neurofibrils are the light microscopic equivalent of the neurofilaments and neurotubules seen in electron microscopy. They are found in large numbers in all parts of the neuron.

The components of the neuropil are not visible in this preparation.

Stain: Bielschowsky pyridine-silver-gold chloride impregnation; magnification: × 900

253 Multipolar Nerve Cells—Cerebral Cortex

Camillo Golgi (1883) developed the method of silver impregnation and with it, he provided the light for a view of a plethora of different structures in and around nerve cells. Silver impregnation shows the cell body and all its processes as a black cell silhouette against a yellow-brown or red-brown background. It is characteristic of the Golgi method to only capture one of several cells and their processes but, in a somewhat capricious way, capture it down to their most minute detail (cf. Figs. 676, 677). These detailed images make the Golgi method invaluable for research into the structure of neurons and the distribution of their synapses, even today. This picture shows two large pyramidal cells from the human cerebral cortex.

Stain: Golgi silver impregnation; x300

251

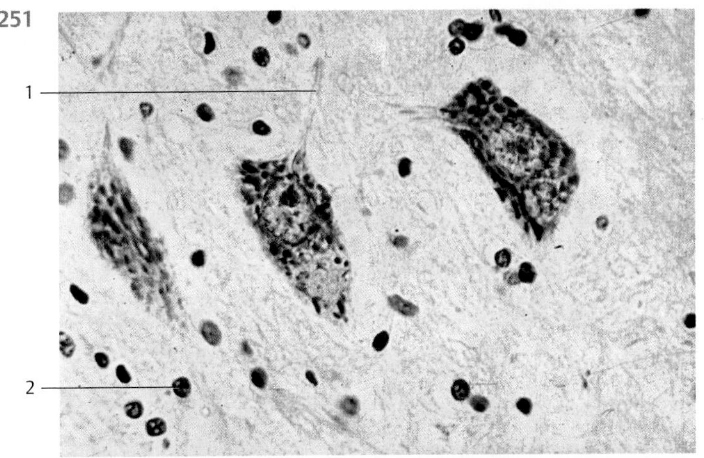

252

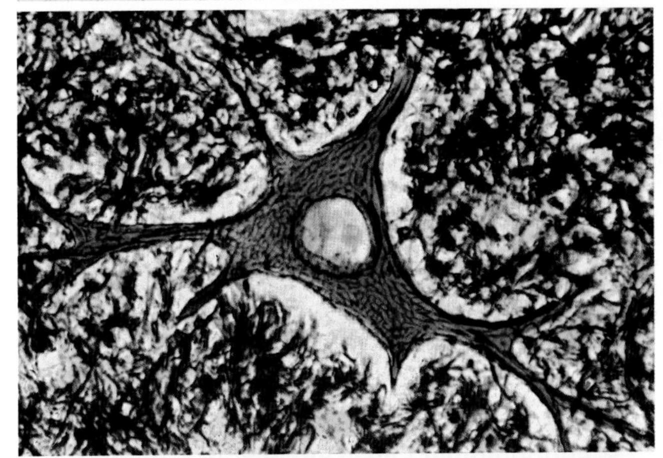

253

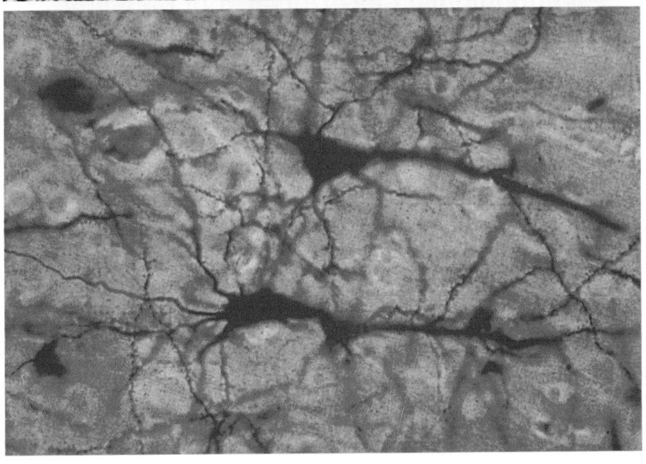

254 Purkinje Cells—Cerebellar Cortex

Purkinje cells (J.E. Purkinje, 1787–1869) are neurons with characteristic attributes They exclusively occur in the cerebellum (cf. Figs. 5, 681, 682). Arranged in rows, Purkinje cells are found in the *stratum neuronorum piriformium* 1 (*stratum gangliosum, Purkinje cell layer*) in the cerebellum (*cortex cerebelli*). The pear-shaped cell bodies are 50–70 µm high and mostly free of pigments. Each cell extends one axon toward the granular layer 2 and projects two, rarely three dendrites 4 toward the molecular layer 3. The dendrites are branched in the way of trellis trees (*trellis cells, espalier cells*). Their processes look like the branches of small trees (*dendrite trees*) and reach up all the way to the cerebellar surface. The branches grow in a plane that stands vertical to the long axis of the cerebellar gyrus.

1 Purkinje cells in the stratum neuronorum piriformium
2 Granular layer (stratum granulosum)
3 Molecular layer (stratum moleculare)
4 Branched dendrites
Stain: Bodian silver impregnation; magnification: × 250

255 Multipolar Autonomic Ganglion Cells

The ganglia of the *autonomous nervous system* contain multipolar cells. Their visceral motor neurons transmit excitations to the intestines, the glands and the vessels. These cells are multipolar ganglion cells of the *plexus myentericus* (*Auerbach*), which form an *intramural web* between the ring musculature and the longitudinal muscles of the intestinal wall (cf. Figs. 220, 432–434, 437). Note the ganglion cell processes, which build the intramural fiber network. The fibers do not have myelin sheaths. They reach to the smooth muscle cells and regulate the rhythmic contractions of the intestinal segments. The dimensions of their cell bodies are uniform. Their lightly stained, large, round nuclei are often in an eccentric position.

Stain: Bielschowsky-Gros silver impregnation; magnification: × 90

256 Pseudounipolar Cell—Dorsal Root Ganglion

The cytoplasm of this ganglion cell contains a large nucleus with a dark-blue stained nucleolus 1 and a yellowish pigment body, which consists of many *lipofuscin granules* of different sizes (cf. Figs. 66–68). The (basophilic) areas in the immediate vicinity of the nuclei (stained blue-violet) call for attention. These are Nissl bodies, which consist of ergastoplasm and free ribosomes (see Figs. 20, 24). A corona of glial cells (*satellite cells*) 2 closely covers the cell body. Their type is that of Schwann cells. They are also present alongside the cell processes. The differently sized crevices between ganglia and satellite cells are artifacts caused by shrinkage (see Fig. 1).
Cells in dorsal spinal nerve root ganglia are pseudounipolar nerve cells.

1 Nucleus with clearly visible nucleolus
2 Nucleus of a satellite cell
3 Nerve fibers
Stain: alum hematoxylin; magnification: × 600

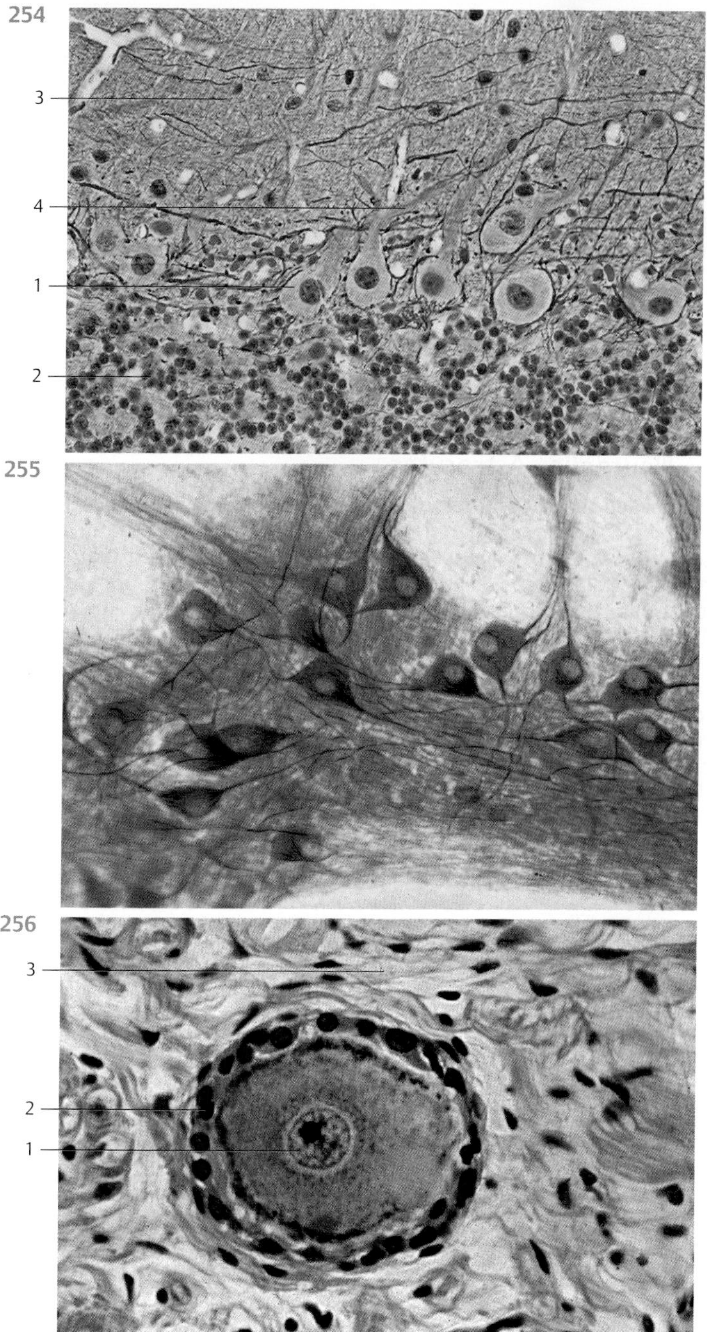
254
3
4
1
2
255
256
3
2
1

257 Neuroglia—Astrocytes

Glial cells (*gliocytes*) are the only cell types in the neuroglial tissue. They occupy the entire space between neurons and separate nerve cells from blood vessels. There are three main cell types: *astrocytes* (*macroglia*), oligodendrocytes and microgliocytes (*mesoglia, Hortega cells*). Astrogliocytes are star-shaped. Their cell bodies have diameters of 10–20 μm and contain large round nuclei with little chromatin. Cell processes of different lengths radiate into the extracellular space. Astrocytes with particularly long and rarely branched processes are called fibrous astrocytes (type I astrocytes). Such an astrocyte is shown in this figure.
An additional characteristic is the presence of cytoplasmic microfilaments. One of the microfilament constituents is the *glial fibrillary acidic protein* (GFAP), which lends itself to immunohistochemical identification.

Stain: Gomori silver impregnation; magnification: × 500

258 Neuroglia—Astrocytes

The branched astrocytes from the lower brain stem look like spiders 1. They are classified as *macroglia*. From the perikaryon radiate a large number of cell processes of different lengths (*protoplasmic astrocytes*). Figure b also shows nerve cells (stained red) 2 and longitudinal, occasionally also transverse cuts through capillaries. The Golgi staining method (a) depicts the structures of isolated astrocytes, while the Held method (b) emphasizes the connection between astrocytes and both the pyramidal cells and vessels.
Astrocytes contain glial fibrils, which are 6–9-nm thick bundles of intermediary filaments. The main building component of these filaments is the *glial fibrillary acidic protein (GFAP)*, which can be identified by immunohistochemistry. The ends of astrocyte processes are widened (astrocyte end-feet) and reach to the surface capillaries. This results in the formation of the *membrana limitans gliae perivascularis.*

1 Astrocytes
2 Pyramidal cells
Stain: a) Golgi silver impregnation; magnification: × 30; b) Held neuroglia method; magnification: × 160

259 Neuroglia—Oligodendrocytes

With a diameter of 6–8 μm, oligodendrocytes are smaller than astrocytes. They have round cell bodies and branched cell processes. The large, chromatin-rich nucleus fills the cell body almost completely. Electron microscopy reveals many ribosomes, microtubules and granular endoplasmic reticulum (rER) in the scarce cytoplasmic space. There are no filaments or glycogen. Among other structures, oligodendrocytes form the myelin sheaths of the central neurons.

Stain: Gomori silver impregnation; magnification: × 380

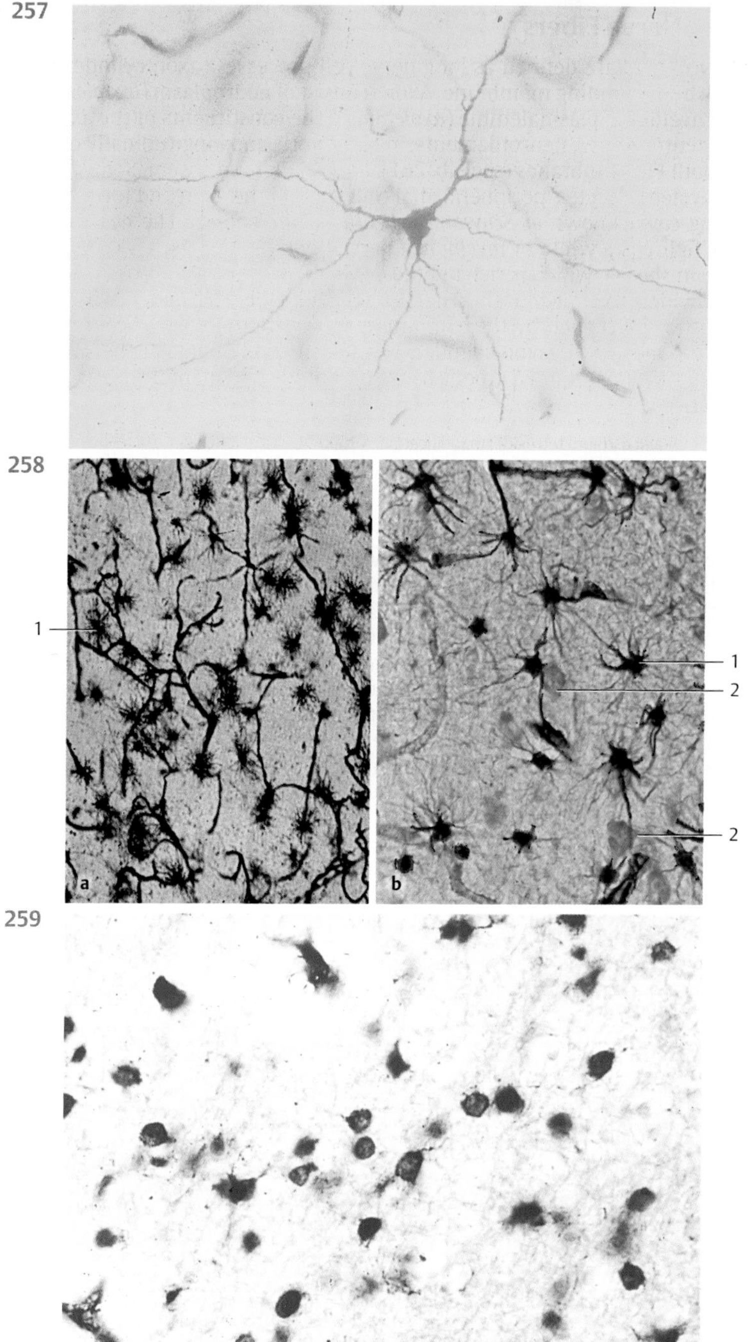
257
258
1
1
2
2
a
b
259

260 Nerve Fibers

Nerve fibers are defined as long nerve cell processes (axon cylinder, axon) with a surrounding membrane. Axons consist of neuroplasm (*axoplasm*) and an enveloping plasmalemma (*axolemma*). The constituents of the axoplasm are neurotubules, neurofilaments, mitochondria and longitudinally oriented smooth ER membranes (see Fib. 261). Nissl bodies are absent. Schwann cells (neurolemmocytes, peripheral glial cells) enfold the axon and form an insulating cover known as *Schwann's sheath* (*neurolemma*). The nerve fiber in this figure is a white or *myelinated* nerve fiber, i.e., the axon is covered by a myelin sheath, which is rich in lipids. Every 0.8 to 1.0 mm, a node of Ranvier subdivides the myelin sheath into segments or internodes. The myelin sheath is blackened by the osmium tetroxide stain. The light central space corresponds to the axon cylinder. The structural elements at the surface of the nerve fiber (stained greenish) are part of the endoneural sheath (Henle's sheath).

Stain: osmium tetroxide; magnification: × 1000

261 Nerve Fibers

The myelin sheath is formed by Schwann cells (*peripheral glial cells*). It consists of several stacked layers of plasma membrane processes that originate with Schwann cells (cf. Figs. 269, 271, 272). The processes end at either side of a Ranvier node. Close to the nodes of Ranvier, the membrane stacks widen and spread out. The ends of the Schwann cell plasmalemma processes 4 attach to the axolemma. The whole area around the Ranvier node is called *paranodium* or *paranodal zone*. The axon only appears to be exposed but is in fact covered by interlocking processes from neighboring Schwann cells and by the basal membrane. Myelinated nerve fiber.

1 Axon or axoplasm
2 Neurofilaments
3 Myelin sheath
4 Plasmalemma stacks of Schwann cells
5 Collagen fibrils
6 Axolemma
Electron microscopy; magnification: × 23 000

262 Sciatic Nerve

Peripheral nerves consist of bundles of either myelinated or unmyelinated nerve fibers 1 that are held together by connective tissue. This cross-section shows numerous fibers of a sciatic nerve 1 enclosed by the perineurium 2 (see Fig. 263). The perineurium is composed of very flat fibrocytes and collagen fibrils. Dense regular connective tissue covers the entire nerve.

1 Fascicle (nerve fiber bundle)
2 Perineurium
3 Epineurium
4 Artery
5 Vein
6 Adipose tissue
Stain: alum hematoxylin; magnification: × 10

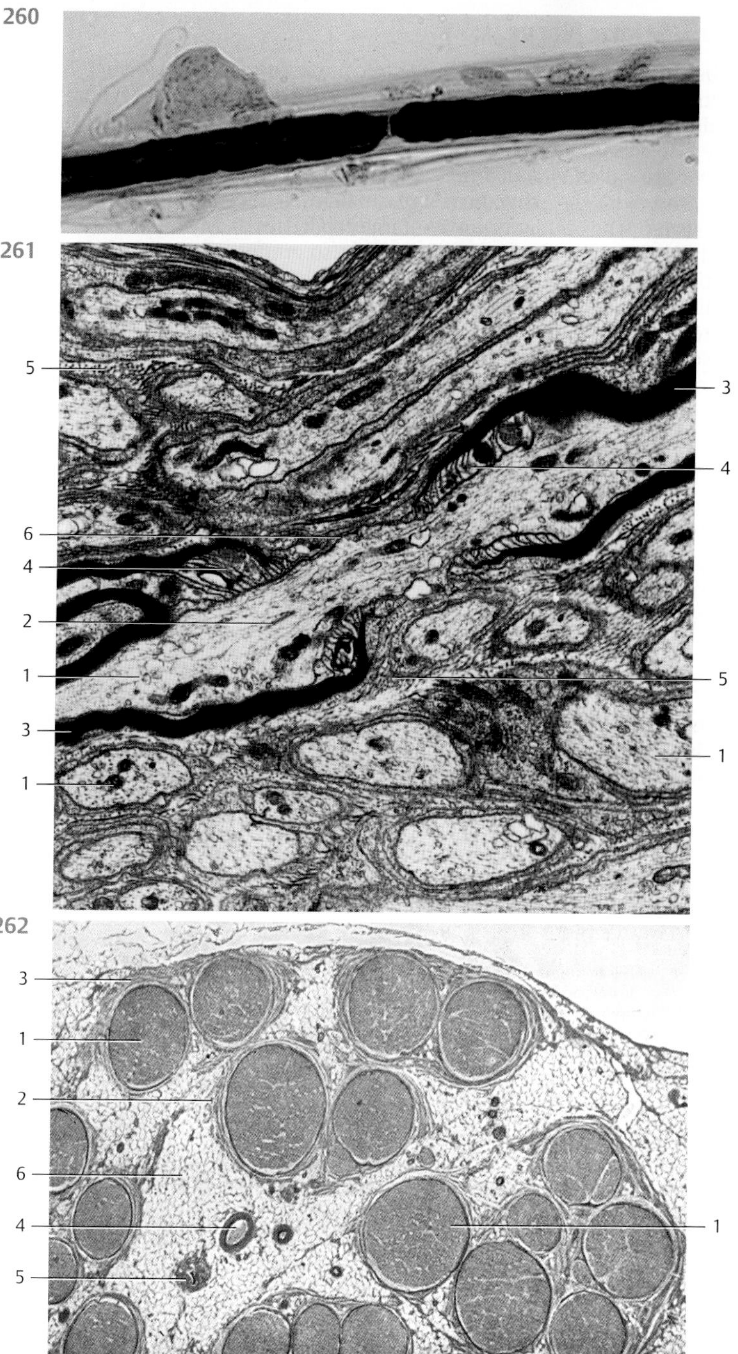
260
261
5
6
4
2
1
3
1
3
4
5
1
262
3
1
2
6
4
5
1

263 Sciatic Nerve

Fiber bundle (*fascicle*) from the sciatic nerve (nervus ischiadicus). The perineurium 1 is a cover of connective tissue around the fascicles (here stained reddish brown). Connective tissue fibers extend from the perineurium into the fascicles where they form septa. The very delicate reticular fibers in the septa are called *endoneurium*. They weave around individual nerve fibers. Together with the Schwann cell plasmalemma, they constitute the *endoneural sheath*. The endoneurium contains capillaries 3. Myelinated nerve fibers 4 have different diameters. There are also groups of thin nerve fibers with little myelin sheathing 5. The myelin sheath is rich in lipids and only slightly stained. The axons appear only as blue-violet dots. Schwann cells and fibrocytes are not visible. Staining of nuclei was not done (cf. Figs. 262, 266–268). Fascicles (nerve fiber bundles) and the perineurium form the peripheral nerve. At its surface is a layer of dense regular connective tissue (*epineurium*) 6. The epineurium seamlessly merges with the surrounding connective tissue (cf. Fig. 262).

1 Perineurium
2 Endoneurium
3 Blood vessel
4 Myelinated nerve fiber
5 Thin nerve fiber with little myelin sheathing
6 Epineurium
Stain: picro-blue black; magnification: × 200

264 Sciatic Nerve

Longitudinal section of fascicles (nerve fiber bundles). The myelinated individual fibers undulate slightly. The spindle-shaped nuclei (stained blue-violet) 1 are part of Schwann cells or fibrocytes in the perineurium. The connective tissue in the perineurium is stained red. The myelinated axons appear light. At the upper edge of the image, the perineurium 2 is cut (cf. Figs. 263, 265–268). This layer mediates an insertion of nerve fibers into the connective tissue that allows for lateral movement. In some places, the epineurium forms thicker layers of connective tissue fibers in a predominantly circular arrangement.

1 Endoneurium
2 Perineurium
Stain: AH = alum hematoxylin; magnification: × 150

265 Sciatic Nerve

Longitudinal section of fiber bundles from the sciatic nerve after staining the myelin sheaths black using osmium tetroxide. Periodically, the myelin sheath shows ring-shaped constrictions called Ranvier nodes (cf. Figs. 260, 261). The axon cylinder is only seemingly exposed at the nodes. Electron microscopy shows that, on the contrary, cytolemma processes from neighboring Schwann cells and a basal membrane (see Fig. 261) cover it. The lightly stained band at the lower edge of the figure is the *perineurium* (cf. Figs. 263, 264).

Stain: 1% osmium tetroxide solution; magnification: × 40

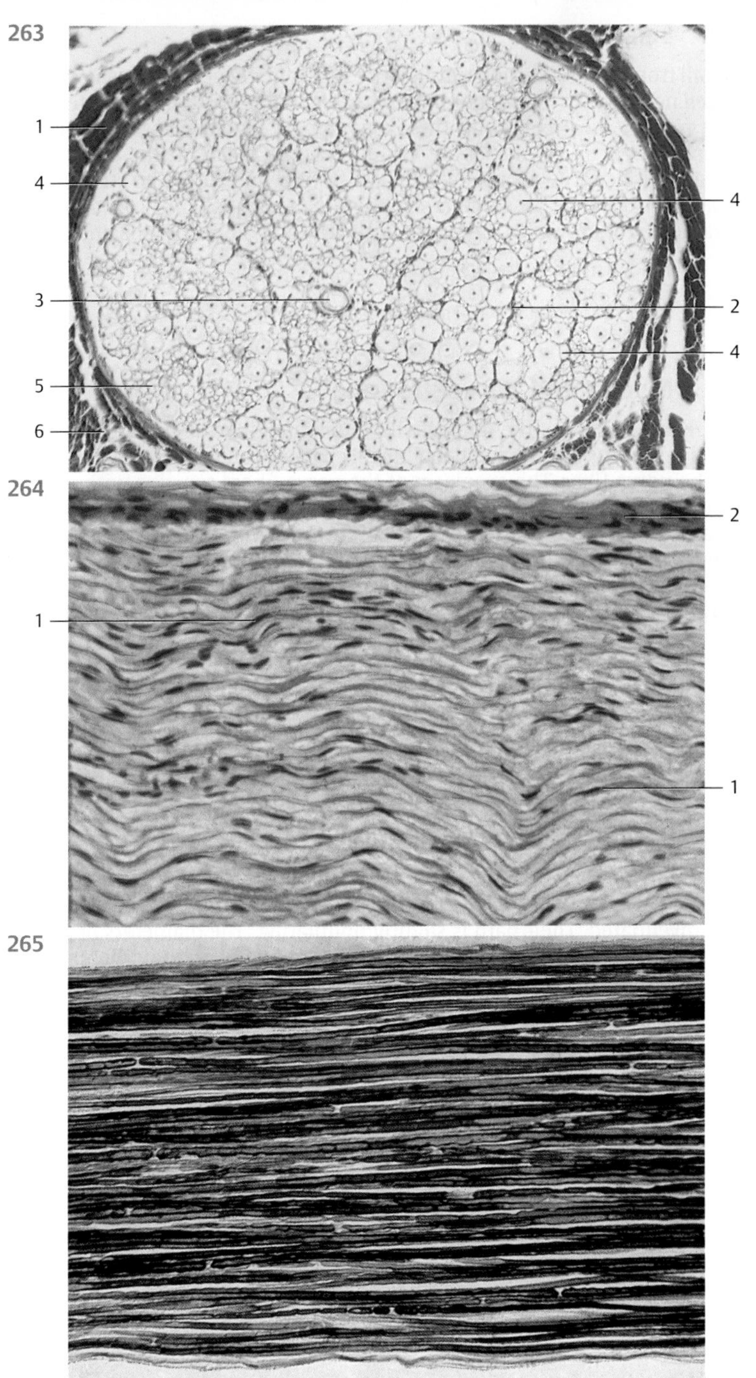
263
1
4
4
3
2
4
5
6
264
2
1
1
265

266 Sciatic Nerve

Detail from a cross-section through the sciatic nerve of a frog. It shows *myelinated* nerve fibers [1] of different sizes after staining with osmium tetroxide. The myelin sheaths around the axons appear as dark rings (rust-colored stain). Schwann cell nuclei are visible in some places at the outer myelin sheath surface. The axoplasm is lightly stained and shows no structural details in this image. In some areas, there is a glimpse of the endoneurium (stained light brown) [2]. Compare with Figs. 263, 265, 267, 269 and 271.

1 Myelinated nerve fibers, cross-section
2 Endoneurium
Stain: 1% osmium tetroxide-lithium carmine; magnification: × 500

267 Myelinated Nerve—Tongue

Myelinated nerve of the tongue with individual fibers of different sizes. The myelin sheaths are stained deep blue. Schwann cell nuclei are located close to the nerve fiber. The axoplasm of the nerve fibers remains without stain. The *endoneurium* between individual fibers contains loose connective tissue (stained light blue). The membranes of the *perineurium* [2] (*perineural epithelium*) envelop the entire fascicle (nerve fiber bundle).
At the top and bottom of the figure are cross-sections through skeletal muscle fibers [3] with nuclei close to the plasmalemma. Several capillaries [4] are cut (cf. Figs. 268).

1 Myelinated nerve fibers, cross-section
2 Perineural membranes
3 Striated muscle fibers
4 Capillaries
Semi-thin section; stain: methylene blue-azure II; magnification: × 300

268 Myelinated Nerve—Tongue

Myelinated nerves [1] in the tongue musculature (cf. Fig. 267). The two larger nerves have been mostly cut longitudinally or tangentially. The nerve fibers are myelinated. Their path is slightly undulating. The diameters of the connective tissue fibers of the endoneurium (stained blue) are different. Every nerve is covered by connective tissue, the perineurium [2]. In the vicinity of the nerves is more or less loosely organized connective tissue [3], which also contains fat cells [4] and vessels.
In the figure in the upper left corner and at the lower edge are striated muscle fibers [5].

1 Myelinated nerves
2 Perineurium
3 Connective tissue
4 Fat cells
5 Striated muscle fibers
Stain: azan; magnification: × 200

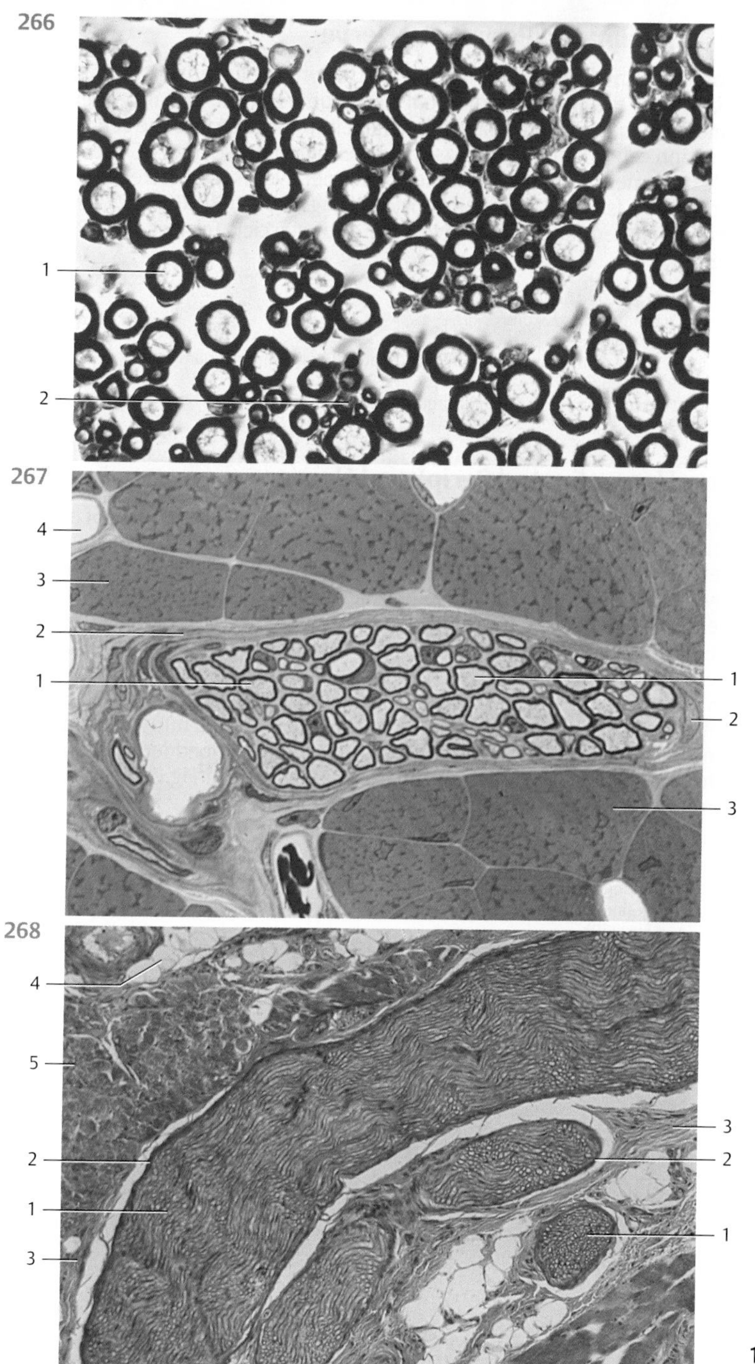
266
1
2
267
4
3
2
1
1
2
3
268
4
5
2
1
3
3
2
1

269 Myelinated Peripheral Nerve

Cross-section of a small peripheral nerve from the adventitia of the trachea. Apart from myelinated individual nerve fibers, there are also a few small bundles of *unmyelinated axons* 2, which have nestled into the cell bodies of Schwann cells 3. In the axoplasm of myelinated nerve fibers 1 are neurotubules and neurofilaments. The loose connective tissue between individual nerve fibers is called endoneurium 4 (cf. Figs. 261, 263, 266, 267). *Perineural epithelium* (perineurium) 5 covers the entire fascicle (cf. Figs. 262–264, 266, 268).

1 Myelinated nerve fibers
2 Unmyelinated axons
3 Schwann cells
4 Loose connective tissue with fine collagen fibrils—endoneurium
5 Perineurium
Electron microscopy; magnification × 4200

270 Unmyelinated Peripheral Nerve

Cross-section of an unmyelinated vegetative nerve from the wall of a human renal pelvis. The axons 1 have different diameters and are not quite completely covered by the *tongue-like processes* of Schwann cells 2. Many axons have sections where their axolemma borders immediately on the basal membrane, which separates the axon from the interstitial connective tissue, the endoneurium 3. The axoplasm contains filaments and microtubules (here cut across their axis) as well as small mitochondria. The image of the nerve in the center of the figure includes the nucleus of a Schwann cell 2. Note: the axons of unmyelinated fibers are not wrapped into the cytoplasmic processes of Schwann cells. Instead, they are embedded (enfolded) in Schwann cell invaginations. Compare this figure with Fig. 273 and with images of myelinated fibers in Figs. 269 and 271.

1 Axons
2 Schwann cell nucleus
3 Endoneural connective tissue fibers, endoneurium
4 Perineural collagen fibrils (perineurium), perineural epithelial cell are not present (cf. Fig. 269)
Electron microscopy; magnification: × 9500

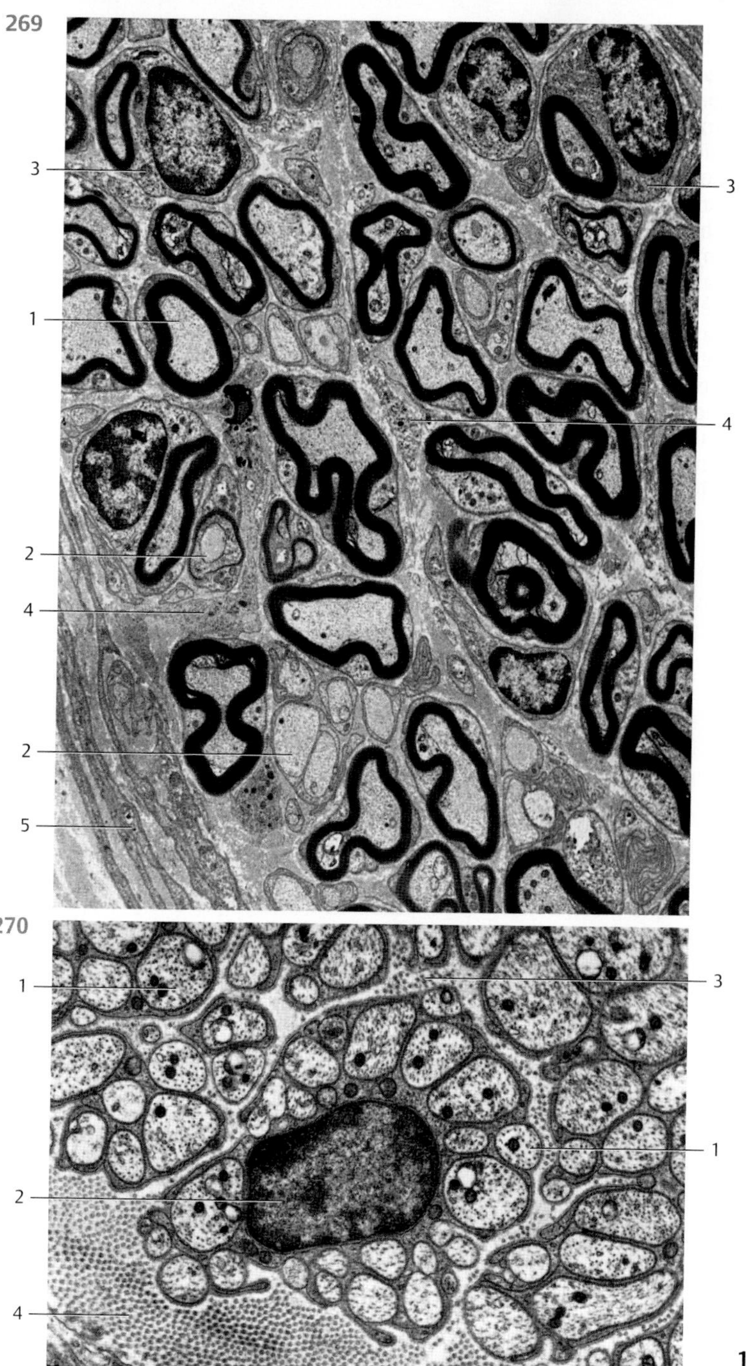
269
3
3
1
4
2
4
2
5
270
1
3
1
2
4

271 Peripheral Nerve

Several myelinated and unmyelinated nerve fibers of the peripheral nerve from the *vomeronasal organ* (*VNO*). Every one of the individual unmyelinated axons is nestled in Schwann cells (*peripheral glial cells*). Schwann cells provide bay-like infolds or grooves at their surfaces as open containments for axons. At their surface, the axons are covered only by the basal membrane [6]. Axons may also be completely covered by plasmalemma folds of the Schwann cells [4]. In this case, the folded part of the Schwann cell plasmalemma is connected to other parts of the plasmalemma via mesaxons [7]. The plasmalemma of an axon is called *axolemma*. In contrast to the cytoplasm of the perikaryon and larger dendrites, there are no Golgi complexes or ergastoplasm in an axon. However, axons do contain smooth endoplasmic reticulum membranes, mitochondria, neurotubules and neurofilaments. The myelin sheath of nerve fibers [1] is covered by the outer Schwann cell cytoplasm [2]. The myelin sheath consists of layers of stacked membranes. Neurofilaments, neurotubules and small round crista-type mitochondria are also found in the axoplasm of the two myelinated nerve fibers. Between nerve fibers, there are collagen fibrils of the endoneurium [8].

1 Myelinated nerve fibers (axoplasm)
2 Outer Schwann cell cytoplasm
3 Schwann cell nucleus
4 Unmyelinated nerve fibers with neurotubules, neurofilaments and mitochondria
5 Basal lamina (basal membrane)
6 Incompletely invaginated axon; here, the axon is covered by the basal membrane
7 Mesaxon
8 Collagen fibrils, endoneurium
9 Cytoplasmic process of an endoneural cell
10 Schwann cell plasmalemma
Electron microscopy; magnification: × 19 000

272 Peripheral Nerve—Myelin Sheath

The *myelin sheath* is formed from Schwann cell processes. The plasmalemma processes encircle the myelinated nerve fibers. The myelin structure is based on a *lipid-protein system (membranes)*, in which lipid and protein lamellae are stacked in concentric layers. The myelin sheath can be stained using osmium tetroxide (cf. Figs. 260, 261, 265, 266, 269). It can also be stained blue-violet with Luxol fast blue. Electron microscopy shows that the myelin sheath is made up of stacked membranes.

The figure shows part of a myelin sheath of a peripheral nerve fiber. The osmiophilic (dark) lines are called *major dense lines*. The intercalated lightly stained lines contain *intermediate lines*. However, these are only visible at higher magnification.

1 Schwann cell
2 Outer mesaxon
3 Inner mesaxon
4 Axoplasm
Electron microscopy; magnification: × 51 000

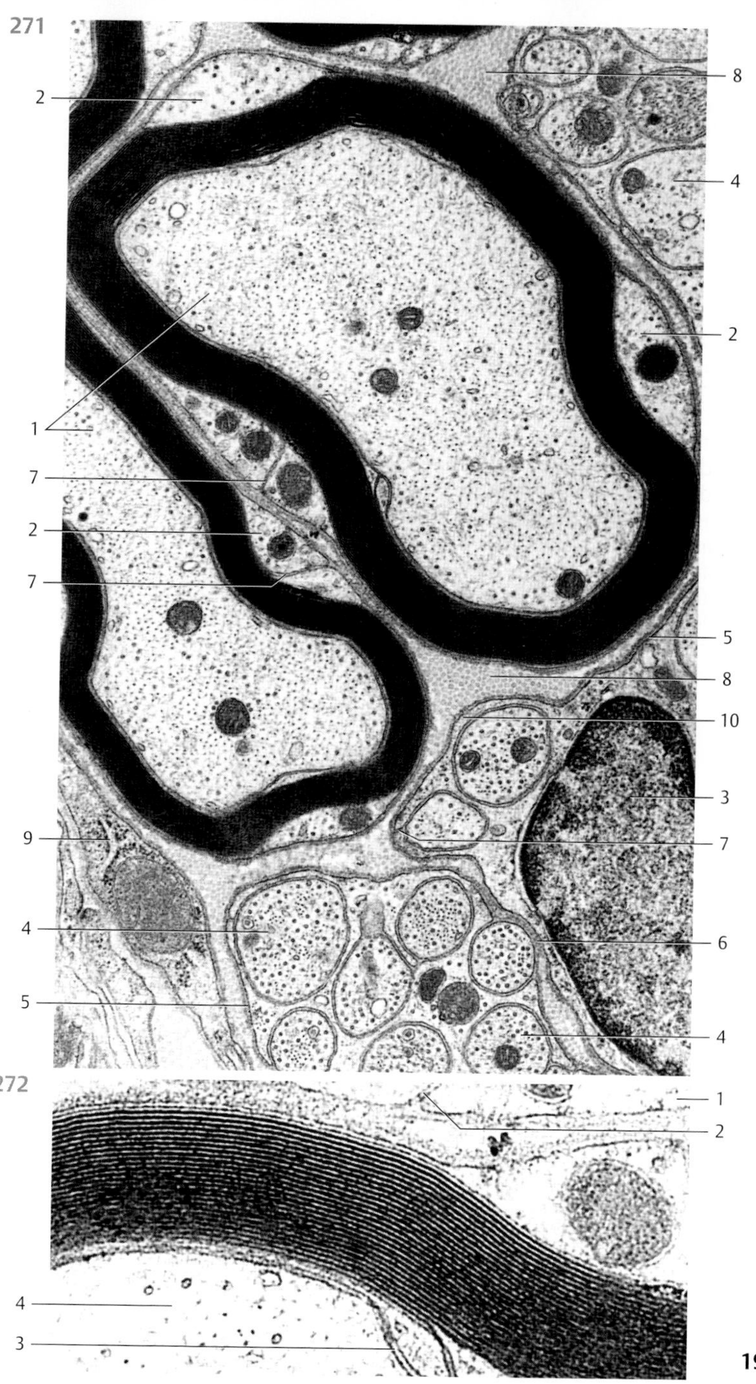
271
2
8
4
2
1
7
2
7
5
8
10
3
9
7
4
6
5
4
272
1
2
4
3

273 Unmyelinated Peripheral Nerve

Small unmyelinated nerve from the uterine myometrium of a sexually mature woman. Among other structures, the neuropil contains only unmyelinated axons of the central nervous system. In the peripheral nervous system, each individual unmyelinated axon is cradled in *Schwann cells* (*peripheral glial cells*) (cf. Figs. 270, 271). The axons of peripheral unmyelinated nerve fibers have diameters between 0.2 and 2.5 µm. They are bedded in Schwann cell invaginations, which look like trenches, grooves or channels. These are open grooves, at the open side only the basal membrane covers the axon. The axons are embedded in invaginations, which are completely lined by the Schwann cell plasmalemma. Mesaxons form connections between the plasmalemma of the large bay-like invaginations and the plasmalemma of the Schwann cell body. Between the outer Schwann cell membrane and the axolemma is a circa 10–20-nm wide intracellular cleft. One Schwann cell is recruited for a maximum of 1.5 µm of axon, then follows the next Schwann cell. In this figure, about 20 unmyelinated axons 2 of different sizes are embedded in a Schwann cell. They are all located in groove-like invaginations, and at their surfaces they are only covered by the *basal membrane* 3. This arrangement precludes mesaxons. At the surface, the tongue-like processes of Schwann cells also border on the basal membrane as well. The basal membrane envelops the entire nerve and separates it from the connective tissue. Axoplasm 2 contains neurofilaments, neurotubules and small, round osmiophilic mitochondria. Schwann cells also contain mitochondria. The nucleus of the Schwann cell is not cut. In the vicinity of the nerve are collagen fibrils 4, which have been mostly cut across their long axis.

1 Cytoplasmic membranes of Schwann cells
2 Axons with axoplasm
3 Basal membrane
4 Collagen fibrils
Electron microscopy; magnification: × 32 000

273

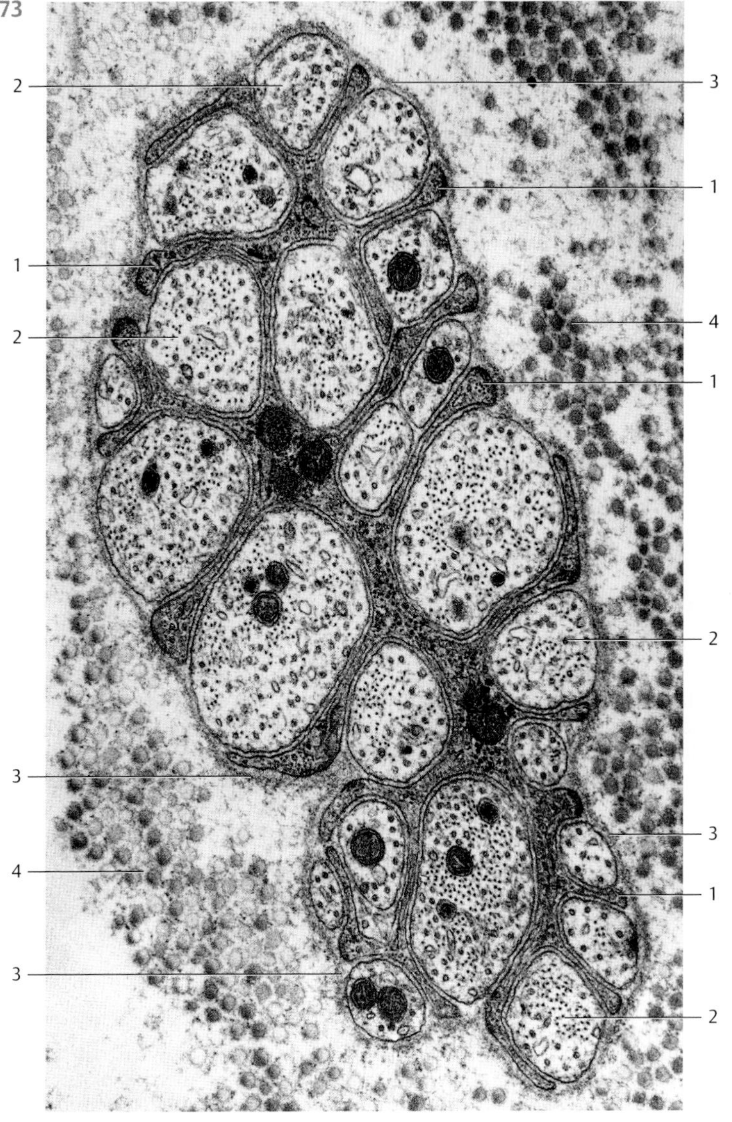

274 Radial Artery

The walls of arteries and veins consist of three layers: the tunica interna (*intima*) [1], the tunica media [2] and the tunica externa (*adventitia*) [4]. There are two types of arteries: conducting and peripheral arteries. Conducting arterial walls contain many elastic fibers and membranes: *elastic arteries*. Peripheral arteries show a special abundance of smooth muscle cells: *muscular or distributing arteries* (see Figs. 275–279). Muscular arteries show the layered character of the walls most impressively. The figure shows a cross-section of the peripheral *radial artery*. Figure 274b shows the tunica intima (top). It is separated from the tunica media [2] by the *tunica elastica interna* [3], a membrane with the appearance of a corrugated sheet. The wide tunica media [2] (stained red in this figure) consists of a densely packed layer of spindle-shaped myocytes in a circular or helical arrangement. The dashed lines in the figure represent the nuclei of the muscle cells. The bottom layers in both figures show the *tunica externa* [4].

1 Tunica intima
2 Tunica media
3 Internal elastic membrane
4 Tunica adventitia
Stain: a) alum hematoxylin-eosin; b) hemalum-orcein; magnification (both): × 120

275 Descending Thoracic Aorta

This cross-section of a thoracic aortic wall exemplifies a typical *elastic artery*. The *tunica intima* [1], followed by the *membrana elastica interna* [2] adjoin the *tunica media*. The tunica media [3] consists of concentric layers of *fenestrated* elastic membranes, which are interspersed with myocytes, fibrocytes, thin collagen fibrils and amorphous substances with a high chondroitin sulfate content (cf. Figs. 276–279). The undulating elastic fibers stand out in vertical sections (cf. Fig. 279). Apart from collagen fibers, the *tunica adventitia* [4] also contains elastic fibers, fibrocytes, adipocytes and *vasa vasorum*.

1 Tunica intima
2 Internal elastic membrane, membrana elastica interna
3 Tunica media
4 Tunica adventitia
Stain: hematoxylin-eosin-resorcin-fuchsin; magnification: × 80

276 Descending Thoracic Aorta

This section across the aortic wall gives a general impression of the number of components and their distribution: elastic membranes (*fenestrated membranes*) are stained white. *Collagen fibers* appear blue and myocytes are stained red. The small, only lightly colored strip on the left represents the tunica intima [2]. The heavily stained band on the outer right is the tunica externa [1]. The tunica media makes up most of the wall. Note: the tunica media is not as clearly distinguished from the neighboring layers, as is the case for a typical muscular artery. The three-layer arrangement is blurred.
Elastic artery (cf. Figs. 275, 277–279).

1 Tunica interna (intima) 2 Tunica externa (adventitia)
Stain: azan; magnification: × 50

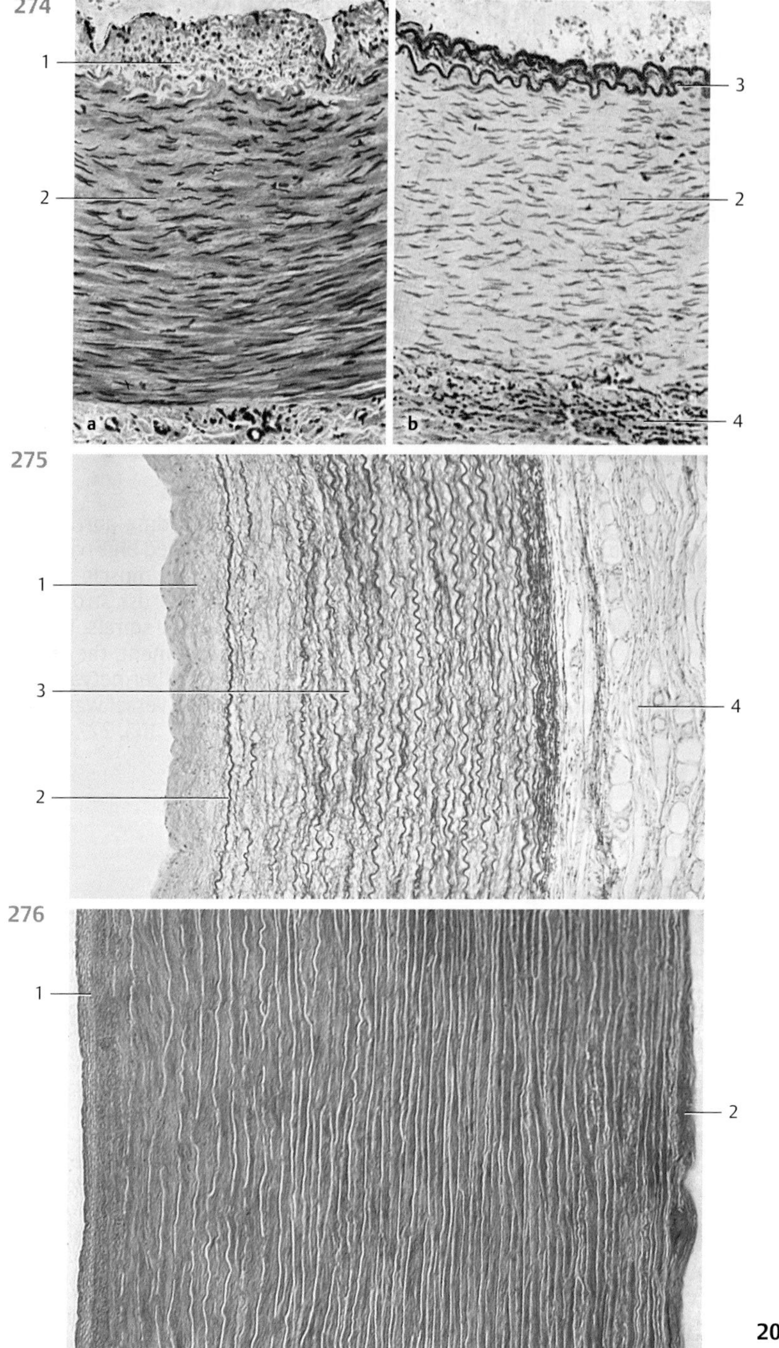
274
1
2
a
b
3
2
4
275
1
3
2
4
276
1
2

277 Descending Thoracic Aorta

The descending aorta, being located close to the heart, is an elastic artery. Due to an abundance of elastic fibers, the aorta and other coronary arteries of elastic type show a yellowish tint, even on the macroscopic level. The elastic components pervade the entire wall. This obscures the borders between layers, which are unlike the distinct borders in muscular arteries (see Figs. 164, 165, 275). The elastic elements take the form of 30–70 concentric layers of *fenestrated elastic membranes* . Their structural details are accessible only in parallel cuts through the aortic wall (cf. Fig. 279).
In this cross-section through the *tunica media* of the aortic wall, the elastic membranes appear as separate, sometimes undulating fibers (cf. Figs. 164–166, 278, 279). The elastic membranes alternate with thin layers of smooth muscle cells (yellow). The latter are *tensor muscles* and originate with the elastic matrix (*elastic muscular systems*). The nuclei have not been stained.

Stain: Weigert's resorcin-fuchsin-picric acid; magnification: × 200

278 Descending Thoracic Aorta

This cross-section of the tunica media from the descending aorta shows strong, in some places undulating *elastic membranes* (stained blue-violet). In a vertical section, they appear as fibers with intertwined muscle cells. At their insertion sites, the muscle fibers create the image of brush strokes. The myocytes encircle the aorta, forming right- and left-handed spirals. This creates a *fishbone pattern* in a cross-section. In this arrangement, the smooth muscle cells can regulate the tensile force of the elastic fiber network. The collagen connective tissue is stained green. A vessel of the vessel wall 1 (*vas vasis*) is visible in the left corner of the image (cf. Figs 164, 165, 277, 279).

1 Vessel with erythrocytes
2 Smooth muscle cells, myocytes
Stain: Masson-Goldner trichrome; magnification: × 400

279 Descending Thoracic Aorta

This parallel section shows the fiber network of the tunica media. It features strong lamellae, homogeneous layers of 2–3-μm thick *elastic membranes* as well as singular elastic fibers. They form tight concentric layers. The *webbed* membranes leave openings in different shapes and sizes and in this way, form *fenestrated elastic membranes*. The number of these fenestrated elastic membranes increases with age (35–40 for a newborn, 65–75 for an adult) (cf. Figs. 164–166, 277, 278). The wall muscles of elastic arteries regulate predominantly the tensile force of the elastic fiber network and, only to a lesser degree, the lumen of the artery.

Stain: Weigert's resorcin-fuchsin-picric acid; magnification: × 300

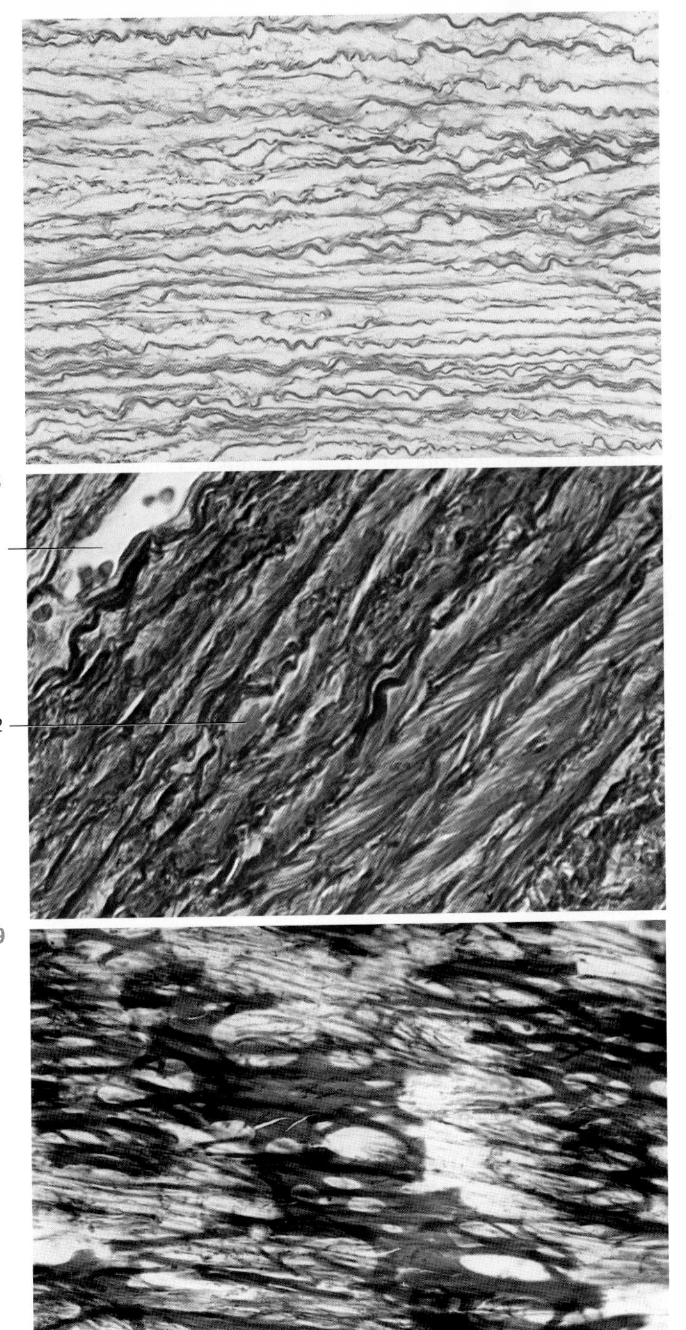
277
278
1
2
279

280 Femoral Artery

Cross-section through the femoral artery with its strong muscles. A clearly visible *internal elastic membrane* [1] separates the tunica intima (left) from the *tunica media* [2]. The smooth muscle cells of the *tunica media* are arranged in tightly threaded spirals. The right part of the photograph shows the tunica externa [3]. The outer layer of the tunica adventitia [4] contains the vessels of the aortic wall (*vasa vasorum*) [5]. Compare with Fig. 275.

1 Internal elastic membrane
2 Tunica media
3 Tunica externa
4 Tunica adventitia
5 Vasa vasorum (vessel of the vessel)

Stain: hematoxylin-eosin; magnification: × 80

281 Testicular Artery

Vertical section through the testicular artery, which is a *muscular-type artery*. The tunica interna or *tunica intima* is the innermost layer in this vessel. Its outer luminal layer of endothelial cells [1] protects against the forces of the bloodstream. Nuclei of endothelial cells are not captured in this section and cytoplasmic structural elements are not recognizable at this magnification. The layer underneath the endothelium is the very thin *lamina propria intima*. It contains collagen fibrils. The following *internal elastic membrane* [2] is clearly defined. In this area, the tunica media consists of four muscle cells [3] with mostly contractile filaments. The nucleus of the muscle cell underneath the elastic internal membrane is visible. There are numerous small mitochondria in the perinuclear space. Collagen fibrils are interspersed with myocytes of the tunica media. A thin *external elastic membrane* [4] separates the tunica media and tunica adventitia [5].

1 Endothelium
2 Internal elastic membrane
3 Tunica media myocytes
4 External elastic membrane
5 Tunica adventitia

Electron microscopy; magnification: × 4000

282 Endothelium

Endothelium from the posterior tibial artery with intermediary filaments [1], plasmalemma invaginations (*caveolae or superficial vesicles*) [2], many intracellular vesicles [3] and *Weibel-Palade bodies* (*Palade granules*, multi vesicular bodies, MVBs) [4] (cf. Fig. 297). Weibel-Palade bodies [4] are membrane-enclosed granules, which contain parallel tubular filaments. They are specialized secretory granules, which contain *von Willebrand factor* and the vasoconstriction peptide *endothelin*, among other factors. Apart from *vimentin intermediary filaments*, the endothelium also contains a contractile filament system (*actin-myosin system*). The two systems can be distinguished using immunohistochemistry.

1 Intermediary filaments
2 Caveolae
3 Vesicles
4 Weibel-Palade body (Palade granules)
5 Lysosomes
6 Intercellular gap
7 Basal membrane
8 Vascular lumen

Electron microscopy; magnification: × 44,200

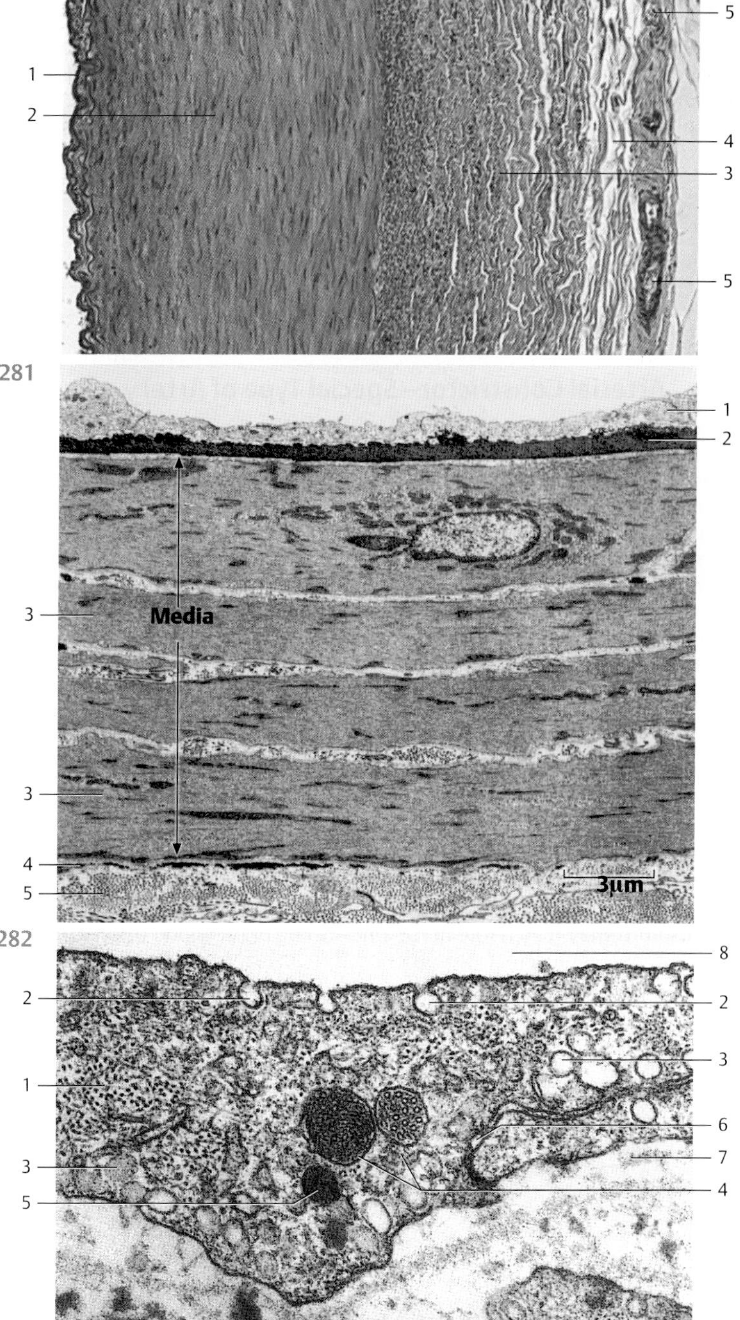
280
1
2
5
4
3
5
281
1
2
3
Media
3
4
5
3µm
282
8
2
2
3
1
6
3
7
4
5

283 Endothelium

Endothelium from the posterior tibial vein with intermediary filaments [1], mitochondria [2] and vesicles [3]. Two endothelial cells, which are clearly separated by an intercellular space [4] overlap like roof shingles. Note the caveolae and the cytoplasmic vesicles [3] in the endothelial cells in the lower part of the photo. Compare with Figs. 281, 282, 289 and 290.

1 Cytoskeleton (filaments)
2 Mitochondria
3 Vesicles
4 Intercellular gap
5 Lysosome
6 Elastic fibers
7 Vascular lumen
Electron microscopy; magnification: × 28 000

284 Arterial Constrictor—Special Type of Artery

Several special structures, such as bulging or lip-shaped prominences [1] can be found in the arterial circulatory system. These occur in most instances close to branching points. There are also constricting arteries, which feature prominences of longitudinal muscle cells at the luminal side of their circular musculature. These muscular prominences look like cushions (muscular tunica intima cushions). The star-shaped lumen owes its form to muscular intima cushions of different sizes [1]. Toward the outside of the vessel, follow several layers of ring muscles [2], which are covered by strong muscle fibers in longitudinal direction [3]. The artery in this figure is from a human spermatic cord.

1 Muscular intima cushion
2 Ring muscle layer
3 Layer of longitudinal muscles
Stain: azan; magnification: × 80

285 Constricting Artery—Special Type of Artery

Close to branching points in the arterial circulatory system, there are often prominences in the shapes of walls, lips or beaks. These arterial prominences or cushions may play a role in the fine-tuning of the blood distribution. The figure shows a muscular prominence [1] in an artery of the psoas muscle. It has caused the endothelium [2] to protrude quite far into the arterial lumen. An elongated nucleus from a muscle cell [3] is visible in the lower part of the photograph. Note the filament system of the *contractile myocyte*, followed by thin processes from fibrocytes along with collagen fibrils.

1 Muscular prominence
2 Endothelium
3 Myocyte
4 Connective tissue
Electron microscopy; magnification: × 7500

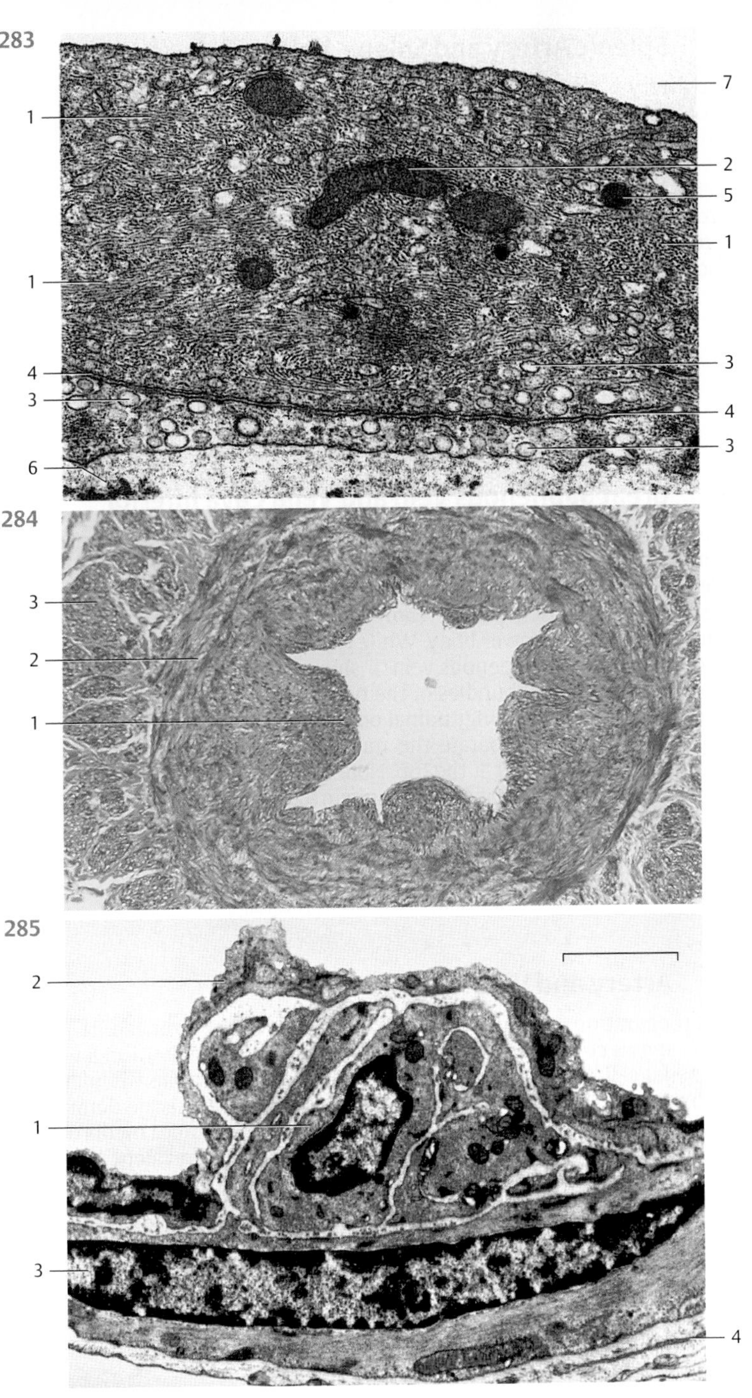
283
1
7
2
5
1
1
4
3
3
4
3
6
284
3
2
1
285
2
1
3
4

286 Splenic Artery and Splenic Vein

The artery is depicted in the upper part, the vein in the lower part of the photo in both figures. The *three-layered structure* is quite apparent in the arterial wall (cf. Fig. 274). This three-layered structure can also be recognized in the venous walls, albeit less clearly. The smooth muscle fibers in the tunica media of the vein 10 are bundled (b). The venous tunica media contains strong elastic networks, which become more prominent after staining with orcein (a). Part of the venous lumen 2 is shown at the lower edges in both micrographs.

1 Arterial lumen
2 Venous lumen
3 Internal elastic lamina
4 Tunica externa of the artery
5 Tunica media of the vein
6 Internal tunica (intima) of the artery
7 Tunica media of the artery
8 Tunica externa of the artery
9 Tunica externa of the vein
10 Tunica media of the vein

Stain: a) alum hematoxylin-orcein, b) hemalum-eosin; magnification (a and b): × 15

287 Great Saphenous Vein and Vena Cava Inferior

The two cross-sections show the vast differences in the ways the structural units are arranged in the venous walls of the *great saphenous vein* (a) and the *inferior vena cava* (b). At the same time, the sections give an impression about the presence of muscle tissue (*yellow*) and connective tissue (*red*) in the large venous walls of the lower body. While the muscle cell bundles of the tunica media of the great saphenous vein 1 show a more or less circular arrangement, the muscle cell bundles of the tunica media of the lower central vein (vena cava) (b) show a longitudinal orientation. Strong septa of collagenous connective tissue 2 separate the muscle cell bundles. In both cases, the tunica interna is located at the top. Note the muscle bundles (yellow) in the tunica externa of the great saphenous vein 3. The inferior vena cava shows a wider connective tissue layer 4 underneath the tunica intima.

1 Tunica media
2 Connective tissue septa
3 Tunica externa
4 Lamina propria intimae

Stain: van Gieson iron hematoxylin-picrofuchsin; magnification: × 15

288 Artery and Vein

This preparation is from the submucosal tissue of the stomach. The micrograph shows cross-sections of a small artery (bottom right) and a vein. The epithelial cell nuclei of the tunica intima protrude into the vascular lumen and make the opening look like an *eyelet* 1. Connective tissue dominates in the tunica media of the venous wall. In contrast, in the tunica media of the arterial wall circular smooth muscle bundles 2 are more prevalent. Folds of the tunica intima form the *venous valves* 3, which extend into the venous lumen (see Fig. 291).

1 Endothelial cell nuclei
2 Circular musculature
3 Venous valve
4 Arteriole (longitudinal cut)
5 Arteriole (cut across the axis)
6 Connective tissue from the submucous coat (stomach)

Stain: alum hematoxylin-eosin; magnification: × 300

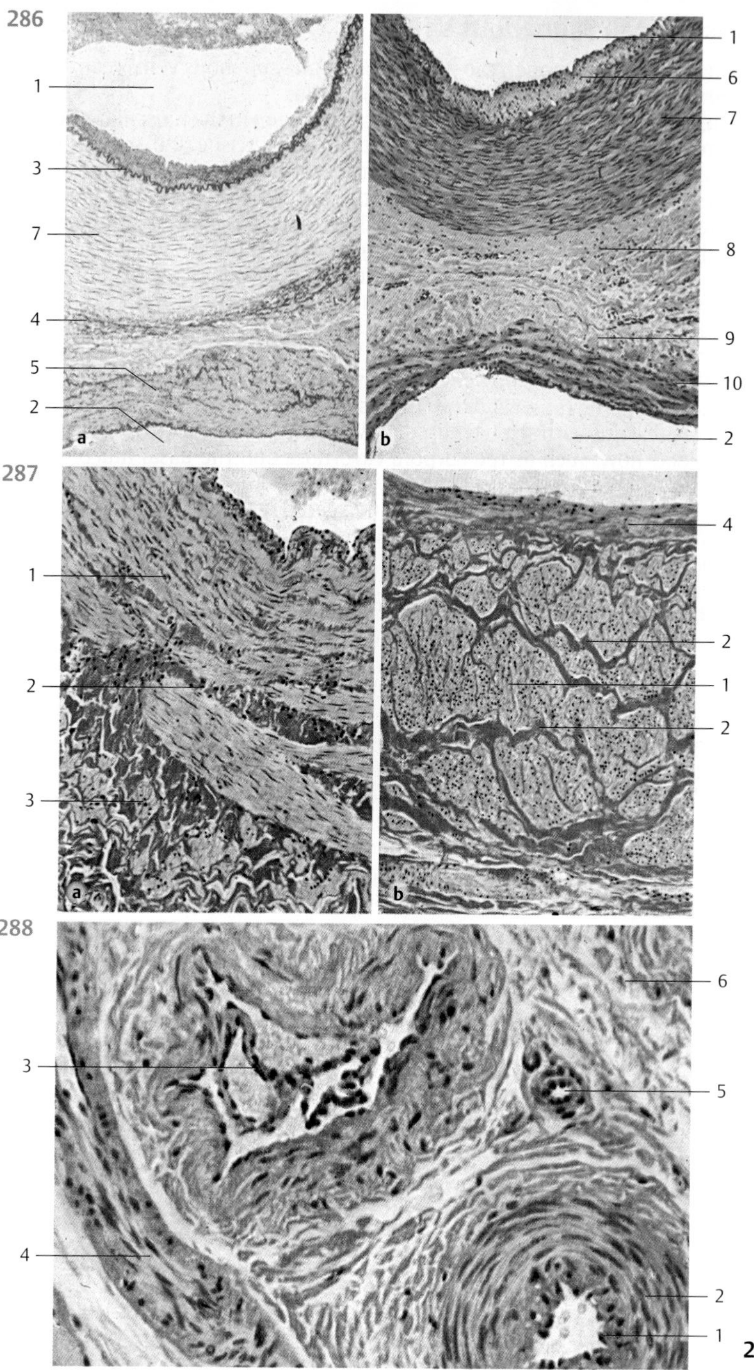
286
1
3
7
4
5
2
a
1
6
7
8
9
10
2
b
287
1
2
3
a
4
2
1
2
b
288
3
4
6
5
2
1

289 Small Saphenous Vein

Vertical section through the wall of the small saphenous vein (*vena saphena parva*) at the knee joint in a 42-year-old man.

The characteristic three-layered structure, as seen in the muscular arteries, is barely visible in veins. The layers of connective tissue and smooth muscle cells in venous walls are woven together without noticeable, distinct borders. In addition, the venous part of the circulatory system displays a considerable morphological variability, which usually is an adaptation to the location of the vein in the body. The walls of the veins of the upper body, for example, consist mostly of connective tissue and only a very thin layer of muscle cells. In contrast, the musculature in the venous walls of the lower body is much more developed. This accommodates the larger *hydrostatic workload* for the leg and pelvic veins. Veins with few muscles occur in parts of the body where the flow regulation via lumen changes is unnecessary, e.g., in the brain, the retina and the sinuses of the dura mater. On the other hand, there are veins with strong muscular walls in organs with strong fluctuations in blood flow, such as the corpora cavernosa and the nasal mucous membranes.

This electron micrograph shows the nucleated sections of two flat, sprawling *endothelial cells* [1]. The layer immediately underneath contains the delicate fibrils of the *lamina propria intimae* [2]. Two spindle-shaped fibrocytes [3] are present between the collagen fibrils. These are followed by cross-sections of slender *myocytes* [4] and collagen fibrils in several alternating layers [5] and [6]. As always, the myocytes display their typical filament structure, even at this magnification (cf. Fig. 622). In the third, fibril-rich connective tissue layer (starting the count from the endothelium, top), there is a darkly stained, largely continuous elastic fiber [7] with bizarre protuberances. Sporadically, very small sections of such elastic fibers [8] occur in other fibril-rich layers as well. The outer venous wall does not have a clearly delimited tunica adventitia because the collagen fibers of the venous wall connect directly with the surrounding connective tissue. Note the collagen fibril bundles are cut across their axis in most instances, i.e., almost all collagen fibrils run longitudinally in the direction of the vein. A three-dimensional reconstruction reveals that the collagen fibrils are arranged in steep spirals.

1 Endothelial cells
2 Lamina propria intimae
3 Fibrocytes
4 Myocytes
5 Collagen fibrils, longitudinal
6 Collagen fibrils, cut across the axis
7 Elastic fiber
8 Elastic fiber material
Electron microscopy; magnification: × 6200

289

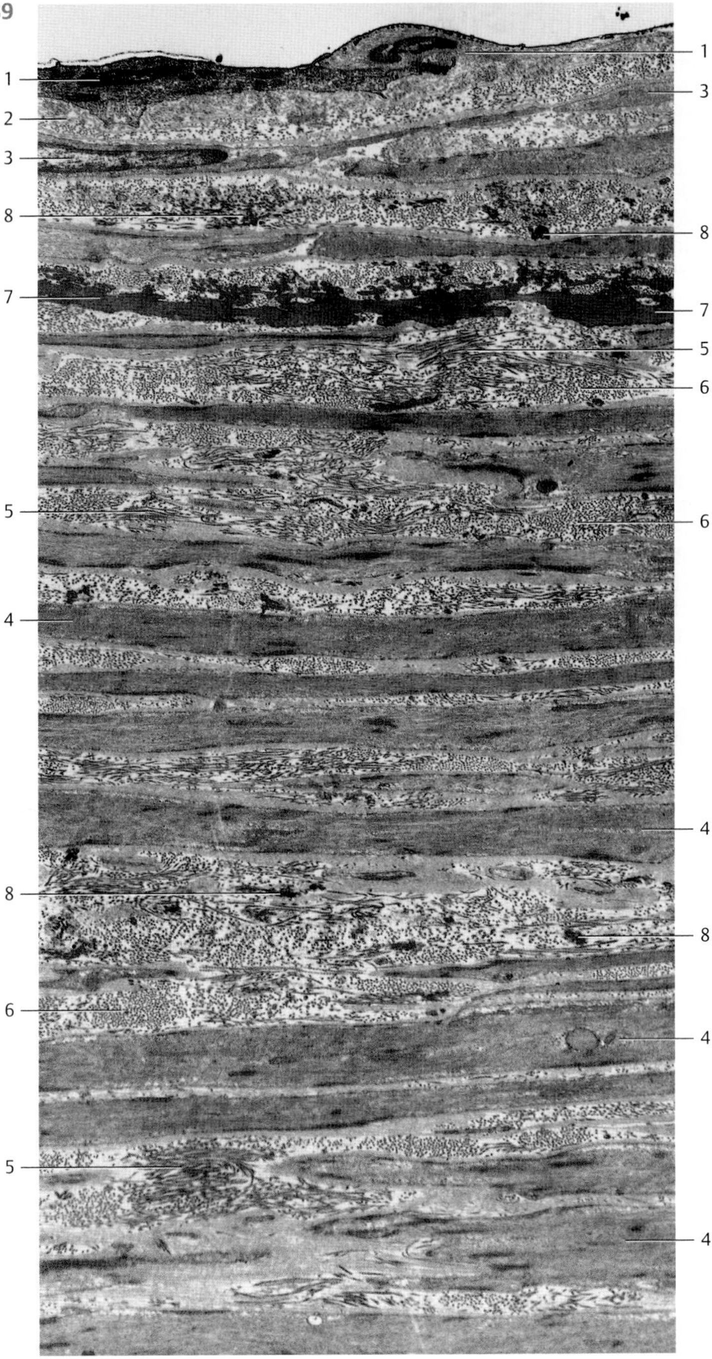

1
1
3
2
3
8
8
7
7
5
6
5
6
4
4
8
8
6
4
5
4

290 Anterior Tibial Vein

Vertical section through the *anterior tibial vein* (section of the wall close to the lumen). Arteries show a typical layered structure. In contrast, this layered structure is much less distinctive in veins. The upper portion of this electron micrograph depicts a flat sprawling *endothelial cell* with its nucleus 1 and underneath the fine fibrils of the *lamina propria intimae* 2. The following layer contains the elastic fibers of the *internal elastic membrane* 3, which are also found in arteries. The layer following the internal elastic membrane contains collagen fibers that have been cut in all planes 4. These layers are followed by the smooth muscle cells 5 of the tunica media. Note that there are also many collagen fibrils between the smooth muscle cells (cf. Fig. 289).

Electron microscopy; magnification: × 6200

291 Venous Valves

One-way valves are present in most veins. They are *folds of the tunica intima*, which protrude into the venous lumen like sails (*leaflet valve, velum*) (see Fig. 288). The leaflet valves can be in the shape of a half-moon or a sickle. Their shapes often remind of a martin's nest 1. Most valves have two flexible leaflets, which freely move with the bloodstream. Valve leaflets are covered on both faces by a layer of endothelium with an underlying network of intersecting collagen fibers. This fiber network is anchored in the venous wall. The space between the venous wall and the outer edge of the velum (leaflet) is called *valve sinus* 2. During normal blood flow through the vein, the leaflets lay against the venous wall, and the valve is open. The leaflet valve prevents the back flow of blood.
Valve of a vein from the orbital sinus (pig).

1 Leaflet valve
2 Valve sinus
3 Endothelium of the orbital sinus
Scanning electron microscopy; magnification: × 180

292 Arteriole

Arterioles are precapillary arteries (*resistance vessels*) with a diameter of less than 0.5 mm. This figure shows a section across the wall of an arteriole from the tunica adventitia of a human urethra. The endothelium is continuous 2. Smooth circular muscles form the underlying *tunica media* 3. Bundles of unmyelinated axons 6 are located in the tunica externa. Contact between two neighboring endothelial cells ↗.

1 Nucleus of an endothelial cell
2 Cytoplasmic process from an endothelial cell
3 Smooth muscle cell with filaments and cell organelles
4 Golgi apparatus of a smooth muscle cell
5 Nucleus of a perivascular fibrocyte
6 Unmyelinated axon
7 Connective tissue of the tunica externa
8 Arteriole lumen
Electron microscopy; magnification: × 8000

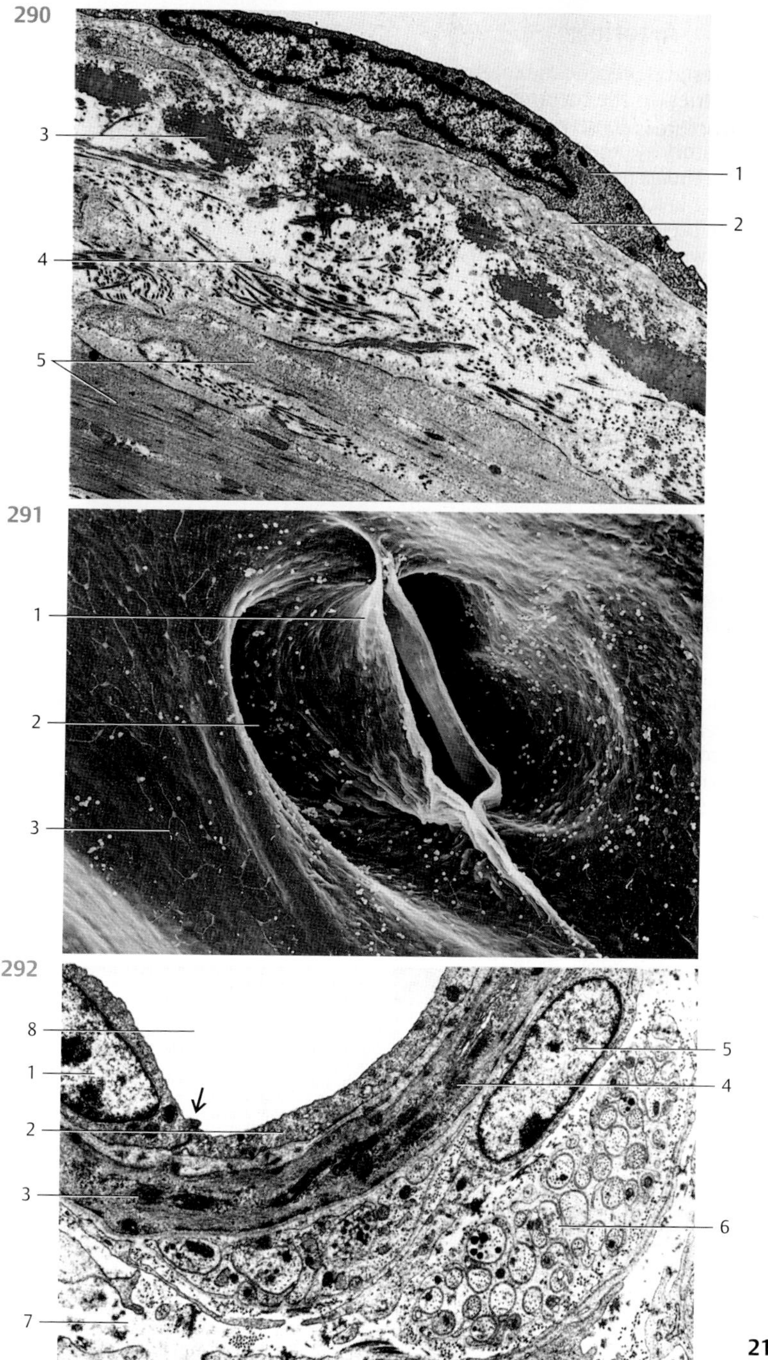
290
3
4
5
1
2
291
1
2
3
292
8
1
2
3
7
5
4
6

293 Arteriole

Arterioles precede the capillaries. They are therefore often called *precapillary* arteries. In the hierarchy of the arterial system, arterioles are the smallest members. Along with the capillaries and venules, they form the terminal circulatory system (*microcirculation*).
The tunica intima of the arterioles consists of endothelium 1 with an underlying layer of connective tissue 2. An internal elastic membrane is usually not present, except occasionally in a fragmented form. The tunica media shows only one layer of muscle cells 3. In this micrograph, the myocytes of the tunica media 3 are mostly cut tangentially or across their axis. This indicates that the myocytes are arranged in a spiral form. Collagen fibrils in different proportions occur between the muscle cells. The tunica adventitia 4 is a narrow layer. It consists of connective tissue cells and collagen fibers.

1 Endothelium
2 Subendothelial connective tissue
3 Myocytes
4 Tunica adventitia
Electron microscopy; magnification: × 3000

294 Microcirculation—Capillaries

Tissue with capillaries serves the metabolic exchange, including the respiratory exchange. All *capillaries* are lined with *endothelial cells*, which can be evaluated by looking on the tissue surface. The images shown here are longitudinal sections. Therefore, they only show the elongated, spindle-shaped endothelial cell nuclei 1. Cells with branched interconnected processes (*pericytes*) 2 populate the outer capillary tube. The capillary from subcutaneous tissue is filled with erythrocytes 3. Figure b shows sprouting capillaries in embryonic connective tissue 4. The diameters of the capillaries vary from 4 to about 15 μm.

1 Endothelial cell nuclei
2 Pericytes
3 Erythrocytes
4 Embryonic connective tissue
Stain: alum hematoxylin-eosin; magnifications: a) × 400, b) × 240

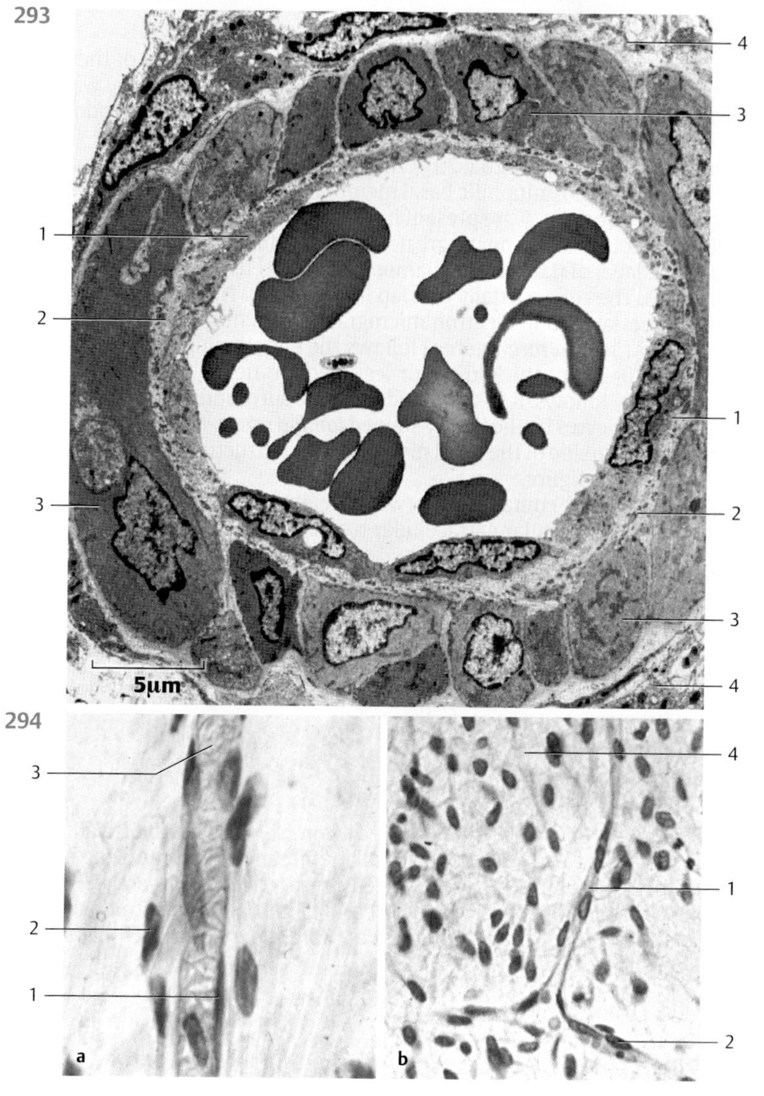
293
4
3
1
2
3
1
2
3
4
5µm
294
3
2
1
a
4
1
2
b

295 Capillaries

Cross-section of a *continuous* capillary from the perineurium of the median nerve. Two endothelial cells 1 take part in building this capillary wall. Their cytoplasm shows small mitochondria, short fragments of rough endoplasmic reticulum membranes, vesicles, filaments and a Palade granule (Weibel-Palade body) 2 (cf. Figs. 282, 297). An erythrocyte is captured in the capillary lumen. A weakly osmiophilic basal membrane 3 underlies the endothelium. Sectioned fibrocytes 4 are present in the immediate neighborhood of the capillary. Endothelial cell nuclei are not visible in this section. The endothelium is a single layer of flat, usually diamond-shaped cells with narrow intercellular spaces. The cells partially overlap like shingles. The basal membrane appears three-layered in electron micrographs. A lightly stained, about 15 nm thick layer (*lamina rara interna*) follows the endothelium. Toward the outer wall, the 20–30 nm thick, more or less electron-dense (*osmiophilic*) *lamina rara densa* 5 follows. It is separated from the surrounding connective tissue and from pericytes by the lightly stained *lamina rara externa*. Pericytes are located at the outside of the basal membrane. The structural details can be seen in the adjacent figure.
Note the cell-cell contacts 7 between neighboring endothelial cells. Also, note the finely granular extracellular matrix 6.

1 Endothelial cells
2 Palade granule (Weibel-Palade body)
3 Basal membrane
4 Fibrocyte processes
5 Lamina densa of the basal membrane
6 Extracellular matrix
7 Cell-cell contacts
Electron microscopy; magnification: × 18 000

296 Capillaries

Continuous capillary (not fenestrated) from the *stratum moleculare* of the feline cerebellar cortex. A strong basal membrane 1 separates the endothelium from nerve tissue 2 and glial cells, respectively. The *pericyte* 3 is also completely enveloped by a separate basal membrane. Pinocytotic vesicles in the endothelium of brain capillaries are rare. Note the sickle-shaped endothelial cell nucleus.

1 Basal membrane
2 Nerve fibers
3 Pericyte
Electron microscopy; magnification: × 10 000

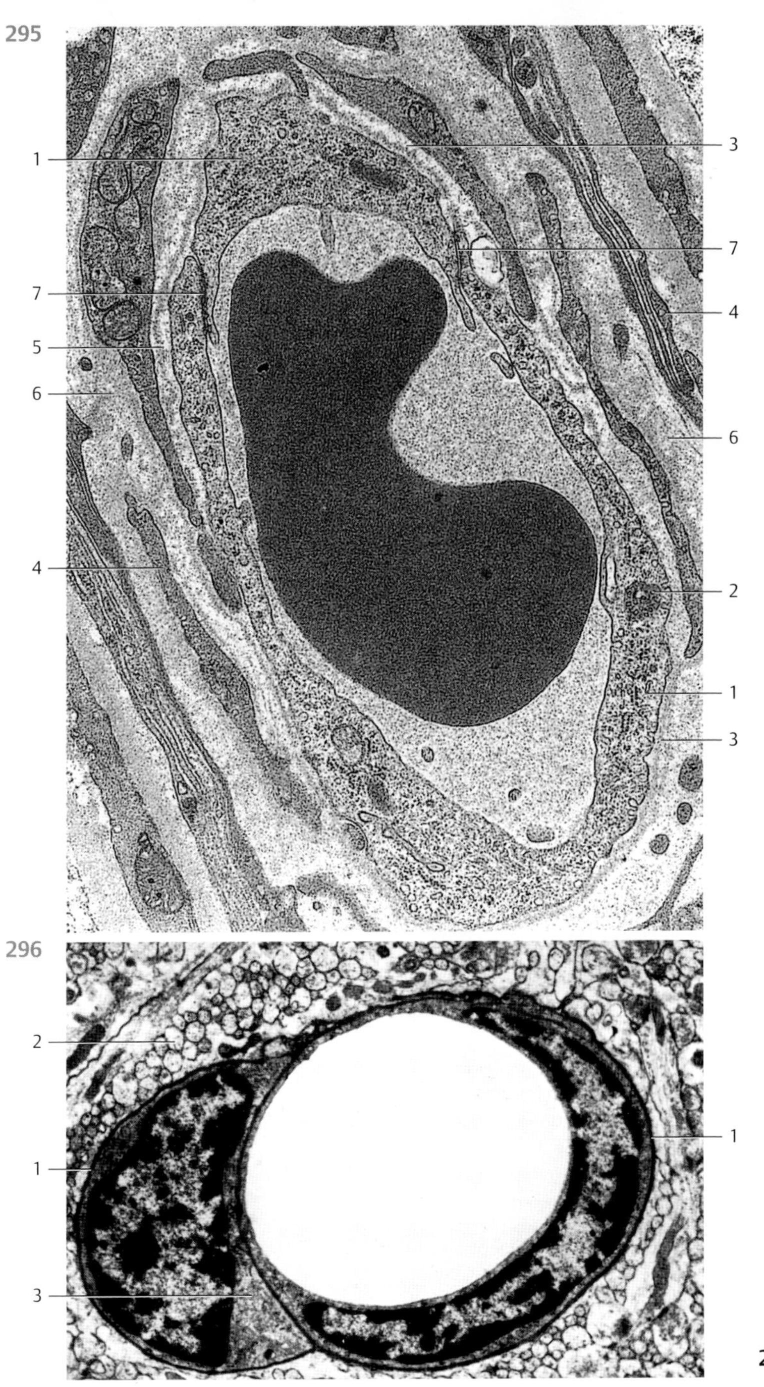
295
1
7
5
6
4
3
7
4
6
2
1
3
296
2
1
3
1

297 Capillaries

Capillaries are lined by a single-layered (simple) endothelium 1 (cf. Figs. 294–296). This figure shows a capillary with a complete layer of endothelial cells, a continuous basal membrane 2 and an incomplete covering with pericytes 3 (cf. Fig. 295). In this case, only a single cell lines the capillary lumen. This is in contrast to the capillary lumen in Fig. 295. However, tongue-like processes from neighboring endothelial cells 4 cover the inner capillary wall in three places (*shingle-type overlapping*).

The cytoplasm of the endothelial cell shown here displays all typical organelles, such as mitochondria, endoplasmic reticulum, Golgi apparatus 5, free and membrane-bound ribosomes, Palade granules (Weibel-Palade bodies, MVBs) 6 and copious *pinocytotic vesicles*. The endothelial cell nucleus 1 is sectioned. The capillary tube is completely covered by a *basal membrane*. Pericyte processes 3 are visible on both sides of the capillary.

Capillary of a skeletal muscle.

1 Endothelial cell nucleus
2 Basal membrane
3 Pericyte sections
4 Processes from neighboring endothelial cells
5 Golgi apparatus
6 Weibel-Palade bodies (Palade granules)
Electron microscopy; magnification: × 18 000

298 Capillaries

This capillary is from the tendon tissue of a rat. A monocyte 2 is located in the capillary lumen (cf. Fig. 144). It is about to leave the capillary (*monocyte diapedesis*). A part of it already protrudes into the connective tissue layer. The endothelial junctions are labeled: ↗.

Note the perivascular connective tissue 4 with fibroblasts 3 and collagen fibrils.

1 Endothelium
2 Monocyte
3 Fibroblast
4 Perivascular connective tissue
5 Section of a pericyte
Electron microscopy; magnification: × 12 800

299 Capillaries

Sector of a *visceral* (*fenestrated*) capillary from an islet of Langerhans from a mouse pancreas (cf. Fig. 300). A diaphragm covers the *fenestration* gaps ↗. For details, see Fig. 300.

1 Capillary lumen (clearance)
2 Fenestrated endothelium
3 Basal membrane
4 Sections of endocrine gland cells
Electron microscopy; magnification: × 18 000

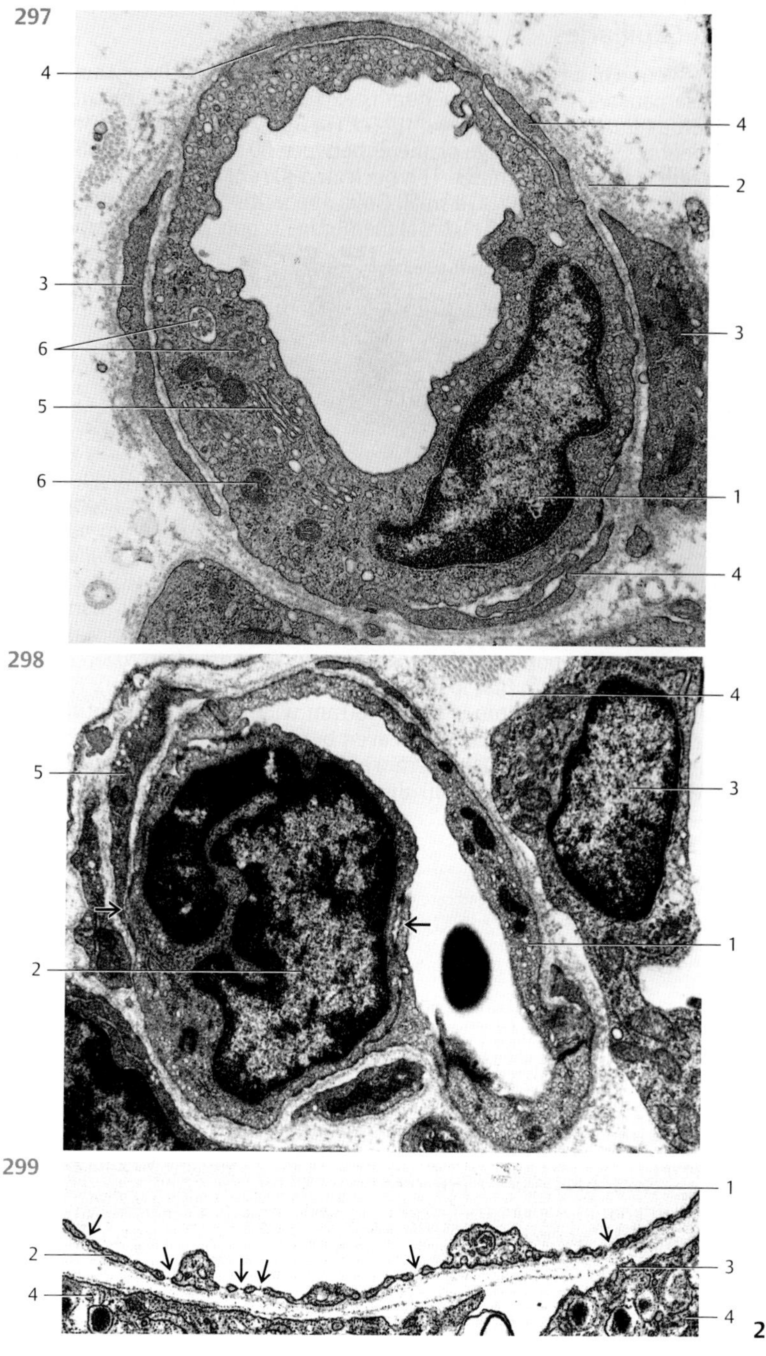
297
4
4
2
3
3
6
5
6
1
4
298
4
5
3
1
2
299
1
2
3
4
4

300 Capillaries

Cross-section of a *visceral* (*fenestrated*) capillary from an islet of Langerhans (mouse pancreas). The endothelium is extremely flat and perforated with numerous small holes (“*windows*”) [1] (cf. Fig. 299). These windows are circular openings with an average diameter between 60 and 70 nm. A delicate diaphragm covers the openings. The nucleated part of the endothelial cell [3] also shows mitochondria [4], a small Golgi apparatus [2] and *caveolae*, among other cell compartments. The basal membrane is only partially visible.

1 Fenestrated membrane with diaphragm
2 Golgi apparatus
3 Endothelial cell nucleus
4 Mitochondria
5 Sections of endocrine cells
Electron microscopy; magnification: × 11 200

301 Capillaries

Capillaries in different locations are built differently. They are categorized according to their structural attributes. There are capillaries with a continuous endothelium and a closed basal membrane (*somatic capillaries, nonfenestrated*). Other arteries have a perforated endothelium (*visceral capillaries, fenestrated*). This figure shows a vertical section through the wall of a renal glomerular capillary. The endothelium is perforated and shows many pores [↗]. In this preparation, it appears to consist of large cytoplasmic islands in a range of sizes. The pores are about 50 nm wide. They are often covered with a 4 nm-thick diaphragm (not in this figure, *open fenestrated artery*). The layer following the endothelium is the 50–60 nm wide *lamina densa* of the continuous basal membrane [4], interleaved by a thin *lamina rara interna*. The lamina densa follows the lamina rara externa and the layer of *podocyte* processes [^]. Podocytes sit like small plugs on the basal membrane (see Figs. 491, 493–496).

1 Capillary lumen
2 Bowman’s space
3 Endothelial cell nucleus
4 Basal membrane
Electron microscopy; magnification: × 10 500

302 Capillaries

Capillaries with fenestrated endothelium (see Fig. 299) must be distinguished from *fenestrated, discontinuous sinusoidal capillaries*. Their endothelial layer shows gaps [2]. The figure shows a section of a liver capillary (*sinusoids of the liver lobule*). The endothelium displays 0.1 to 1.0 μm-wide gaps [↗]. Exchanges between capillary lumen and the *Disse space* [3] (*spatium perisinusoideum*) proceed via this *discontinuous endothelium*. There is no basal membrane. The surfaces of the liver cells (*hepatocytes*) next to the Disse space are covered with microvilli of different sizes. There are reticular and collagen fibers present in the Disse space (cf. Fig. 449). With a diameter of 30–50 μm, discontinuous sinusoidal capillaries are wider than other types of capillaries.

1 Capillary lumen
2 Endothelium
3 Disse’s space
4 Liver cell cytoplasm
Electron microscopy; magnification: × 8500

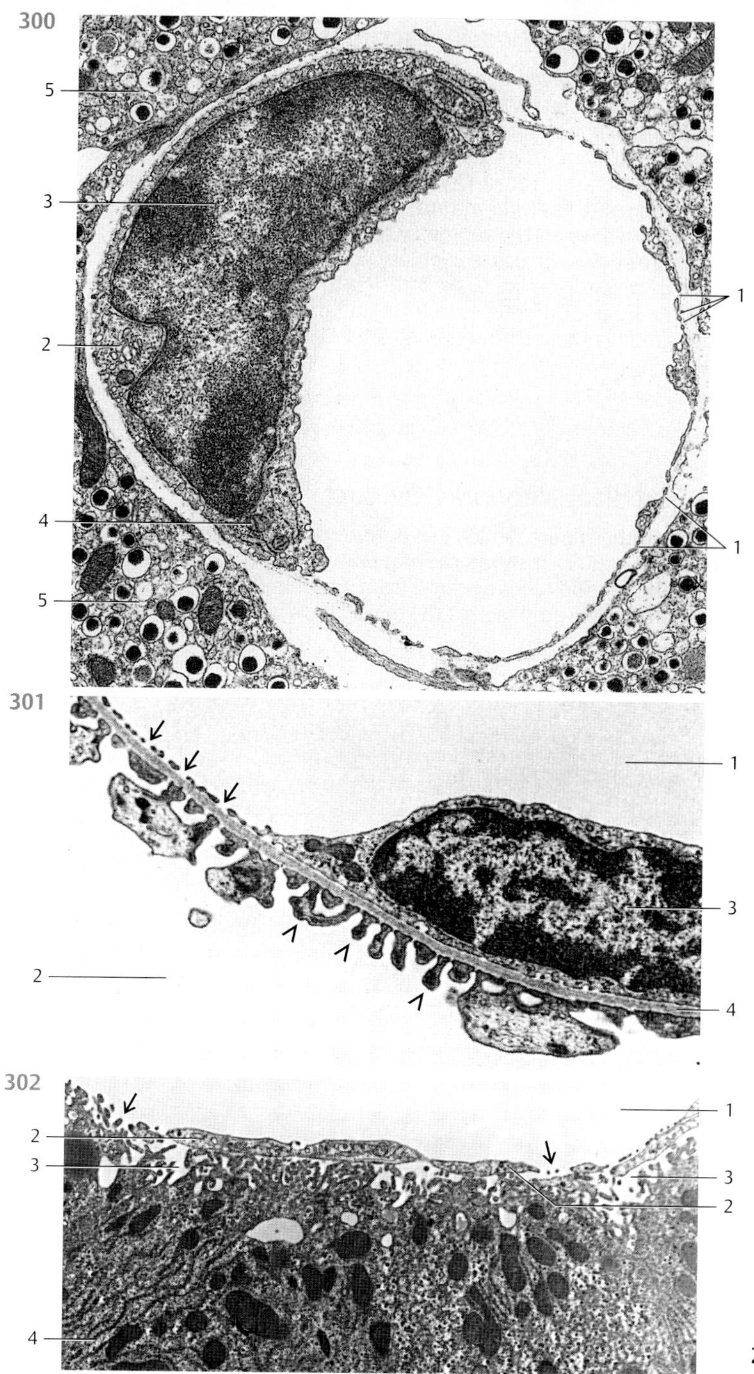
300
5
3
2
4
5
1
1
301
1
3
2
4
302
2
3
4
1
3
2

303 Capillary Network—Lacrimal Gland

The capillary bed of an organ can be made visible using one of several injection techniques, and its three-dimensional structure can then be examined by scanning electron microscopy. In this instance, the arteries that go to the head of a cat were filled with a resin, which was allowed to harden at a defined temperature range. Organic materials were than removed using acid or alkaline solutions (*maceration*). This procedure creates a *corrosion preparation,* which leaves the geometry of the capillaries intact.
This figure shows the dense capillary network in the lacrimal gland of a cat. Note the branching of the larger arteries 1. Veins 2 are visible in the bottom left of the figure. Differences in form and orientation of the endothelial cell nuclei, among other attributes, indicate whether a vessel is an artery or vein.

1 Arteries
2 Veins
Scanning electron microscopy; magnification: × 85

304 Capillary Network—Oviduct

This is another figure, which exemplifies the dense capillary network of an organ (cf. Fig. 303). It shows the elaborately vascularized (capillarized) fimbria of the uterine tube (oviduct) from a rabbit. The corrosion cast preparation impressively emphasizes the dense, tight-meshed capillary network.

Corrosion preparation; scanning electron microscopy; magnification: × 40

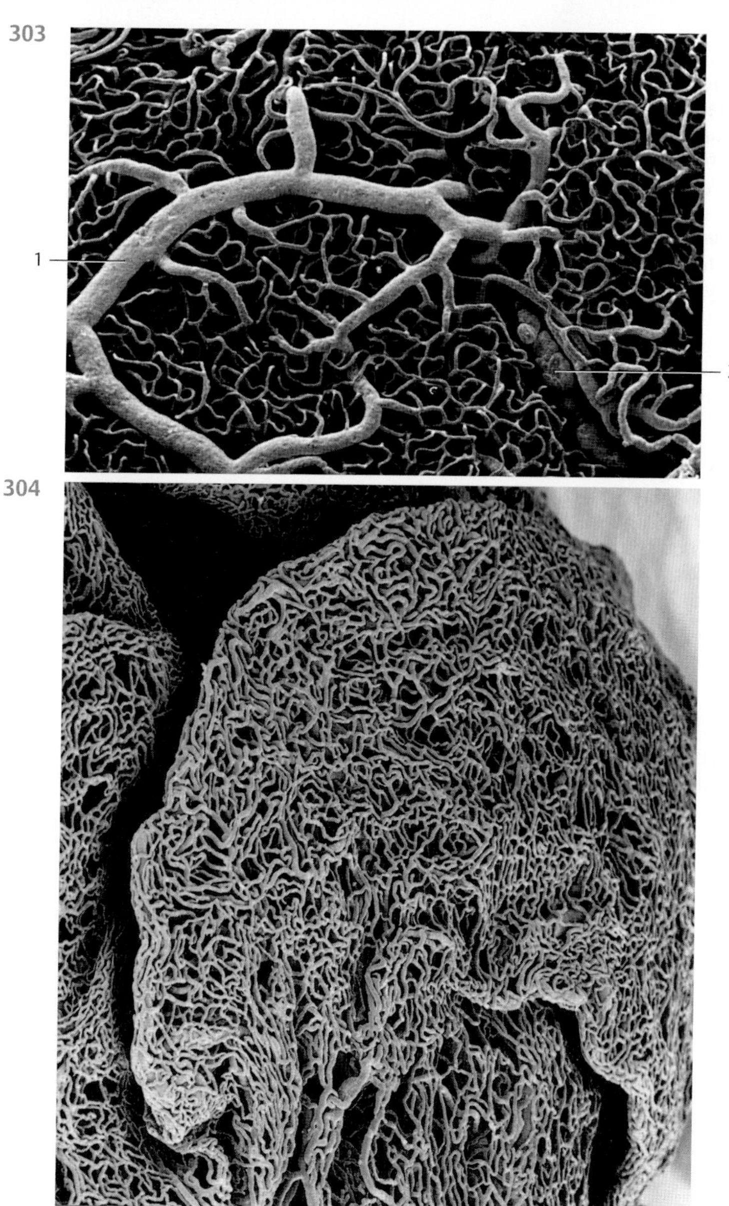
303
1
2
304

305 Arteriovenous Anastomoses

The connection between the very small arteries and venules is not always made via the capillary network but in many cases, via immediate contractile *shunts*. These *anastomosis* vessels reroute the bloodstream directly from the arterial high-pressure circulation to the venous low-pressure system, thus circumventing the capillary network. In humans, arteriovenous anastomosis vessels occur in large numbers in the extremities. They are known as *Masson's organs* or *Hoyer -Grosser organs* (*glomus neuromyoarteriale, anastomosis arteriovenosa glomiformis*). These organs show specific forms of epithelial myocytes.

Longitudinal muscle bundles already exist on the arterioles where the shunts originate. The connection between artery and vein consists of *winding tubules* 1 with thick walls (about 40–60 µm) and narrow lumina (10–30 µm). Unmyelinated nerve cells often weave around these looping coils of vessels. A layer of connective tissue separates the shunt vessels and nerve cells from the surrounding tissue.

This figure shows such a shunt structure. The presence of a strong layer of *epithelioid* muscle cells under the epithelial layer emphasizes the shunts. Epithelioid muscle cells are fibril-free. Their cytoplasm is only slightly stained with the procedure used here. The by-pass canals (shunts) do not have an internal elastic membrane (*tunica elastica interna*).

Human fingertip.

Stain: hematoxylin-eosin; magnification: × 200

306 Lymph Capillaries

Lymph capillaries form as collecting tubes from tissue canals in the interstitial space. Lymph capillaries are very small vessels without valves. They usually form drainage systems. Lymph capillaries have extremely thin walls. Their walls consist of only one layer of lymphatic endothelial cells, which are flattened like wallpaper. There is no basal membrane. Instead, electron microscopy shows a layer of matted 10 nm-thick filaments underneath the epithelium in its place. From these felted filaments emerge anchor filaments, which reach to the endothelial cells of the lymph capillary on one side and to the connective tissue on the other side. The matted subendothelial fibers are *collagen fibers, types IV* and *VI*, among others.

The adjacent lymph capillary from the nasal mucous membrane (rat) contains several lymphocytes. Labels ↗ indicate easily recognizable subendothelial matted fibers.

Lymph capillaries turn into *collector lymph vessels*. Their walls contain a basal membrane and contractile myocytes. Collector lymph vessels also contain valves (cf. Fig. 327)

1 Endothelium
2 Endothelial cell nucleus
3 Connective tissue cells (fibrocytes)
Electron microscopy; magnification: × 4000

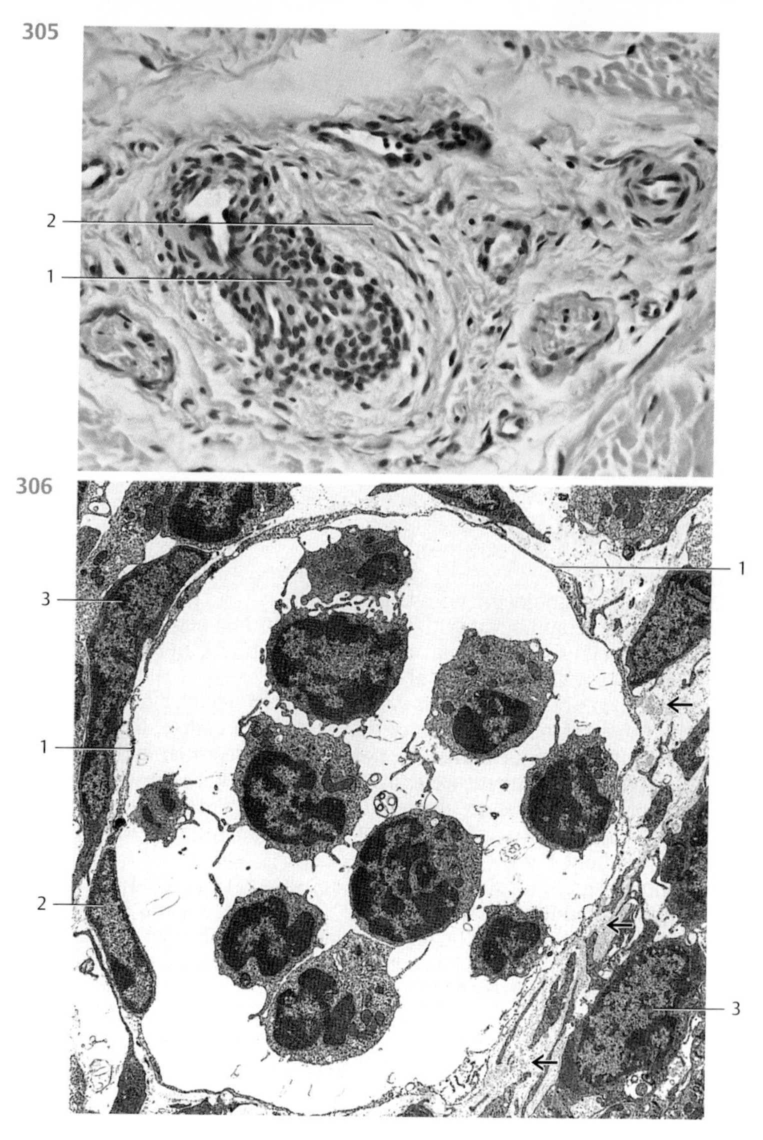
305
2
1
306
3
1
2
1
3

307 Bone Marrow

The biogenesis of the different blood cells in the bone marrow (*medulla ossium*) of adults occurs simultaneously and in close spatial proximity. The number of precursor cells accounts for the variability in form and character of cells in the bone marrow. Numerous capillaries are present in the reticular connective tissue stroma. They are enlarged to sinusoids and measure about 50–70 µm.
In the reticular spaces occur mostly myeloid progenitor cells, but also macrophages and local adipocytes. They form the *marrow parenchyme*. This figure shows a section of the human bone marrow (*iliac crest*). The eosinophilic promyelocytes [1] are particularly easy to recognize. However, a more precise description of the different cell types requires higher microscopic resolution.

1 Eosinophilic promyelocyte
2 Neutrophilic promyelocyte
3 Proerythroblast
4 Adipocytes
Stain: Pappenheim (May-Grünwald, Giemsa); magnification: × 320

308 Blood Smear

Granulocytes:
a) Neutrophilic granulocyte with banded nucleus.
b) Neutrophilic granulocyte with banded nucleus and beginning segmentation of the nucleus. The cytoplasm is stained light pink and contains azurophilic granules with a diameter of about 0.5 µm.
c) Two neutrophilic granulocytes with segmented nuclei. Fine threads connect the three segments in each of the nuclei. The coarse, heavily stained chromatin bodies are located at the peripheral nuclear membrane.
d) Neutrophilic granulocyte, excessively segmented with five segments.
e) Eosinophilic granulocyte (*eosinophil*) with segmented nucleus. The cell body is filled with coarse eosinophilic (= acidophilic) granules with a diameter of about 1 µm.
f) Eosinophilic granulocyte. The nucleus consists of two round segments.
g) Basophilic granulocyte (*basophil*).
h) Basophilic granulocyte. The large nuclei of basophils take up most of the cell body. The cytoplasm contains granules (stained dark violet) of different sizes, which sometimes cover the nucleus.
Lymphocytes:
i) Small lymphocyte. The large eccentric nucleus with large chromatin bodies is lobed and fills the cell body almost completely.
j) Lymphocyte. The large nucleus hardly displays any structural details. It leaves room for only a small seam of cytoplasm.
k) Large lymphocyte. The eccentric, round nucleus shows coarse bodies. Note the wide seam of cytoplasm.
l) Medium-sized lymphocyte with cytoplasmic azurophilic granules.
Monocyte:
m) Monocyte (*mononuclear phagocyte*). The nucleus is lobed. Its chromatin has a layered structure. The cytoplasm stains grayish-blue and contains small azurophilic granules.

Stain: Pappenheim (May-Grünwald, Giemsa); magnification: × 900

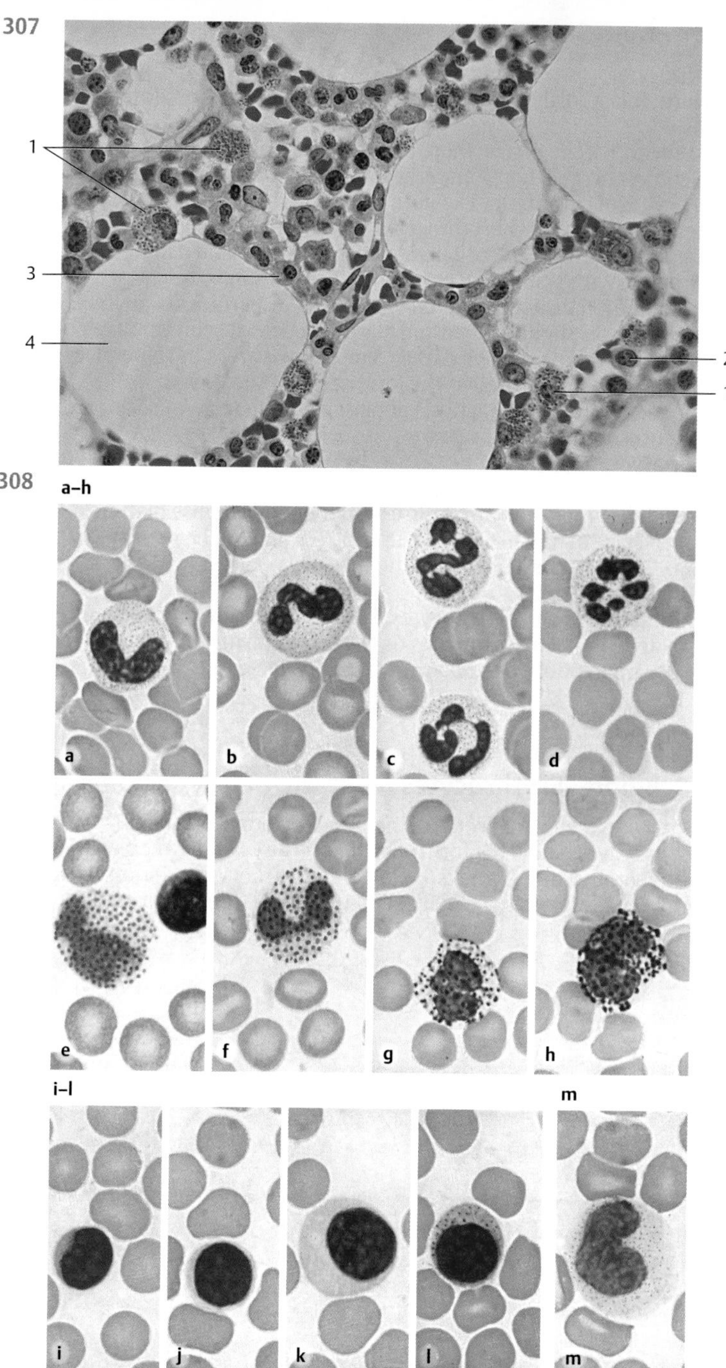
307
1
3
4
2
1
308
a–h
a
b
c
d
e
f
g
h
i–l
m
i
j
k
l
m

309 Blood Smear

Erythrocytes:

a) Normoblast (orthochromatic erythroblast). Ejected or almost ejected nucleus.

b) At the top of the image, there is a proerythroblast and a macroblast with a polychromatic cell body underneath it. The macroblast nucleus shows a coarse web of chromatin. The normoblast on the right has a pyknotic homogeneous nucleus. Two erythrocytes with basophilic spots are found in the center of the image. The cell underneath is nipped and damaged. Lower left: macroblast with spoke-like chromatin distribution.

c) Basophilic megaloblast (*promegaloblast*) in pernicious anemia. The nucleus is large, is slightly lobed and features a delicate chromatin web. The cytoplasm (light blue) shows darker blue stained areas in some places. A mature macroblast is located at the lower edge of the image.

d) Blood smear with a diagnosis of pernicious anemia. Anisocytosis and poikilocytosis of the erythrocytes.

Megakaryocyte:

e) Mature granular megakaryocyte. Large, lobed, polyploid nucleus. Finely granulated cytoplasm with diffuse border (sternal biopsy material). Megakaryocytes have diameters of more than 50 μm and can be seen at low magnification. Their precursor cells are the megakaryocytes.

Thrombocytes:

f) Thrombocytes and erythrocytes. Thrombocytes are pinched-off cells from megakaryocytes, the giant cells of the bone marrow. A megakaryocyte can produce up to 8000 thrombocytes (*thrombopoiesis*) (cf. Figs. 312, 313).

Stain: Pappenheim (May-Grünwald, Giemsa); magnification: × 900

310 Blood—Erythrocytes

Erythrocytes (red blood cells) of mammals do not have nuclei (cf. Figs. 309a–d). Erythrocytes show the form of biconcave disks with a median diameter of 7.5 μm (*normocytes*). At the outer edge, an erythrocyte is 2.5 μm thick. The biconcave shape is easily recognized in this figure. It leads to an enlarged surface.

Scanning electron microscopy; magnification: × 6500

309

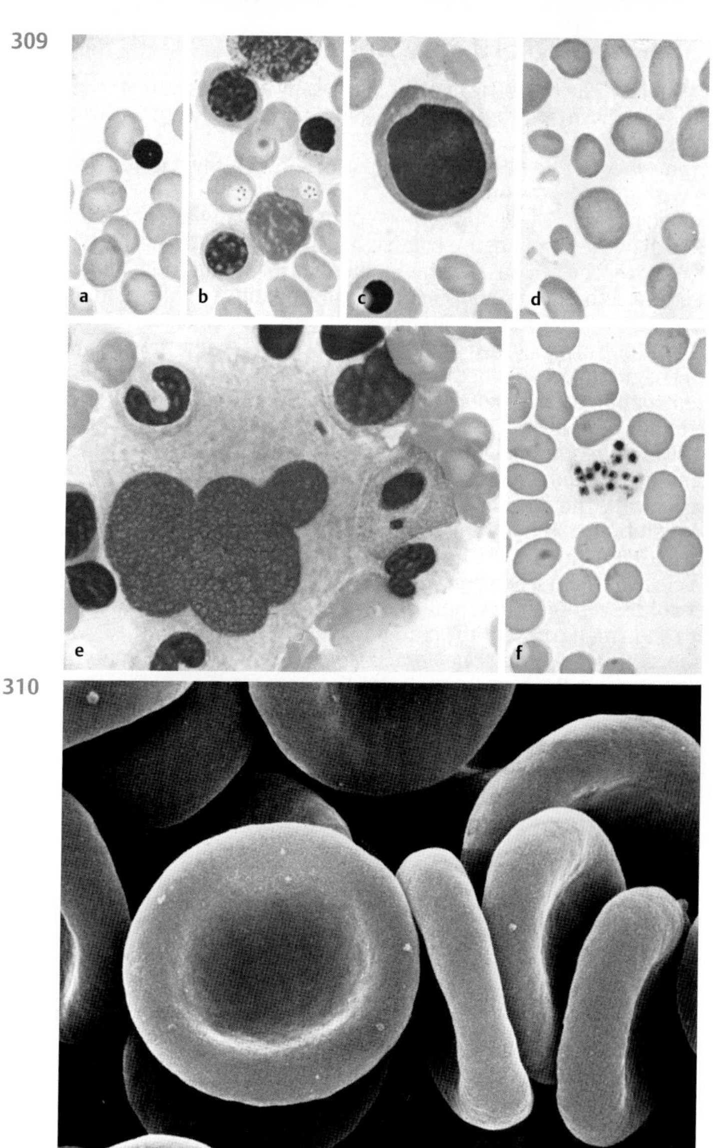

310

Blood—Sternal Biopsy Smear

a) Myeloblast. The eccentric nucleus leaves only a small seam of strongly basophilic cytoplasm without granules. Note the web-like chromatin structure and the nucleoli.
b) Promyelocyte. The basophilic cytoplasm shows a fine granulation. A nucleus with nucleolus is present.
c) Promyelocyte. The cytoplasm shows only slight granulation. The nucleus is smaller than the one in figure b. It has a coarse structure (myelocyte?).
d) Myelocyte. The cell has become smaller during maturation. It has an oval, coarsely structured nucleus. The cytoplasm contains specific granules.
e) Basophilic myelocyte with granules (stained dark violet).
f) Eosinophilic myelocyte or metamyelocyte, respectively, the nucleus showing the beginnings of a lobed structure. There are eosinophilic granules.
g) Neutrophilic metamyelocyte. The slightly basophilic cytoplasm shows neutrophilic granules.
h) Neutrophilic granulocytes with banded nuclei and coarsely structured chromatin. The cell bodies show beginning granulation.
i) Plasma cell. The nucleus is small and shows hyperchromatosis of the nuclear membrane. The chromatin bodies have a circular symmetry (*wheel-spoke nucleus*). The basophilic cell body shows a lighter stained cytocentrum (area close to the nucleus) (cf. Fig. 145 b).
j) Reticulum cell with basophilic cell body, cytocentrum, numerous fat vacuoles and small coarsely structured nucleus.
k) Proerythroblast (*pronormoblast*), a normoblast above it. Proerythrocytes are the largest cells in erythropoiesis (diameter 14–17 μm). Their nuclei display a finely meshed chromatin structure. The basophilic cytoplasm reacts slightly polychromatic.
l) Proerythroblast (center image), macroblast (top), neutrophilic granulocyte with rod-shaped nucleus (right bottom). Note the oxyphilic cytoplasm of the macroblast.
m) Macroblast with almost homogeneous pyknotic nucleus. The cytoplasm is still slightly polychromatic.
n) Mitosis (*equatorial plate*) in a proerythroblast. The cytoplasm is basophilic.
o) Mitotic macroblast.

Stain: Pappenheim (May-Grünwald, Giemsa); magnification: × 900

311

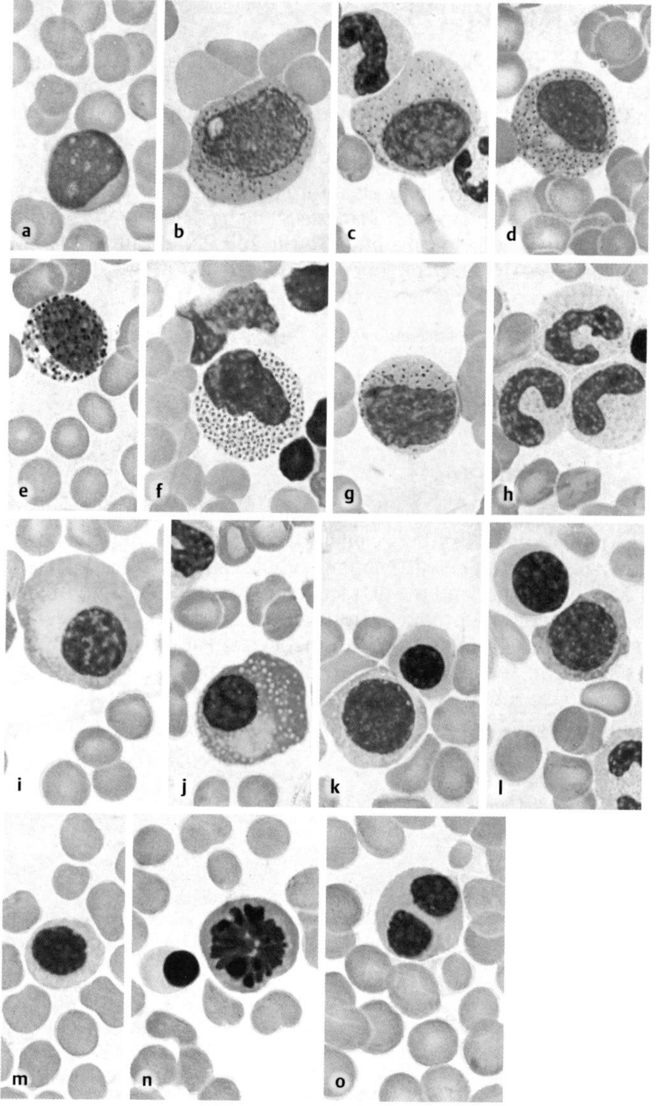

312 Thrombocytes

At about 3 μm, thrombocytes are the smallest of the blood cells. They are created as the megakaryocyte disintegrates (see Fig. 309e). Thrombocytes do not have a nucleus. In streaming blood, thrombocytes have the shape of biconcave disks. In vascular endothelium, they attach to damaged structures and in this way seal the vessels. In the process, thrombocytes are activated, change their shape and release secretory products 2, 3. One important sign of this activation is the formation of *pseudopodia*. The secretory products not only stimulate blood clotting, but also the subsequent processes of inflammation and repair. Electron micrographs usually show thrombocytes as spindle-shaped cells in cross-sections.

1 Peripheral bundle of microtubules
2 α-granules
3 Serotonin-containing granule (dense body)
Electron microscopy; magnification: × 27 600

313 Thrombocytes

The equatorial section shows the array of organelles. Particularly prominent are the many α-granules 1 as well as the sections through the open tubular systems 2. The latter consist of many tubules and vacuoles, which interconnect with each other and the extracellular space. This system influences the release of secretory products from stored secretory granules and is instrumental in the activation of thrombocytes. The peripheral layer also attracts attention. It contains a bundle of microtubules and somewhat thicker, electron-dense tubules 3, which are involved in the regulation of the Ca^{++} concentration and the prostaglandin metabolism.

1 α-granules
2 Open system of canaliculi
3 Peripheral bundles of microtubules and electron-dense tubules
4 Mitochondrion
5 Golgi apparatus
6 Pseudopodium
Electron microscopy; magnification: × 27 600

312

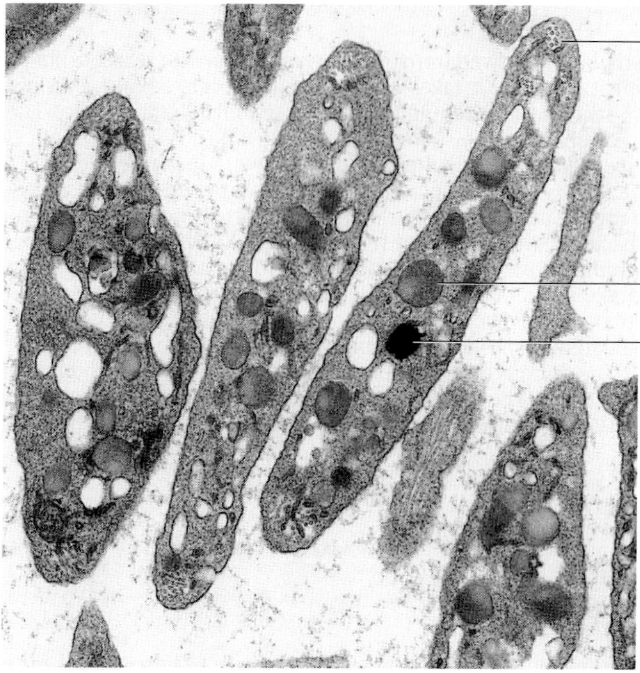

1
2
3

313

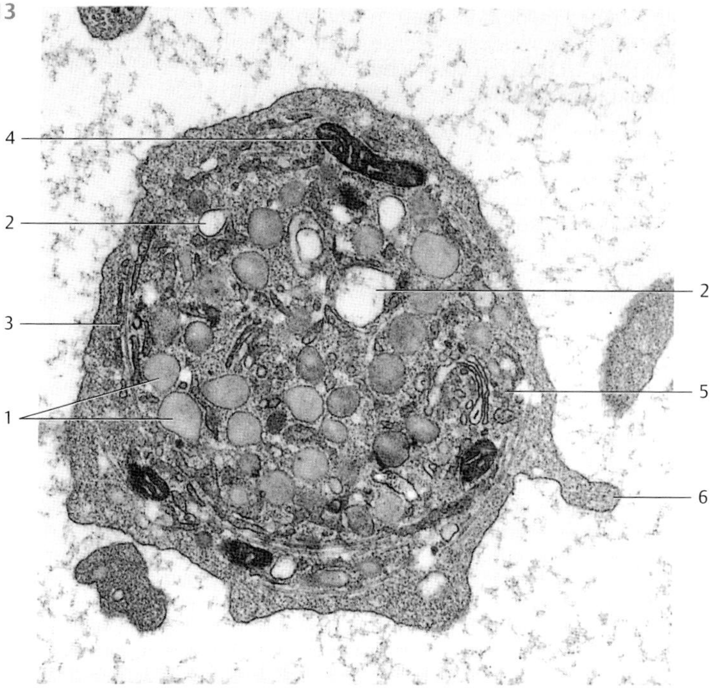

4
2
2
3
5
1
6

314 Thymus

The thymus is derived from the *pharyngeal pouch*. In relationship with other lymphatic organs, it takes a central, superordinate place. In a histological cross-section, the infantile thymus is seemingly built of lobes. Each lobule consists of a *cortex* 1 (stained blue-violet), which is rich in lymphocytes, and the *medulla* (stained lighter and reddish) with lower cell density 2. Vascularized connective tissue 3, 4 fills the spaces between lobules. It also pushes into the organ, up to the border between cortex and medulla, forming septa (trabeculae). Meshworks of reticulum cells (*epithelial reticulum cells, lymphoepithelial organ*), not fibers, form the supportive structures for cortex and medulla. The reticular cells have arisen from entodermal epithelium. Small lymphocytes (*T-lymphocytes*) predominate underneath the cortex. The medulla contains mostly lymphoblasts, lymphocytes and epithelial reticulum cells. The thymus also contains mast cells, macrophages and *interdigitating dendritic cells*. The literature often describes six different types of epithelial cells. Lymph follicles with germinal centers do not exist in the thymus.

1 Cortex
2 Medulla
3 Blood vessels
4 Connective tissue
Stain: alum hematoxylin-eosin; magnification: × 10

315 Thymus

Higher magnification of a thymus lobule with heavily stained cortex 1 and lighter stained medulla 2. Mature T-lymphocytes are densely packed in the cortex. They are much less dense in the medulla. On the right, the figure shows the vascularized connective tissue capsule 3 (cf. Fig. 314). The medulla contains *Hassall corpuscles* 4 (see Figs. 316, 317).

1 Cortex
2 Medulla
3 Capsule
4 Hassall corpuscles (bodies)
Stain: alum hematoxylin-eosin; magnification: × 80

316 Thymus

Large *Hassall corpuscle* 1 in the medullary thymus from a child. The figure shows the concentric layering of the reticulum cells particularly well (cf. Fig. 317). Note the somewhat larger epithelial reticulum cells in the medulla, which interconnect via their cell processes and form a meshwork. There are fewer lymphocytes in that area. The sectioned blood vessels 2 are filled with erythrocytes. The thymus is equipped with a *blood-thymus barrier*, which is restricted to the cortex.

1 Hassall corpuscle
2 Capillary
Stain: alum hematoxylin-eosin; magnification: × 400

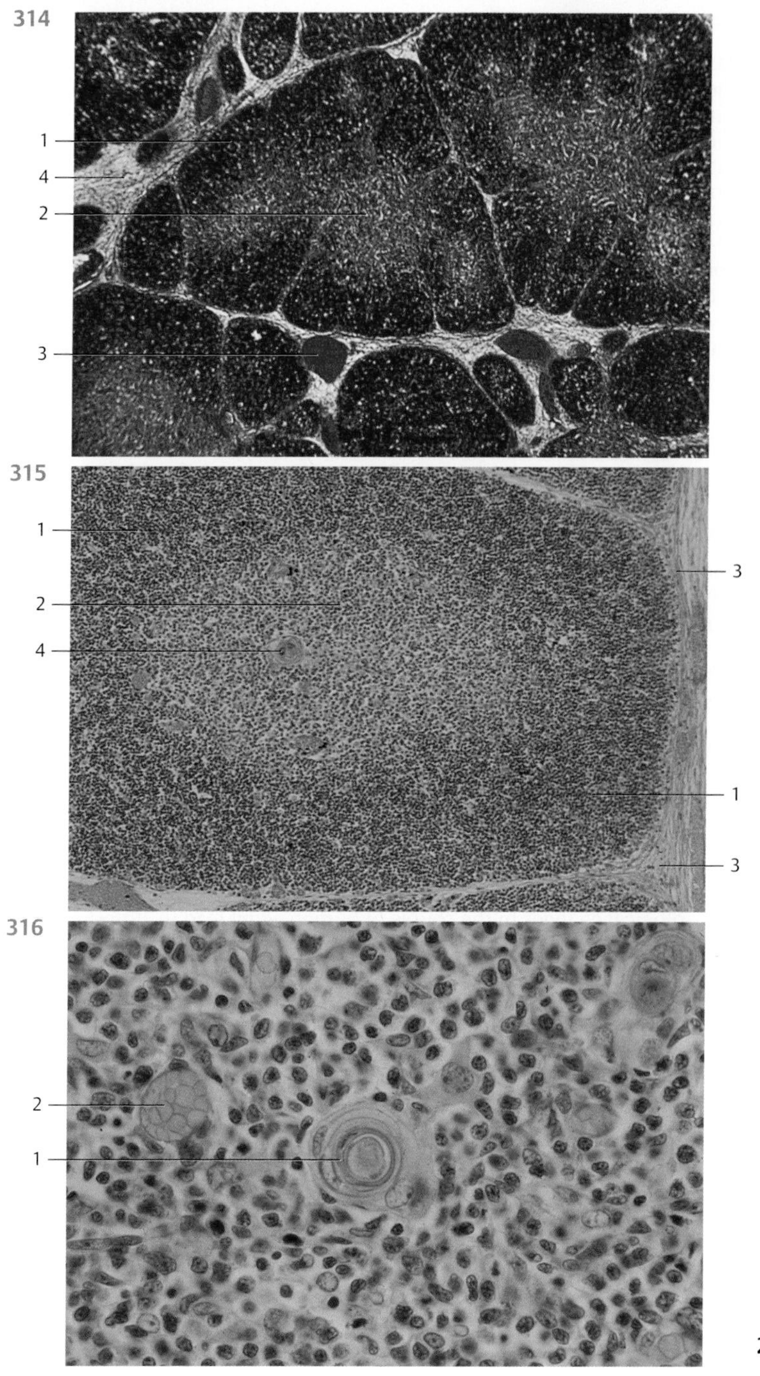
314
1
4
2
3
315
1
2
4
3
1
3
316
2
1

317 Thymus

Hassall corpuscles 2 are characteristic elements of the thymus medulla. They consist of several concentric layers of reticulum cells in an arrangement reminiscent of an onion. The reticulum cells often show hyaline degeneration. Therefore, they occasionally look homogeneous and stain intensely with eosin. Cysts may form as well. A remarkably enlarged epithelial reticulum cell usually occupies the center of the Hassall corpuscle. Medulla cells form a layer around this center. The diameter of Hassall corpuscles is 20–500 µm (cf. Figs. 315, 316). Their function is unknown. They may arise from ectodermal tissue because analytical data show prekeratin and keratin in their cells, similar to the cells of the epidermis.

Several epithelial thymus cells biosynthesize substances, which presumably have hormone character. Known, well-defined substances are *thymosin*, *thymopoietin* and *thymulin*, among others.

1 Hassall corpuscle
2 Cortex
Stain: alum hematoxylin-eosin; magnification: × 240

318 Thymus

The specific thymus tissue organization slowly disappears in puberty (*puberty involution*). In the adult thymus, lobules are no longer present. Then the fatty involution ensues (*age involution*), which initially affects the cortex more than the medulla. Finally, the residual thymus organ consists mainly of degenerated medullary tissue strands. Note the enormous increase in adipose tissue 1 (cf. Fig. 319).

1 Adipose tissue
2 Medulla with Hassall corpuscle
3 Residual cortex tissue
Stain: alum hematoxylin-eosin; magnification: × 30

319 Thymus

Physiological changes in the course of human aging lead to almost complete degeneration of the thymus (*age involution*). In the process, the cortex 1 becomes deplete of lymphocytes. The strands of tissue in the medulla become smaller and reticular connective tissue invades from the outside, to be replaced by adipose tissue 2. The result of this involution process is a residual thymus with mostly adipose tissue (*adipose thymus organ*) (cf. Fig. 318). At this stage, only scarce remnants of the specific organ tissue are left.

1 Residual thymus, cortex
2 Adipose tissue
3 Hassall corpuscles
Stain: alum hematoxylin-eosin; magnification: × 10

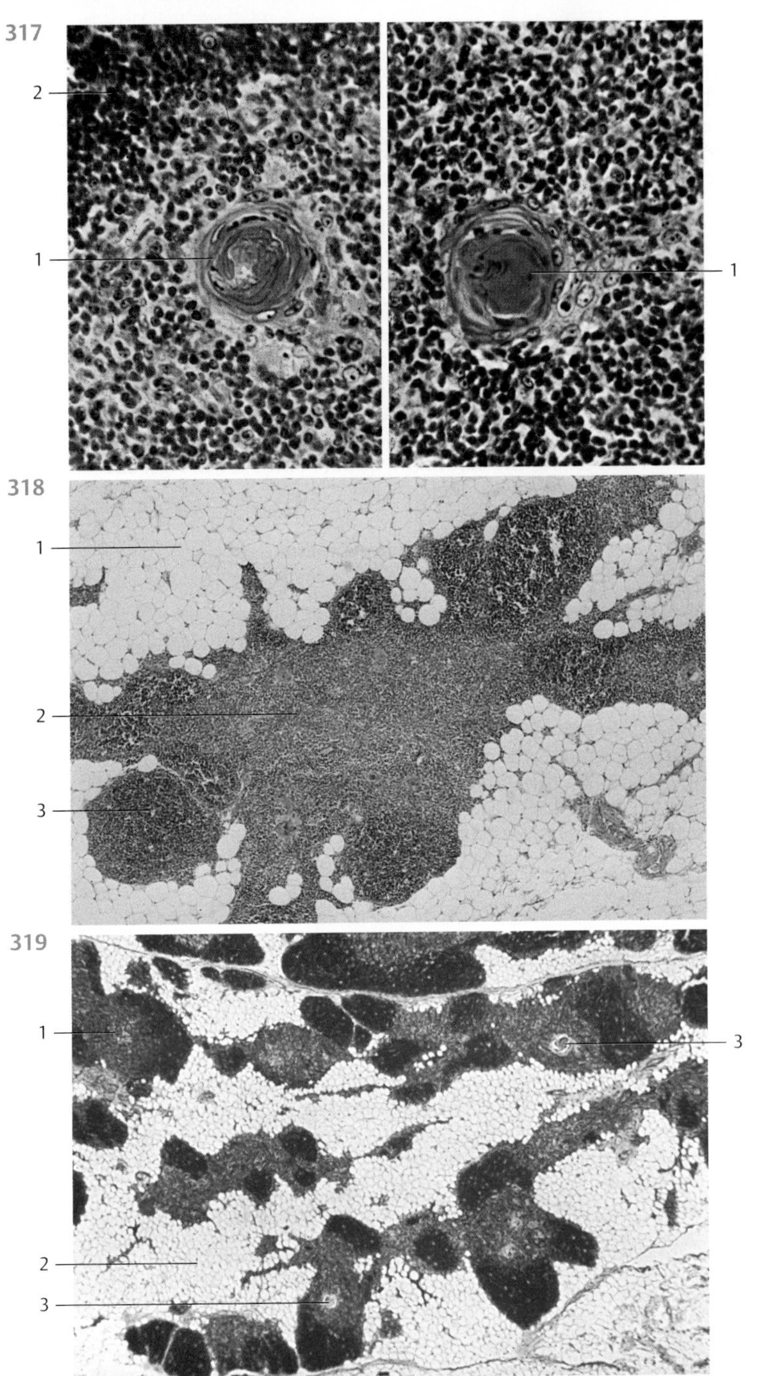
317
2
1
1
318
1
2
3
319
1
3
2
3

320 Lymph Nodes

Lymph nodes, *nodi lymphatici*, are oval or bean-shaped organs. They function as biological filters in the lymphatic circulation. Their sizes may range between several millimeters to more than 2 centimeters. They are encapsulated by connective tissue collagen fibers 1. Connective tissue divisions from the capsule, the trabeculae, extend into the interior node. Sporadic myocytes are found inside the capsule. Trabeculae form the basic skeleton of the organ. The finer network of reticulum cells and the argyrophilic fibers (reticular fibers) is interspersed with this skeleton. The web contains considerable numbers of lymphocytes and macrophages (*lymphoreticular organ*). Lymph nodes consist of the cortex 2 and inner medulla 3. Blood vessels enter at the hilus region, and efferent lymph vessels (vasa efferentia) from the lymph node exit at the hilus. Several afferent lymph vessels (vasa afferentia) pierce the capsule and bring lymph into the lymph node. The figure very clearly shows the heavily stained cortex and the lighter medulla. In the cortex, we see a large number of nodular follicles with germinal centers (*lymphatic nodules*). Please, note the central medullary sinus 4 (cf. Figs. 321–326). Human inguinal lymphatic node.

1 Capsule
2 Cortex with secondary follicles (lymphatic nodules)
3 Medulla
4 Medullary sinus
Stain: alum hematoxylin-eosin; magnification: × 20

321 Lymph Nodes

A small lymph node from a rabbit was injected with Indian ink. It is possible to clearly recognize the strong connective tissue capsule 1, the heavily stained cortex 2 with lymphatic nodules and the lighter medulla 3 as well as the finer branches of the arteries, which extend from the hilus region to the trabeculae, the medulla and, finally, to the cortex.

1 Capsule
2 Cortex
3 Medulla
Tissue injection with Indian ink; stain: hemalum-eosin; magnification: × 5

322 Lymph Nodes

Section of a lymph node. The surface is encased in a strong connective tissue capsule 1. Lymph vessels close to the lymph nodes (vasa afferentia) pierce this capsule and enter the outer cortical sinus (sinus marginalis) 2, which is clearly accentuated as a lighter crevice between capsule and cortex with only a few lymphocytes. The marginal sinus is connected to the radial structure of the trabecular sinus, which ultimately leads to the central medullary sinus 3 with its wider lumen. Lymphocyte-rich areas, named primary noduli, populate the cortex 4. The small piles of darker granules are carbon inclusions.

1 Capsule
2 Marginal sinus
3 Medullary sinus
4 Cortex
Stain: hemalum-eosin; magnification × 20

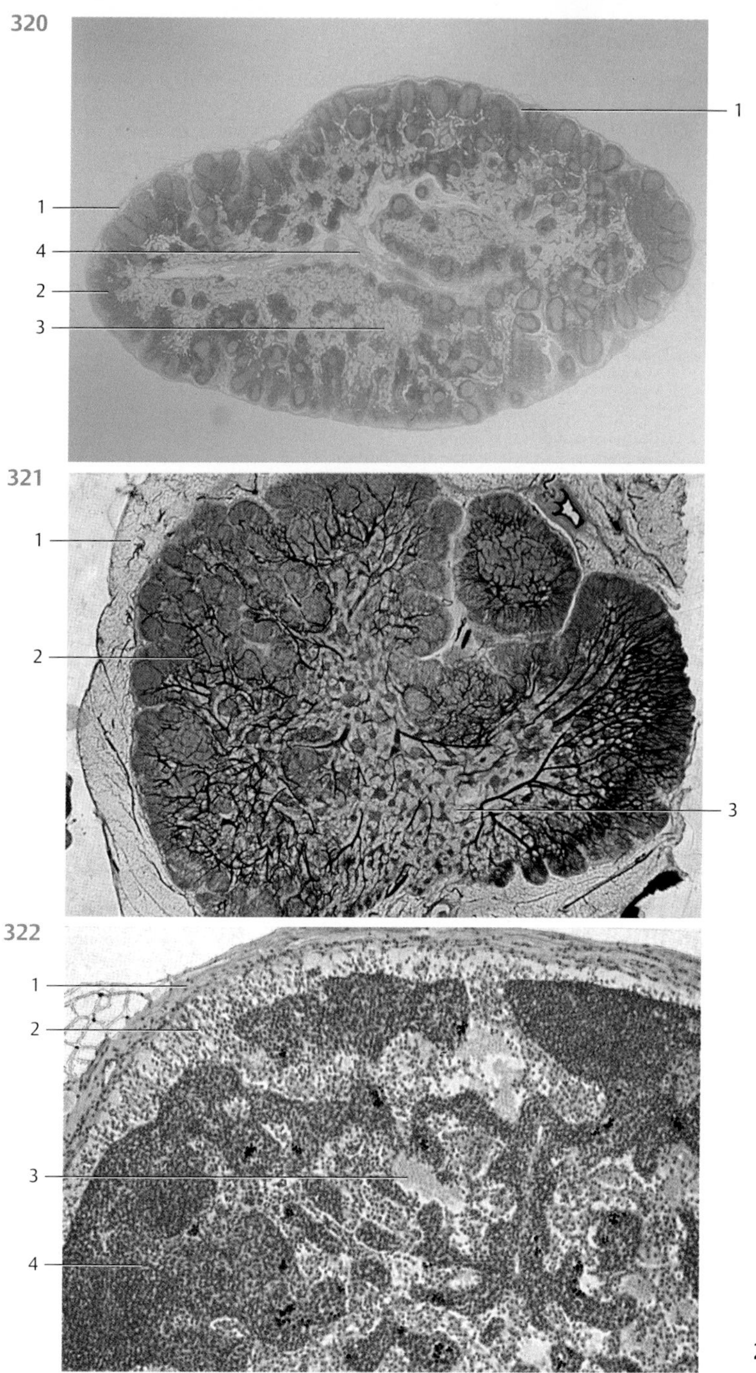
320
1
1
4
2
3
321
1
2
3
322
1
2
3
4

323 Lymph Nodes

Outer region of a lymph node from the human axilla, with a relatively tough connective tissue capsule 1, marginal sinus 2 and cortex 3 (cf. Figs. 321, 322, 324). Reticulum cells (*sinus reticulum*) and reticulum fibers are clearly visible in the *marginal sinus*. They traverse the marginal sinus and form a loose meshwork. Note the subcapsular cells, named mantle cells, which are similar to endothelial cells. Intermediary sinuses, which push through the compact cortical tissue, connect the marginal sinuses with the wide medullary sinuses. Lymphocytes are densely packed underneath the marginal sinus. They form a *secondary follicle* with a lymph corona 4 and a germinal center 5.

1 Capsule
2 Marginal sinus
3 Cortex
4 Lymph corona of the secondary follicle
5 Germinal center
Stain: alum hematoxylin-eosin; magnification: × 200

324 Lymph Nodes

Outer zone of a human inguinal lymph node. The marginal sinus (*sinus marginalis*) wraps around the lymph node immediately underneath the capsule 1 like a shell (cf. Figs. 320–323). Numerous afferent lymph vessels (*vasa afferentia*) discharge into this marginal sinus. Reticulum cells with many cytoplasmic processes span the marginal sinus. Delicate collagen and reticulum fibers (here stained light blue) lend mechanic support to the cells. A *follicle* with many lymphocytes (a *lymphatic nodule*) 3 is shown in the lower half of the figure (see Fig. 325).

1 Capsule
2 Marginal sinus
3 Lymph follicle
Stain: azan; magnification: × 400

325 Lymph Nodes

The lymphocytes in the outer layer of the cortex occur condensed in ovoid or round nodes, called follicles or *noduli lymphatici* (see Fig. 320). These follicles are the B-lymphocyte regions of the lymph node. The regions with T-lymphocytes are the diffusely delimited paracortical zones. Cortical nodes solely consist of densely packed small and medium-sized lymphocytes. They are called *primary follicles*. This preparation presents a *secondary follicle*. Apart from small lymphocytes, it contains in its center large cells with basophilic cytoplasm (*centrocytes* and *centroblasts*). These regions inside a follicle are called *germinal centers* 1. They arise from primary follicles during *immunogenesis*. A lymphocyte barrier (corona) 2 (cf. Fig. 323) surrounds the germinal center of a secondary follicle. It predominantly consists of small lymphocytes. Sporadically, plasma cells occur in the lymphocyte corona.

1 Germinal center
2 Lymphocyte corona (barrier)
Stain: azan; magnification: × 200

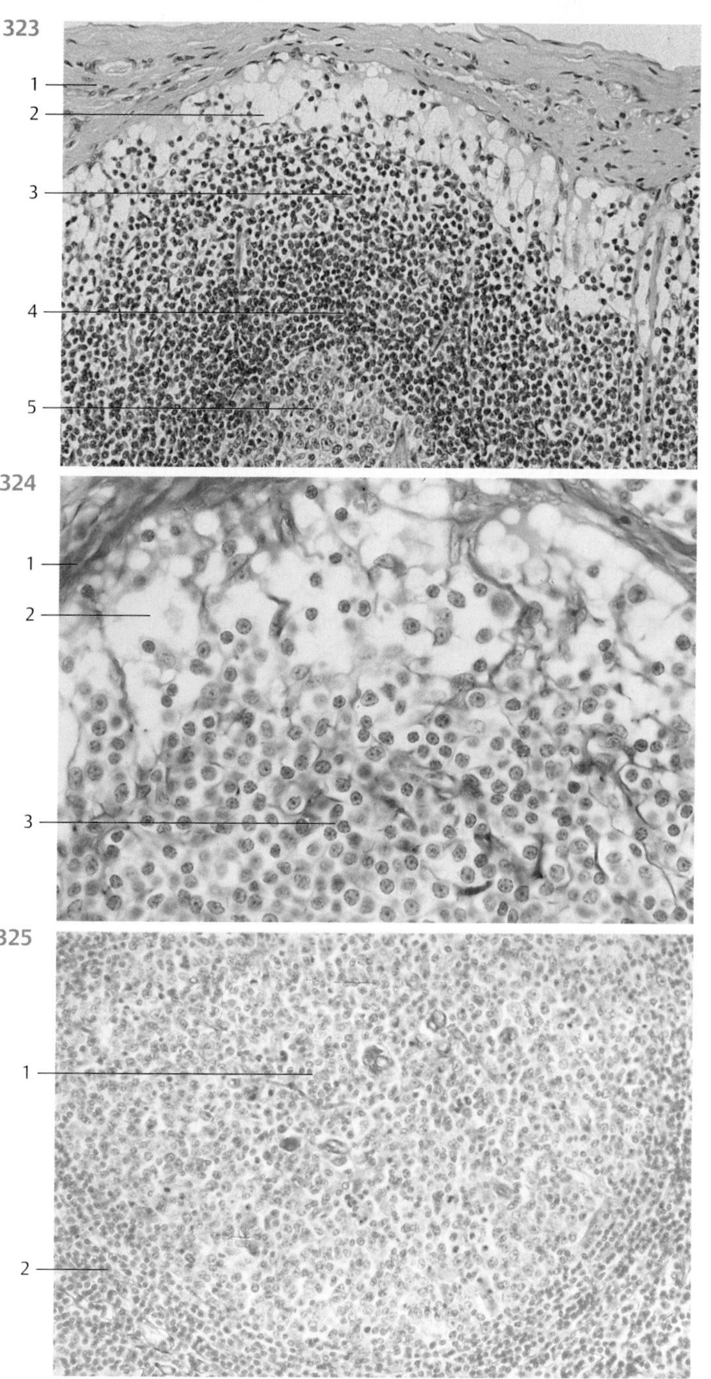
323
1
2
3
4
5
324
1
2
3
325
1
2

326 Lymph Nodes

Section of a medullary sinus from a feline lymph node. The medullary sinuses are located between medullary cords (cf. Figs. 320, 322). They connect to the marginal sinus via intermediary sinus (see Figs. 323, 324). Reticulum cells traverse the medullary sinus as well as the other lymph node sinuses. This creates a bow net system. Note the lacy web of the reticulum cells (stained light blue). Their structure is sponge-like. Lymphocytes, often macrophages, occasionally monocytes and plasma cells occur in the meshwork.

Stain: azan; magnification: × 400

327 Lymph Vessels—Collector Lymph Vessels

Lymph vessel 1 remind of thin-walled veins. They are lined by an endothelium (*lymph endothelium* 3, cf. Fig. 306), which itself is covered by a delicate layer of connective tissue. There is no basal lamina (cf. Fig. 306). With increasing size, the vessel wall also contains smooth muscle cells (*transport vessels*). Lymph vessels are equipped with overlapping flap valves and intralymphatic funnel valves (*lymphatic valve*) 2. The freely moving valve flaps stream with the lymph fluid (b). In the direction of the lymph flow, there are the following segments: extravascular lymph vessels, lymph capillaries, which usually form networks (*rete lymphocapillare*), precollector lymph vessels (diameter ca. 100 µm), *collector lymph vessels* (diameter 150–600 µm), lymphatic trunks and lymphatic ducts.
This specimen is from the splenic capsule of a bovine fetus.

1 Lymph vessels
2 Intralymphatic (funnel) valve
3 Lymphatic endothelial cells
Stain: alum hematoxylin-eosin; magnifications: a) × 120; b) × 240

328 Spleen

The spleen is the largest lymphatic organ in the human body. It is enveloped by a collagen fiber capsule 1, which has a covering of *peritoneal epithelium* (top of the figure). Irregularly arranged connective tissue cords traverse the organ, starting at the outer capsule. They are named splenic trabeculae 2 (almost unstained in this preparation) and contain the trabecular blood vessels. Richly vascularized reticular connective tissue occupies the space between splenic capsule and trabeculae. The abundance of blood explains the name red spleen pulp 3 for the flexible reticular web. The pulp contains splenic follicles 4 (stained darker blue), which in their entirety represent the *white pulp*. This white pulp forms a reticular tissue with many lymphocytes, which surrounds the vessels like a sheath. Many of these vessels are cut longitudinally in this preparation.

1 Capsule
2 Spleen trabeculae with trabecular vein
3 Red splenic pulp
4 Splenic nodule with central artery
Stain: alum hematoxylin; magnification: × 4

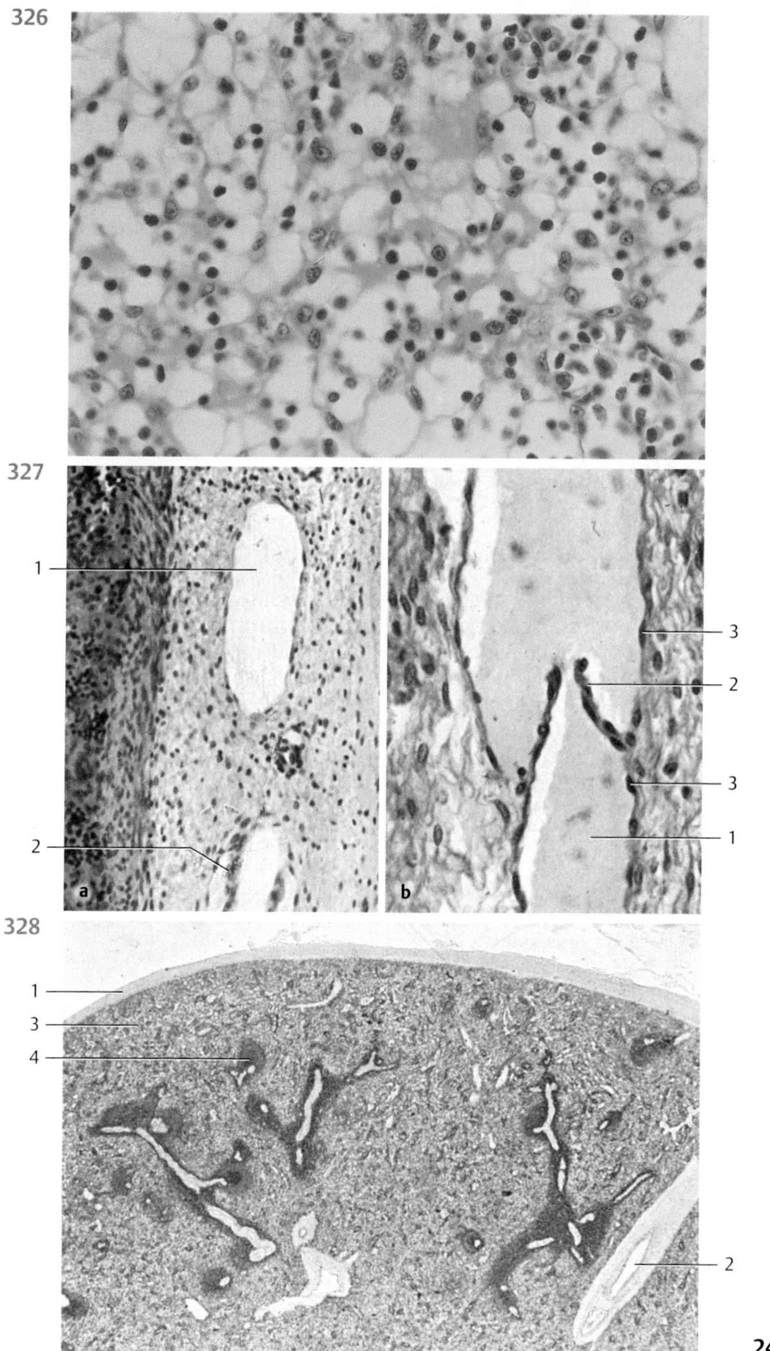
326
327
1
2
a
b
3
2
3
1
328
1
3
4
2

329 Spleen

This section shows part of a feline spleen with a splenic follicle (*spleen follicle; periarterial lymphocyte sheath*), which contains the follicular or central artery [1]. The central artery splits into 25–50 arterioles, sometimes still inside the follicle, but mostly at the exit point. The arterioles spread out like a brush or tree (*brush arterioles, penicillus*) [2]. The penicillar arterioles are covered by a spindle-shaped sheath [3] (*Schweigger-Seidel sheath, ellipsoid*) shortly after they have split off the central artery (*sheath arterioles*). The sleeve-like sheaths are hard to find in a human spleen. However, in a feline spleen they appear as prominent small follicles. They consist of dense reticular connective tissue and macrophages. The lighter stained and loosely structured areas are part of the red splenic pulp [4]. The feline spleen was perfused with physiological saline solution before specimen preparation.

1 Splenic follicle
2 Brush arteriole
3 Sleeve-like sheath
4 Red splenic pulp
Stain: methyl blue; magnification: × 10

330 Spleen

The parenchyme of the spleen consists of the white pulp (= *all lymphoreticular arterial sheaths, T-cell region*) and the red pulp [1]. This figure shows white pulp as part of a round lymph follicle (*folliculus lymphaticus splenicus*). It features a prominent *germinal center* [2]. The branches of the trabecular artery run through the follicle and are now called *follicular artery* [3] or *central artery*. There are usually two to three follicular arteries. They traverse the arterial sheaths eccentrically, especially when secondary follicles with germinal centers (B-cell regions) are present, as is the case here. A barrier of small lymphocytes surrounds the germinal center [2], which is called *corona* or *mantle zone* [4]. The area around the splenic follicle represents red pulp [1] (cf. Fig. 329).

1 Splenic red pulp
2 Germinal center of a spleen follicle
3 Follicular (central) artery
4 Corona or mantle zone
Stain: alum hematoxylin-eosin; magnification: × 100

331 Spleen

From follicular arterioles (penicillar arterioles) derive terminal capillaries, which continue in the surrounding splenic sinuses, except the marginal sinus. There, they supply anastomosing venous sinuses. Terminal capillaries can only be studied in the perfused spleen. The wall of a splenic sinus is built in the form of a grid. It consists of elongated sinus endothelium and argyrophilic fibers in a circular arrangement. The figure provides a view of the surface of the reticular connective tissue. The typical network can be seen in the top half of the figure.

Stain: alum hematoxylin; magnification: × 800

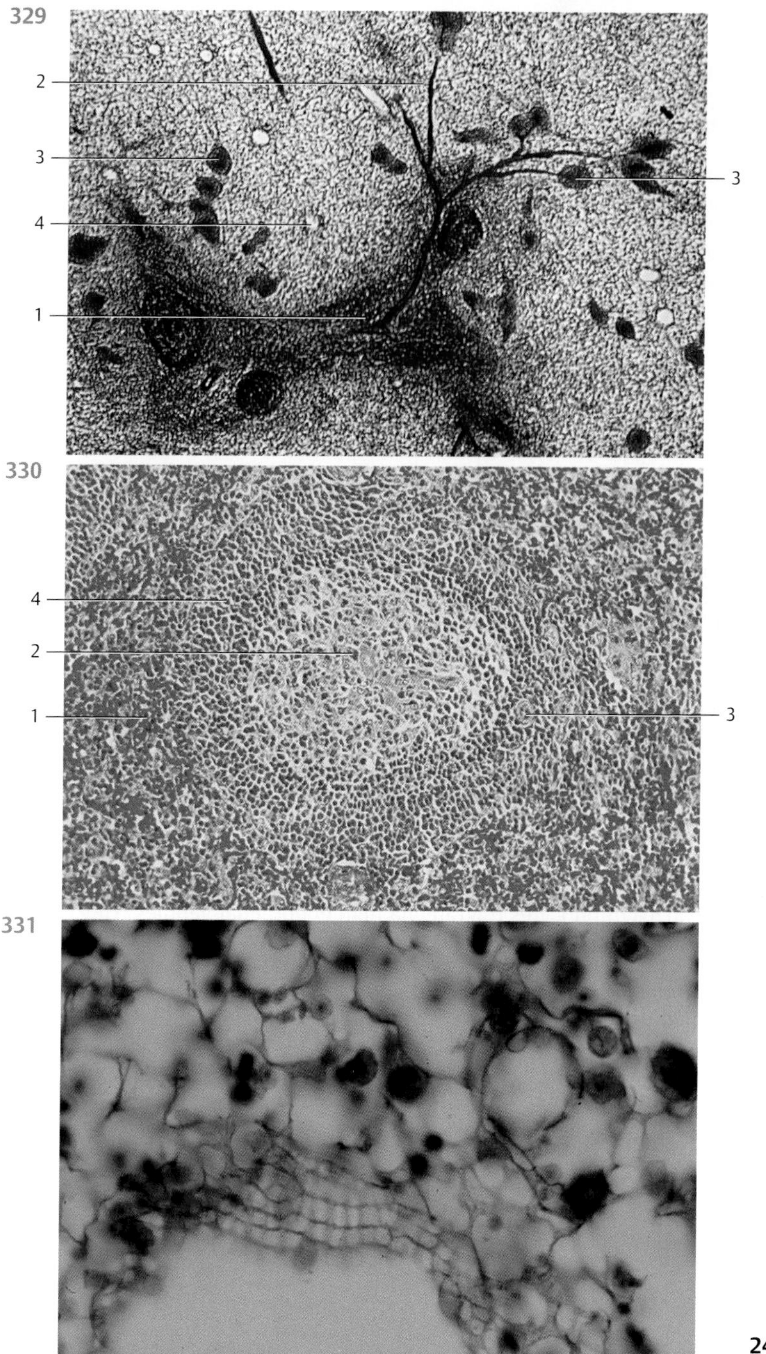
329
2
3
4
1
3
330
4
2
1
3
331

332 Spleen

This figure shows the distribution of B- and T-lymphocytes in the spleen. As shown by immunohistochemistry, B-lymphocytes (stained blue) are located mostly in follicles 1 and the marginal zone 1. The lymphatic arterial sheath 3, that is predominantly the area around the central artery, contains only few B-lymphocytes ↗.
The section following the one described in (a) shows the localization of T-cell receptors (red). They are found in large numbers in the lymphatic arterial sheaths 3. Apart from many macrophages, there are also B- and T-lymphocytes in the splenic red pulp 4.

1 Follicles
2 Marginal zone
3 Lymphatic arterial sheath
4 Red pulp. The darts show the central arteries.
Magnification: × 60

333 Lymph Nodes

This figure shows the distribution of B- and T-lymphocytes in lymph nodes. Immunohistochemistry reveals that B-lymphocytes (stained blue) occur mostly in the cortex 1 and the medulla 2. The paracortical region contains only a few B-lymphocytes, which migrate along with T-lymphocytes from the high endothelial venules 4 into the lymph node.
T-cell receptors (red) were traced in the section next to the one described in (a). They are found in the paracortex 3 in large numbers.

1 Cortex
2 Medulla
3 Paracortex
4 High endothelial venule
Magnification: × 250

334 Lymph Nodes

B- and T-lymphocytes migrate via high endothelial venules (HEV) into the lymph node. Labeled lymphocytes were injected intravenously and traced after 15 minutes using an immunohistochemical procedure (stained brown). B-lymphocytes were also identified (stained blue). This figure indicates that immediately after injection B-lymphocytes (brown and blue, darts) as well as T-lymphocytes (brown) migrate from the blood into the lymph nodes via HEV (traced with a dashed line).

Magnification: × 60

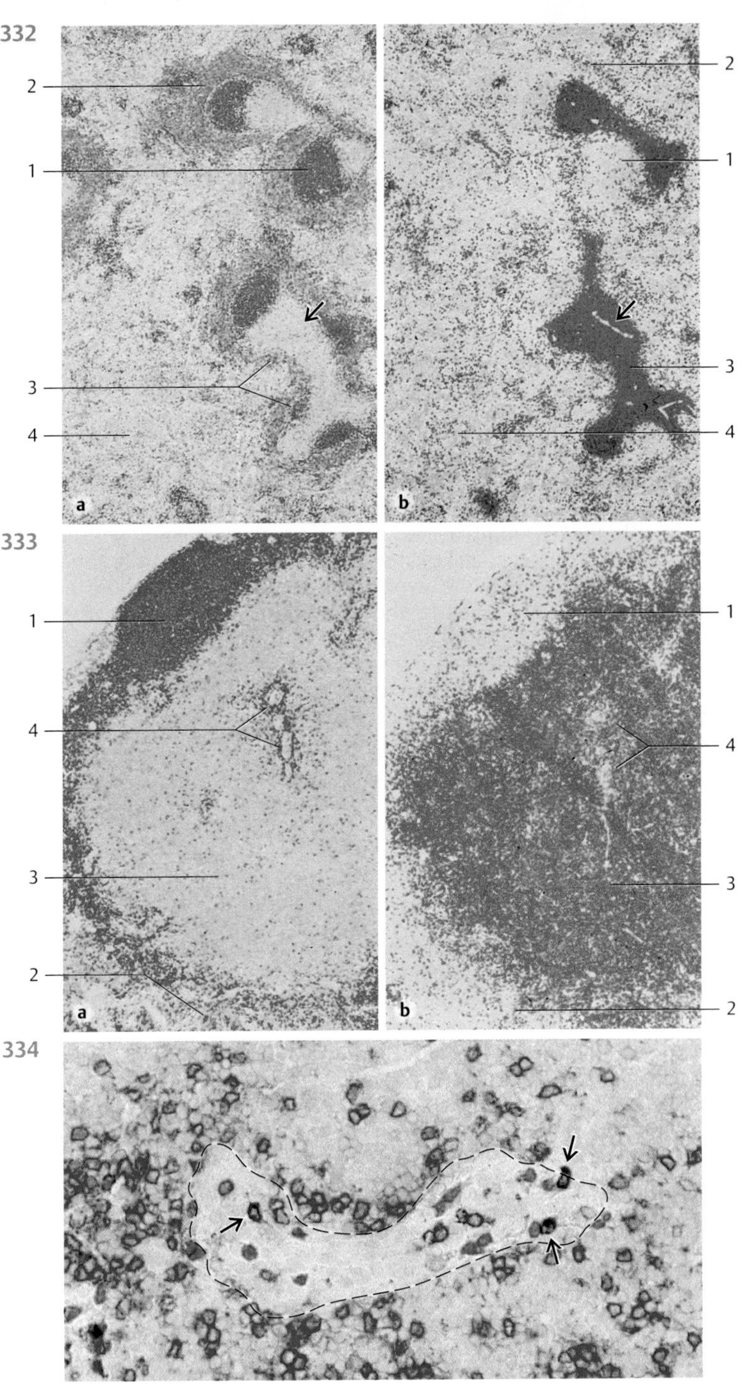
332
2
1
3
4
a
b
2
1
3
4
333
1
4
3
2
a
b
1
4
3
2
334

335 Palatine Tonsil

The palatine tonsils are covered by the mucous membranes of the oral cavity [1] (multilayered nonkeratinizing squamous epithelium). The tonsils show about 15–20 deep, often branched crypts [2] (*fossulae tonsillares*). The crypts extend deep into the lymphoreticular tissue of the tonsil. A wall of lymphoreticular tissue with secondary follicles (see Fig. 336) surrounds each crypt. A connective tissue capsule separates the palatine tonsil from the surrounding and the Killian muscle. In the figure, at the right and left, the muscles of the palatopharyngeal arch [3] are cut.

1 Epithelium of the oral cavity
2 Tonsillar crypts
3 Killian muscle, musculature of the palatopharyngeal arch
4 Connective tissue capsule
Stain: azan; magnification: × 10

336 Palatine Tonsil

Longitudinal section of a crypt from the palatine tonsil with the adjacent layer of lymphoreticular tissue, which is part of the lamina propria of the mucous membrane. The multilayered nonkeratinizing squamous epithelium [1] at the mouth of the crypt and the tonsillar surface shows hardly any lymphocytes. Only in the depth of the crypt [2] is the squamous epithelium infiltrated by lymphocytes. Consequently, the epithelium there is more loosely organized and the structural integrity of the epithelium diminished (cf. Fig. 337). The germinal centers [3] display an incomplete layer that looks like a cap [4] with the top directed toward the crypt. This layer consists of small lymphocytes (B-lymphocytes). The T-cell region is located in the interfollicular zone [5].

1 Multilayered nonkeratinizing squamous epithelium from the oral mucous membranes
2 Crypt
3 Germinal center
4 Follicle cap (B-lymphocyte cap)
5 Interfollicular areas
Stain: alum hematoxylin-eosin; magnification: × 12

337 Palatine Tonsil

Longitudinal section of the *tonsillar crypt* [1]. In the center of the figure, the structure of the multilayered nonkeratinizing squamous epithelium [2] of the oral mucous membranes is completely obliterated by lymphocytes [3]. It now has the structure of a sponge. The underlying lymphoreticular tissue [4] follows without clear demarcation. The multilayered squamous epithelium to the right and left is for the most part intact. Only a few small, heavier stained lymphocytes reside in this part of the layer. The epithelium of the adjacent crypt wall (top of the figure) appears unchanged. Inflammation (tonsillitis) may cause increased scaling of epithelial cells. This, and the increased presence of leukocytes and microorganisms of the oral cavity, can lead to tonsillar plugs (*detritus plugs*, tonsillar abscess). Occasionally, these will calcify and form tonsillar stones (cf. Fig. 336).

1 Tonsillar crypt
2 Multilayered nonkeratinizing squamous epithelium
3 Lymphocyte immigration and leukocytic diapedesis
4 Lymphoreticular tissue
Stain: azan; magnification: × 200

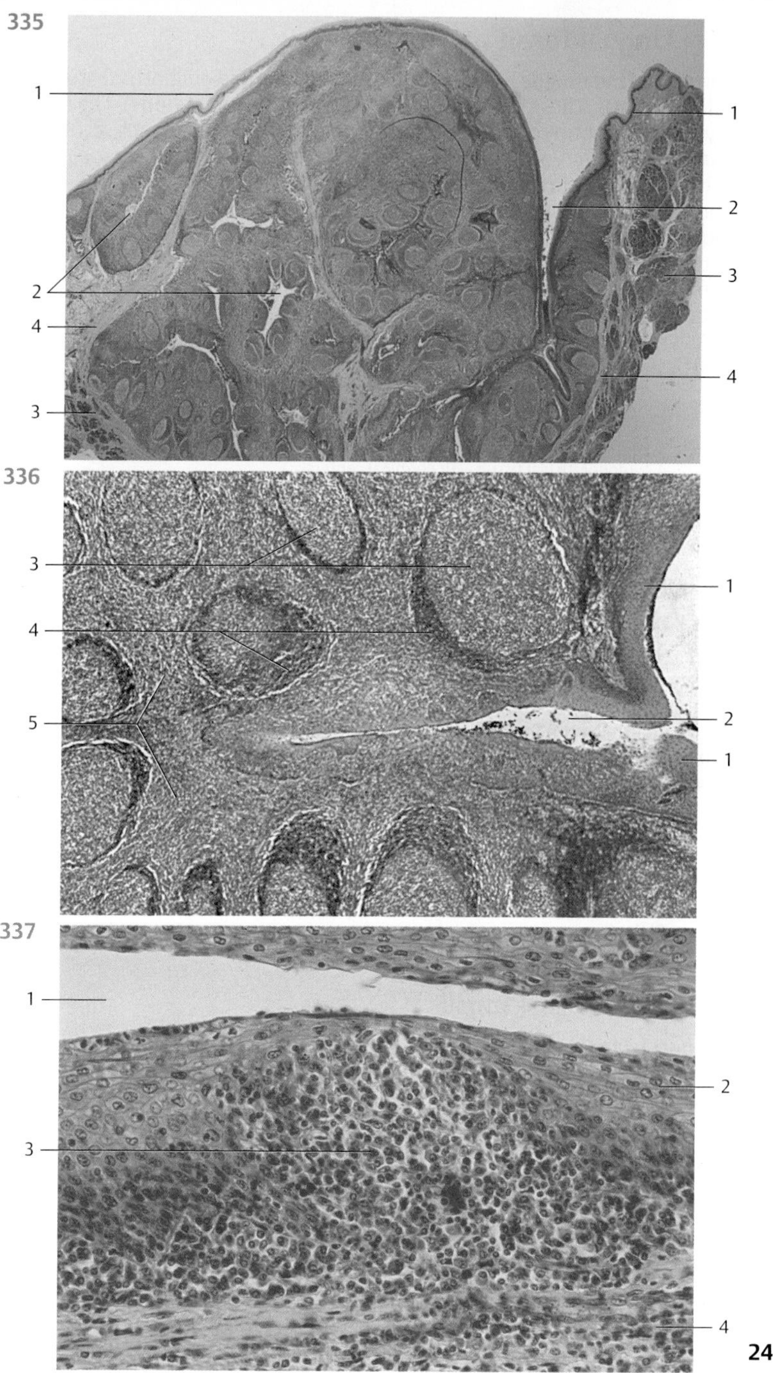
335
1
1
2
2
3
4
4
3
336
3
1
4
2
5
1
337
1
2
3
4

338 Lingual Tonsil

The root of the tongue between sulcus terminalis and epiglottis features tonsillar crypts ①. These are short narrow caverns (invaginations). The tonsillar crypts may continue in the secretory ducts of mucous glands ② or have a blind end. The crypts are lined by multilayered nonkeratinizing squamous epithelium and surrounded by lymphatic tissue.
The figure shows the multilayered squamous epithelium ③, which covers the root of the tongue and its crypts (invaginations, caverns) ①. The lymphoreticular tissue (stained deep blue) ④ underneath the epithelium is part of the lamina propria. Numerous more lightly stained areas are found in the lymphoreticular tissue. These are secondary follicles. The lymphoreticular tissue is separated from the surrounding tissue by a more or less complete connective tissue capsule ⑤.

1 Tonsillar crypts
2 Mucous glands of the root of the tongue, glandulae linguales posteriores
3 Epithelium of the lingual mucous membrane
4 Lymphoreticular tissue with germinal centers
5 Connective tissue capsule
Stain: alum hematoxylin-eosin; magnification: × 14

339 Lingual Tonsil

This vertical section through the root of the tongue shows the lingual follicles ① (see Fig. 338). The top part of the figure reveals the multilayered nonkeratinizing squamous epithelium of the root of the tongue ② and the underlying lymphoreticular tissue ①. Striated muscle fibers of the lingual musculature ④ are visible in the lower half of the image. The muscle cells are interspersed with the lobules of the posterior lingual mucous glands ⑤. The connective tissue is stained blue.

1 Lymphoreticular tissue
2 Epithelium of the root of the tongue
3 Crypt
4 Tongue musculature
5 Mucous glands
Stain: azan; magnification: × 12

340 Pharyngeal Tonsil

In contrast to the palatine and lingual tonsils (see Figs. 335–339), the epipharyngeal tonsil has a *multilayered ciliated epithelium* ①. Islands of multilayered squamous epithelium may interrupt it. This nonciliated epithelium may contain lymphocytes (cf. Fig. 337) as well. The mucous membrane forms sagittal folds, i.e., the surface is enlarged not by invaginations and tonsillar pits, but by the formation of microfolds. As in the palatine tonsil, there is a layer of lymphoreticular tissue ② with germinal centers immediately under the epithelium. The connective tissue is stained blue.

1 Multilayered stratified ciliated epithelium with goblet cells
2 Lymphoreticular tissue
3 Crypt between two microfolds of the mucous membrane
Stain: azan; magnification: × 25

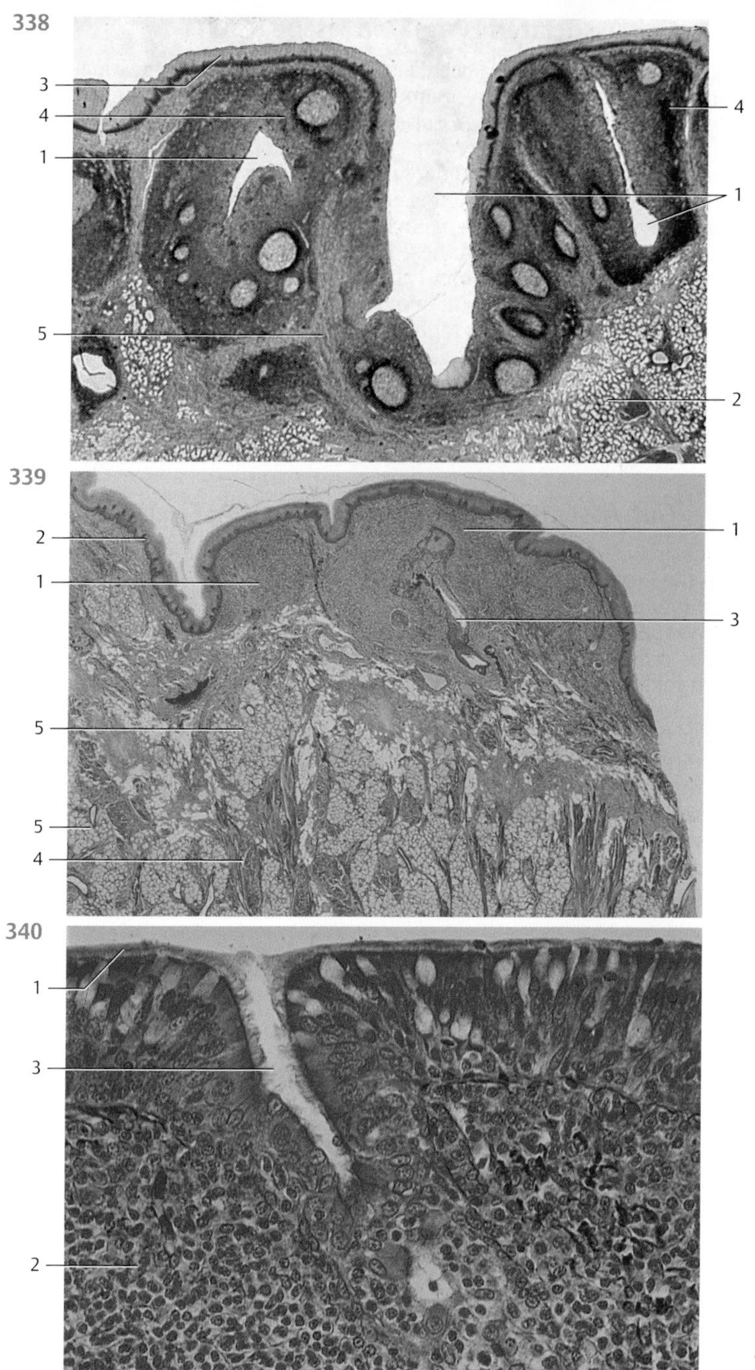
338
3
4
1
5
4
1
2
339
2
1
5
5
4
1
3
340
1
3
2

341 Gut-Associated Lymphoid Tissue (GALT)

Organized lymphatic tissue occurs in the walls of the gastrointestinal tract in multiple forms. The collective name for such lymphatic cell aggregates in the intestinal walls is GALT (*gut-associated lymphoid tissue*).
This cross-section of an appendix shows a lot of lymphatic tissue with secondary follicles ① in the submucosal tissue. Groups of T- and B-lymphocytes bulge into the intestinal lumen over each follicle. These regions are named *domes* or *dome areas* ②. Normal mucous membranes of the large intestines with crypts ③ exist between these dome areas (cf. Figs. 342, 343). A region between the follicles with densely packed small lymphocytes and postcapillary venules with high endothelium is called *interfollicular* region ④.
Vermiform appendix from a rabbit.

1 Lymph follicles, secondary follicles
2 Dome area
3 Mucous membrane of the large intestine
4 Interfollicular region
5 Tunica muscularis
Stain: azan; magnification: × 18

342 Gut-Associated Lymphoid Tissue (GALT)—Dome Areas

Dome areas ② bulge from the lymphatic tissue ① of the submucosal tissue into the intestinal lumen. In comparison with the epithelium from mucous membranes of the large intestines ③, the epithelium over the dome areas shows special attributes: there are no *microvilli*, *crypts* or *mucous-producing goblet cells*. Instead of microvilli, these specialized epithelial cells show microfolds at their surfaces (microfold cells, M-cells) (see Fig. 343). M-cells can take up antigenic materials from the lumen and transport it to the lymphatic tissue.
M-cells cannot be identified using histological routine preparations and light microscopy. M-cells from a rabbit contain a lot of *vimentin* as a component of intermediary filaments. It was therefore used here as a marker for the presence of M-cells. The immunohistochemical localization of vimentin produced black precipitates in the epithelium.
Vermiform appendix of a rabbit.

1 Lymph follicles
2 Dome areas
3 Mucous membrane from the large intestine
4 Tunica muscularis
Stain: immunohistochemical localization of vimentin; differential interference contrast imaging; magnification: × 80

343 Gut-Associated Lymphoid Tissue (GALT)—M-Cell

Dome epithelium from the *Peyer patches* (*plaques*) of the small intestines. The *M-cells* ① are interspersed with enterocytes ②. The basolateral cell surfaces form pocket-like invaginations. These pockets contain lymphocytes ③ and sometimes macrophages. Enterocytes ② show a continuous brush border of microvilli ④ (cf. Figs. 73, 75–77). In contrast, M-cells have an irregular apical surface without mucus. M-cells initiate the immune response.
Porcine small intestines.

1 M-cell
2 Enterocytes
3 Lymphocyte
4 Enterocyte microvilli
Electron microscopy; magnification: × 580

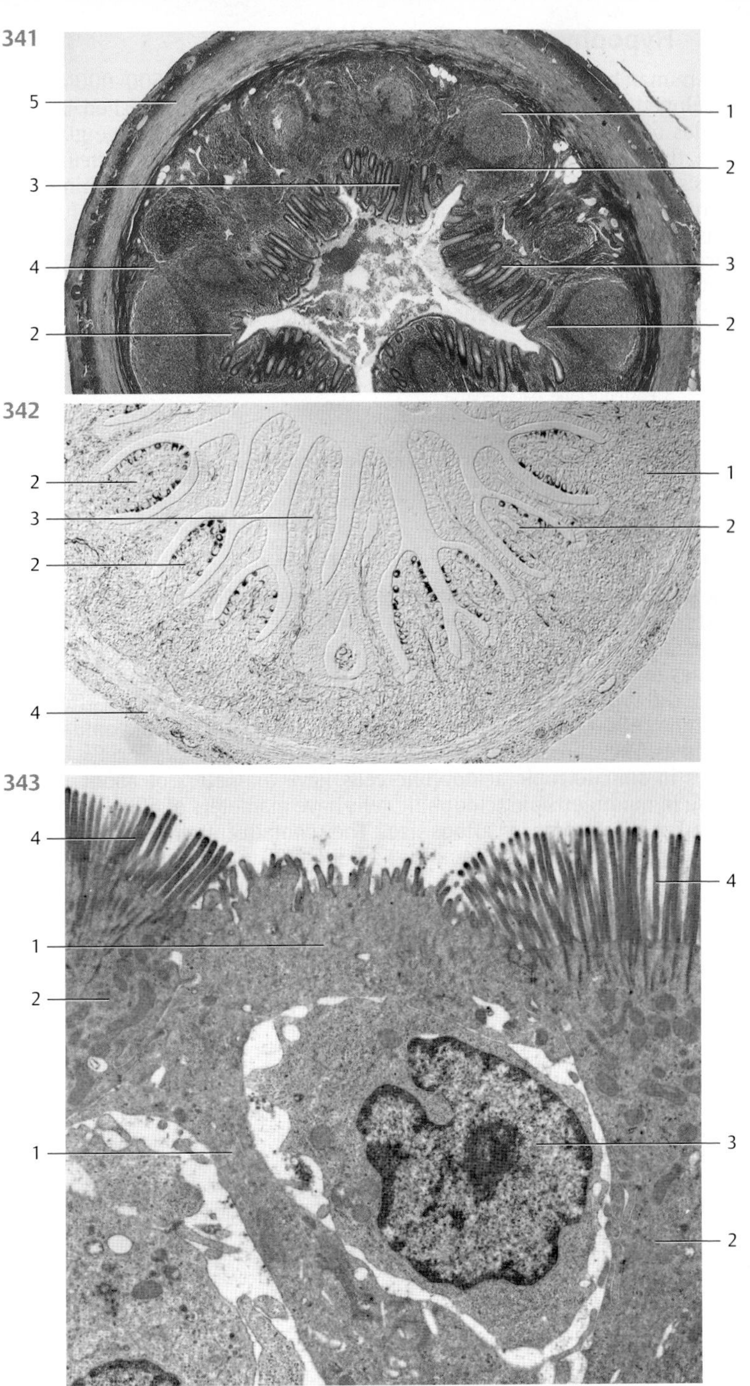
341
5
1
3
2
4
3
2
2
342
2
1
3
2
2
4
343
4
4
1
2
1
3
2

344 Hypophysis—Pituitary Gland

The human hypophysis (*hypophysis cerebri*) weighs about 600–900 mg. It is enveloped by a thin connective tissue capsule 1. Distinguished by their modes of development and detail structure, there are the large glandular lobe, the *adenohypophysis* 2, and the smaller cerebral lobe, the *neurohypophysis* 3. The adenohypophysis (anterior lobe, pars distalis) continues toward the cranium as tubular part of the hypophysis cerebri (pars infundibularis) 4. The infundibulum 5 connects the neurohypophysis (posterior lobe, pars nervosa) to the diencephalon. The *intermediary lobe* 6 between anterior and posterior lobes is part of the adenohypophysis. This sagittal section distinctly shows these different parts of the hypophysis.

1 Capsule
2 Anterior lobe, pars distalis
3 Posterior lobe, pars nervosa
4 Infundibular lobe, pars infundibularis
5 Infundibulum with eminentia mediana
6 Intermediary lobe with colloid cysts (adenohypophysis)
Stain: azan; magnification: × 7

345 Adenohypophysis—Anterior Lobe

The *anterior lobe* of the adenohypophysis (*pars distalis*) consists of cords and nests of different types of epithelial cells. These are surrounded by reticular fibers and wide blood sinuses. The cells are grouped according to their affinities to dyes as *acidophilic* 1, *basophilic* 2 or *chromophobic* 3 cells. The three cell types can be distinguished in this figure without much effort. Acidophilic cells 1 are round and contain a dense (acidophilic) population of granules. There are *somatotropic* and *mammotropic acidophilic* cells. The granules in somatotropic acidophilic cells have diameters of about 300 nm, those in mammotropic acidophilic cells have diameters of 600–900 nm. Basophilic cells 2 come in various sizes. They contain granules. There are *gonadotropic basophilic* cells (granule size: 300–400 nm), *thyrotropic basophilic* cells (granule size: 60–160 nm), *adrenotropic basophilic* cells (granule size: 200–500 nm), *lipotropic basophilic* cells (granule size: 200–500 nm) and *melanotropic basophilic* cells (granule size: 200–400 nm). According to current opinion, the chromophobic cells 3 do not participate in the biosynthesis of hormones. They are very likely precursors of hormone-producing cells.

1 Acidophilic cells
2 Basophilic cells
3 Chromophobic cells
4 Capillary
Stain: hematoxylin (Carazzi)-eosin; magnification: × 320

346 Adenohypophysis—Anterior Lobe

Section of the anterior lobe (pars distalis) from the adenohypophysis. Compare this micrograph with Fig. 345. The legend includes both commonly used terminologies.

1 α-cells (acidophilic)
2 β-cells (basophilic)
3 δ-cells
4 γ-cells (chromophobic)
5 e-cells
Stain: azan; magnification: × 400

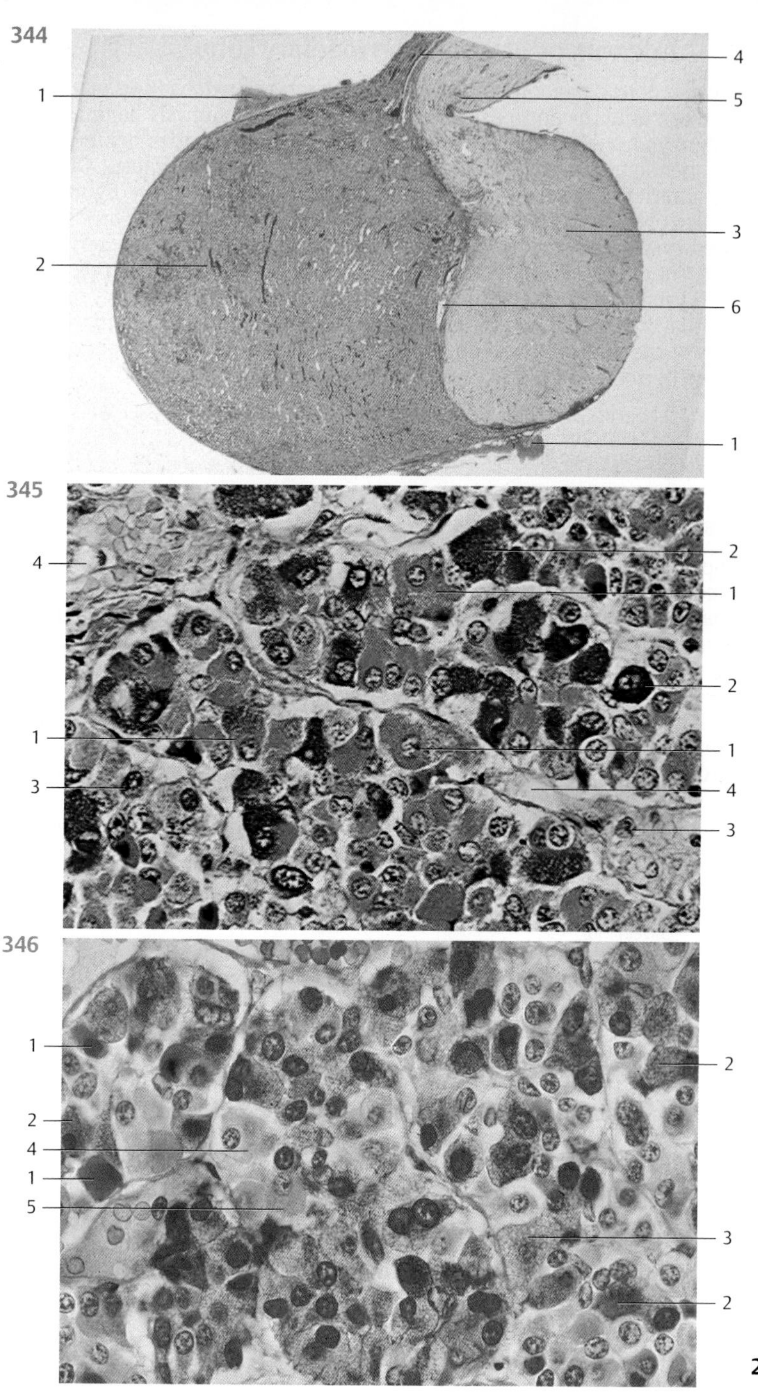

Endocrine Glands

347 Adenohypophysis—Intermediary Lobe

Because of its developmental origin, the intermediary lobe (*pars intermedia*) between anterior and posterior lobes 1 of the hypophysis belongs to the adenohypophysis (cf. Fig. 344). The intermediary lobe constitutes about 3% of the adenohypophysis. The details of its structure are very complex. Groups of the anterior lobe cells 3 are captured in the lower part of the figure. Basophilic cells may enter the dorsal hypophysis (*basophil invasion*). Colloid-filled cysts (*colloid cysts*) 2 are conspicuous elements in the intermediary lobe. They derive from the hypophyseal pouch (*remnant of the Rathke pouch*). The cysts may be lined by a single-layered epithelium or sometimes by a multilayered stratified epithelium at different levels of differentiation. The cells of the intermediary lobe synthesize *melanotropin* (melanocyte stimulating hormone, MSH).

1 Posterior lobe (pars nervosa)
2 Colloid cysts
3 Cells of the adenohypophysis

Stain: azan; magnification: × 80

348 Neurohypophysis

The neurohypophysis consists of the posterior lobe (*pars nervosa*) and the infundibulum, including the eminentia mediana (see Fig. 344).
The constituent cells of the neurohypophysis are neuroglia cells (*pituicytes, protoplasmic glial cells*), numerous unmyelinated nerve fibers, which stem from neurosecretory neurons of the hypothalamus, connective tissue and vessels. Routine staining procedures reveal a dense matted layer of fibers (a) or a woven meshwork of fine, unmyelinated nerve fascicles 1 (cross-sectioned or cut longitudinally). The meshwork of the nerve fascicles contains pituicytes and wide capillaries. Figure (b) shows numerous basophilic cells 2, which have invaded from the intermediary lobe (*basophil invasion*) into the posterior lobe. Two main neurosecretory systems exist; their morphological and biochemical attributes are different.

1 Bundles of unmyelinated nerve fibers
2 Basophilic cells, invaded from the intermediary lobe
3 Vein

Stain: alum hematoxylin-eosin; magnifications: a) × 40; b) × 100

349 Pineal Gland—Epiphysis Cerebri

The pineal gland has a conical shape. Its surface is covered by the *pia mater*. Connective tissue septa 1 originate at the pia mater and subdivide the parenchyme into incompletely separated lobes of different sizes. The pineal gland consists of *pinealocytes* (*modified photoreceptor cells*), interstitial cells and glial cells (*astrocytes*). The interstitial cells often form structures in the same way that epithelial cells do. Degeneration of the pineal gland proceeds throughout human life. It leads to the formation of a gritty substance (*acervulus*), brain sand. In this figure, the gritty substance 2 takes the form of stacked lamellae (stained red or blue), which consist of pebbles of organic substances as well as calcium and magnesium salts.

1 Connective tissue septa
2 Gritty substance of the pineal gland (acervulus)

Stain: azan; magnification: × 150

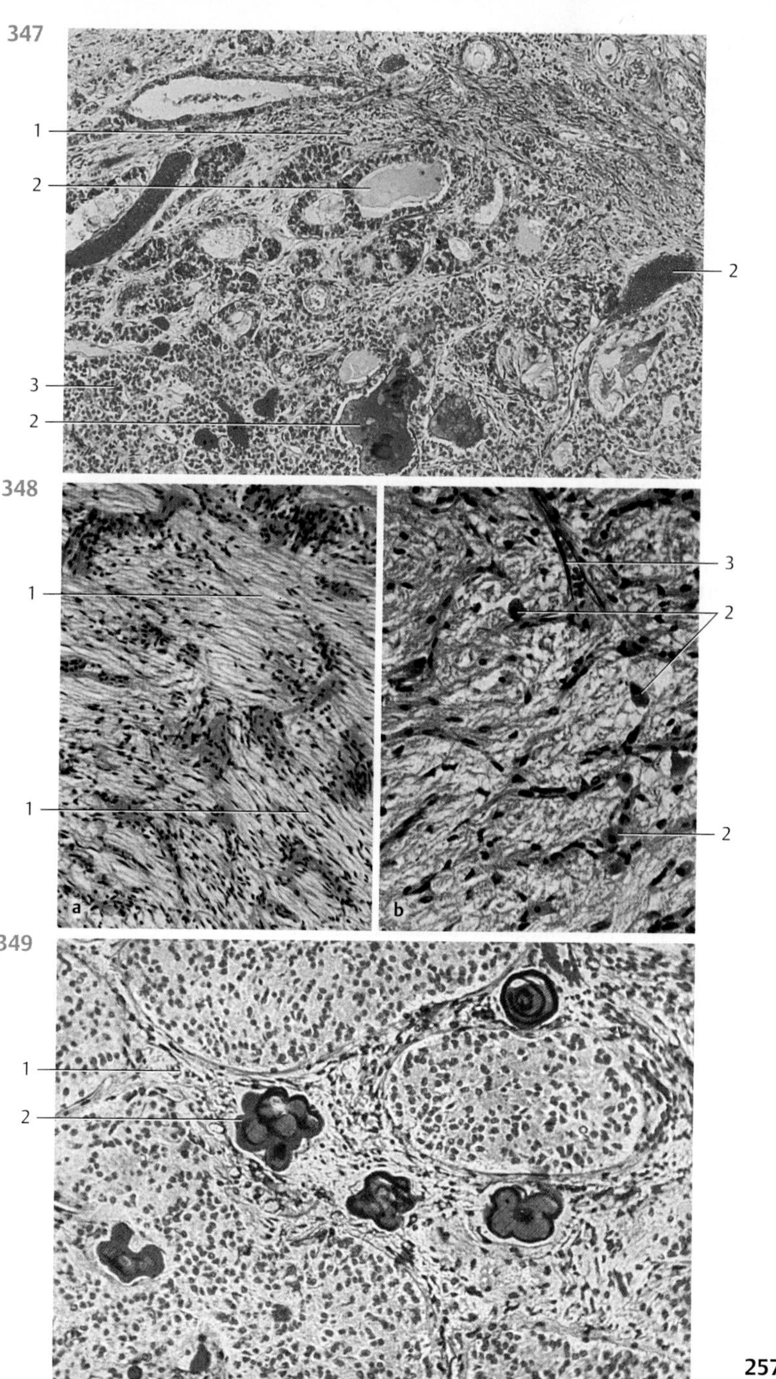
347
1
2
2
3
2
348
1
1
a
b
3
2
2
349
1
2

350 Pineal Gland—Epiphysis Cerebri

The specific cells of the pineal gland are the *pinealocytes* 1. They usually have a bizarre geometry, although some may appear rounded or polygonal. Their nuclei have little chromatin. Pinealocytes have numerous branched cell processes with synaptic ribbons in close proximity to blood vessels. As is the case in the neurohypophysis, there are nerve-blood contact zones. In addition, the epiphysis contains contact neurons in the pineal recess. The pinealocytes 1 in this figure are embedded in a meshwork of glial cells 2.

1 Pineal cells
2 Meshwork of glial cells
Stain: azan; magnification: × 400

351 Adrenal Gland—Glandula Suprarenalis

The furrowed surface of the adrenal gland (suprarenal gland) is encased in a vascularized connective tissue capsule 1. The adrenal gland consists of the *cortex* 2 and the *medulla* 3. The zona reticularis 4 of the cortex is emphasized as a heavily stained dark band. This band makes the border between cortex and medulla particularly obvious in this preparation. A large muscular vein 3 in the medulla is cut (cf. Fig. 357).
Cortex and medulla are of different phylogenetic origin and have distinct functions within the organ.

1 Organ capsule
2 Cortex
3 Medulla with vein
4 Zona reticularis
5 Adipose tissue
Stain: alum hematoxylin-eosin; magnification: × 4

352 Adrenal Gland—Glandula Suprarenalis

The adrenal gland is enveloped by a fiber-rich connective tissue capsule 1. Above it, there is a layer of vascularized loose connective tissue with many adipocytes. The *zona glomerulosa* 2 is the outermost narrow layer of the cortex. The epithelial cells in this zone have formed round aggregates or nests. The underlying cells are part of the wide *zona fasciculata* 3. The cells are arranged in lightly stained strands and columns. The *zona reticularis* 4 follows without demarcation. It is a loose web-like tissue (cf. Fig. 353c), which borders on the medulla. Part of the ectodermal medulla 5 is visible on the right of this figure.

1 Capsule
2 Zona glomerulosa
3 Zona fasciculata
4 Zona reticularis
5 Medulla
6 Medullary vein
Stain: azan; magnification: × 25

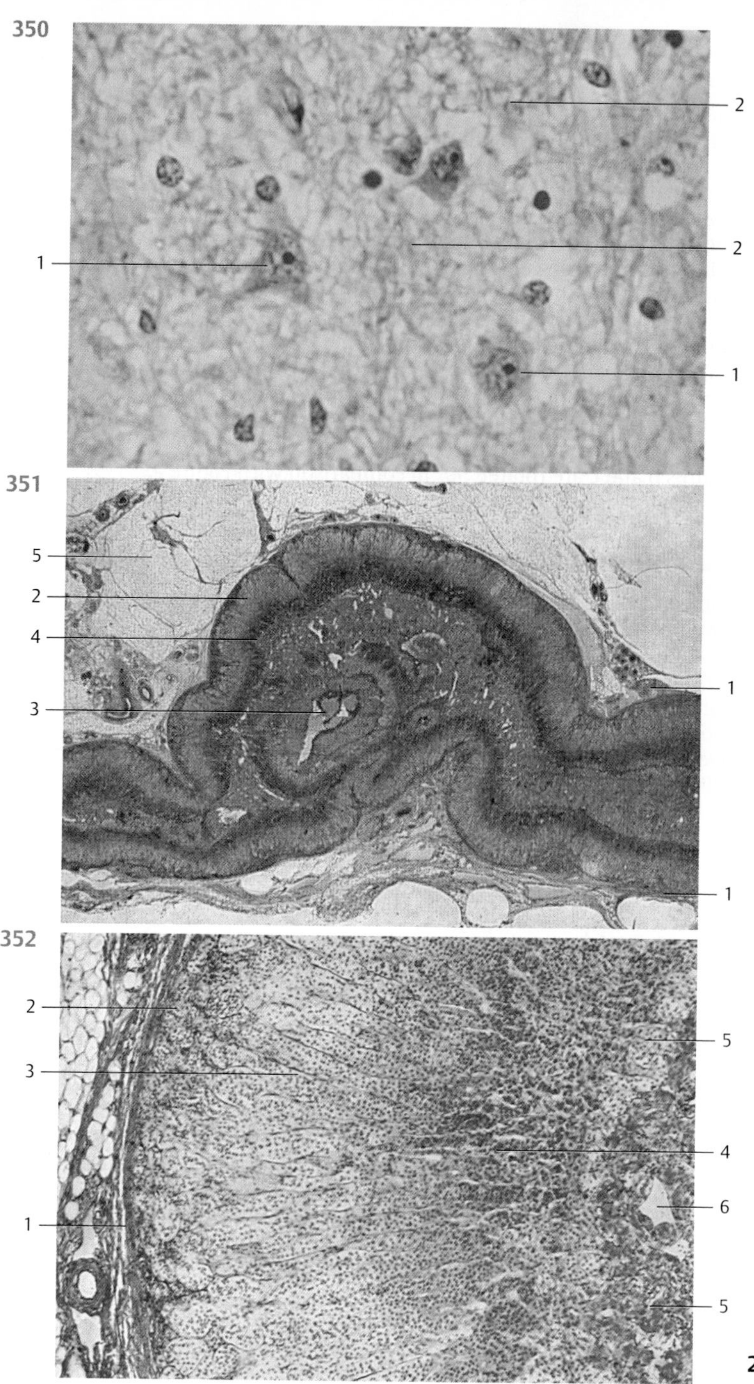
350
2
2
1
1
351
5
2
4
3
1
1
352
2
3
1
5
4
6
5

353 Adrenal Gland—Glandula Suprarenalis

a) *Zona glomerulosa, zona multiformis.*
The fiber-rich organ capsule can be found at the left edge of the microphotograph. The round or oval groups of cells and cell nests in the following cortical layer are the glomeruli. The right part of the figure shows part of the zona fasciculata.
b) *Zona fasciculata.*
The top half of the figure shows the large columnar cells, which are only lightly stained. The cells are evenly filled with small lipid droplets (honeycomb structure, spongiocytes). The cell cords in the lower part of the image are more loosely arranged. The cells are smaller and contain pigments. The pigments make the cells appear darker.
c) *Zona reticularis.*
The sizes of cells in this layer may vary. Its cell cords are arranged in a loose web-like structure. Sinusoid blood vessels and strong connective tissue trabeculae are found between cells.
Figures b and c are rotated 90° in comparison with Figure a.

Stain: azan; magnification: × 100

354 Adrenal Gland—Glandula Suprarenalis

The connective tissue capsule 1 of the adrenal gland contains nerves and blood vessels. The small rounded groups of cells of the *zona glomerulus* are located underneath it (cf. 353a). The large round nuclei of the glomerular cells are heavily stained. The lipid droplets in the cells have been removed during preparation. This has left empty, vacuole-like spaces in the place of fat droplets in the acidophilic cytoplasm (cf. Fig. 63). Strands of delicate connective tissue start at the organ capsule and continue between the glomerular cells. They contain wide sinusoid blood vessels 2. Note the button-shaped endothelial cells, which push into the lumen.
Cells in the zona glomerulosa mostly biosynthesize mineral corticoids, which predominantly regulate the potassium and sodium balances. The most important mineral corticoids are aldosterone and deoxycorticosterone.

1 Connective tissue capsule
2 Sinusoids
Semi-thin section; stain: methylene blue-azure II; magnification: × 800

355 Medulla of the Adrenal Gland

The medulla of the *suprarenal gland* is derived from *sympathochromaffin* tissue. It is therefore a *sympathetic paraganglion*. The polygonal cells 1 are arranged in cords and show a fine granulation. Due to their affinity to chromium salts, the cells are often called *chromaffin* or *pheochrome* cells. Their secretory granules contain adrenaline or noradrenaline. The medullary cell nests (cell clusters) 1 are pervaded by large, strong muscular veins 2 (cf. Fig. 357). All cells of the medulla have immediate access to capillaries and venules. The medulla contains autonomous multipolar sympathetic ganglion cells 3, either singly or as clusters. Unmyelinated nerve fibers are seen at the left edge of the figure.

1 Cords of chromaffin medullary cells
2 Medullary veins
3 Multipolar ganglion cells
4 Cushion of smooth muscle cells, smooth muscle prominence
Stain: alum hematoxylin-eosin; magnification: × 40

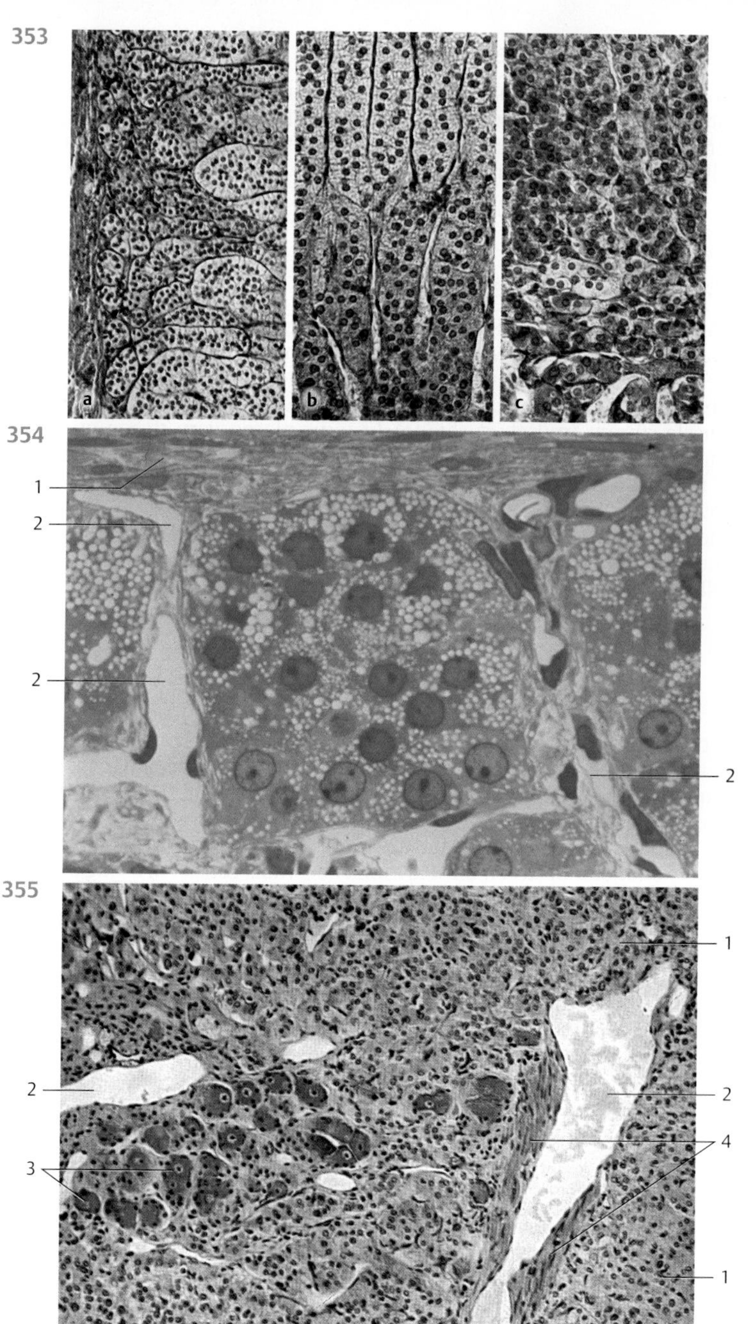

Endocrine Glands

356 Medulla of the Adrenal Gland

Most of the medullary parenchyme of the adrenal gland (suprarenal gland) consists of *chromaffin* or *pheochrome cells*. There are also multipolar sympathetic ganglion cells [1] with long cell processes and satellite cells. Ganglia cells occur singly or in small clusters.

Stain: azan; magnification: × 400

357 Medulla of the Adrenal Gland

The adrenal gland is a richly vascularized organ. There are connections between the vascular networks of the cortex and medulla. Having passed the medullary sinuses, the venous blood accumulates in the throttling veins, which are characterized by irregularly arranged subendothelial longitudinal muscle strands (muscle cushions). In some places, very strong underlying muscles may cause the venous walls to bulge into the lumen. The contraction of muscles underneath the tunica intima presumably throttles the blood flow in the capillaries, which supply the surrounding tissue.
The figure shows a throttling vein in the adrenal medulla and its powerful muscle bulges [1]. Note the cross-sectioned smooth muscle cells. The muscle cells run parallel to the longitudinal axis (cf. Figs. 284, 285).

Stain: hematoxylin-eosin; magnification: × 80

358 Thyroid Gland

In contrast to other endocrine glands, the thyroid gland stores large amounts of its hormone-containing secretory product in the extracellular space. Consequently, the ultrastructure with its irregular lobes and follicles looks more like that of an exocrine gland.
The follicles of the thyroid gland are round, ovoid or tube-like hollow organs with a diameter between 0.1–0.8 mm. Their walls consist of a single-layered epithelium (see Fig. 362). The height of this epithelium depends on the functional status of the follicle. The epithelium is isoprismatic (cuboidal) in the inactive thyroid gland and the spaces are filled with secretory product (colloid) (a). The secretory product contains the thyroid hormones T_4 and T_3 in an inactive, glycoprotein-bound form. The height of the epithelium increases with increasing secretory activity (b). The follicles here are free of colloid.
The epithelial cells of thyroid follicles have a polar structure. The apical surface is covered with microvilli of various lengths (see Figs. 361, 362). This is the site where secretory vesicles are released or retrieved by the cell. Note that the thyroid follicles are surrounded by vascularized connective tissue (stained blue) (cf. Figs. 160, 362). Parafollicular cells (C-cells) (see Fig. 361) are found in the epithelium. They have no contact to the colloid bodies.

Stain: azan; magnification: × 300

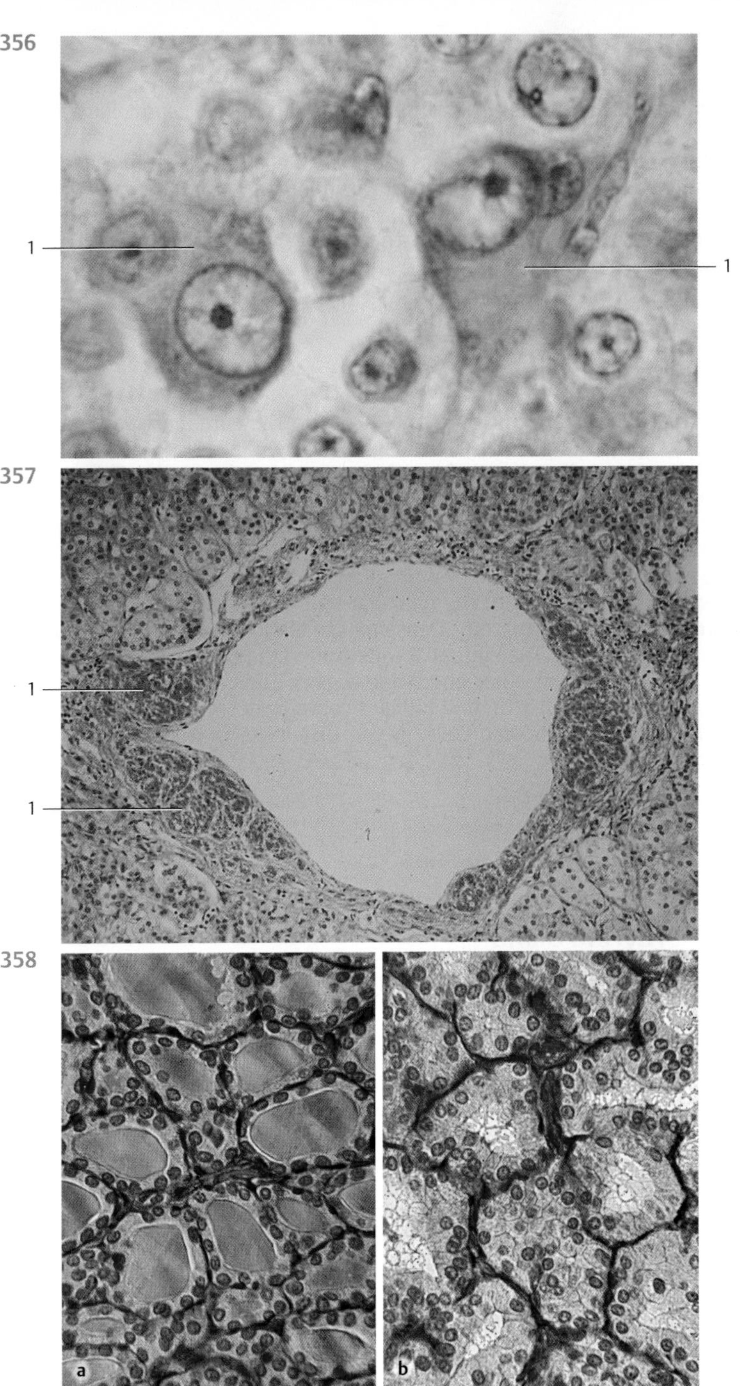

Endocrine Glands

359 Thyroid Gland

Thyroid follicles are lined by a single-layered isoprismatic (cuboidal) epithelium with round nuclei. Their lumina contain *homogeneous colloid* material (cf. Fig. 358a). The clearly defined cells are lightly stained. A capsule with an outer and inner lamina encloses the thyroid gland, as seen in other organs. Strands of connective tissue start at the inner lamina and pervade the gland. This creates a lobular structure. A basal membrane and a dense meshwork of fenestrated capillaries and sympathetic nerve fibers encircle the thyroid follicles.

Stain: iron hematoxylin; magnification: × 200

360 Thyroid Gland

Thyroid follicles are mostly round or ovoid. They are encased by a single-layered epithelium 1 of various heights (cf. Figs. 358–362). First, a liquid secretion of low viscosity is released into the follicular lumen. This secretory product is called *colloid* (mostly thyroglobulin) 2. It is the carrier for thyroid hormones. *Colloid secretion* leads to the storage of thyroid hormones inside the follicle (thyroid hormone is entrapped in a thyroglobulin scaffolding). In the process, the heights of the epithelial cells decrease (see Fig. 358, 359). The basal lamina underneath the follicular epithelium can only be seen on the level of electron microscopy. Dense nets of blood and lymph capillaries surround the follicles. The epithelial cells around the capillaries are fenestrated 3, as is the case in other endocrine organs. The connective tissue 4 (see Fig. 160) between the thyroid follicles contains nerve fibers. C-cells 6, also known as parafollicular cells, occur dispersed in the epithelium (see Fig. 361).

1 Follicular epithelium
2 Colloid
3 Fenestrated capillaries
4 Connective tissue
5 Connective tissue cells
6 C-cells

Electron microscopy; magnification: × 2300

361 Thyroid Gland

This figure shows a section from the wall of a thyroidal follicle. Four follicles 1 are cut. Their lumina are filled with colloid 2 (cf. Figs. 359, 360). Microvilli extend from the epithelial surfaces into the follicle lumina. The cytoplasm contains regions with elaborate ergastoplasm 3, Golgi complexes 4 and secretory granules. The cell on the right displays the entire nucleus. There is a web of terminal bars (terminal complexes) at the apicolateral surfaces of epithelial cells, which border at the follicular lumen. A large C-cell (*parafollicular cell*) 5 is seen in the lower part of the figure. C-cells originate with the ultimobranchial body and have developed as part of the thyroid gland. Their important attribute is the presence of secretory granules. The granules have diameters of 100 to 180 nm and contain the hormone calcitonin. Calcitonin consists of 32 amino acids.

1 Follicular epithelium
2 Colloid
3 Ergastoplasm
4 Golgi apparatus (complexes)
5 C-cell
6 Connective tissue

Electron microscopy; magnification: × 5520

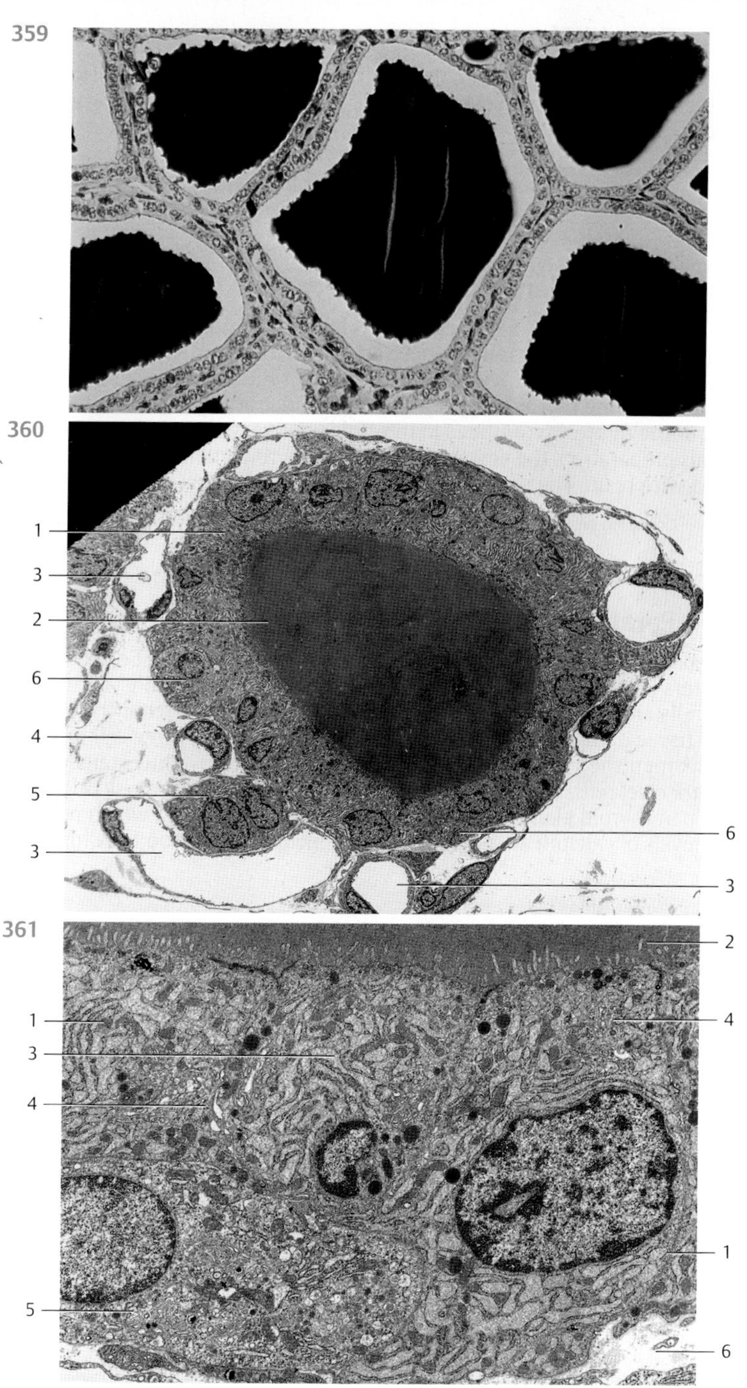

359
360
1
3
2
6
4
5
3
6
3
361
2
1
4
3
4
1
5
6

362 Thyroid Gland

This view into three sectioned thyroid follicles shows the polygonal follicular epithelial cells. They are covered with short microvilli. There are residual secretory products.

1 Cut surface of the follicular epithelium
2 Vascularized connective tissue lining of the follicle (cf. Fig. 160)
Scanning electron microscopy; magnification: × 1800

363 Thyroid Gland—Capillary Network

An extraordinarily rich vascularization is the common characteristic of all endocrine organs. A capillary network encircles the thyroid follicles (see Fig. 360). This figure provides a vivid image of the capillary network at the surface of feline thyroid follicles. An interlobular artery is seen in the lower part of the figure. It continues in interfollicular vessels.
In this preparation, the vessel system of the thyroid gland was only partially filled with resin. The capillary network is in reality much more elaborate.

Corrosion preparation (cf. Fig. 303, 304); scanning electron microscopy; magnification: × 250

364 Parathyroid Gland

The parathyroid glands (*glandulae parathyroideae*) consist of epithelial cell clusters that are about as big as a wheat kernel. They are richly vascularized. Fat cells and an occasional colloid-containing follicle interrupt the parathyroid tissue organization. Based on their affinity to dyes, three cell types can be distinguished in light microscopy: 1, *clear chief cells* (lightly stained cells); 2, *dark chief cells;* and 3, *oxyphilic cells* (*chromophilic cells, Welsh cells*).
The parathyroid glands biosynthesize *parathormone* (PTH), which regulates the levels of calcium and phosphate ions, including the blood calcium level.

1 Oxyphilic cell
2 Main light cell
3 Connective tissue
Stain: azan; magnification: × 400

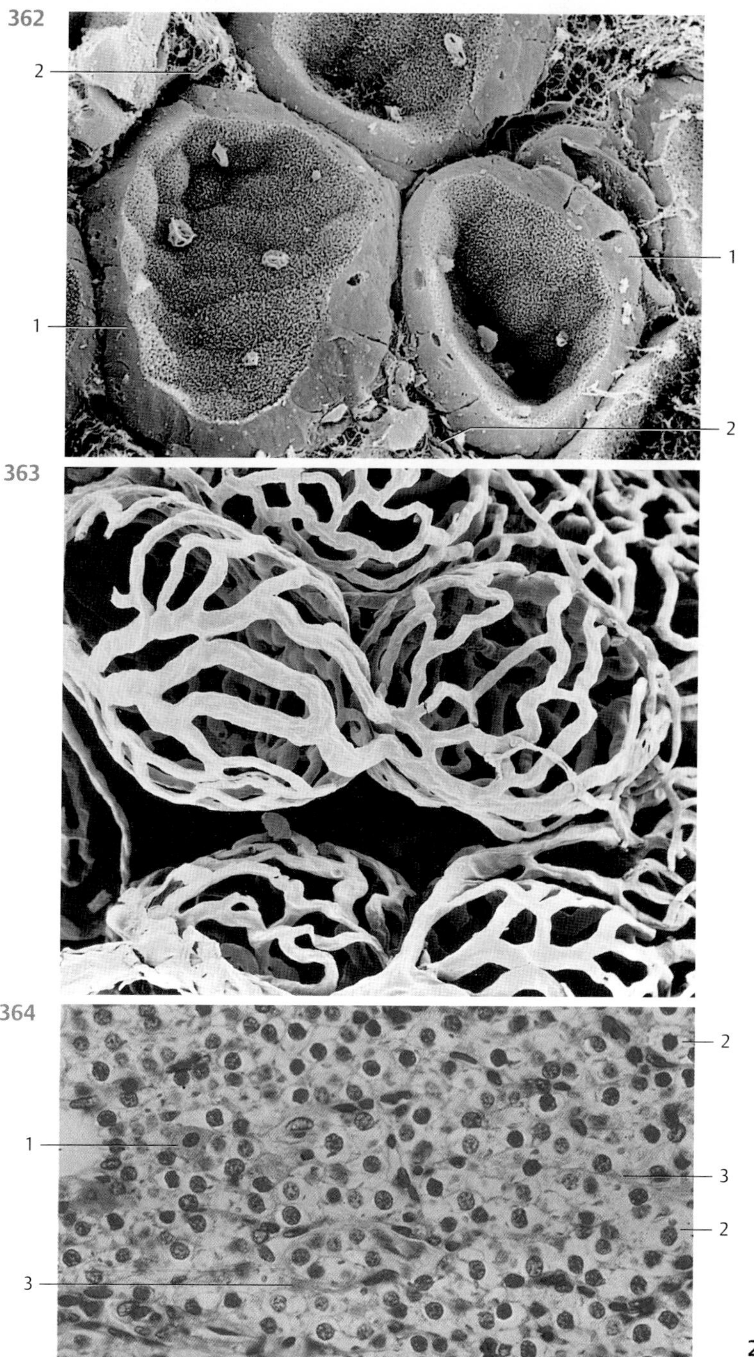
362
2
1
1
2
363
364
2
1
3
2
3

365 Pancreatic Islets of Langerhans

Clusters of endocrine cells are found in a sea of pancreatic exocrine cells. They are clusters of vascularized epithelium, called the *islets of Langerhans* (Paul Langerhans, 1847–1888), or simple islet cells. Exocrine pancreatic cells and islet cells have different structures and stain differently (see Fig. 455, 457, 459). There are three types of islet cells, α-, β- and δ-cells (A-, B- and D-cells. In figure (a), the α-cells 2 are stained red (their secretory product is *glucagon*) and the β-cells 3 are stained blue (they secrete *insulin*). About 60–80% of the islet cells are β-cells, i.e., the insulin-producing cells predominate. Figure (b) shows *necrotic islet cells* after parenteral administration of Alloxan. There are still α-cells 2 at the periphery. The lighter stained regions represent necrotic β-cells 4 with almost completely degenerated nuclei. There are acini 1 of the exocrine pancreas adjacent to the necrotic islet (cf. Fig. 366).

1 Serous acinar cells, exocrine pancreas
2 α-cells (A-cells)
3 β-cells (B-cells)
4 Necrotic β-cells
5 Fat cells
Stain: a) Ivic; magnification: × 64; b) alum hematoxylin-eosin; magnification: × 100

366 Pancreatic Islets of Langerhans

Section of a human pancreas with an *islet of Langerhans* (cf. Fig. 18, 365). Islet cells do not contain zymogen granules. Therefore, they always appear lighter after staining than the exocrine cells. The acinar cells of the eccrine gland 1 contain secretory granules in their apical region. The acidophilic granules are stained blue. There is loose connective tissue around the eccrine gland cells. The connective tissue contains larger blood vessels.

1 Acini of the exocrine pancreas
2 Capillaries within the islet organ
3 Vessels of the exocrine pancreas
Semi-thin section; stain: methylene blue-azure II; magnification: × 400

367 Pancreatic Islets of Langerhans

The entire endocrine portion of the pancreas consists of Langerhans islets (*insulae pancreaticae*). The islets consist of cords of cells, which form an irregular network. This network is extensively vascularized so that virtually every islet cell is connected to the bloodstream. Five cell types can be defined for the cell cords: α-, β-, δ-, PP- and D_1-cells. α-, β- and δ-cells produce the following polypeptide hormones: α-cells secrete glucagon, β-cells secrete insulin and δ-cells secrete somatostatin. About 5–7% of the cells are δ-cells. This figure shows the α-cells of a Langerhans islet using fluorescence-labeled antibody to glucagon. The yellow fluorescence indicates that the α-cells mostly reside at the islet periphery. There are also fluorescent α-cells in the duct epithelium. None of the other islet cells are stained and neither is the exocrine portion of the pancreas. The PP-cells biosynthesize the pancreatic polypeptide.

Fluorescence microscopy, × 150

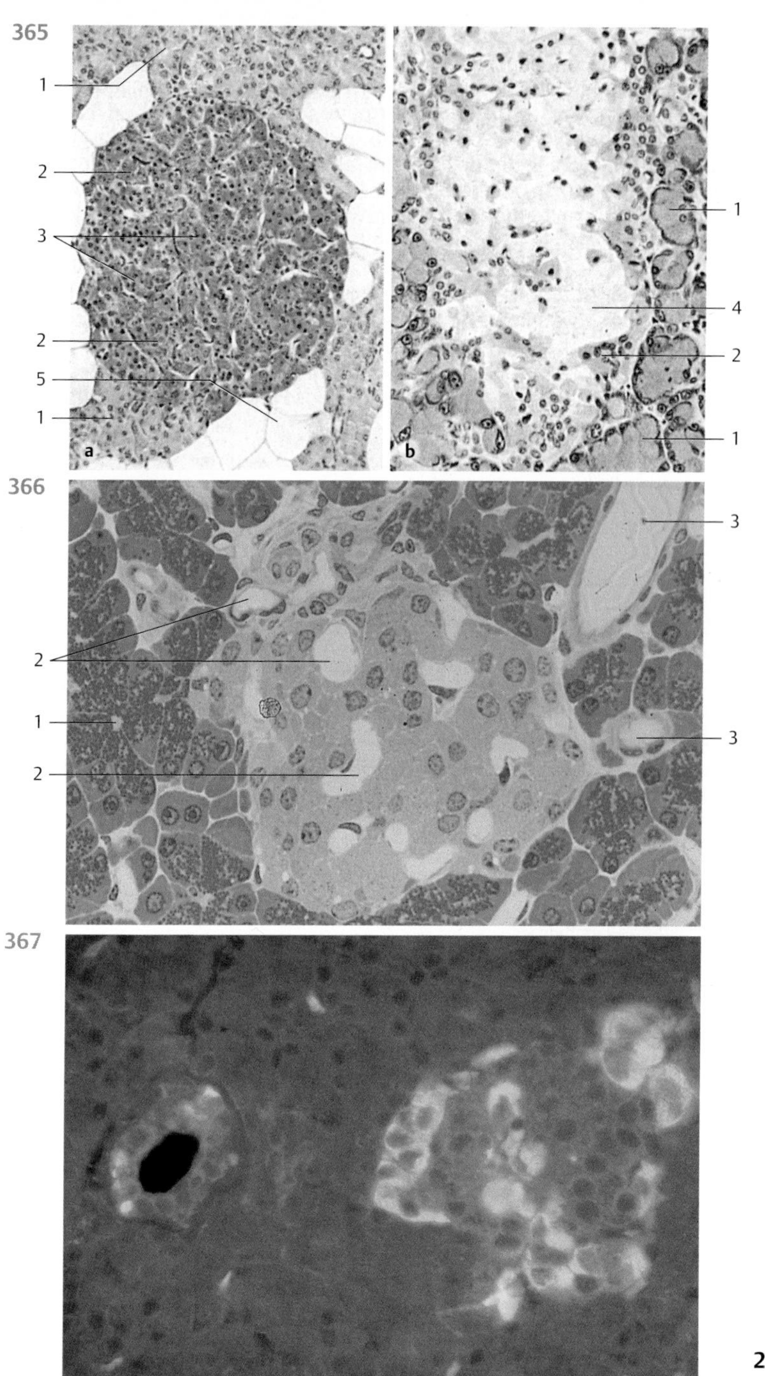
365
1
2
3
2
5
1
a
1
4
2
1
b
366
3
2
1
2
3
367

368 Pancreatic Islets of Langerhans

There are at least five different cell types in the islets of Langerhans. Each type biosynthesizes a different hormone (see Fig. 365, 367). This section shows three cell types: α-*cells*, β-*cells* and δ-*cells*. The α-cells biosynthesize *glucagon*. The average diameter of the hormone-containing granules (α-*granules*) is 300 nm. In electron microscopy, they show an electron-dense center, which is surrounded by a narrow, less electron-dense halo. About 80% of all islet cells are insulin producing β-*cells* 2. Their secretory granules (β-granules) are surrounded by a membrane. The sizes of β-*granules* vary, and they come in different geometrical forms (*polygonal crystalloid*). The granules always show a lighter halo. δ-*Cells* 3 occur mostly in the center of the islet. They biosynthesize the hormone *somatostatin*. Their secretory granules measure about 320 nm. Somatostatin containing secretory granules are not as electron-dense as β-granules. Note the close proximity of islet cells and capillaries 4.

1 α-cells
2 β-cells
3 δ-cells
4 Capillaries
Electron microscopy; magnification: × 3100

369 Pancreatic Islets of Langerhans

δ-Cell (*somatostatin cell*) 1 from the Langerhans islet of a mouse. About 5% of all islet cells are δ-cells. They are usually located at the end of an islet cell cord. δ-Cell granules have diameters of about 320 nm. They are not as electron-dense as the granules from α- or β-cells, and do not have the characteristic light halo of β-granules (cf. Fig. 368). The content of the δ-cell granules is either homogeneous or shows a very fine granulation.
Somatostatin inhibits the secretion of insulin and glucagon. Glucagon stimulates the release of pancreatic somatostatin. In contrast, insulin inhibits somatostatin release.

1 δ-cell
2 δ-cell granule
3 β-cells
4 Nucleus
Electron microscopy; magnification: × 10 000

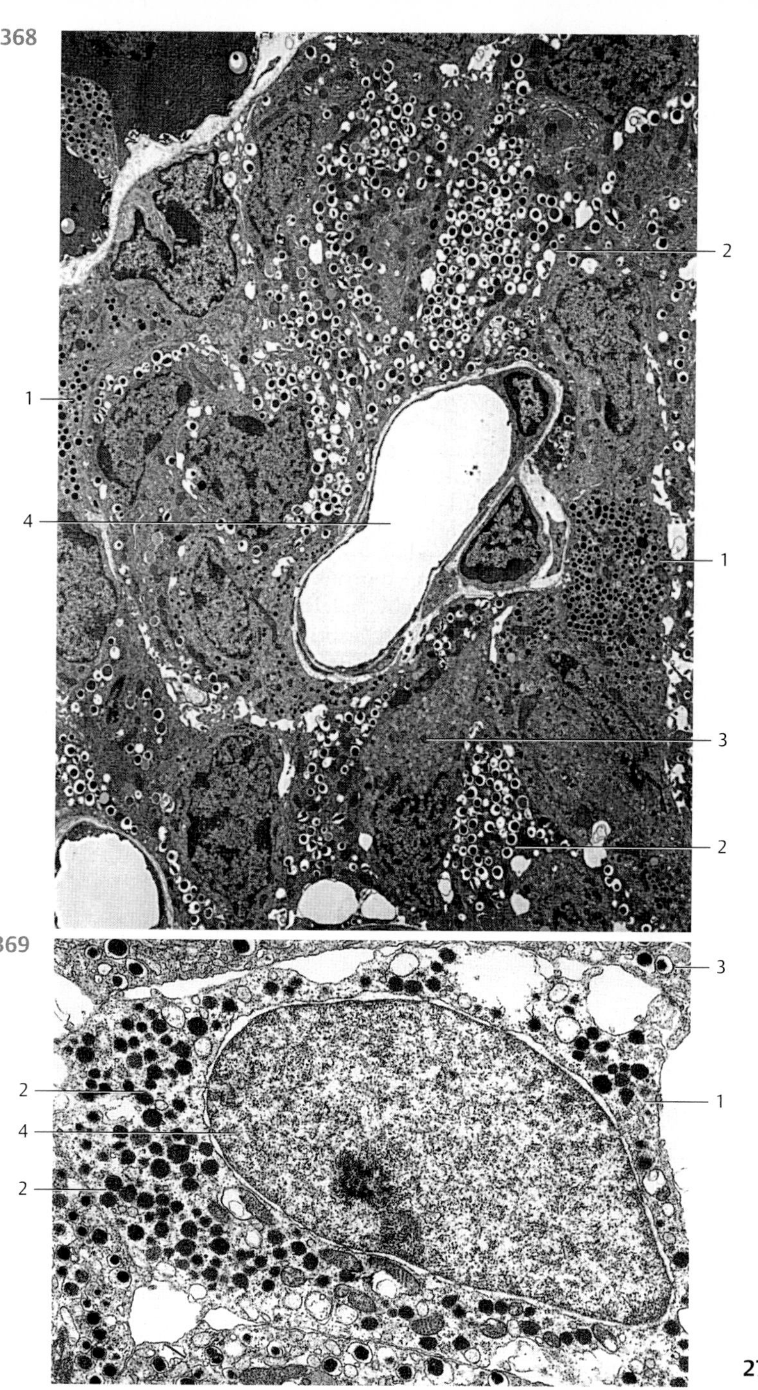
368
2
1
4
1
3
2
369
3
2
4
1
2
Endocrine Glands

370 Oral Cavity—Nasal Cavity

Frontal section through the head of a human embryo. The crown–rump length is 80 mm. The palate is closed.

1 Telencephalon
2 Eye
3 Nasal septum
4 Nasal cavity
5 Superior nasal concha
6 Middle nasal concha
7 Inferior nasal concha
8 Palate
9 Tongue
10 Oral cavity
11 Tooth germ—mandible (cf. Figs. 388–391)
Stain: Masson-Goldner trichrome; magnification: × 10

371 Lips—Labia

The outer lips are covered by skin [1] (*pars cutanea, multilayered stratified nonkeratinizing squamous epithelium*), hair, sebaceous glands and sweat glands. The mucous membrane [2] of the vestibulum oris (*pars mucosa, multilayered stratified nonkeratinizing squamous epithelium, seromucous salivary glands*) covers the inner part of the lips. The transition from the outer to the inner epithelium is made in the vermilion border [3] (*pars intermedia*). This sagittal section of a human adult lip shows the characteristic epithelial covering: the outer skin is on top, mucous membranes are in the lower part. The vermilion border is on the right. A plate of connective tissue and striated muscle fibers [4] (*orbicularis oris muscle*) forms the middle part of the pecten. The orbicular ring muscle abruptly turns outward in the region of the vermilion border (*pars marginalis of the ring muscles*) [4]. The fibers of the orbicular ring muscle are cut vertical to their long axis. Note the clearly defined cell groups of the *seromucous labial glands* [5]. The keratinization and pigmentation of the epithelium is marginal in the vermilion border. Therefore, the color of blood shines through the epithelium. Note the thick multilayered nonkeratinizing epithelium on the mucous membrane side of the lips. Hair shafts and sebaceous glands are seen on the outer (skin) side [1].

1 Skin, pars cutanea
2 Mucous membrane, pars mucosa
3 Vermilion border
4 Marginal part of orbicularis oris muscle
5 Labial gland
Stain: hematoxylin-eosin; magnification: × 15

372 Tongue—Lingua

This frontal section of the tongue from a human newborn shows the arrangement of the musculature (cf. 233). The dorsal tongue (*dorsum linguae*) is in the top part of the figure. The larger vessels are filled with Indian ink. The three-dimensional grid formed by the inner musculature can easily be discerned in the center of the figure. Distinct muscle fibers run in longitudinal [2], transverse and vertical direction (*M. longitudinalis, verticalis* and *transversus linguae*; cf. Fig. 373).

1 Lingual artery
2 Inferior longitudinal muscle of tongue
3 Genioglossus muscle
4 Submandibular duct
5 Geniohyoid muscle
6 Mucous membrane of the dorsal tongue with lingual papilla
7 Aponeurosis of the tongue
Indian ink injection; stain: van Gieson picric acid; magnification: × 12

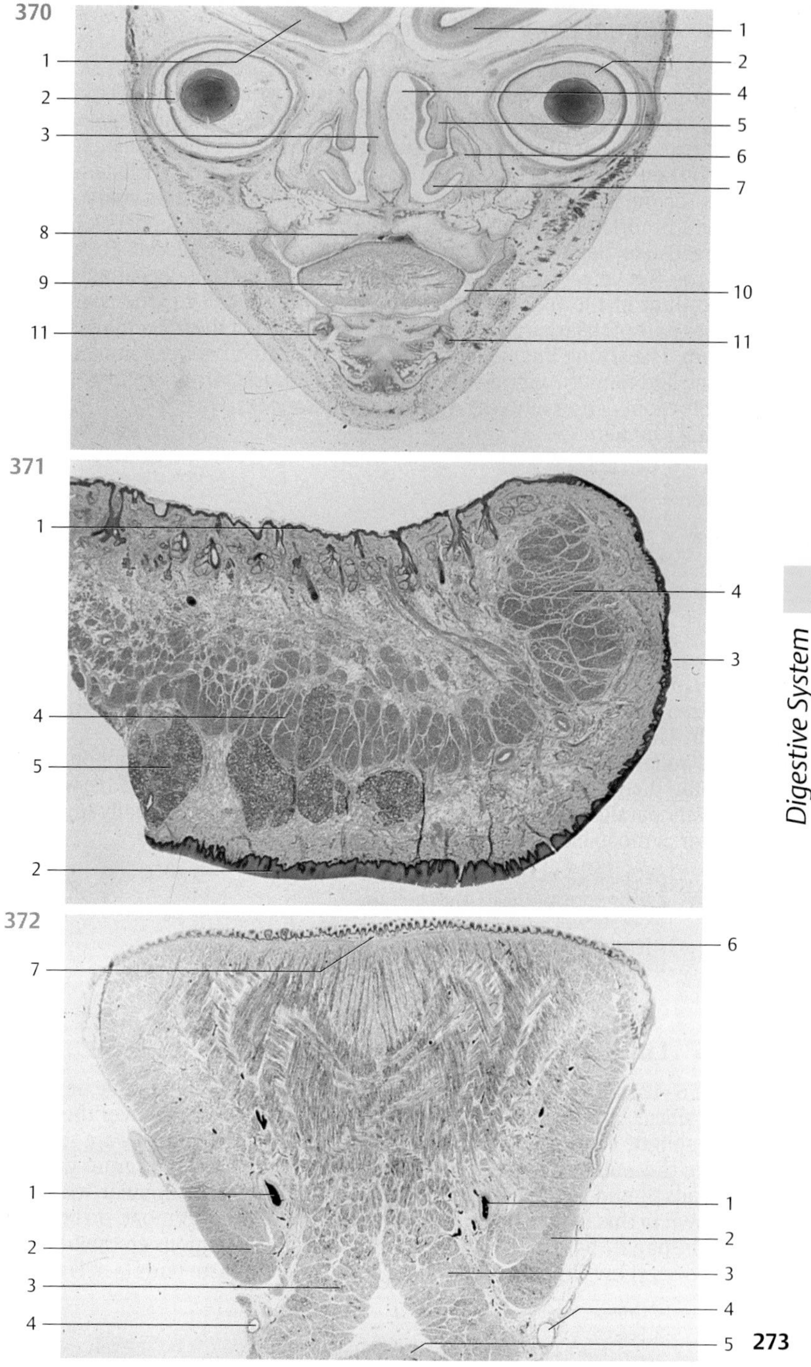
370
1
2
3
8
9
11
1
2
4
5
6
7
10
11
371
1
4
5
2
4
3
372
7
1
2
3
4
6
1
2
3
4
5

373 Lingual Papillae—Filiform Papillae

The mucous membranes everywhere on the tongue are a multilayered stratified squamous epithelium and may have many forms. The dorsal tongue displays raised mucous membrane epithelium called lingual *papillae*. These come in all kinds of forms and structures. The base of the papillae is formed by the lamina propria mucosae. This figure shows that the papillae subdivide into secondary papillae, which appear toward the throat as arcuate, sometimes fimbriated lappets. The keratinized epithelium lappets of *filiform* (thread-like) *papillae* 1 are constantly scuffed off and replaced. They give the tongue the velvety appearance. Scuffed-off epithelial cells, along with the mycelium of the fungus *Leptothrix buccalis*, form the tongue coating. The lower part of the figure shows the regular pattern of the *inner tongue musculature*. The strong lingual aponeurosis 2 is located between mucous membrane and tongue muscles. The lingual aponeurosis forms a rigid (kinetically stable) connection with the mucous membrane (cf. Fig. 372).
Feline tongue.

1 Filiform papilla
2 Lingual aponeurosis
3 Vertical muscle of the tongue
4 Transverse muscle of the tongue
Stain: alum hematoxylin-eosin; magnification: × 10

374 Lingual Papillae—Filiform and Vallate Papillae

Toward the throat oriented *filiform papillae* 1 of a feline tongue. The keratinized points are intact. Filiform papillae are well developed in many animals. They give their tongues a grating quality (see Fig. 373).
The *vallate papillae* 2 on the posterior third of the feline tongue are less evenly distributed than on a human tongue. They are found between the mostly parallel rows of filiform papillae, which will occasionally tower over them. A moat-like groove surrounds the vallate papillae.

1 Filiform papillae (thread-like)
2 Vallate papillae (round, knob-like)
3 Circular wall
4 Moat-like groove, moat or furrow
Scanning electron microscopy; magnification: × 4 .5

375 Lingual Papillae—Vallate Papillae

The 6–12 vallate papillae at the border to the root of the tongue and before the *sulcus terminalis* (groove) (*papillae vallatae*) barely rise over the level of the tongue's mucous membrane 1. The *wall-enclosed papillae* are separated from the wall by a narrow moat. The secretory ducts of the serous gustatory glands 3 end at the bottom of the groove (moat). Their lobular structure is shown in this figure. The ducts connect with the groove (moat) on both sides of the papilla base 4. The multilayered stratified squamous epithelium of the grooves shows lighter spots. These correspond to taste buds (see Fig. 662).

1 Groove, moat
2 Secretory ducts
3 Ebner's glands
4 Papilla base
Stain: alum hematoxylin-eosin; magnification: × 10

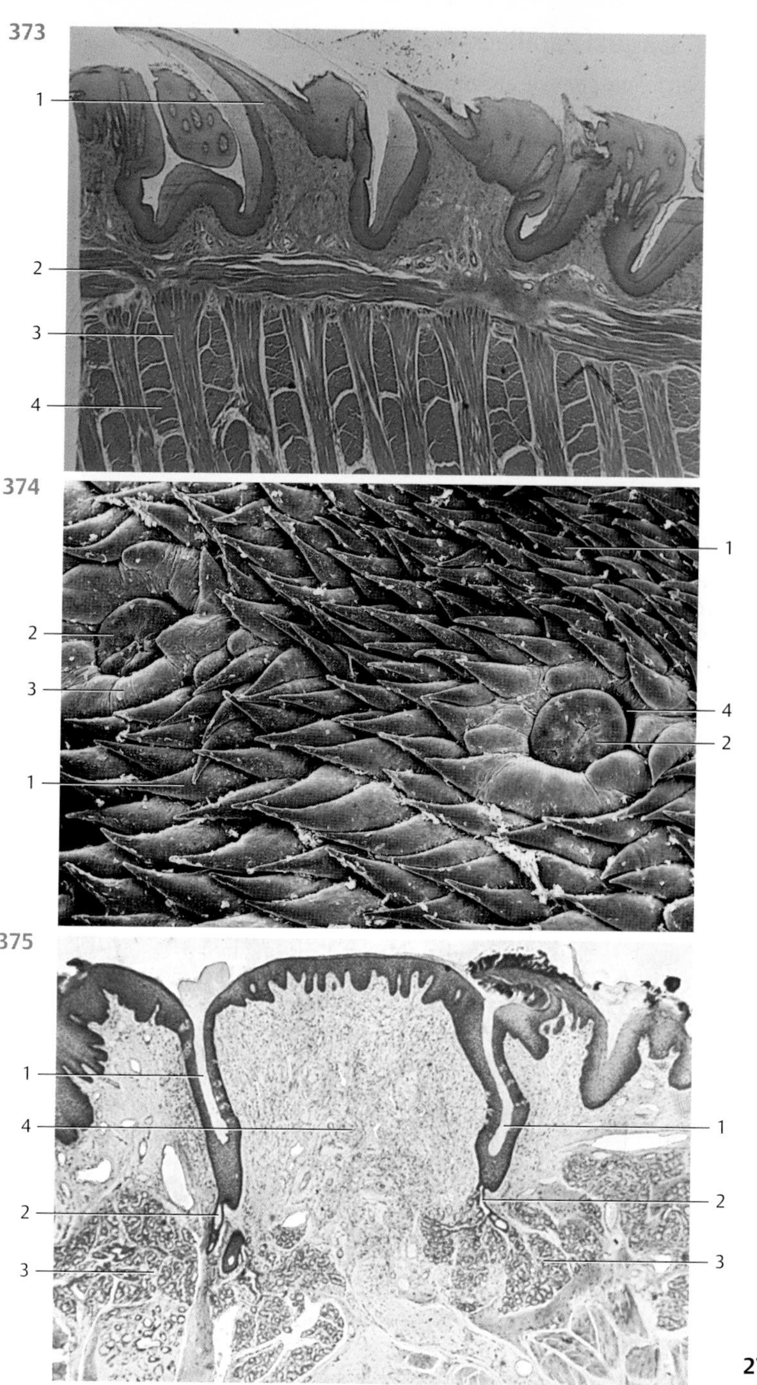
373
1
2
3
4
374
1
2
3
1
4
2
375
1
4
2
3
1
2
3

376 Lingual Papillae—Foliate Papillae

Human *foliate papillae* are well developed only in children. However, rabbits possess dense fields of foliate papillae at the posterior lateral edges of the tongue. This preparation shows rabbit foliate (leaf-like) papillae. The surface folds are separated from each other by deep grooves (cf. Fig. 377). The foliate papillae are supported by several parallel connective tissue cords ⊡1. The multilayered stratified epithelium contains *taste buds* ⊡2 (cf. Fig. 662). The ducts of serous gustatory glands ⊡3 end at the bottom of the deep grooves. Two small groups of glands ⊡3 are present in the subepithelial connective tissue ⊡4. They are located in close proximity to the striated skeletal muscle fibers ⊡5 of the tongue.

1 Connective tissue cords
2 Taste buds
3 Serous gustatory glands
4 Lamina propria
5 Striated lingual musculature
Stain: van Gieson iron hematoxylin-picrofuchsin; magnification: × 80

377 Lingual Papillae—Foliate Papillae

The lingual vessels initially follow the patterns of the inner lingual musculature. Then, having traversed the tightly structured aponeurosis, they spread into the mucous membrane. The vessel terminals form a densely woven network, which ends in a capillary web area. Each secondary papilla has a capillary loop ⊡3 (cf. Fig. 376).
The lower part of the figure shows the striated lingual musculature ⊡2. Serous glands have not been sectioned.

1 Multilayered stratified squamous epithelium
2 Lingual musculature
3 Capillary loop (ansa)
Stain: alum hematoxylin-eosin after injection with Indian ink; magnification: × 15

378 Lingual Glands—Posterior Lingual Glands

Groups of mucous glands (glandulae radices linguae) in considerable numbers exist in the area of the lingual root, *radix lingua*, under the *lingual tonsil* (see Figs. 338, 339). The clustered mucous glands are not restricted to the tunica mucosa but extend deeper between the muscle fiber bundles. The glandular ducts end in the canals of the lingual follicles. Connective tissue septa (trabeculae) (stained blue) and sectioned striated muscle fibers ⊡1 are present between the glandular lobes. The nuclei (stained red) in the basal cell region and the cytoplasm with its honeycomb structure (cf. Fig. 130) are characteristic of mucous glands. The secretory ducts have wide lumina.
The paired seromucous anterior lingual gland (*Nuhn's gland*) is located close to the tip of the tongue.

1 Striated skeletal musculature of the tongue
2 Artery
Stain: azan; magnification: × 100

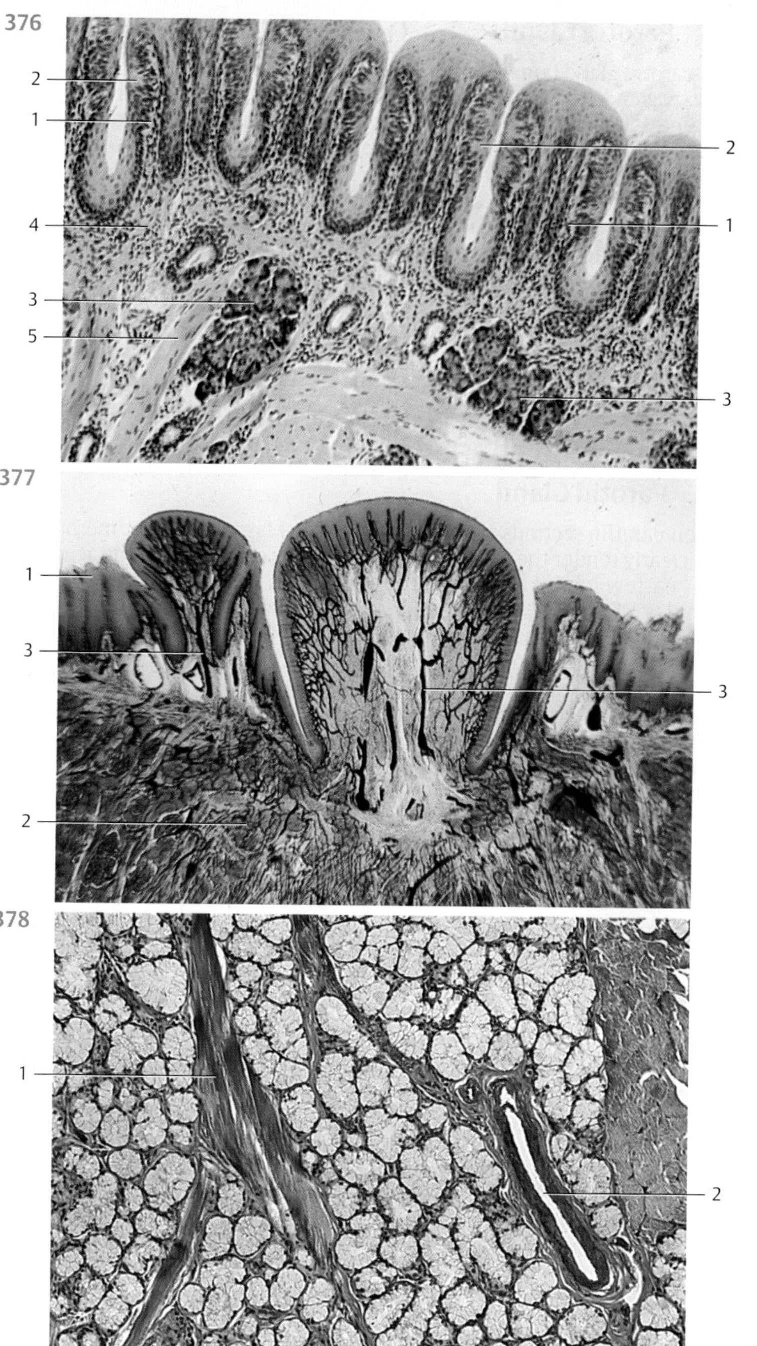
376
2
1
4
3
5
2
1
3
377
1
3
3
2
378
1
2

379 Parotid Gland

The parotid gland (*glandula parotidea*, or short *parotis*) is the largest human salivary gland. It is a purely serous gland with long, branched secretory ducts. The entire length of the secretory duct is always contained in the glandular lobe. Groups of fat cells 2 occur between the wide serous acini 1. The nuclei of serous acinar cells are round and located in the basal cell region. Their cytoplasm is finely granulated (see Fig. 129). A long intercalated duct 3 traverses the center of the image from top left to bottom right. There are also cross-sectioned intercalated ducts 4. The ducts are lined by an isoprismatic (cuboid) epithelium (see Figs. 380, 381).

1 Serous acini
2 Fat cells
3 Intercalated duct, cut longitudinally
4 Intercalated duct, cross-sectioned
Stain: alum hematoxylin-eosin; magnification: × 200

380 Parotid Gland

When paraffin sections are stained using the Masson-Goldner method, they will clearly render the cone or pyramid-shaped cell groups of the acini 1 and their narrow lumina. The acinar cell cytoplasm contains slightly acidophilic granules (cf. Figs. 379, 381). A sectioned salivary or striated duct 2 is visible in the lower right half of the image. The oval nuclei of the pseudostratified columnar epithelial cells are located in the central or basal cell regions. A basal striation is visible underneath the nuclei (see Fig. 90). It is caused by involutions of the basal plasmalemma and densely packed mitochondria between the membrane pleats (cf. Fig. 91). A longitudinally section of an intercalated duct 3 is visible in the right part of the figure, another duct is cross-sectioned 4 (cf. Figs. 379, 381). Note the sparse connective tissue (stained green) and the numerous adipocytes 5.

1 Serous acini
2 Salivary duct, cross-sectioned
3 Intercalated duct, cut longitudinally
4 Intercalated duct, cross-sectioned
5 Adipocytes
Stain: Masson-Goldner trichrome; magnification: × 200

381 Parotid Gland

The epithelium of serous acini 1 consists of nearly pyramid-shaped cells with central or basal cell nuclei. The supranuclear or apical cell region of the serous acinar cells is filled with secretory granules (stained blue). The number of granules varies with the secretory activity. A cross-sectioned intercalated duct 2 is shown in the center of the figure. Spindle-shaped, flat myoepithelial cells (cf. Figs. 379, 380) surround it. There are fibrocytes and capillaries in the loose connective tissue between acini. Compare with Figs. 127 and 129.

1 Serous acinus
2 Intercalated duct with myoepithelial cells
Semi-thin section; stain: methylene blue-azure II; magnification: × 200

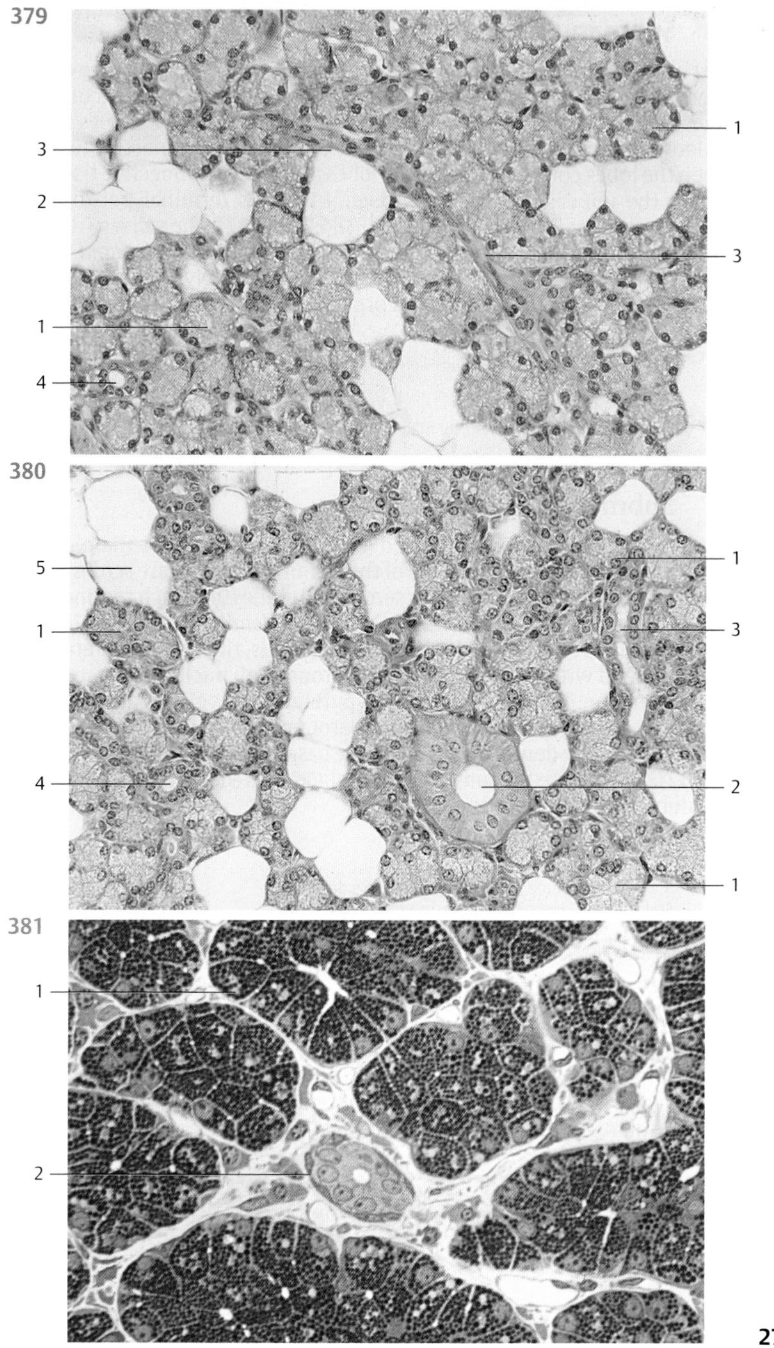
379
1
3
2
3
1
4
380
5
1
1
3
4
2
1
381
1
2

382 Submandibular Gland

The *submandibular gland* is a mixed (seromucous) gland. The figure displays several lobes that are separated by connective tissue septa (trabeculae). The larger ducts, the blood and lymph vessels and the vegetative nerves traverse the loose interlobular connective tissue [1]. The fibrous connective tissue between the lobes continues inside the lobes as reticular connective tissue. The lobe in the upper layer contains several mucous terminal portions with serous demilunes [2] (cf. Figs. 132, 383, 384, 386, 387). The salivary ducts are stained bright red. The branched ducts in the *submandibular gland* are particularly long and elaborate [3]. The preparation is heavily stained with eosin. Note that the submandibular gland predominantly contains serous acini [4].

1 Interlobular connective tissue
2 Mucous terminal portion with serous demilune (Ebner's or Giannuzzi's demilune)
3 Salivary duct
4 Serous acini
Stain: alum hematoxylin-eosin; magnification: × 40

383 Submandibular Gland

The *submandibular gland* is a mixed (*seromucous*) gland; for the most part, however, it is a *serous* gland. Some of the terminal portions are *serous acini* [1], others are *mucous tubules* [2] with serous demilunes [3], which remind of half moons or lunar sickles (*Ebner's* or *Giannuzzi's demilunes*, cf. Figs. 132, 382, 384, 386, 387). As observed for the parotid glands, the serous secretory cells can be stained with acidophilic dyes. The round cell nuclei are located in the basal cell region. The tubular cells from purely mucous glands are distinct because they are stained lighter than the serous cells. The flat nuclei of mucous gland cells appear dense and reside in the basal or basolateral cell regions (cf. Fig. 132). Again, note the salivary serous gland cells (demilunes) at the end of the mucous gland tubules.

1 Serous acini
2 Mucous tubules
3 Serous demilune (Ebner's or Giannuzzi's demilune)
Stain: alum hematoxylin-eosin; magnification: × 240

384 Submandibular Gland

The mucous glands can be emphasized using histochemical staining procedures. The *mucous secretory tubules* [1] in this section are stained with Alcian blue. In the image, the blue stain distinguishes them from the serous acini [2]. The nuclei are stained with nuclear fast red. The combination of dyes in this preparation does not stain the interlobular connective tissue.

1 Mucous tubules
2 Serous acini
Stain: Alcian blue at pH 2.5, nuclear fast red; magnification: × 120

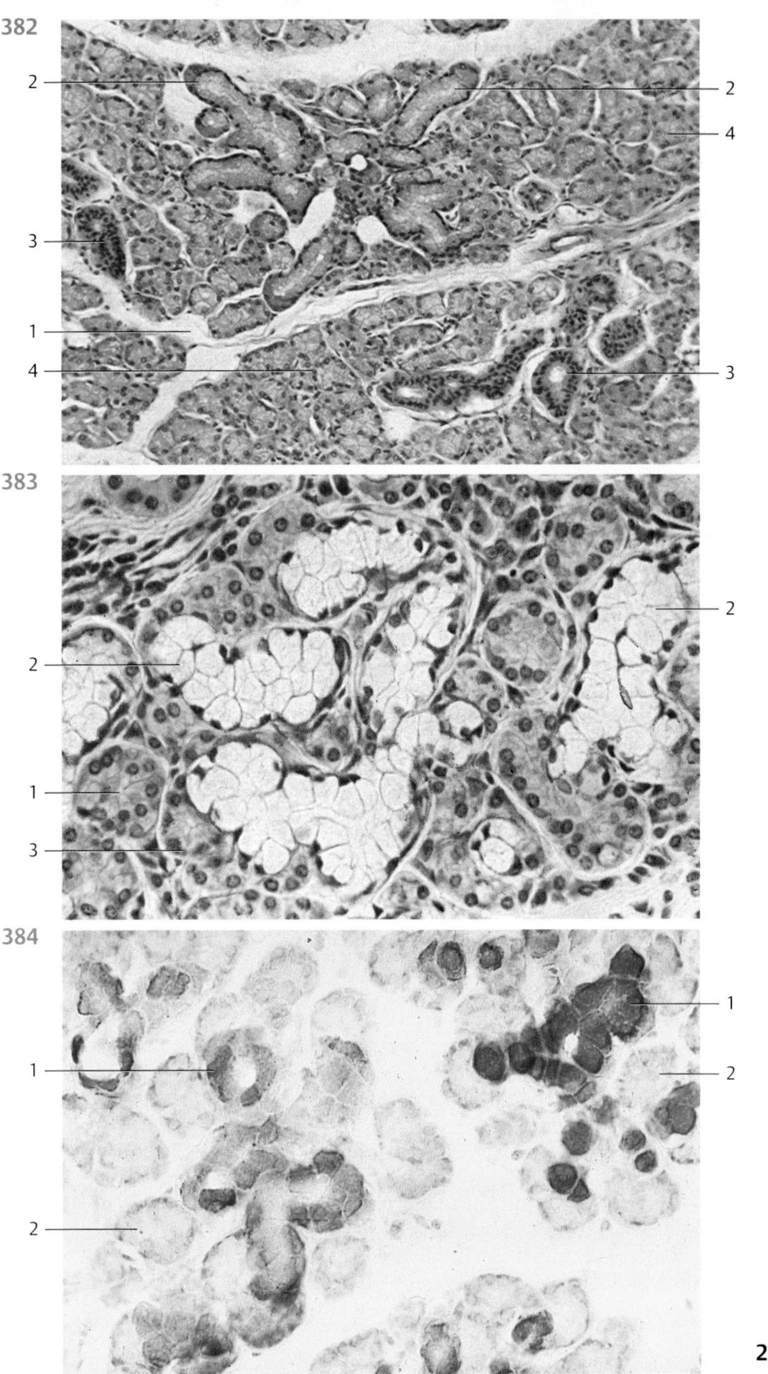
382
2
2
4
3
1
4
3
383
2
2
1
3
384
1
1
2
2

385 Sublingual Gland

The sublingual gland is a mixed, i.e., *seromucous gland*. Mucous glands predominate. The *intercalated and striated ducts* are exceptionally short. Different segments cannot be defined for these ducts and histological preparations of them are rare.
This preparation shows the lobe of a sublingual gland with typical mucous tubules 1. Most of them are cross-sectioned (cf. Figs. 383, 384, 386, 387). There is also fibrous, relatively coarse interlobular connective tissue 2 with several ducts 3. The ducts are lined by a two-layered pseudostratified columnar epithelium (see Fig. 386).

1 Mucous glands
2 Interlobular connective tissue
3 Salivary ducts
4 Intercalated duct
Stain: azan; magnification: × 80

386 Sublingual Gland

The mixed, *seromucous sublingual* gland contains mostly mucous gland tubules 1. The tubules often branch out, as they do in this figure. There are serous demilunes 2 at the ends of the tubules (cf. Fig. 382–384). The tubules are filled with mucus and often distended. Note the different shapes of the nuclei. In cells from mucous glands 1, the nuclei are mostly small and spindle-shaped. The nuclei of serous gland cells 3 are large and round. The nuclei of mucous and serous cells, both are in basal positions (cf. Fig. 387). An interlobular duct 4 embedded in coarse connective tissue 5 is seen at the left edge of the figure. A vein 6 is located underneath the duct. Intercalated ducts are not sectioned.

1 Tubules of mucous glands
2 Serous half-moon (demilune)
3 Serous acinus
4 Interlobular connective tissue
5 Salivary duct
6 Vein
7 Striated duct, salivary duct
Stain: alum hematoxylin-eosin; magnification: × 120

387 Sublingual Gland

The sublingual gland consists of a group of about 50 single glands, each with its own duct; 10–12 sublingual ducts end on a mucous membrane fold, called the sublingual fold *(plica sublingualis)*.
This figure shows a section of the seromucous sublingual gland, which consists mostly of mucous glands. The mucous tubules 1 are branched. There are serous caps at the end of each tubule 2 (*Ebner's or Giannuzzi's demilunes*) (cf. Figs. 132, 382–384, 386). The lightly stained cells in the tubules of the mucous glands show a honeycomb structure. Their spindle-shaped nuclei are located in the basal regions of the cells. In contrast, the cytoplasm of the serous demilune cells is stained red. The nuclei in these cells are round.

1 Mucous tubules
2 Serous demilunes
Stain: hematoxylin-eosin; magnification: × 400

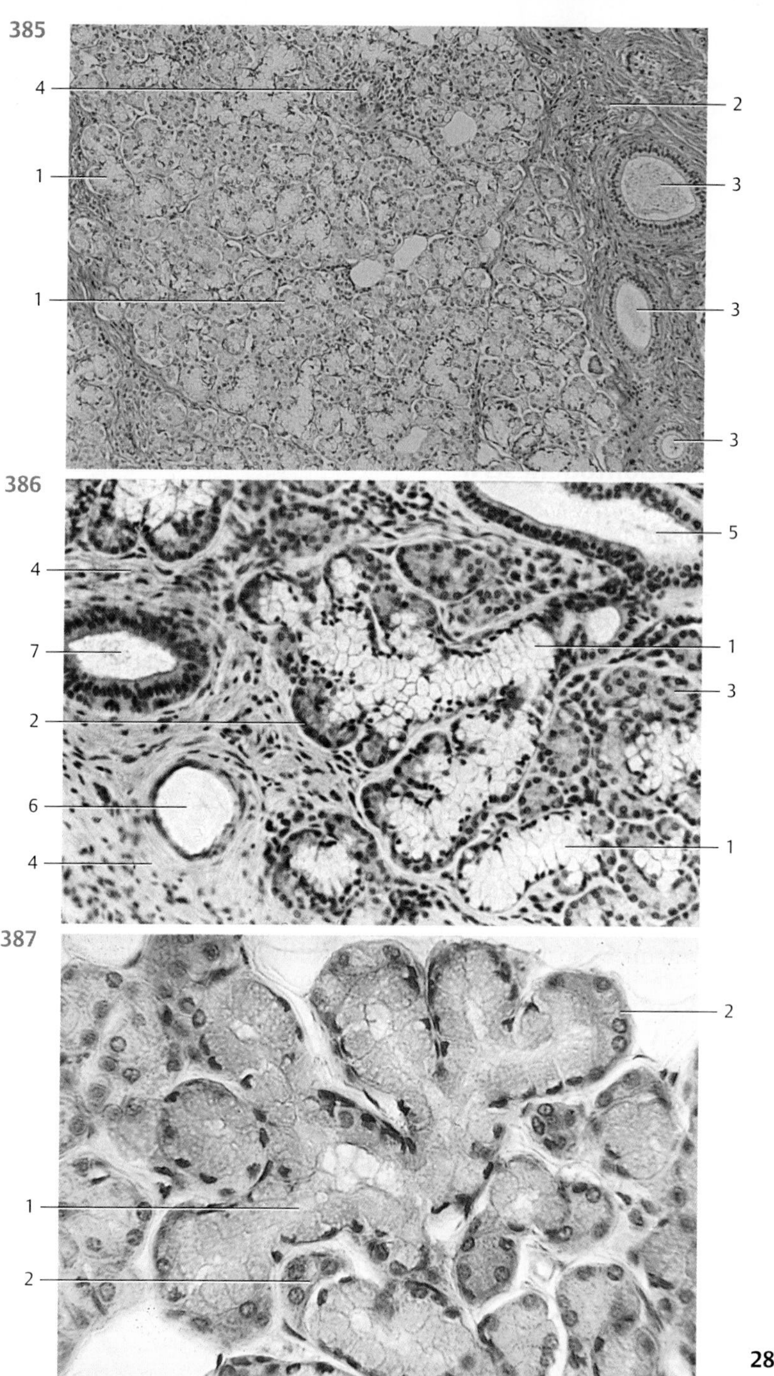

Digestive System

388 Odontogenesis I

Ectoderm and *mesoderm* partake in odontogenesis. The development of teeth starts in the 5th week of pregnancy. The fetal crown-rump length at this stage is about 7–10 mm. At this time, the multilayered nonkeratinizing squamous epithelium 1 proliferates and forms a narrow layer, which corresponds to the line of the adult jaw. Concomitantly, the epithelium fuses with the underlying jaw mesenchyme. This figure shows an early stage of the tooth germ in the form of the dental lamina 2 and the permanent teeth ridge 3, which are both oriented toward the inside. Fetus (crown-rump length = 2.8 cm).

1 Proliferated oral epithelium
2 Dental lamina
3 Permanent teeth ridge
4 Enamel organ
5 Jaw mesenchyme
6 Oral cavity
Stain: hematoxylin-eosin; magnification: × 80

389 Odontogenesis II

The adjacent mesenchyme around the *tooth germ* has condensed to the *dental papilla* 1. The beginning separation of the *dental sac* 2 and the dense population of cells in the dental papilla are already discernible. The multilayered *internal enamel epithelium* 3 is located at the inner surface of the cap enameloid. The layer of cells, which borders on the surrounding mesenchyme 5, forms the *external enamel epithelium* 4 at the outer surface of the cap enameloid (cf. Fig. 390). Fetus (crown-rump length = 3.2 cm).

1 Dental papilla
2 Dental sac
3 Internal enamel epithelium
4 External enamel epithelium
5 Jaw mesenchyme
6 Proliferated epithelium of the oral cavity
7 Dental lamina
8 Permanent teeth ridge
9 Stellate reticulum
Stain: hematoxylin-eosin; magnification: × 80

390 Odontogenesis III

Bell stage of the enamel organ. The *enamel organ* consists of the external 1 and internal 2 enamel epithelium. The stellate reticulum (*pulpa enamelea*) 3 is located inside the nonvascularized enamel organ 3. At the outer convex surface of the enamel organ, the external enamel epithelium 1 separates the stellate reticulum from the dental sac 4. The internal enamel epithelium 2 covers the inward dwelling part of the bell and supplies the *ameloblasts* (*enameloblasts, adamantoblasts*). The enameloblasts are pseudostratified columnar cells, which can be up to 70 μm high. The condensed mesenchyme in the area of the inward dwelling part of the bell is the *dental papilla* 5. The mesenchyme cells (dental papilla), which border at the inner enamel epithelium, are *odontoblast* progenitor cells. Odontoblasts biosynthesize dentine. The strong epithelial strand above the bell is the permanent teeth ridge 6. Fetus (crown-rump length = 8 cm).

1 External enamel epithelium
2 Internal enamel epithelium
3 Stellate reticulum
4 Dental sac
5 Dental papilla
6 Permanent teeth ridge
7 Multilayered nonkeratinizing squamous epithelium
Stain: alum hematoxylin-eosin; magnification: × 20

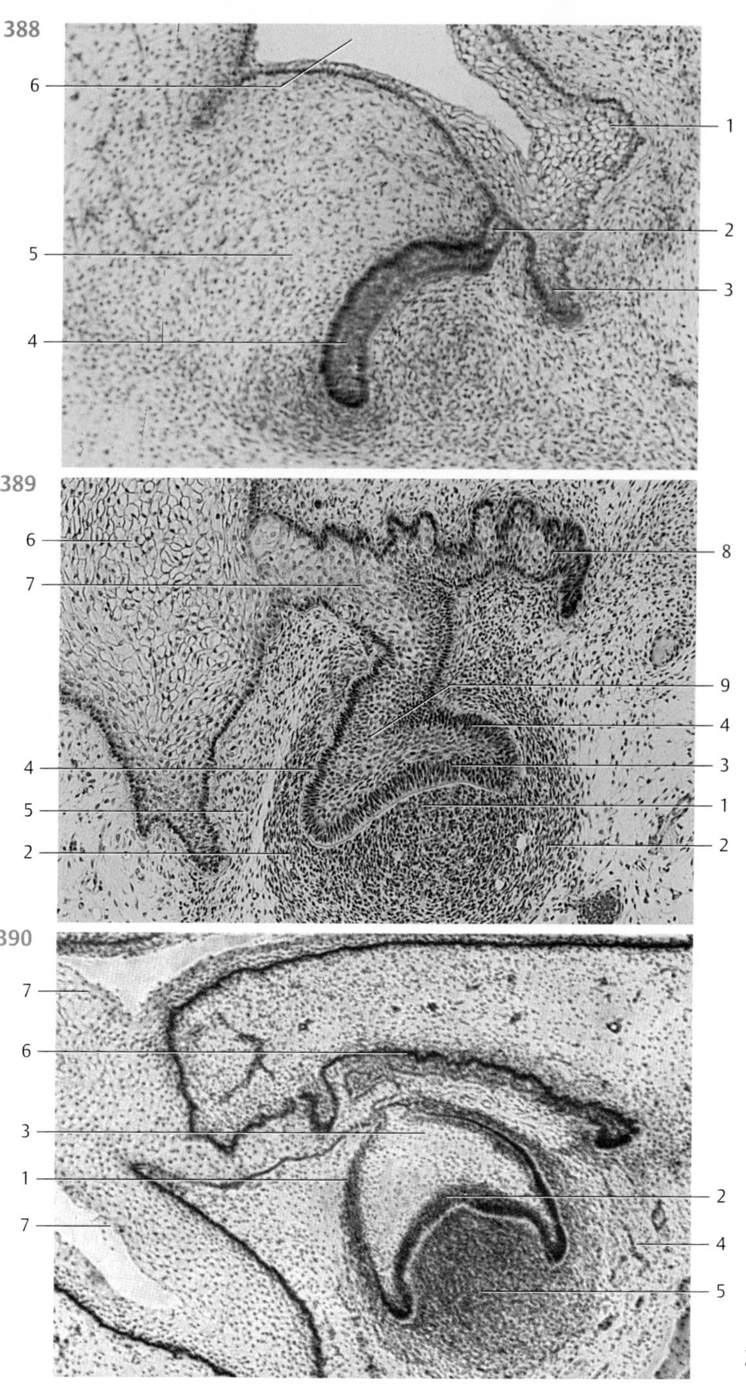

Digestive System

391 Odontogenesis III

Frontal section through the head of a hamster fetus on the 15th day of gestation. The *bell-shaped enamel organs* 5 in the upper and lower jaws are fully developed (cf. Fig. 390). Note the vessels, which are filled with Indian ink.

1 Oral cavity
2 Tongue
3 Palate
4 Nasal cavity
5 Bell-shaped enamel organ
6 Lower jaw
Indian ink injection; stain: iron hematoxylin; magnification: × 20

392 Odontogenesis—Enamel Organ

Tooth germ of a human fetus in the 5th month of pregnancy. The metachromatic intercellular substance inside the nonvascularized enamel organs has increased and has pushed the epithelial cells away from each other. This creates the stellate reticulum (*pulpa enamelea*) 1, in which cells of reticular character 4 form a web-like structure. The stellate reticulum at the outer convex surface of the enamel organ is separated from the adjacent connective tissue of the dental sac 3 by the external enamel epithelium 2 (cf. Figs. 390, 395).

1 Stellate reticulum
2 External enamel epithelium
3 Connective tissue of the dental sac
4 Epithelial cells of the stellate reticulum
Stain: hematoxylin-eosin; magnification: × 200

393 Air-Filled Ground Dental Section, Unstained

Figure (a) shows osteocytes in the fibrous bone of the tooth enamel. The osteocytes feature long cytoplasmic processes. Figure (b) depicts the ground section of the crown of a tooth with the enamel (top) and dentine (bottom). There is a clear border between both the hard substances. Dentine is traversed by air-filled, parallel *dentine canals* 1. Their ends may branch and fan out like bushels. The dentine canals cause a radial striation of the dentine. The long odontoblast processes are located in the dentine canals. They are also called *Tomes fibers*. The odontoblast processes reach to the enamel border or the cement border, respectively. In contrast to enamel, dentine is a living tissue. The odontoblasts are able to produce new dentine throughout life. The tooth enamel is covered by an about 1 μm-thick fibrous *enamel cuticle* 2. Noncalcified areas of dentine are called interglobular dentine 4 or *Tomes granular layer*.

1 Dentine canals
2 Enamel cuticle
3 Enamel prisms (prisma adamantina)
4 Interglobular dentine
Ground tooth sections; magnifications: a) × 250; b) × 50

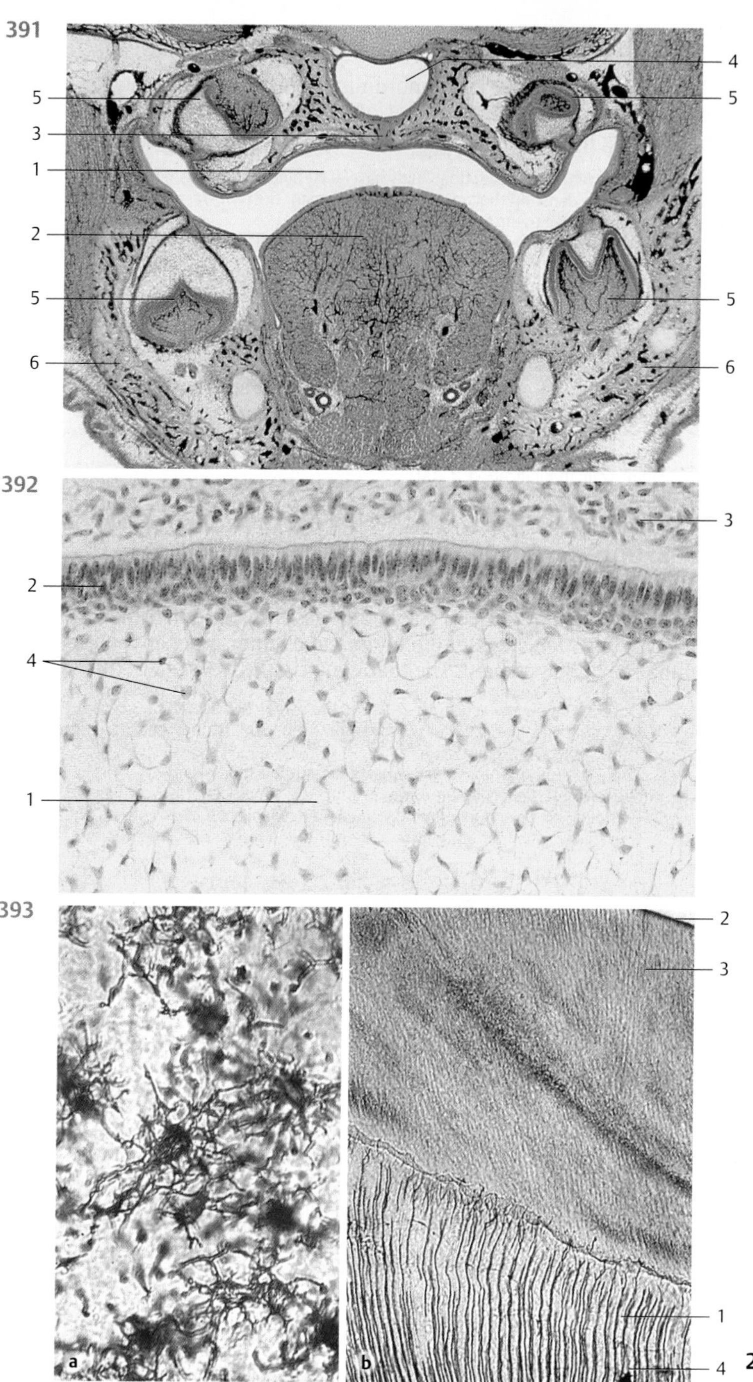
391
4
5
5
3
1
2
5
5
6
6
392
3
2
4
1
393
2
3
1
a
b
4

394 Odontogenesis

Vertical section through the primordium in the feline lower jaw (cf. Fig. 395). The figure shows the development of dentine and tooth enamel. There are the following layers:

1 *Stellate reticulum*. Interstitial fluids have accumulated and pushed apart the cells of the originally dense epithelium of the enamel organ. The now star-shaped cells form a reticular connective tissue (see Fig. 392).
2 The *internal enamel epithelium* initially borders on the mesenchyme of the dental papilla (see Fig. 390). It consists of pseudostratified columnar ameloblasts (adamantoblasts, enameloblasts) (see Fig. 395).
3 *Enamel*. The enamel cap (stained dark red) is generated by ameloblasts.
4 *Dentine* (stained red). Predentine is already mineralized.
5 *Predentine* (stained blue) is a soft intercellular substance that is rich in fibrils and comparable to the osteoid.
6 *Odontoblast* layer. The pseudostratified columnar cells are responsible for the formation of dentine.
7 *Dental papilla* and *stellate reticulum*, respectively, consist of very delicate fibrous connective tissue. Their star-shaped, branched cells are probably fibroblasts.

Stain: azan; magnification: × 200

395 Odontogenesis

Enamel and dentine can be particularly well demonstrated showing an incisor in the 5th fetal month. At the end of development, dentine is a 1–5–nm wide layer between stellate reticulum and enamel, and between stellate reticulum and dental cement. The following tissues are seen in this figure:

1 Loosely arranged mesenchyme cells and the connective tissue fibers of the *dental sac*.
2 A layer of densely packed cells of the stellate reticulum (*stratum stellate, stratum intermedium*).
3 Single-layered columnar *ameloblasts* (adamantoblasts).
4 The enamel (stained light red) was produced by ameloblasts.
5 The following layer consists of dentine (stained violet). It clearly shows fine light lines. These are *dentine canals*, which contain the odontoblast processes, also called *Tomes fibers* (cf. Fig 393b).
6 A layer of not yet mineralized dentine follows (*predentine*, stained blue) (see Fig. 394).
7 A layer of dentine-forming *odontoblasts* is located underneath the predentine. Their cytoplasmic processes appear prominently as fine dark lines.

Stain: azan; magnification: × 500

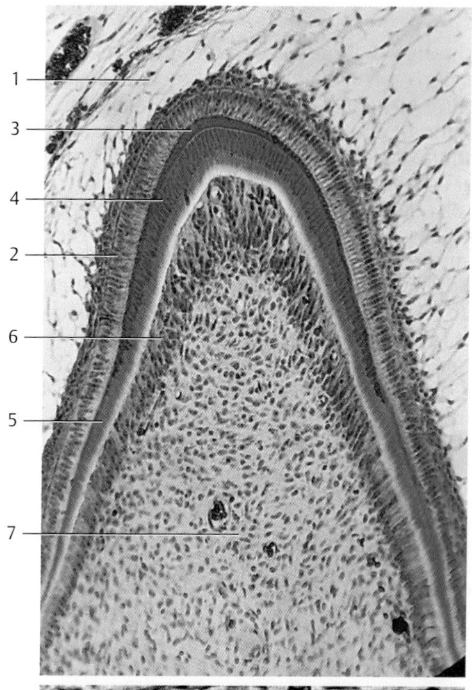

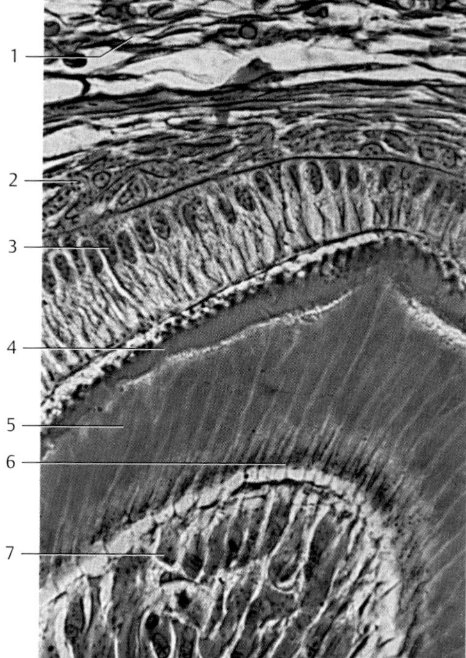

Digestive System

396 Teeth

Cross-section through the roots of two teeth and their *alveoli*. The roots are covered with *dental cement* 1 and are anchored in the jaw. The *periodontium* 2 connects dental cement and the walls of the alveoli. The morphological and functional unit of dental cement, periodontium and alveolar bone 3 is called *parodontium*. This unit holds the tooth. The periodontium 2 consists of dense regular collagen fibers, known as Sharpey's fibers. They attach to the dental cement on one side and the alveolar bone on the other. The dense collagen fibers of Sharpey's fibers contain fibrocytes. The gums (*gingiva*) 4, which border on the alveolar part (*pars alveolaris mandibulae*), are seen in the top part of the figure. The gums are the mucous membranes in the oral cavity, which do not contain glands. They consist of particularly dense connective tissue and are covered by a multilayered, mostly keratinized, squamous epithelium 5.
The main mass of a tooth is dentine 6, which surrounds the tooth cavity 2. The cavity contains dental pulp, a connective tissue with delicate fibers and star-shaped cells (*pulp fibrocytes*).

1 Dental cement
2 Periodontium
3 Bone of the alveolar wall
4 Dense connective tissue of the gums (gingiva)
5 Multilayered squamous epithelium of the gums
6 Dentine
7 Dental pulp
Stain: hematoxylin-eosin; magnification: × 10

397 Soft Palate and Uvula

The mucous membranes of the hard palate continue toward the pharynx as soft palate (*palatum molle*) with the velum (*velum palatinum*) and the *uvula*. A multilayered nonkeratinizing squamous epithelium covers the velum and the uvula at the side of the oral cavity. It folds on the side of the nasal cavity. The figure shows part of a longitudinal section of the uvula at its root, i.e., close to the velum. The multilayered columnar respiratory epithelium 1 contains goblet cells (stained blue). It covers the strong basal membrane 2. Mucous glands 3 can be recognized in the subepithelial connective tissue. Their ducts 4 are lined with columnar epithelium.

1 Respiratory epithelium
2 Basal membrane
3 Mucous glands
4 Salivary ducts
Stain: azan; magnification: × 400

398 Soft Palate and Uvula

Muscle fibers from the velum extend into the uvula. Some clusters of mucous glands of the uvula are located in this web of muscle fibers. Sporadically, there are also small tonsil-like structures in the uvula. The striated muscle fibers of the uvula (*muscle of the uvula*) branch out in an almost regular pattern. *Circumferential muscles* are also found (cf. Fig. 237).
Longitudinal section through the uvula with striated muscle fibers 1 and mucous glands 2. The connective tissue is stained blue.

Stain: azan; magnification: × 400

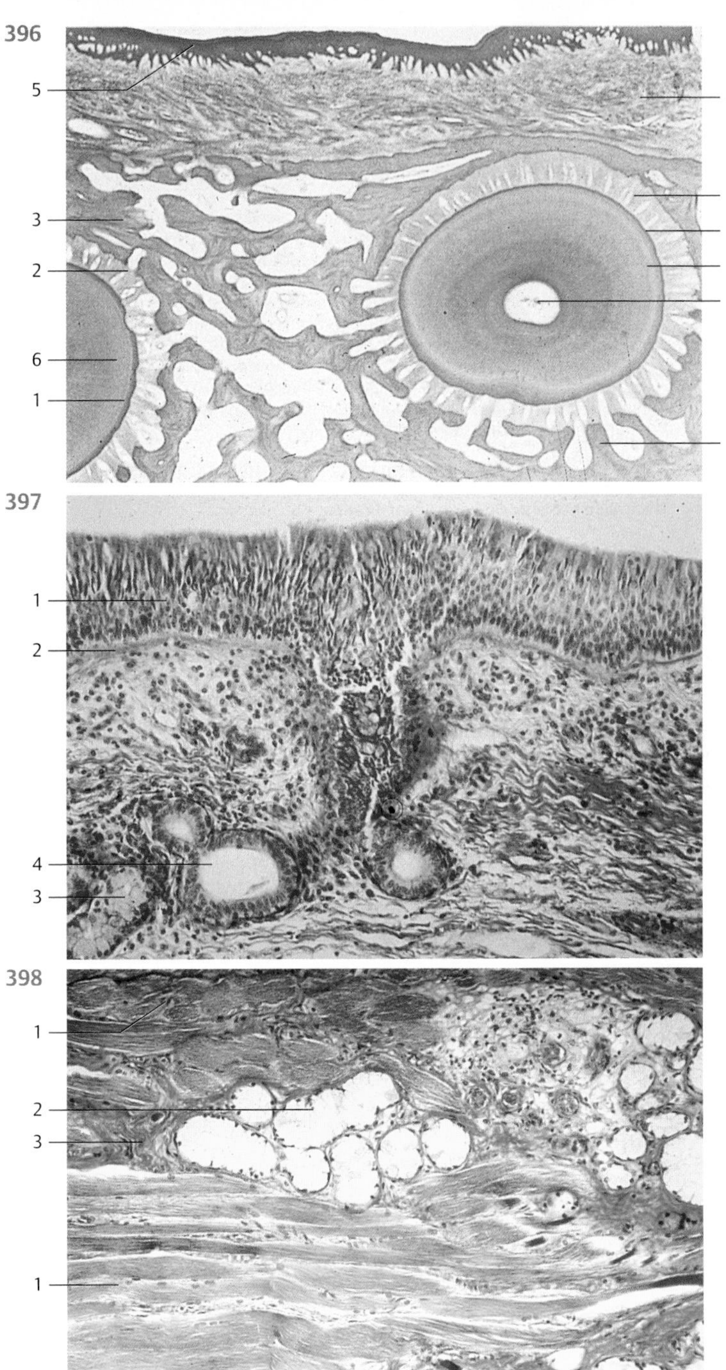

Digestive System

399 Esophagus

This cross-section of the thoracic part of the esophagus shows all layers of the intestinal walls (*esophagus, stomach, small and large intestines*). There are the following layers:

1 Lamina epithelialis mucosae (epithelial part of the mucous membrane): multilayered nonkeratinizing squamous epithelium
2 Lamina propria mucosae: predominantly fibrous reticular connective tissue
3 Lamina muscularis mucosae: the smooth muscle cells of this layer show a helical configuration. A layer of striated muscle fibers surrounds the star-shaped lumen. Most muscle bundles are cross-sectioned
4 Tela submucosa: this wide layer consists of loosely arranged collagen fiber bundles and an elastic fiber meshwork. It contains clusters of glands (see Figs. 400, 401)
5 Tunica muscularis with inner circular layer and outer longitudinal layer (stratum circulare and stratum longitudinale). The entire intestinal tunica muscularis can be divided into an inner circular layer and an outer longitudinal layer of muscle cells
6 Tunica adventitia. Loose, fibrous connective tissue makes up the tunica adventitia. It surrounds and structurally supports the esophagus

Layers 1, 2 and 3 form the tunica mucosa (mucous membrane).

Stain: alum hematoxylin-eosin; magnification: × 5

Digestive System

400 Esophagus

This cross-section of the esophageal wall shows the high, multilayered nonkeratinizing stratified squamous epithelium [1]. With 300–400 µm, the epithelium is of remarkable height. The *lamina propria mucosae* [2] underlies the epithelium. Its rich collagen fiber and elastic fiber meshwork contains a lymph follicle [3]. The strong *lamina muscularis mucosae* [4] is composed of smooth muscle cell bundles of different sizes. These are cross-sectioned. Two clusters of glands (*glandulae esophageae*) [6] are visible in the wide, richly vascularized *submucosal tissue* [5]. The lower part of the figure shows a salivary duct, which ends between mucous membrane papillae. The tunica muscularis [6] (right half of the figure) is up to 2 mm thick and consists of the inner circular layer and the outer longitudinal layer of muscle cells (*stratum circulare et longitudinale*). The tunica adventitia with blood vessels is visible in the right corner of this figure [8].

1 Lamina epithelialis mucosae
2 Lamina propria mucosae
3 Singular follicle
4 Lamina muscularis mucosae
5 Tela submucosa (submucosal tissue)
6 Esophageal glands
7 Tunica muscularis
8 Tunica adventitia

Stain: alum hematoxylin-eosin; magnification: × 30

401 Esophagus

This micrograph shows the esophageal mucous membrane (tunica mucosa) at higher magnification (cf. Fig. 399, 400).

1 Lamina epithelialis mucosae: multilayered nonkeratinizing squamous epithelium
2 Lamina propria mucosae: connective tissue containing fine fibers
3 Lamina muscularis mucosae
4 Esophageal glands

Stain: azan; magnification: × 80

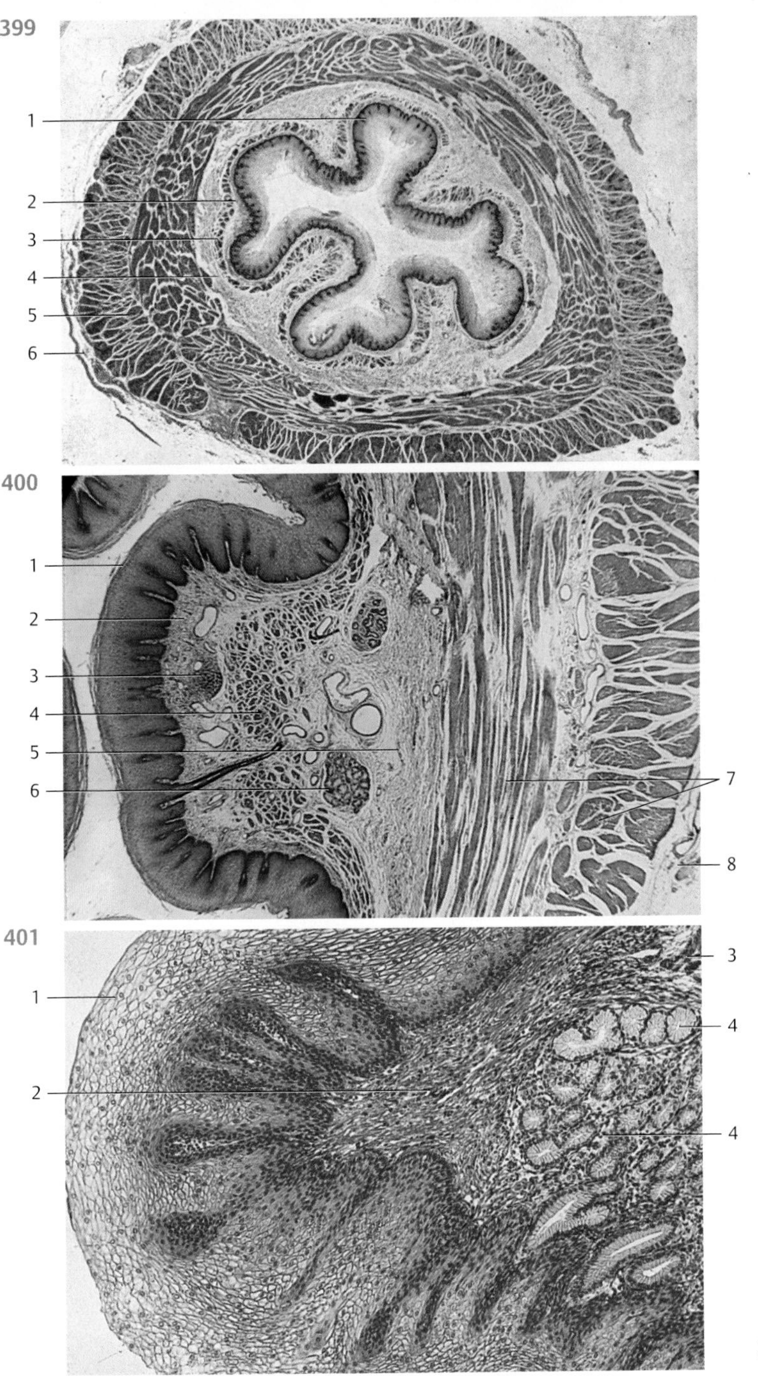
399
1
2
3
4
5
6
400
1
2
3
4
5
6
7
8
401
1
2
3
4
4

402 Esophagus—Cardia—Esophagogastric Junction

Transitional tissue between esophagus (right) and the gastric cardia of the stomach (left). The mucous membranes of the esophagus end and those of the stomach begin. The multilayered nonkeratinizing squamous epithelium 1 of the esophagus ends abruptly at the border to the single-layered columnar epithelium of the gastric mucous membranes. The pars cardiaca (short cardia) of the stomach features cardiac glands 2 with elaborately branched tubules in irregular shapes. Occasionally, they have ampullary extensions 3. The mucus-producing cardiac glands consist of only one cell type. There are no parietal or background cells. The lamina muscularis mucosa 4 is visible at the lower edge of the figure.

1 Multilayered nonkeratinizing squamous epithelium of the esophagus
2 Cardiac glands
3 Distended tubule
4 Lamina muscularis mucosae
5 Foveolae gastricae
Stain: azan; magnification: × 40

403 Pars Cardiaca—Cardiac Glands

The pars cardiaca is a 2–3 cm ring-shaped strip of mucous membranes at the stomach entrance (see Fig. 402). A single-layered columnar epithelium covers the surface of the mucous membranes, including that of the foveolae (foveolae gastricae) 1 (cf. Fig. 407). The foveolae continue in the deeper, sometimes winding tubules of the mucous cardiac glands 2 in the mucous membrane. The lamina muscularis mucosae 3 can be seen at the right edge of the figure. Note the large lymph follicle 4. The cardiac glands release alkaline mucus and the enzyme lysozyme.

1 Gastric foveolae
2 Cardiac glands
3 Lamina muscularis mucosae
4 Lymph follicle
5 Lamina propria mucosae
Stain: azan; magnification: × 80

404 Corpus of the Stomach—Gastric Glands

The corpus and fundus of the stomach (*corpus and fundus ventriculi*) contain the *gastric glands* 1. The glands are about 1.5–2.0 mm long, rarely branched tubules, which will split in two shortly before they reach the lamina muscularis mucosae. The tubules are densely packed. Their lumina are only 3–6 µm wide. *Chief or zymogenic cells, parietal or oxyntic cells, neck mucous cells and enteroendocrine* cells form the lining of the secretory tubules (cf. Fig. 405–410). The parietal cells (stained red) are prominent in this figure. Note the short *gastric pits (foveolae gastricae)* 2. Their deepest point marks the beginning of the gastric glands, which consist of a gland isthmus, the neck, the main body and a fundus.

1 Gastric glands
2 Gastric pits
Stain: alum hematoxylin-eosin, x80

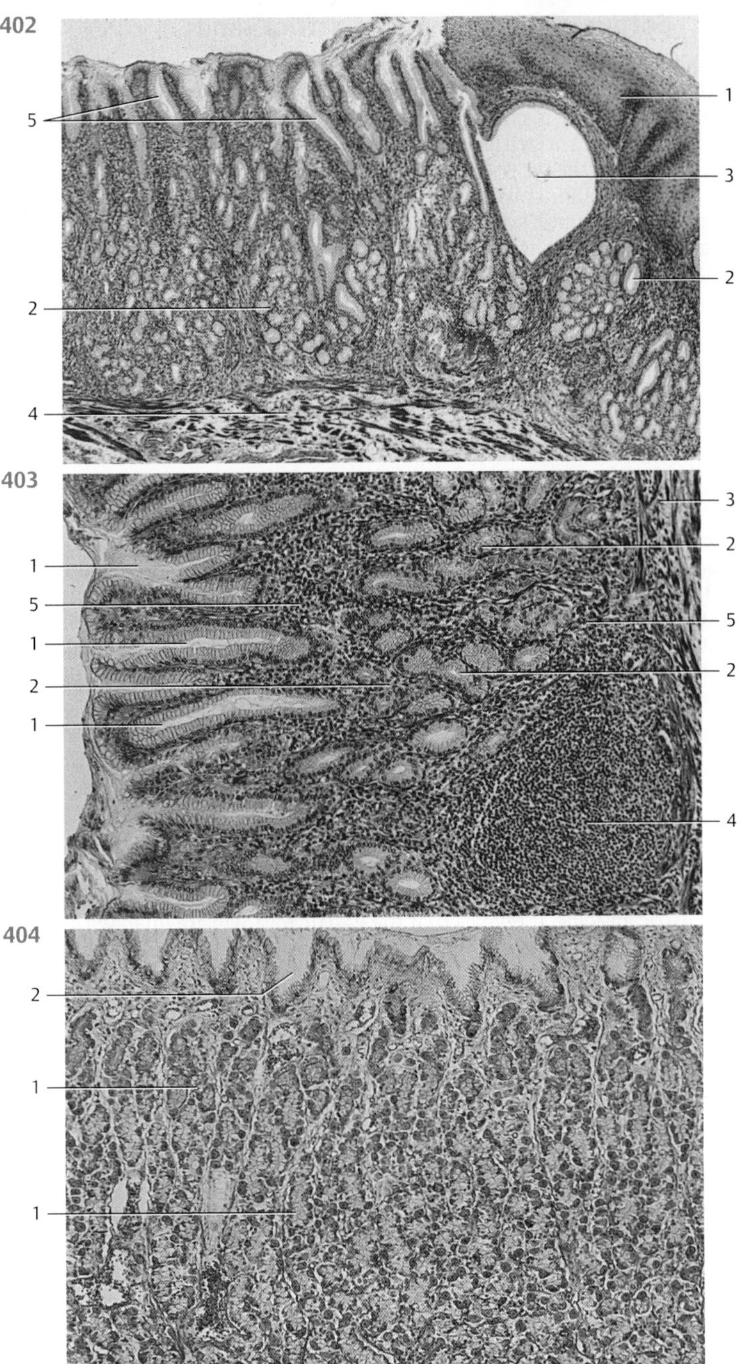

Digestive System

405 Corpus of the Stomach—Gastric Glands

As shown in this vertical section through the mucosa and submucosal layer of the gastric corpus region, the surface of the mucous membrane, including *foveolae gastricae*, is covered by a single-layered columnar epithelium 1. This covering or surface layer of cells sequesters alkaline mucus (cf. Fig. 407). The tubules of the gastric glands (*glandulae gastricae propriae*) 2 lead into the pits. The glands consist of moderately branched tubules, which widen at their ends. The tubules are about 1.5 μmm long and extend to the *lamina muscularis mucosae* 3. Little room is left for the lamina propria. The highly vascularized *submucosal tissue* is shown as a parallel strand at the bottom edge of the figure.

1 Lamina epithelialis mucosae
2 Gastric glands
3 Lamina muscularis mucosa
4 Tela submucosa (submucosal tissue)
Stain: alum hematoxylin-eosin; magnification: × 50

406 Corpus of the Stomach—Gastric Glands

The *parietal cells* are rich in crista-type mitochondria. *Succinate dehydrogenase* (SDH) is a marker enzyme for mitochondria. Here, it has been utilized in an immunotopochemical procedure to selectively emphasize the mitochondria-rich parietal cells. This figure also demonstrates that parietal cells in the gastric glands are unevenly distributed. Note the dense layer of parietal cells in the neck of the gland. The small band at the lower edge of the picture is the lamina muscularis mucosae.

1 Lamina muscularis mucosae
Histochemical localization using the enzyme succinate dehydrogenase; magnification: × 65

407 Fundus of the Stomach—Gastric Foveolae

The mucous membrane has been cut parallel to the tissue surface through the *gastric foveolae*. It reveals that the gastric foveolae are lined with columnar epithelium 1. The epithelial nuclei are located in the basal cell region. The *lamina propria mucosa* 2 is visible between the foveolae. The single-layered columnar epithelium 1 consists of PAS-positive cells, which secrete mucus. The mucus forms a viscous protective barrier against the hydrochloric acid and lytic enzymes in the stomach. This prevents the autodigestion of the mucous membrane. Note: the single-layered columnar epithelium covers the entire inner stomach surface, including the gastric foveolae (cf. Figs. 402–405).

1 Columnar epithelium
2 Lamina propria mucosae
3 Lumina of the gastric foveolae
Stain: alum hematoxylin-orcein; magnification: × 300

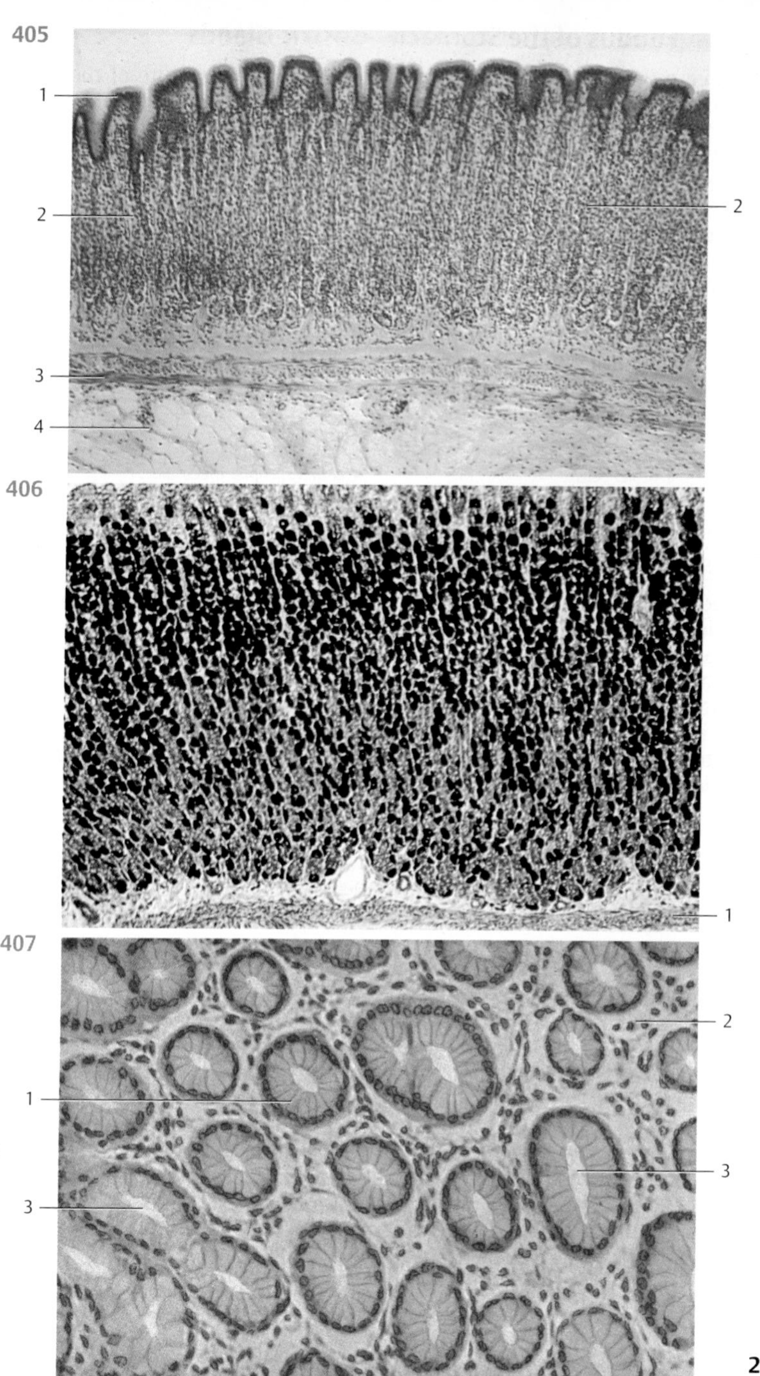
405
1
2
2
3
4
406
1
407
2
1
3
3

408 Fundus of the Stomach—Gastric Glands

Three different types of merocrine cells build the structure of the gastric gland lumina.
1. *Chief cells.* It is easiest to locate them in the glandular body or fundus.
2. *Parietal (covering) cells.* They are particularly numerous in the neck part of the gland.
3. *Neck mucous cells* (predominantly in the neck of the gland).
The figure shows *mucus producing* neck cells 1 (stained dark blue), chief cells 2 (stained muddy blue, *pepsinogen* producing cells), and almost homogeneous *parietal cells* 3 (stained light blue, *acid producing cells*). The latter often outnumber the other cells. The parietal cells contain large, rounded nuclei. Cells and fibers of the *lamina propria mucosae* 4 spread out between the gastric glands.
Semi-thin section, parallel to the surface of the mucous membrane (cf. Fig. 409).

1 Neck mucous cells
2 Chief cells
3 Parietal cells (covering cells)
4 Lamina propria mucosae
Semi-thin section; stain: methylene blue-azure II; magnification: × 400

409 Fundus of the Stomach—Gastric Glands

Because parietal cells 1 are so rich in mitochondria, they heavily stain with acidic dyes, such as eosin, Congo red, benzyl fast red (*acidophilia*). In this cross-section of gastric gland tissue, the cells have a distinctly different appearance when compared with the strongly acidophilic parietal cells (stained brilliant red) (cf. Fig. 408). The large, pyramid-shaped parietal cells often appear triangular in a cross-section. The chief cells 2 display the characteristics of protein-synthesizing cells. They biosynthesize *pepsinogen* and *lipase*. The neck mucous cells 3 look almost identical to chief cells with the staining method used here.

1 Parietal (covering) cell
2 Chief cell
3 Neck mucous cell
4 Lumen of the glands
Stain: hemalum-eosin; magnification: × 400

410 Pyloric Part of the Stomach—Pyloric Glands

In contrast to the gastric glands of the corpus and fundus of the stomach, the tubules of the pyloric glands (*pylorus = pars pylorica ventriculi*) branch out and form coils only deep in the mucous membrane (cf. Fig. 405). The *gastric foveolae (little dents)* 1 are deeper than the foveolae in the *mucous membrane of the gastric corpus and fundus*. The glandular tubules undulate considerably and may therefore be sectioned in different planes relative to their axis. The columnar surface epithelium also covers the funnel-shaped gastric foveolae 1. Pyloric glands exclusively consist of mucous cells (*mucous pyloric glands*, here lightly stained). Routine preparations usually show a cytoplasmic honeycomb structure. The nuclei are located in the basal cell region. Note the following layers of the intestinal wall.

1 Gastric foveolae
2 Lamina muscularis mucosae
3 Submucosal tissue
4 Tunica muscularis
5 Lamina propria mucosae
6 Gland fundus
Stain: alum hematoxylin-eosin; magnification: × 16

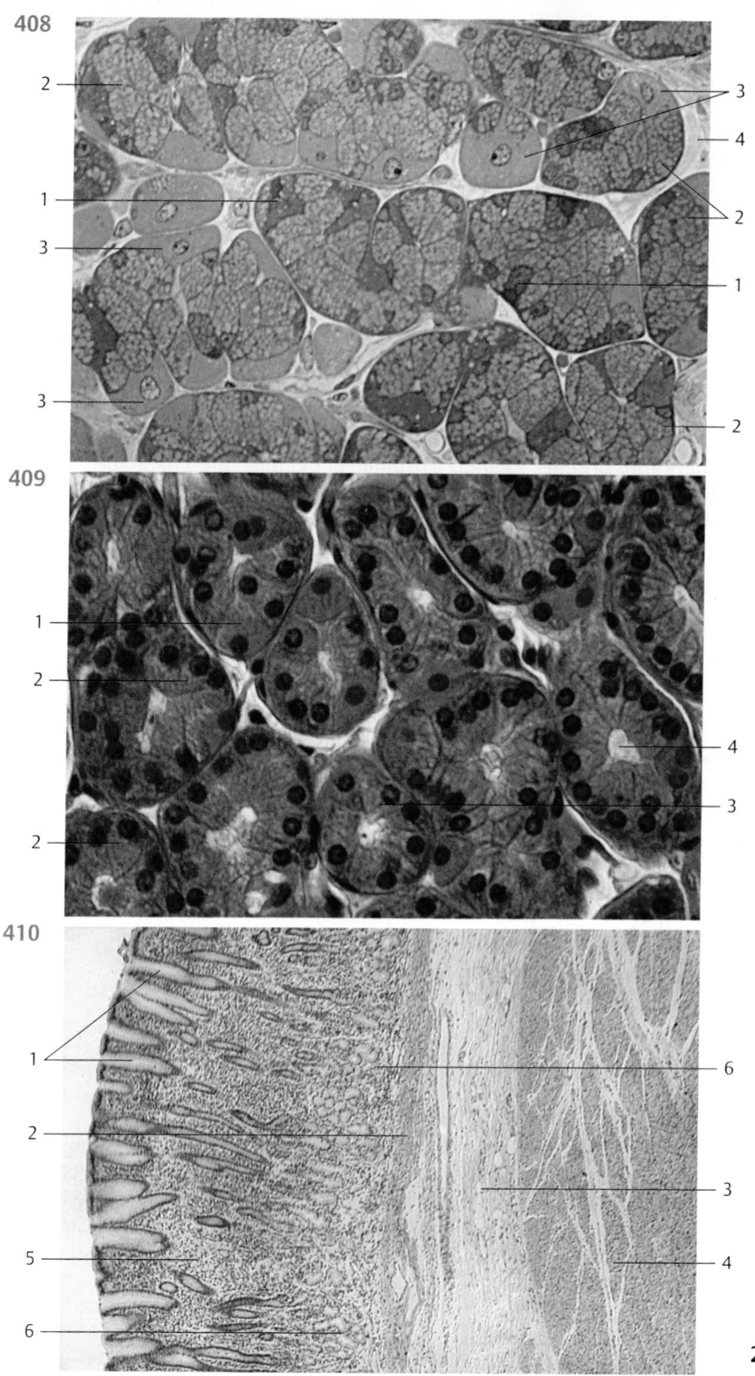
408
2
1
3
3
3
4
2
1
2
409
1
2
2
4
3
410
1
2
5
6
6
3
4

411 Small Intestine—Duodenum

The tissue surface in the duodenum, as in the rest of the upper small intestine, shows circular folds called *plicae circulares* or Kerckring's folds 1. Circular folds form an impressively articulated relief in the duodenum. They are part of the mucous membranes and the submucosal tissue 2 and can be up to 8 mm high. The tunica muscularis 3 is not a part of the plicae. This section shows two looped folds 1. The *tunica muscularis* 3 and the *tunica serosa* 4 can be seen in the lower left of the figure. The surface of the Kerckring folds features *intestinal villi* 5 in different shapes and sizes (*villi intestinales*). They are 0.5–1.5 mm high and about 0.15 mm thick. Intestinal villi are covered with a columnar epithelium (*enterocytes, absorptive cells*) (see Fig. 73). Smooth muscle cells reach from the lamina muscularis mucosae to the *lamina propria* of the villi. The finger-shaped villi are therefore protrusions from the mucous membranes. Tubular canals extend from the cell surface at the bottom of the invaginations between microvilli to the lamina muscularis mucosae. These are the *intestinal glands of Lieberkühn*, also called crypts of Lieberkühn. *Brunner's glands* 6 (*duodenal glands*) are characteristic of the duodenum. They are located in the submucosal layer. The glands with their winding tubules remind of the pyloric glands.

1 Kerckring's folds
2 Submucosal tissue
3 Tunica muscularis
4 Tunica serosa
5 Villi
6 Brunner's glands (duodenal glands)
Stain: alum hematoxylin-eosin; magnification: × 5

412 Small Intestine—Duodenum

Longitudinal section of the duodenal wall of an adult human. It shows the *plicae circulares* (*Kerckring folds*) and *Brunner's glands* 1 in the submucosal tissue 2. The plicae circulares are densely covered with villi 3 in the shape of leaves or tongues. The defining characteristic of the duodenum are the *duodenal glands* (*Brunner's glands*) in the submucosa. The *tunica muscularis* 4 with its inner circular layer and outer longitudinal layer parallels the lower edge in the figure.

1 Brunner's glands
2 Submucosa
3 Villi on the plicae circulares
4 Tunica muscularis with inner stratum circulare and outer stratum longitudinale
5 Tela subserosa and tunica serosa
Stain: azan; magnification: × 13

413 Small Intestine—Duodenum

Partial section of *Kerckring's fold* with tunica mucosa and tela submucosa 1. The surface epithelium contains goblet cells (cf. Fig. 108, 415). A cluster of *Brunner's glands* 2 is seen in the submucosal layer. Their nuclei are localized in the basal part of the cell. The cytoplasm is only lightly stained. Strong collagen fiber bundles (stained blue) are visible between the cross-sectioned glands (cf. Figs. 411, 412, 415).

1 Tela submucosa
2 Duodenal glands (Brunner's glands)
3 Lamina propria mucosae
Stain: azan; magnification: × 80

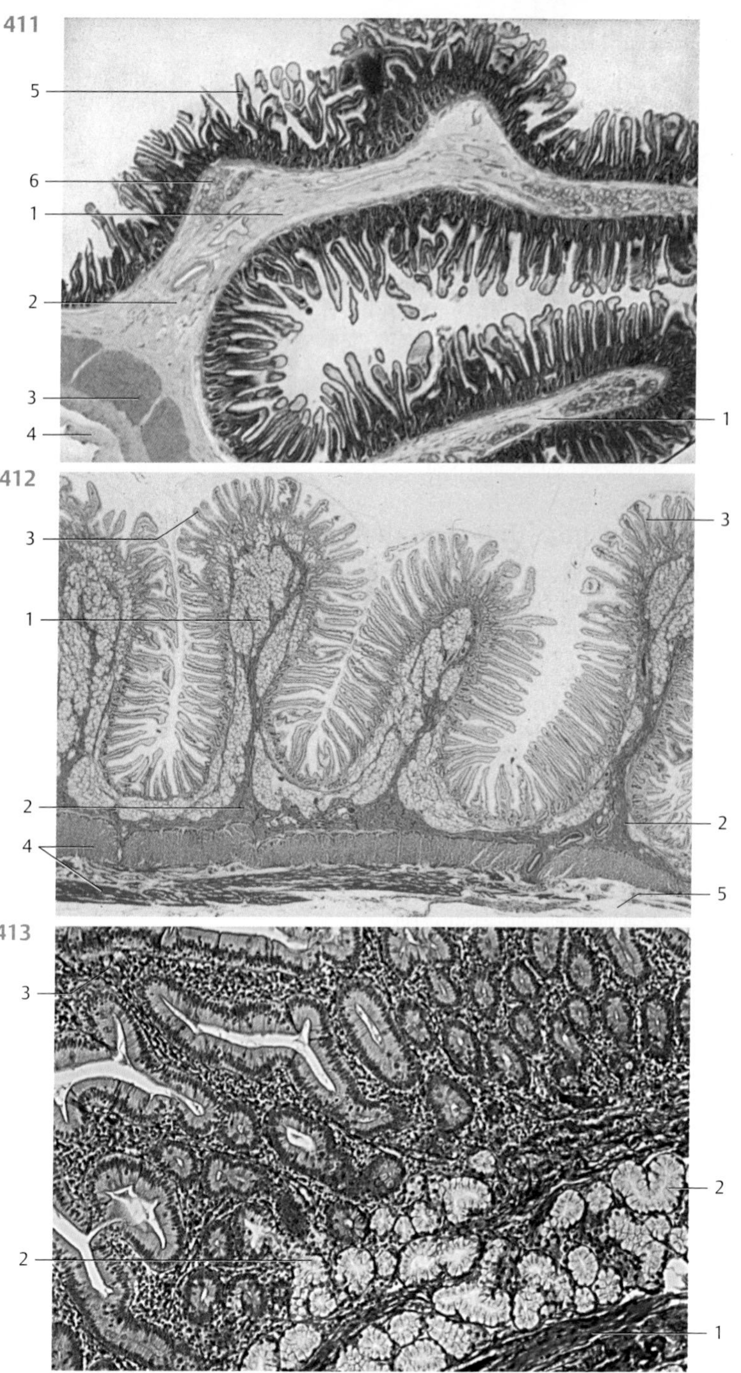

Digestive System

414 Small Intestine—Duodenum

Enlargement of a detail from Fig. 412. It shows the villi of a Kerckring valve. The tall *circular folds* are densely covered with villi 1, which may be long and slender or wide and leaf-like. The villi are enveloped by a single-layered columnar epithelium (*enterocytes*) with interspersed goblet cells (see Fig. 415, 416). The tubular canals of the intestinal glands (*Lieberkühn glands, crypts of Lieberkühn*) extend from the bottom of the dents between villi to the lamina muscularis mucosae 3. The intestinal glands are tubular, partially branched invaginations of the intestinal epithelium. Their depths range between 200 and 400 µm. The tubules undulate, and therefore may be sectioned in different planes. The *submucosa* with Brunner's glands and vessels are visible on the right side of the figure. Brunner's glands are branched, winding tubuloalveolar glands.

1 Villi
2 Crypts (glands) of Lieberkühn
3 Lamina muscularis mucosae
4 Artery in the submucosa
5 Brunner's glands
6 Lamina propria mucosae
Stain: azan; magnification: × 80

415 Small Intestine—Duodenum

Longitudinal section of the *surface epithelium* 1, which covers two villi on opposite sides of the intestinal lumen. The slender columnar cells (*enterocytes*) clearly show a *brush border* (see Figs. 73, 75–78, 108, 109) at their apical surface (directed toward the intestinal lumen). The *microvilli*, which make up the brush border, are 1.2–1.5 µm long and 0.1 µm thick. On average, about 2500–3000 microvilli protrude from an epithelial cell. The elongated nuclei are located in the basal third of the enterocytes. There are occasional goblet cells in the epithelium. Their secretory products (mucus) are stained blue. Note the discontinued brush border around the goblet cells (cf. Fig. 108).
Enterocytes are 15–30 µm high and 5–10 µm wide. Note the smooth muscle cells in the lamina propria mucosae.

1 Enterocytes
2 Lamina propria mucosae (connective tissue of the villi)
3 Intestinal lumen (clearance)
Stain: azan; magnification: × 200

416 Small Intestine—Duodenum

Parallel section through the duodenal mucous membrane. It shows the *crypts* (*glands*) *of Lieberkühn*. The diameter of these crypts is smaller than that of the villi. The tubular epithelial dells (foveolae) are cross-sectioned in this figure. They have diameters of about 200–400 µm and are located in the cellular *lamina propria mucosae* 1. Apart from the surface cells, the epithelium of the crypts also contains typical goblet cells. Their secretory product is stained blue. Note the lightly stained emptied cells. *Paneth cells* (see Fig. 417) and *endocrine cells* (see Fig. 422) are other cell types in the intestinal surface epithelium, along with enterocytes and goblet cells. Note the oval nuclei in the basal part of the enterocytes (cf. Figs. 414, 415).

1 Lamina propria mucosae
2 Lumen of a crypt (gland)
Stain: azan; magnification: × 200

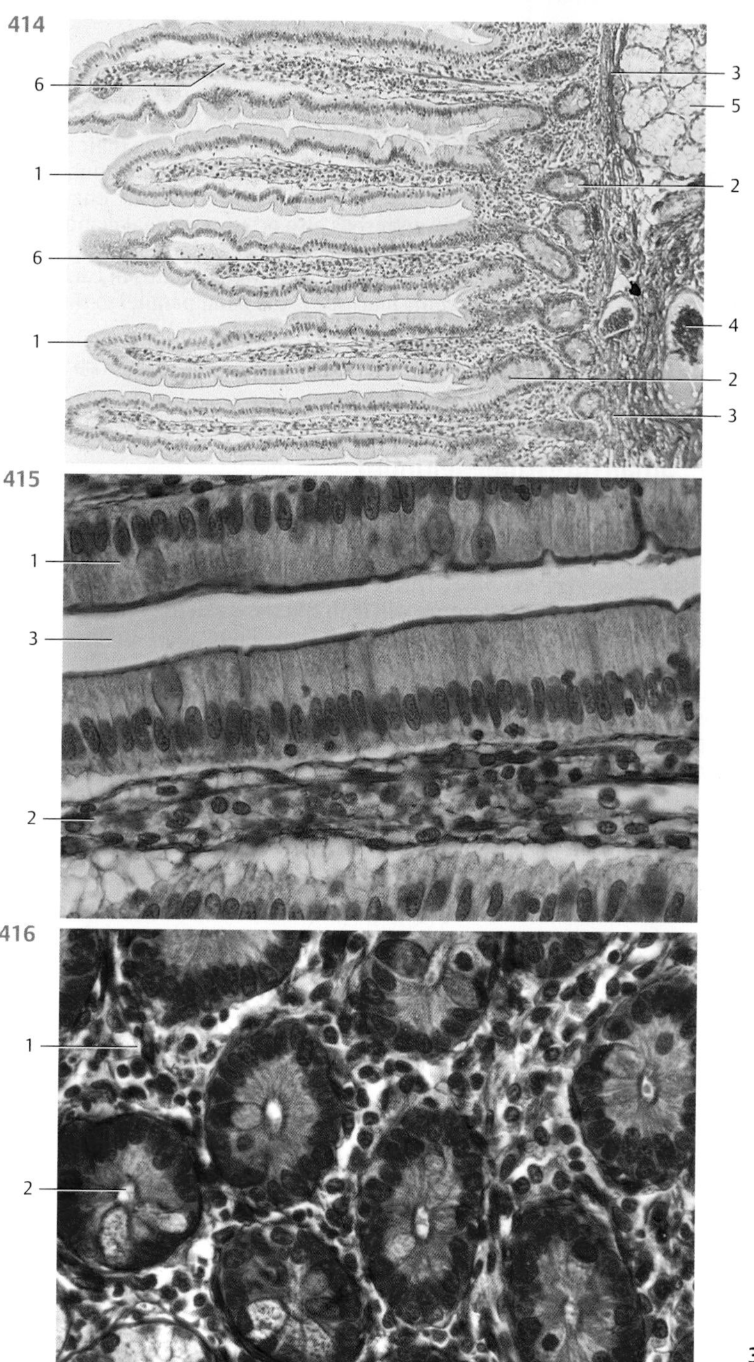

Digestive System

417 Small Intestine—Duodenum—Paneth Cells

Clusters of cells with apical granulation are found in the intestinal epithelium at the fundus of the crypts (see Fig. 414). These cells were named *Paneth cells* (*Paneth cell glands*) after Joseph Paneth (1857–1890) who first described them. They are also called *oxyphilic granule cells* in reference to their staining characteristics 1. Paneth cells are exocrine glands. Their granulation is caused by secretory granules, which contain the bacteriolytic enzyme *lysozyme* or several *peptidases*. Paneth cells also occur in jejunal glands. They are found in larger numbers in the lower ileum and the vermiform appendix. This micrograph clearly shows two Paneth cells in the fundus of each of the two crypts. The *lamina muscularis mucosae* is the band parallel to the lower edge of the picture.

1 Paneth cells
2 Lamina propria mucosae
3 Goblet cells
Stain: azan; magnification: × 400

418 Small Intestine—Jejunum

This longitudinal section of the jejunal wall from an adult human shows six circular plicae (*Kerckring's folds*) 1. Compare the form of these plicae with those of the duodenum and note that there are no *Brunner glands* in the submucosa 2 (see Figs. 411–414). This preparation is from the upper section of the jejunum where the plicae are still high and show a dense microvilli brush border (*villi intestinales*) 3. The villi of the small intestines are protrusions from the *tunica mucosa*. Therefore, they consist of the surface epithelium, the *lamina propria mucosae* and sporadic smooth muscle cells from the lamina muscularis mucosae. As the jejunum continues toward the ileum, the circular plicae stand lower and become sparse. The density of their villi decreases as well (see Figs. 423, 424).

1 Circular plica (fold)
2 Submucosa
3 Villi of the small intestine, villi intestinales
4 Tunica muscularis with an inner circular layer and an outer longitudinal layer of muscle cells
Stain: hematoxylin-eosin; magnification: × 14

419 Small Intestine—Jejunum

Longitudinal section of the jejunal wall from an adult human. The picture shows the outer membrane between two circular plicae. Therefore, no Kerckring folds are present (see Figs. 418, 420). Closer toward the ileum, the distances between plicae widen. Note the configuration of the villi 1. The unbranched tubular *intestinal glands* (*Lieberkühn glands, crypts of Lieberkühn*) 2 are present between shorter villi. The band of the tunica muscularis 4 is demonstrated parallel to the lower edge of the figure. The circular layer shows vertical, heavily stained bands (red). These are artifacts. Cutting has pushed the tissue components together.

1 Intestinal villi
2 Crypts of Lieberkühn
3 Tela submucosa
4 Tunica muscularis
Stain: azan; magnification: × 25

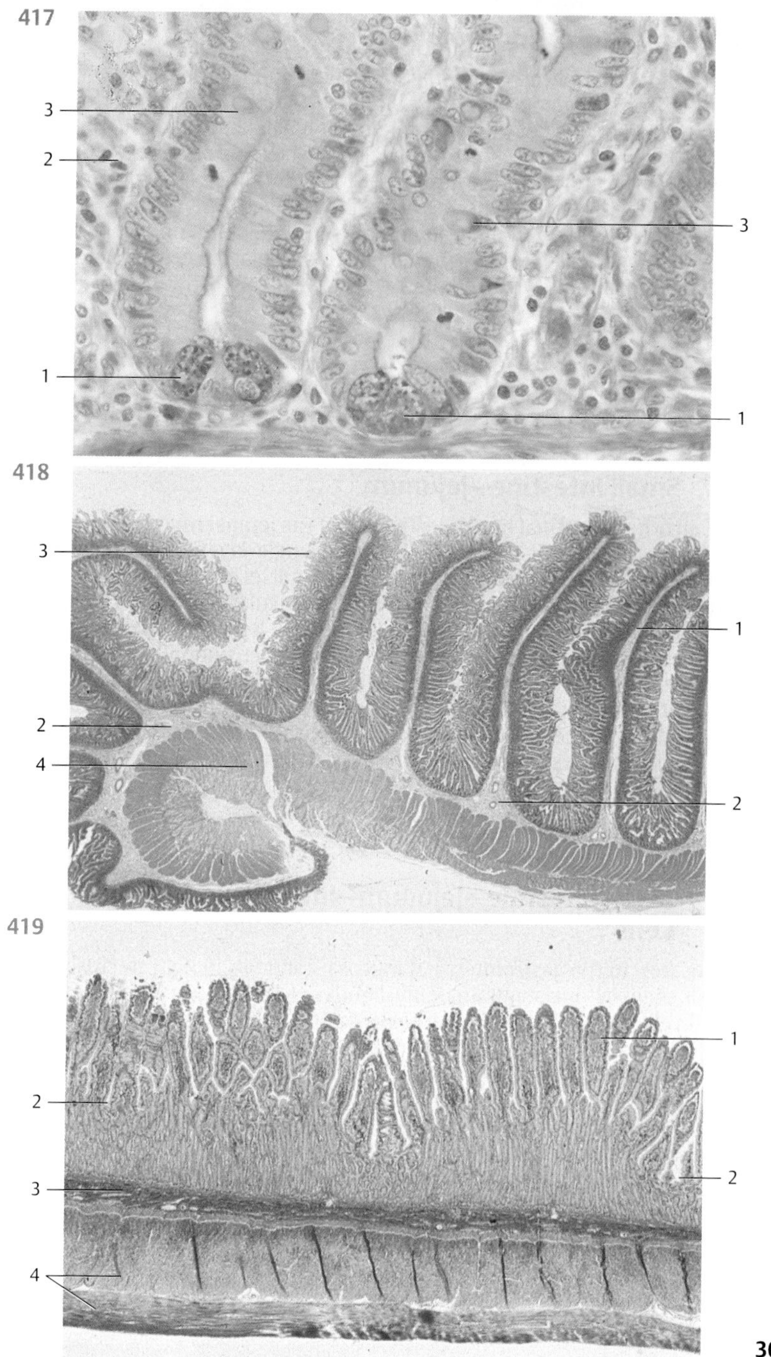
417
3
2
1
3
1
418
3
1
2
4
2
419
1
2
3
4
2

420 Small Intestine—Jejunum

The high jejunal plicae (*Kerckring's folds*) are supported by the connective tissue of the *tela submucosa*. The submucosa 1 of the looped fold runs parallel to the lower edge of the photomicrograph. The density of microvilli that cover the plicae decreases toward the ileum. The long, often flattened villi 2 look like fingers or clubs. The number of goblet cells increases toward the distal side. Note the short crypts 3 with copious *Paneth cells* (cf. Fig. 417). Brunner's glands do not occur in the jejunum (cf. Fig. 419). The connective tissue of the villi 4 contains free cells, lymphocytes and plasma cells, macrophages, eosinophilic granulocytes and mast cells (cf. Fig. 413–416).

1 Tela submucosa
2 Villi intestinales
3 Crypts
4 Lamina propria mucosae (connective tissue of the villi)
Stain: azan; magnification: × 80

421 Small Intestine—Jejunum

Like all other intestinal mucosae, the villi of the jejunal mucosa in this longitudinal section (cf. Figs. 418, 420) feature a single-layered columnar surface epithelium (enterocytes). As always, the oval nuclei of the enterocytes are located in the basal cell region (cf. 415). The reticular connective tissue lines the lamina propria on the inner face of the villi. Its meshwork contains free cells, such as lymphocytes, plasma cells and eosinophilic granulocytes, among others. The inner part of the villi features a dense capillary network, lymphatic vessels and smooth muscle cells 1, which traverse the villi along their long axis. The muscle cells originate with the *lamina muscularis mucosae*. Their activities generate the rhythmic contractions of the villi.

1 Smooth muscle cells
Stain: alum hematoxylin-eosin; magnification: × 100

422 Small Intestine—Jejunum—Intestinal Enteroendocrine Cells

Some cells in the gastrointestinal mucosa stand out in light microscopy because their cytoplasm stains only lightly. Their secretory granules in the basal cell region are also remarkable. They can be emphasized by staining with chromium-silver salts and are therefore named *enterochromaffin* cells (compare the cells with Paneth cells in Fig. 417). These cells produce hormones and their entire population forms the *gastroenteropancreatic system* (*GEP*). About 19 GEP cell types have been defined to date. They produce 18 peptide hormones and serotonin.
In the jejunal epithelium in this figure, one cell stands out because its basal region is stained intensely brown. This cell contains *gastrin inhibitory peptide* (*GIP*). The staining is based on the PAS reaction using an antibody to GIP. Electron microscopy reveals that secretory granules are the cause for the intense brown staining of the basal cytoplasmic region.

Specimen; magnification: × 400

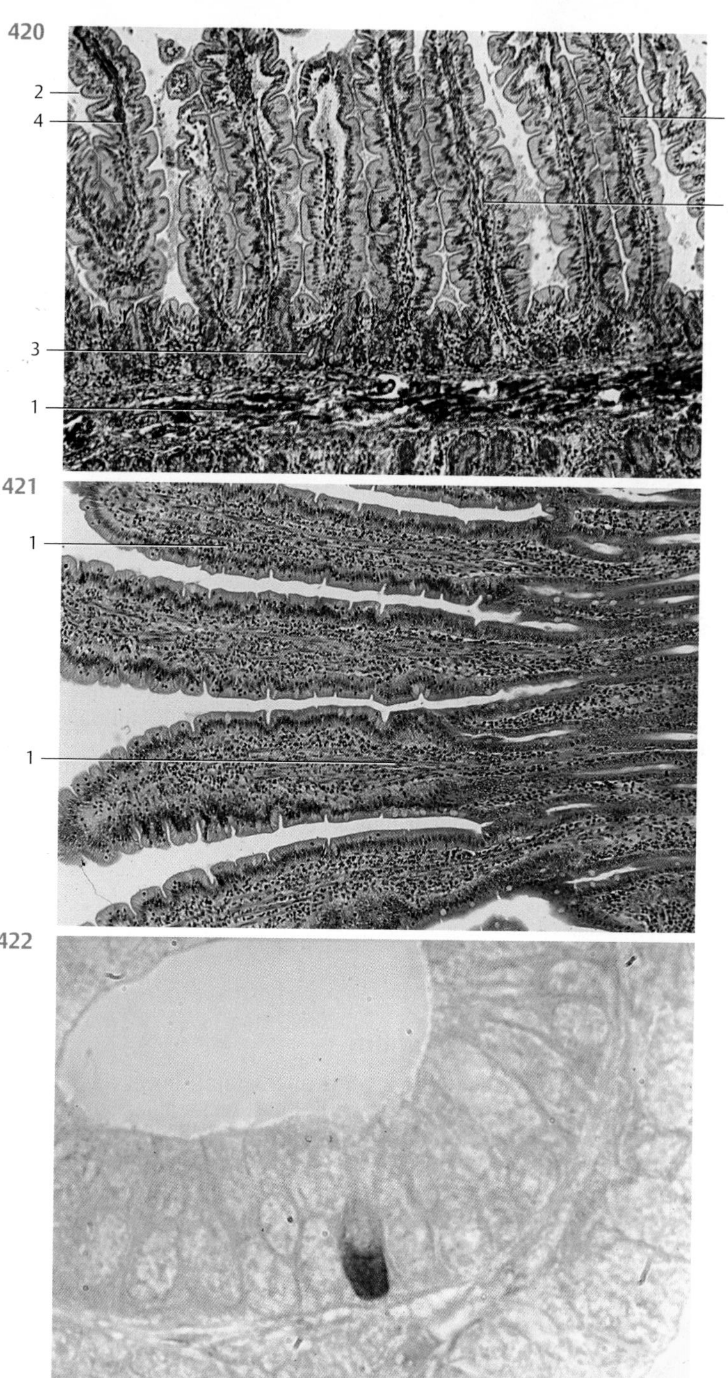
420
2
4
4
2
3
1
421
1
1
422

423 Small Intestine—Ileum

Compared with the adjacent small intestine, there is only little surface enlargement in the ileum. This is the major difference between both tissues. The circular plicae are lesser in height, and there are fewer and fewer of them until they are completely absent. In the process, the villi also become shorter and scarcer than in the jejunum.

The figure shows a longitudinal section through the ileum. None of their circular folds are part of this micrograph. Some villi are branched, some show somewhat odd shapes 1. There are small crypts at the bottom of the spaces between the villi. The development of the lymphoreticular organs in the form of lymphatic nodules (*noduli lymphatici aggregati* 2, *Peyer's plaques*) is remarkable. Peyer plaques or glands pervade the connective tissue of the mucosa and the entire submucosa. Note the missing villi over the Peyer plaques. This is the only location where M-cells are found in the epithelium (see Figs. 341–343). The lower edge represents the thin tunica muscularis (cf. Figs. 419, 424).

1 Villi
2 Lymphatic nodules (noduli lymphatici aggregati)
3 Tunica muscularis
Stain: iron hematoxylin (Masson-Goldner trichrome); magnification: × 20

424 Small Intestine—Ileum

Cross-section of iliac mucosa, including villi 1 and *solitary lymphatic nodules* 2, which occur predominantly as *Peyer plaques* (*patches*) in the tela submucosa 3 opposite the attachment of the mesentery. The tunica muscularis 4 is stained gray-yellow.

All solitary and aggregated lymphatic follicles form the gut-associated lymphoid tissue (GALT). As always, villi are absent from the mucosa in the areas of the summits 5 over lymphatic follicles (cf. Figs. 341–343, 431).

1 Villi
2 Lymphatic follicles
3 Tela submucosa
4 Tunica muscularis
5 Summit over a lymphatic follicle
Stain: hematoxylin-picric acid; magnification: × 8

425 Small Intestine—Jejunum

Normal mucosa from a dog (beagle). The micrograph shows villi, some are long and round, others are more flattened, almost rectangular. Small grooves subdivide the villi surface into smaller areas. The small dells in some places are probably caused by goblet cells.

Villi and crypts enlarge the surface area of the small intestinal mucosa about 7- to 14-fold. The mucosa of the small intestine measures about 4.5 m^2.

Scanning electron microscopy; magnification: × 80

423

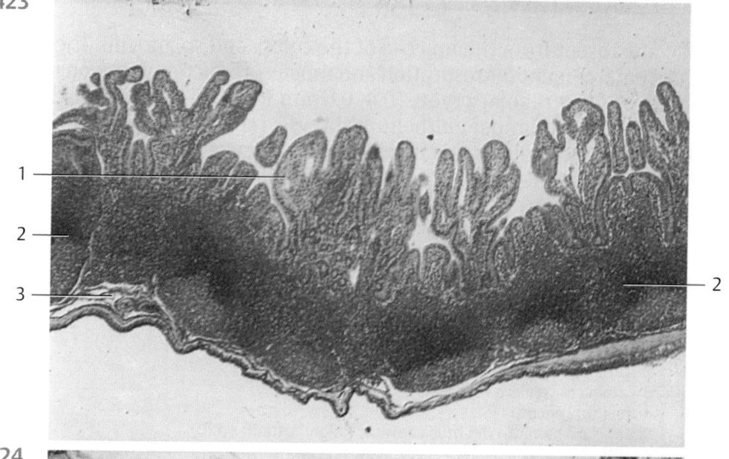

424

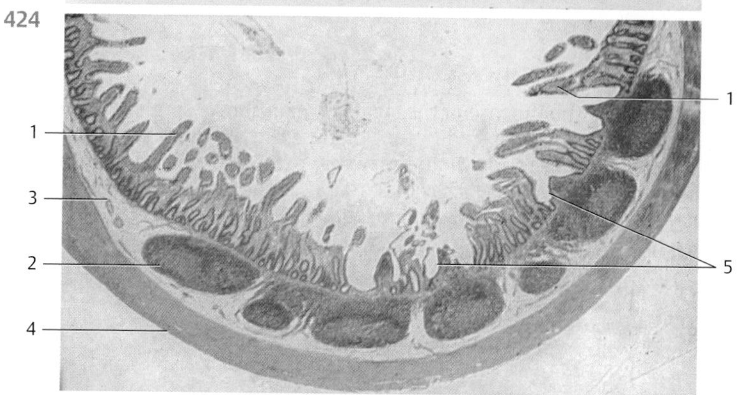

425

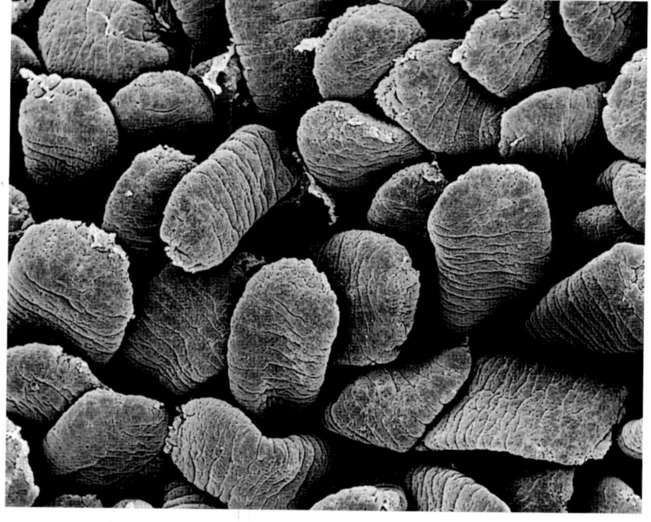

426 Large Intestine—Colon

Plicae are absent from the mucosa of the colon, and so are villi. The needed surface enlargement for resorption and mucus production relies on the large number of deep tubular crypts (0.4–0.6 mm long) 1 in close proximity of each other. The columnar epithelium shows a remarkable number of mucus producing goblet cells. In this figure, the presence of goblet cells is indicated only by small red dots. All other epithelial cells, i.e., the enterocytes of the mucosa, are covered with a *brush border.* There are also *enteroendocrine cells* and undifferentiated stem cells in the wall of the crypts. Sporadically, brownish *hemosiderin inclusions* are found in the lamina propria mucosae 2. There is the lamina muscularis mucosae 3 underneath the crypts, followed by submucosal tissue 4 (see Fig. 427).

1 Crypts
2 Lamina propria mucosae
3 Lamina muscularis mucosae
4 Tela submucosa
Stain: alum hematoxylin-mucicarmine; magnification: × 120

427 Small Intestine—Colon

This section of the mucosa of the *sigmoid colon* shows single tubular glands 1, which have been cut in different planes. The only lightly stained goblet cells appear oval or round. Note the highly vascularized lamina propria mucosae 2. The tunica muscularis mucosae 3 is thicker than that of the small intestines. Two larger vessels are present in the submucosal tissue 4 (cf. Figs. 426, 428, 429).

1 Crypts
2 Lamina propria mucosae
3 Lamina muscularis mucosae
4 Submucosal tissue with large vessels
Semi-thin sections; stain: methylene blue-azure II; magnification: × 100

428 Large Intestine—Colon

These two figures show parallel sections through the mucosa of the colon. The crypts 1 in the micrograph have been cross-sectioned. Enterocytes and goblet cells 3 are arranged around the tubular *Lieberkühn glands* (cf. Figs. 108, 122, 123, 125). The goblet cells are stained red using mucicarmine. They stain only lightly with hematoxylin-eosin. The cells between the cross-sectioned tubules belong to the highly vascularized, cellular lamina propria mucosae 2, which shows accumulations of yellow-brown hemosiderin pigments (cf. Fig. 426).
The mucosa of the colon resorbs water and provides mucus for the movement of the thickened colon content.

1 Lumen of crypt
2 Lamina propria mucosae
3 Goblet cells
Stain: a) alum hematoxylin-eosin; b) hemalum-mucicarmine; magnification: × 250 for a) and b)

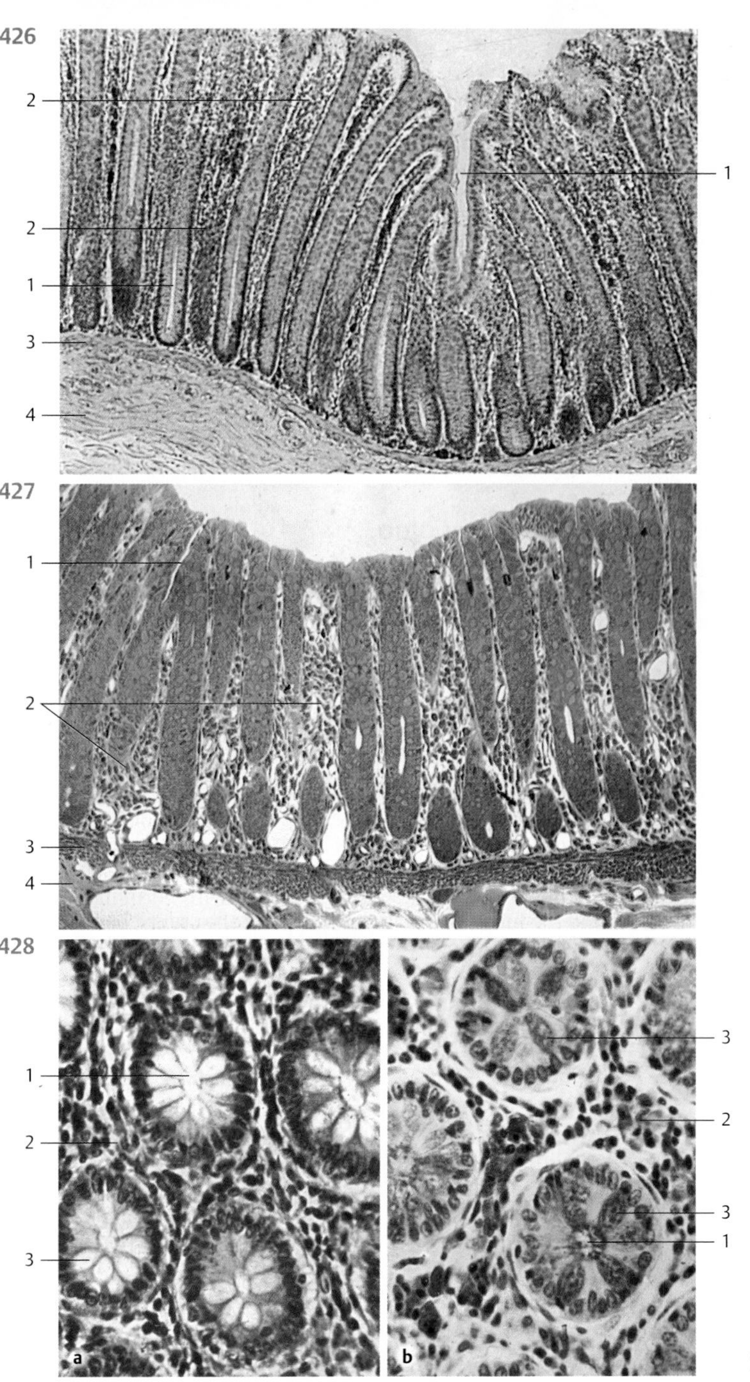
426
2
1
2
1
3
4
427
1
2
3
4
428
1
2
3
a
3
2
3
1
b

429 Large Intestine—Colon

This figure shows the *tunica mucosa* of the colon, which has been cut parallel to the tissue surface (cf. Figs. 123, 428). The lumina of the crypts are only slits 1. Goblet cells are stained intensely blue. The vascularized connective tissue of the *lamina propria mucosae* 3 is seen between the cross-sectioned tubules of the glands.

The about 0.4–0.6 mm deep crypts are arranged in a remarkably regular pattern. This can be seen in mucosa sections, which run parallel to the surface (see Fig. 428), or when looking onto the surface (see Fig. 430). Compare this with the vertical sections of the mucosa from the colon in Figs. 426 and 427. As an exception, the crypts of the appendix are arranged irregularly (see Figs. 341, 431).

1 Lumina of crypts
2 Goblet cells
3 Lamina propria mucosae
Semi-thin section; stain: methylene blue-azure II; magnification: × 400

430 Large Intestine—Colon

View of the mucosa of the ascending colon from a rat, which shows the crater-shaped openings of the crypts. The epithelium appears irregular when viewed from the top. The velvety covering consists of short villi. Compare with Figs. 428 and 429.

Scanning electron microscopy; magnification: × 750

431 Vermiform Appendix

Cross-section through the entire appendix and *mesenteriolum* (at the lower left 1 of the figure). The micrograph presents all layers of the intestinal wall. Note that the crypts 2 are arranged in a less regular pattern. In some places, crypts are missing entirely (cf. Figs 426, 427). The copious presence of lymphatic tissue is impressive. Large lymph follicles with germinal centers 3 occur all around the lumen. They in part supplant the crypts, but they are restricted to the mucosa. However, lymph follicles can break through the lamina muscularis mucosae and extend into the tela submucosa 4 (cf. Fig. 341). Epithelial crypts and lymphoreticular tissue form a functional unit ("intestinal tonsil"). The fiber components of the submucosal tissue continue in the mesenteriolum 1. The next layer is the tunica muscularis 5. The epithelium of the mucosa 2 consists mostly of columnar cells that are covered with an apical brush border. They resemble the enterocytes of the small and large intestines. The height of the villi is reduced only for the epithelium of the crypts. The villi at the fundi of the crypts are only small stumps.

1 Mesenteriolum
2 Mucosa with crypts
3 Lymph follicles with germinal centers
4 Tela submucosa
5 Tunica muscularis
Stain: hematoxylin-eosin; magnification: × 3

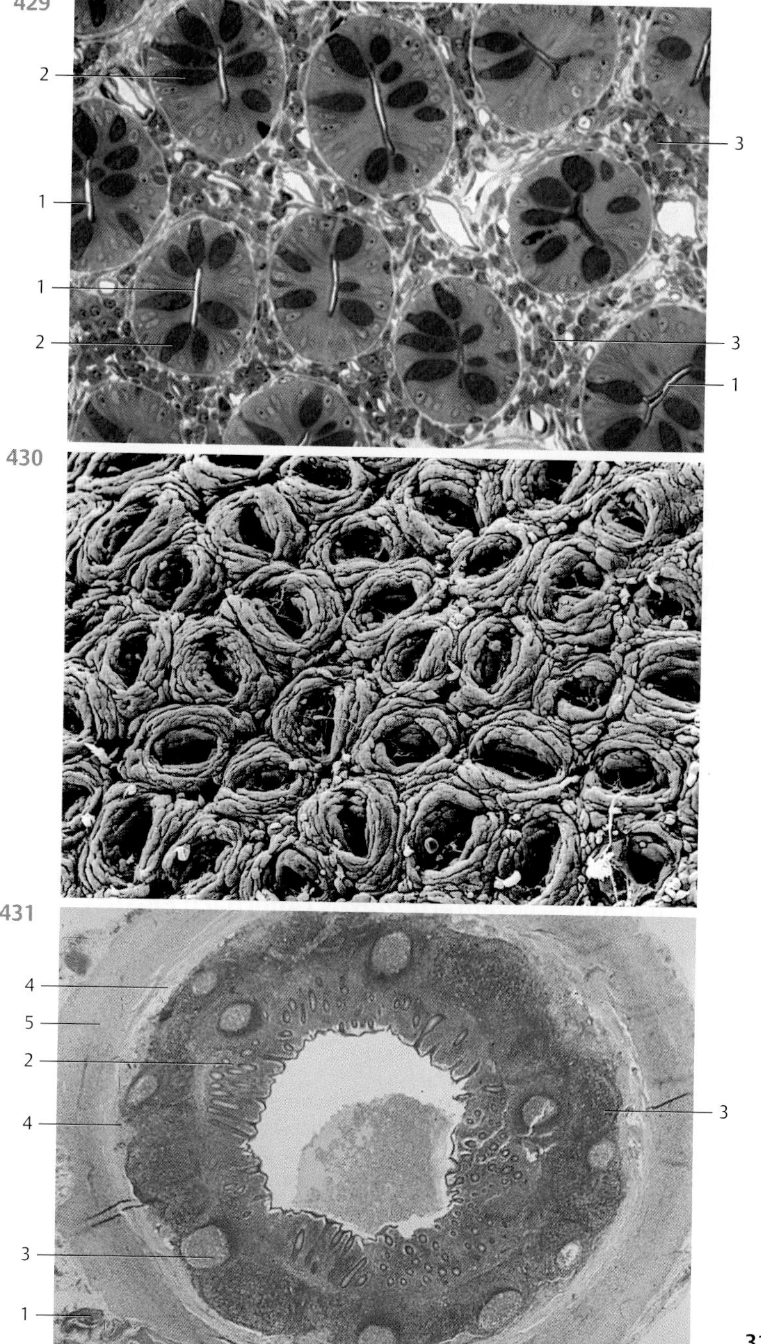

Digestive System

432 Jejunum—Myenteric Plexus (Auerbach Plexus)

This longitudinal section of the jejunal *tunica muscularis* shows the inner circular layer 1 (top) and the outer *longitudinal layer* 2 (bottom), followed by the *tunica serosa* 3. The voluminous ganglion cells of the myenteric plexus (Auerbach plexus) 4 are situated in the loose connective tissue between the two muscle layers (cf. this section with Figs. 220, 433 and 434). The *myenteric (Auerbach) plexus* otherwise consists of a network of autonomous nerve fibers. The densities of these networks may be regionally different (see Fig. 437). They are part of the intrinsic intramural nervous system (*organ-specific nervous system, enteric nervous system* (*ENS*).

1 Circular layer of the tunica muscularis (cf. Figs. 433, 434)
2 Longitudinal layer of the tunica muscularis (cf. Figs. 433, 434)
3 Tunica serosa
4 Ganglion cells of the myenteric plexus (cf. Figs. 220, 433)
Stain: alum hematoxylin-eosin; magnification: × 180

433 Stomach—Myenteric Plexus (Auerbach Plexus)

The myenteric plexus (*Auerbach plexus*) consists of *ganglion cells* that are surrounded by *glial cells* and a wide-meshed network of *nerve fibers* (cf. Fig. 437). This vertical section through the stomach wall fundus shows ganglion cells 1 with lightly stained, large nuclei, glial cells 2 with small, intensely stained nuclei and undulating nerve fibers 3 (cf. Fig. 434). The circular muscle layer 4 is shown in the top part of the microphotograph. The longitudinal muscle layer is represented in the lower part 5.

1 Ganglion cell of the myenteric plexus
2 Nucleus of a Schwann cell
3 Nerve fibers
4 Circular layer of the tunica muscularis
5 Longitudinal layer of the tunica muscularis
6 Capillaries
Semi-thin section; stain: methylene blue-azure II; magnification: × 240

434 Jejunum—Myenteric Plexus (Auerbach Plexus)

The myenteric plexus (Auerbach plexus) 3 is found in the intestinal tunica muscularis between the inner circular layer 1 and the outer longitudinal layer 2 (see Figs. 399, 400, 432, 433). It is part of a connective tissue layer of different widths. The myenteric plexus consists of a network of nerve fibers, as well as ganglion cells and glial cells. The nerve fiber network is visible in light microscopy (see Fig. 437).
This cross-section of the jejunum shows only unmyelinated nerve fiber bundles 4 in the connective tissue layer between the two muscular layers.

1 Circular layer of the tunica muscularis
2 Longitudinal layer of the tunica muscularis
3 Myenteric plexus (Auerbach plexus)
4 Unmyelinated nerve fibers
Electron microscopy; magnification: × 4600

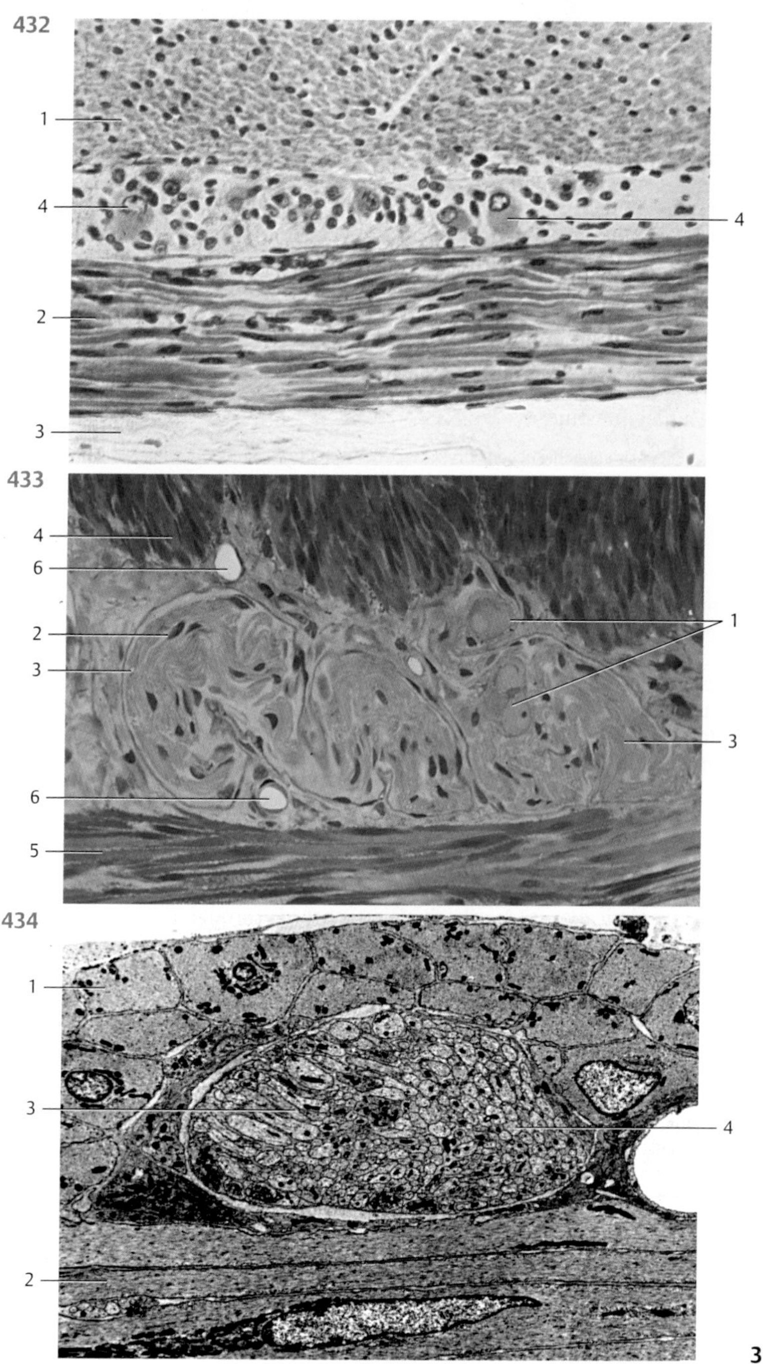
432
1
4
4
2
3
433
4
6
2
3
1
3
6
5
434
1
3
4
2

435 Jejunum—Mucosal Plexus

All neurons and glial cells in the gastrointestinal tract from the esophagus to the inner anal sphincter, including gallbladder, extrahepatic gall ducts and the pancreas are part of the enteric nervous tissue (*ENS, intramural nervous system*). The extrinsic innervation of the gastrointestinal tract is mediated by the *sympathetic* and *parasympathetic nervous system*, i.e., by afferent and efferent nerve paths, which connect the ENS and CNS. The ENS consists of several spread out nerve fibers (plexus), which are located in different layers of the intestinal wall. In principle, there is a *plexus mucosus* (without nerve cells), a *plexus submucosus internus* (Meissner plexus) and *externus* (Schabadasch plexus) and a *myenteric plexus* (Auerbach plexus). Whole-mount preparations and immunohistochemistry methods allow it to three-dimensionally render each type of the ENS plexus (compare the sections in Figs. 432–434). The adjacent figure displays a mucous plexus of a villus from the porcine small intestines.

Stain: immunohistochemistry to trace gene product 9.5 (PGP 9.5); magnification: × 250

436 Colon—Inner and Outer Submucosal Plexus, Meissner Plexus and Schabadasch Plexus

The submucosal networks of nerve fibers are situated in different layers of the submucosal tissue. The *internal submucosal Meissner plexus* is located underneath the lamina muscularis mucosae toward the lumen. The *external-submucosal Schabadasch plexus* borders on the circular layer of the tunica muscularis. When compared with the *myenteric plexus* (cf. Fig. 437), the submucosal plexus has more delicate nerve fiber strands and smaller ganglia. Human colon.

Stain: immunochemistry to trace protein gene product 9.5 (PGP 9.5); magnification: × 30

437 Colon—Myenteric Plexus (Auerbach)

The *myenteric plexus* (*Auerbach plexus*) spreads through the thin connective tissue between the circular and longitudinal layers of the tunica muscularis. Predominantly, the nerve cells (*ganglion cells*) are found in the nodal points (*ganglia*) of the nerve fiber meshwork. The ganglia are interconnected via broad nerve fiber bundles (*primary nerve strands*), which forms a prominent *primary web. Secondary strands* extend from the primary strands. They are not quite as broad and rarely contain nerve cells. The numerous thin tertiary strands should be considered extensions of the primary and secondary nerve strands. They branch out in the neighboring muscle layers.
Human colon. Compare this preparation with those described in Figs. 432–434.

Stain: immunochemistry to trace protein gene product 9.5 (PGP 9.5); magnification: × 30

435

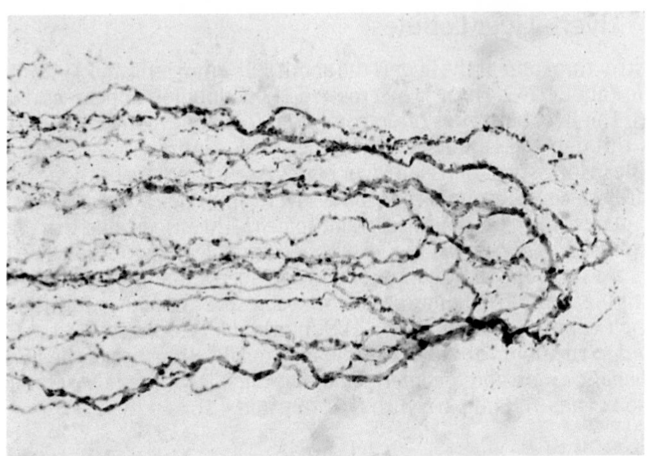

436

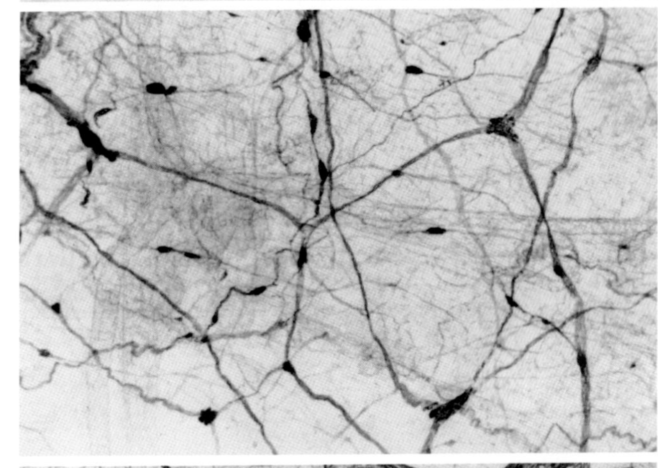

437

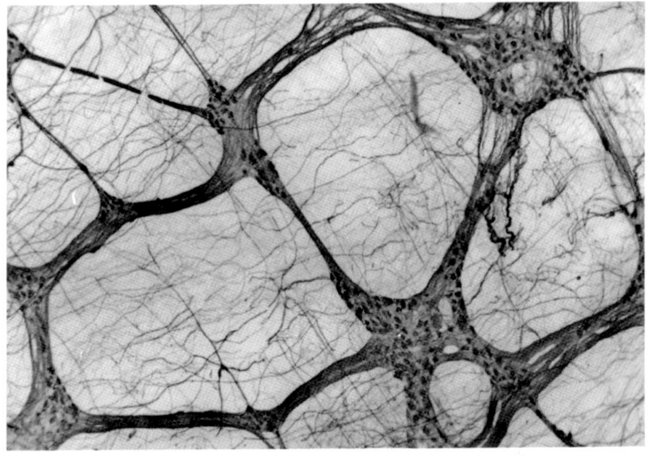

438 Liver—Liver Lobules

The structural unit of the liver is the about 1.5–2 mm long and 1–1.2 mm wide *lobule* (about 2–2.4 mm^2). In cross-sections, lobules appear as polygonal areas. The liver surface is often compared to a honeycomb. The *central vein* runs through the center of the lobule (*vena centralis*) 1. *Hepatocytes* assemble to long strips of tissue (liver plates), which radiate from the periphery toward the central vein of the lobule. Liver capillaries meander between the liver plates (*liver sinusoids, vasa sinusoidea*). This ascertains that liver cells are exposed to an arterial blood supply from at least two sides. The liver lobules are surrounded by connective tissue fibers (stained blue). The connective tissue at the triangular points between several lobules forms a capsule (*Glisson capsule, Glisson triad*). The interlobular connective tissue is connected to the fibers of the hepatobiliary capsule. Branches of the *portal vein*, the *hepatic artery* and the *interlobular bile ductules* are regularly found in the Glisson triads 2. Compare with Figs. 439 and 441. Porcine liver.

1 Central vein
2 Glisson triad
Stain: azan; magnification: × 40

439 Liver—Portal Triad

This section shows a Glisson triad (portal triad). The large clearing at the top of the figure represents a section through the interlobular branch of the *portal vein* 1. Two interlobular arteries 2 (*branches of the hepatic artery*) are visible in the connective tissue underneath the interlobular vein. A sectioned *bile ductule* 3 (*ductus interlobularis*) is situated between the two arteries. The bile duct wall contains isoprismatic (cuboid) epithelium). Liver cords (laminae) (cf. Fig. 442) surround the triad. Note the lymphatic vessel 4.

1 Branch of the portal vein
2 Branch of the hepatic artery
3 Interlobular bile ductule
4 Lymphatic vessel
Stain: alum hematoxylin-eosin; magnification: × 120

440 Liver—Kupffer Cells

The inner surfaces of the liver sinusoids 1 are lined with fenestrated epithelium (see Figs. 447–449). Kupffer cells 2 are other fixed cells in this lining. Because of their often star-like shape, they used to be called “stellate cells of Kupffer” (Karl Wilhelm von Kupffer, 1829–1902). However, the cells may vary in shape. Kupffer cells have very long cytoplasmic processes that sometimes traverse the entire sinusoid. The cells are able to phagocytose, and they are considered macrophages. After staining of vitamin C, the Kupffer cells in this micrograph appear dark. Do not confuse Kupffer cells with the lipocytes or Ito cells in the perisinusoidal regions of Disse’s space. The central vein 3 is seen at the top right of the figure.

1 Sinusoids
2 Kupffer cells (macrophages)
3 Central vein
Stain: Giroud-Leblond; nuclear staining with carmine red; magnification: × 300

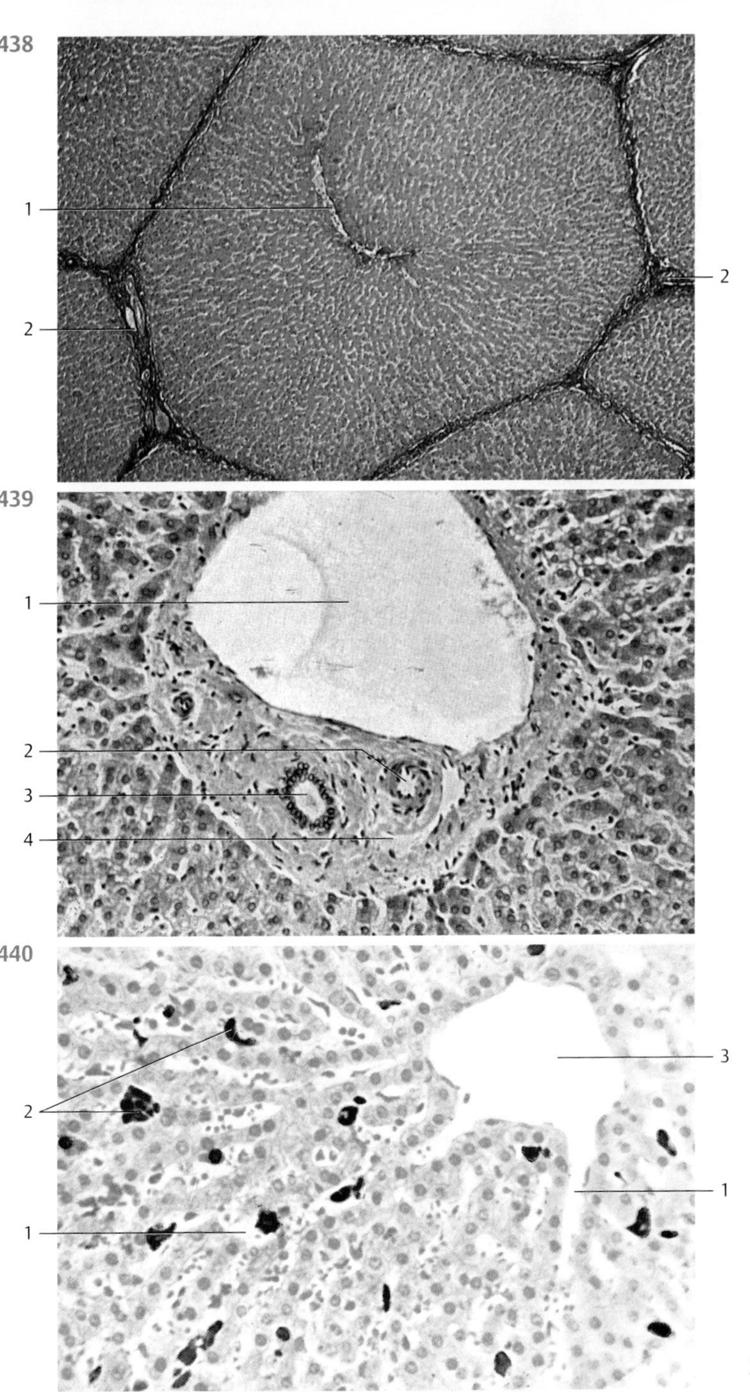

Digestive System

441 Liver—Portal Triad

The liver sinusoids are supplied with blood by vessels, which derive from the *portal vein* and the *hepatic artery*. The latter run parallel with the interlobular bile ductules (*ductuli biliferi*) 1 in the portal canals. Together they are known as portal triad (Glisson triad). The triads assemble where several hepatic lobules meet (see Fig. 438). This figure shows the *portal triad* (cf. Fig. 439). The large vessel is a branch of the portal vein 2. Next to it, there is the branch of the hepatic artery 3. It contains several erythrocytes. Several *interlobular bile ductules* are found in the periportal connective tissue. The ductules are covered by an isoprismatic (cuboid) epithelium. The portal triad is surrounded by hepatocyte cords (laminae) and sinusoids 4, which occasionally contain erythrocytes. Many hepatocytes contain deep blue stained granules of different sizes. These are fat droplets. Rat liver.

1 Bile ductules
2 Interlobular vein
3 Interlobular artery
4 Liver sinusoid
Semi-thin section; stain: methylene blue-azure II; magnification: × 400

442 Liver—Liver Lobules

Semi-thin section of a liver lobule from a rat. The center clearance represents the central vein (tributary of hepatic vein). The entrance of the *liver sinusoids* in the central vein can be seen in several places ↗. Note the thin endothelium of the central vein. The lumina of some liver sinusoids show erythrocytes. The nuclei of the liver cells clearly display nucleoli. The cytoplasm appears finely granulated (cf. Figs. 441, 443).

Semi-thin section; stain: methylene blue-azure II; magnification: × 200

443 Liver—Liver Sinusoids

Semi-thin section showing the central portion of a *liver lobule*. The top part of the figure still displays the lumen of the central vein 1 and its endothelial lining. *Liver sinusoids* end in the central vein ↗. Wide liver sinusoids (capillaries) run between hepatocyte cords (laminae). They are about 400–500 μm long and of various widths (6–15 μm). The artery walls consist of epithelium and *Kupffer cells* 2. The endothelial cells are flat and have openings and pores: *fenestrated endothelium* (see Fig. 302). They do not have a basal membrane. Disse's space is defined between hepatocyte surface and the endothelial cells of the sinusoid walls (see Figs. 446–449). It contains reticular fibers, a few connective tissue cells and adipocytes. Some Kupffer cells are part of the liver sinusoid walls. More frequently, however, the Kupffer cells are located on the surfaces of endothelial cells. Kupffer cells are macrophages and can phagocytose. They are part of the *mononuclear phagocyte system* (cf. Fig. 440).

1 Central vein
2 Kupffer cells in a liver sinus
Semi-thin section; stain: methylene blue-azure II; magnification: × 400

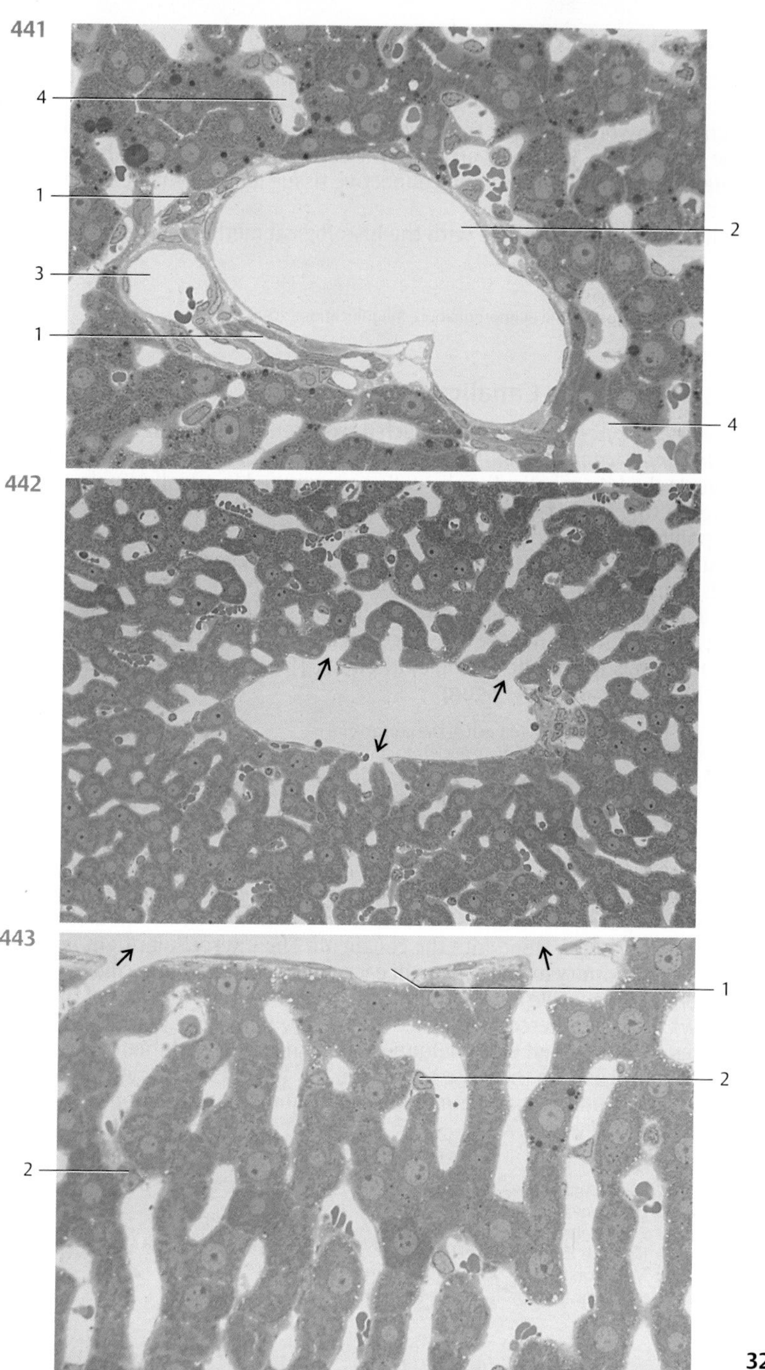
441
4
1
3
1
2
4
442
443
1
2
2

444 Liver—Reticular Fibers

In the *Disse space* of the hepatocyte cords (laminae) run argyrophilic fibers. These are *reticular fibers* as well as collagen I, III and V fibers, which form a tight meshwork. The fiber meshwork weaves around the liver sinusoids and the central vein. The fibers attach to the connective tissue of the *hepatic capsule*. Scaffoldings of fibers and connective tissue lend mechanical support to the liver.
Cell borders are not visible with the histological method used here.

1 Liver cells
2 Fiber meshwork
Stain: Hortega silver impregnation; magnification: × 500

445 Liver—Bile Canaliculi

The hepatocytes produce bile, which is excreted through intercellular canals (*bile canals, canaliculi biliferi*). Metal impregnation, among other methods, reveals the bile canaliculi. Liver cells are arranged in usually single-layered, intersecting laminae. Because of the regular pattern formed by the octagonal or polyhedral hepatocytes, the structure is called a *muralium*. The bile canaliculi appear to be arranged in a zigzag pattern in the intercellular spaces in this muralium, following the pattern of the hepatocyte plates. The intercellular *bile canaliculi* continue in the periportal bile ductules (ductules of Hering). These empty into the bile ducts (see Figs. 339, 441). The bile ducts are lined with isoprismatic cuboid epithelium. The *interlobular vein* [1] is shown in the lower part of the figure.

1 Interlobular vein (branch of the portal vein)
Golgi silver impregnation; nuclei are stained with carmine red; magnification: × 150

446 Liver—Bile Canaliculi and Space of Disse

Bile canaliculi [1] and cytoplasm of two neighboring rat hepatocytes. Bile canaliculi begin as larger intercellular crevices between hepatocytes. The canaliculi are spaces, which are surrounded and delimited by hepatocytes. Hepatocyte microvilli extend into the canaliculi. The intercellular tight junctions in close proximity to bile canaliculi each consist of a *zonula occludens, zonula adherens* and *macula adherens* (*terminal complex*). The right part of the figure shows that the intercellular space opens into Disse's space [2]. Slender processes of fenestrated endothelium [4] limit the sinusoid lumen [3]. There are reticular fibrils [5] in the Disse space (see Fig. 444, 449). The cytoplasm of hepatocytes contains many mitochondria [6] and small osmiophilic glycogen granules (cf. Figs 447, 448).

1 Bile canaliculi
2 Disse's space
3 Lumen of a sinusoid vessel
4 Fenestrated sinus endothelium
5 Reticular fibrils, cross-sectioned
6 Mitochondria
Electron microscopy; magnification: × 10 600

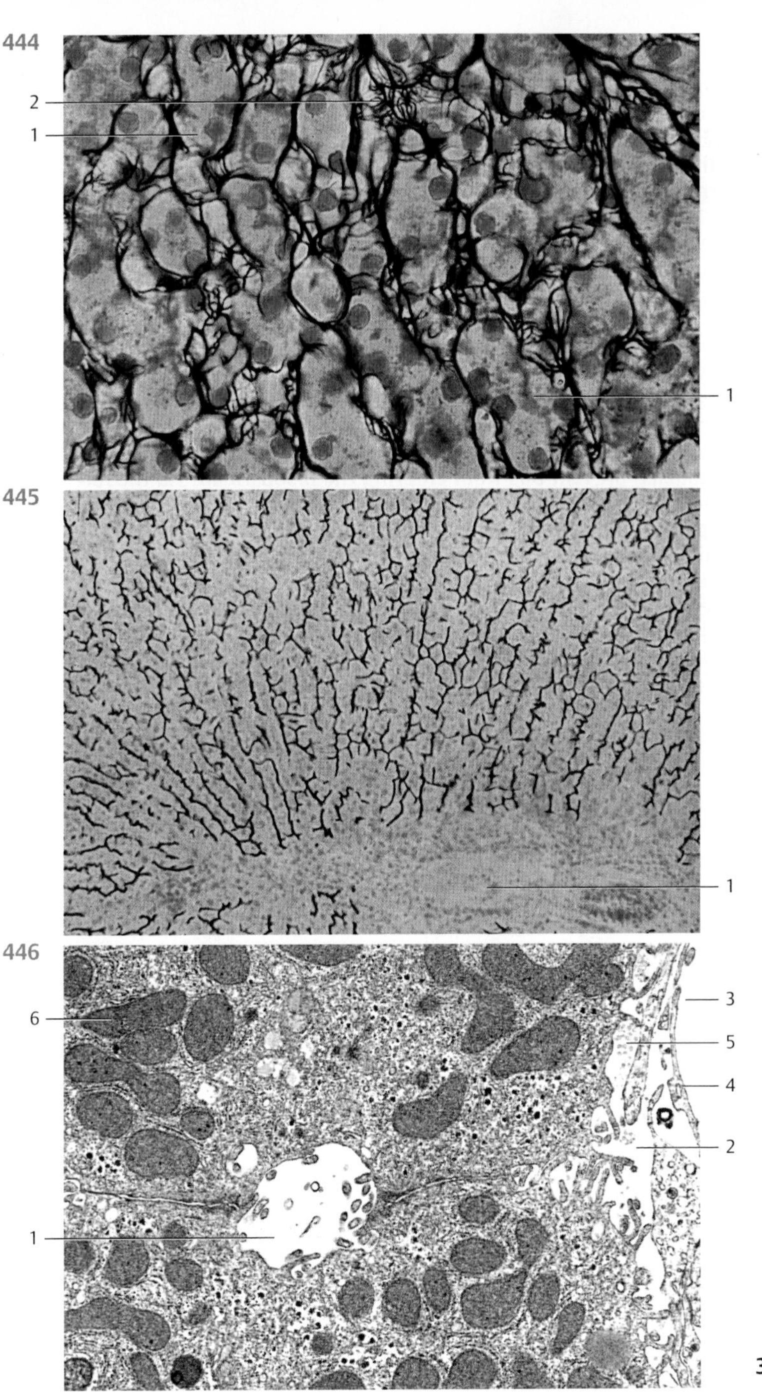
444
2
1
1
445
1
446
6
1
3
5
4
2

447 Liver—Hepatocytes

Hepatocytes are polyhedral cells with diameters of 20–30 µm. They form cords (or laminae) of hepatocytes, which run in the direction from the periphery of a liver lobule to the central vein. In this arrangement, at least one cell surface of each hepatocyte borders on a sinusoid vessel [1]. Hepatocytes form microvilli on their surfaces, which face a sinusoid. The microvilli are of various lengths and reach into the Disse space [4]. Microvilli enlarge the hepatocyte surfaces. The sinusoid endothelium is fenestrated ↗. Therefore, blood can directly flood the Disse space (see Figs. 446, 448, 449) and is in direct contact with hepatocytes. This ascertains an effective exchange of metabolites. The *bile canaliculi* [2] are spaces between hepatocytes. The canaliculi have no wall or endothelium of their own. Processes from surrounding hepatocytes delimit them. These processes too are covered with microvilli (cf. Figs. 446, 448). The cell membranes of hepatocytes that border on the bile ductules run mostly straight. The bile canaliculi are only about 20 nm wide. They open to the Disse space. Tight junctions (*terminal complex with zonula occludens*) prevent bile from entering the bloodstream via the intercellular space (see Fig. 446).

Hepatocytes have large, round central nuclei [3]. They are in many cases polyploid and their sizes vary accordingly. The cell nuclei usually appear light in electron microscopy and show chromatin bodies and one or two nucleoli. The cytoplasm of hepatocytes contains numerous crista-type mitochondria, elaborate membranes of the smooth and rough endoplasmic reticulum, Golgi complexes, lysosomes, peroxisomes, fat droplets and glycogen granules.

1 Liver sinusoids with fenestrated endothelium ↗
2 Bile canaliculi
3 Nuclei
4 Disse's space
Electron microscopy; magnification: × 4000

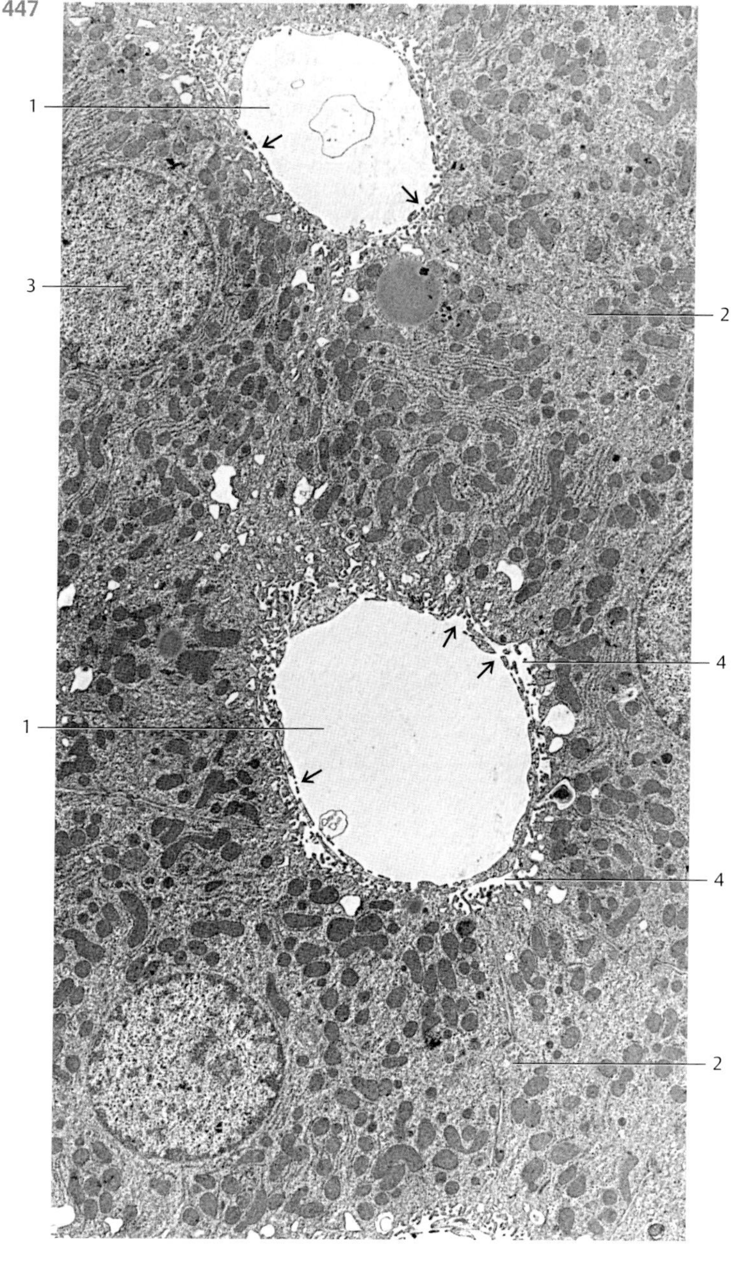
1
3
2
4
1
4
2

448 Liver—Hepatocytes

Hepatocytes (*liver parenchyme cells*) have a diameter of about 20–30 µm with several surface structures. The side of the hepatocyte that faces the Disse space ③ is covered with microvilli, which protrude into the perisinusoidal space (see Fig. 449). The spaces between hepatocytes enlarge and form bile canaliculi (*canaliculi biliferi*) ④ (see Fig. 446). Short microvilli from the hepatocytes protrude into the bile canaliculi as well. The hepatocyte plasmalemma contains a Mg^{2+}-ATPase, which is present exclusively in this region. Hepatocyte nuclei are large and round. They contain 1–2 nucleoli. The cytoplasm contains about 2000 mitochondria per hepatocyte and copious smooth (agranular) endoplasmic reticulum in the entire perinuclear space. There are also membranes of the rough endoplasmic reticulum (rER) and free ribosomes. Some portions of the ergastoplasm form basophilic bodies, which are visible in light microscopy after staining. Golgi complexes are frequently found adjacent to bile canaliculi ④. They are involved in the formation and excretion of bile. Hepatocytes also contain lysosomes and peroxisomes. Glycogen granules are typical for liver cells. Hepatocytes of older people may contain *lipofuscin* granules.

1 Lumen of a liver sinusoid
2 Fenestrated endothelium
3 Disse's space and hepatocyte microvilli
4 Bile canaliculi (cf. Fig. 446)
Electron microscopy; magnification: × 8300
Pointers:
Liver glycogen, see Fig. 64, 65
Liver peroxisomes, see Fig. 48
Liver MVBs (multivesicular bodies), see Fig. 50

448

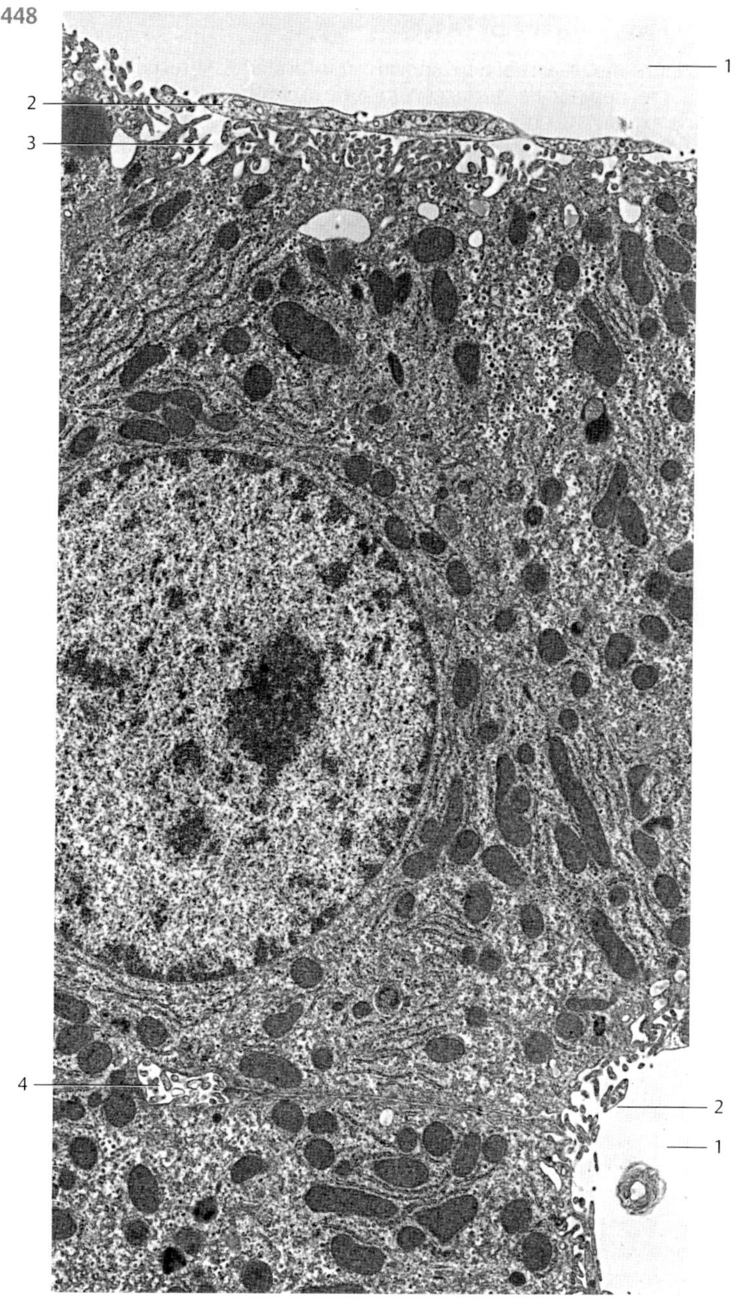

449 Liver—Space of Disse

The figure shows part of a hepatocyte. It is located next to a liver sinusoid [1]. From the hepatocyte surfaces protrude irregularly shaped microvilli [2], which extend into the *Disse space* [3] (*perisinusoidal space*) (cf. Figs. 446–448). Microvilli considerably enlarge the hepatocyte surface. The Disse space is about 0.3–0.5 µm wide and contains delicate collagen fibrils [3] (here cross-sectioned). Reticular fibers can be seen in light microscopy (cf. Fig. 444). The fenestrated sinusoidal endothelium [4] does not have a basal membrane, although its structural components, laminin, fibronectin and several proteoglycans, have been detected and immunochemically identified in the Disse space. Note the large mitochondria [5].

1 Liver sinusoids
2 Microvilli
3 Disse's space with fibrils
4 Fenestrated endothelium
5 Mitochondria
Electron microscopy; magnification: × 23 000

450 Liver—Injection Preparation

This injection preparation of a rabbit liver shows the vascular bed. The liver was filled via the *portal vein* with a red gelatin solution. At the same time, the *hepatic vein* was perfused with a blue gelatin solution via the *vena cava* inferior.
There are two larger vessels, which are filled with red gelatin solution. They are branches of the portal vein [1]. The vessels with the blue gelatin solution on the left side of the figure are *central veins* [2]. The vessels with the differently stained gelatin solutions meet in the periportal field. The network of dye-filled vessels indicates the extent of vascularization by the liver sinusoids (cf. Fig. 451). This vascular plexus spans the liver lobule.

1 Branches of the portal vein
2 Central veins
Dye double-injection; magnification: × 80

451 Liver—Corrosion Preparation

A rat liver was filled with Mercox resin via the portal vein. When the resin had hardened, the liver was macerated. This corrosion preparation shows the resin-filled *central vein* [1] and the *liver sinusoids*, which radiate from it (cf. Figs. 442, 443). The vessels span the hepatocytes of the liver lobule (cf. Fig. 450).

1 Central vein
Scanning electron microscopy; magnification: × 250

449

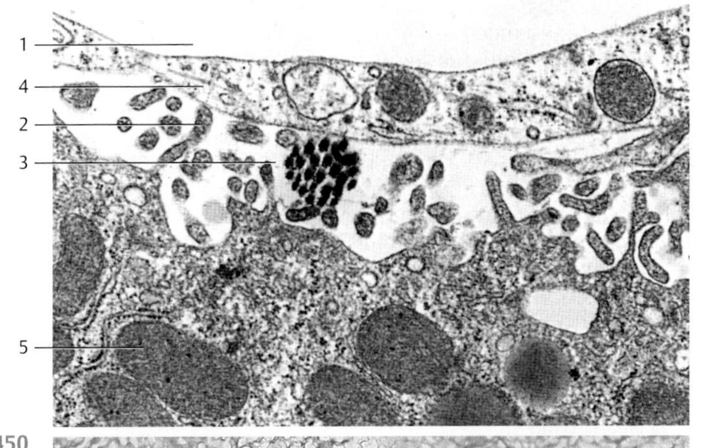

450

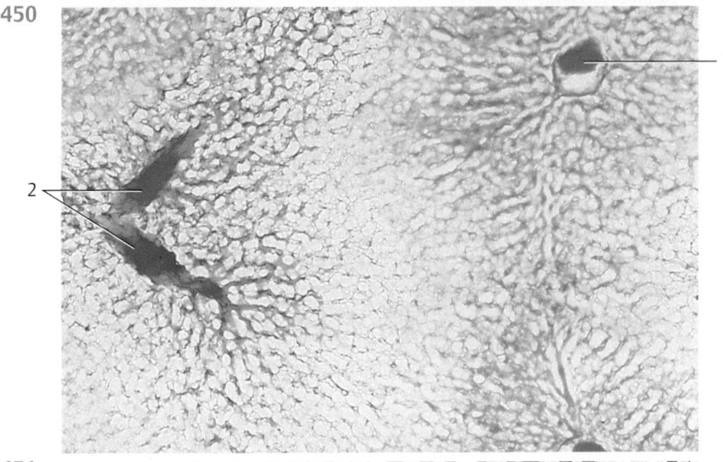

451

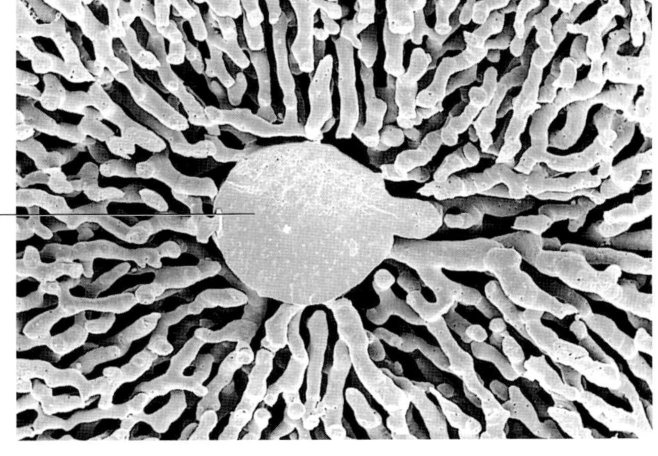

452 Gallbladder—Vesica Fellea sive Biliaris

Section of the tunica mucosa 1 from a human gallbladder. The mucous layer shows characteristic folds (*plicae*) 2, which alternate with wide bays or foveolae. The folds may branch and display various shapes. There are deep mucous membrane crypts 3 in some places (*cryptae tunica mucosae, Rokitansky-Aschoff crypts*). The mucous membrane is covered by a single-layered columnar epithelium with short microvilli. The ellipsoid cell nuclei are located in the basal cytoplasmic region. The epithelial cells form tight terminal complexes (junctions), focal desmosomes and nexuses (cf. Fig. 95, 97). The fibrous lamina propria 4 is loosely built and contains fibroblasts as well as copious free cells. The tunica muscularis is not captured in this figure. It consists of a network of connective tissue fibers and helical smooth muscle cells. Sporadically, there are also small mucous glands (*glandulae tunicae mucosae*) predominantly in the neck region of the gallbladder.

1 Tunica mucosa
2 Mucosal folds (plicae)
3 Mucosal crypts
4 Lamina propria
Stain: Masson-Goldner trichrome; magnification: × 80

453 Gallbladder—Vesica Fellea sive Biliaris

View of the surface of a feline gallbladder mucosa.
A web of connective tissue cords raises mucosa folds of different heights and irregular shapes 1 (cf. Fig. 452). A single-layered columnar epithelium covers the mucosa, including the folds. At this magnification, the epithelial surface relief and the brush border are just visible. Note the openings of the mucosa crypts 2 (cf. Fig. 452).

1 Mucosa folds
2 Openings to the mucosa crypts
Scanning electron microscopy; magnification: × 110

454 Common Bile Duct

The common bile duct (*ductus choledochus*) has a diameter of about 0.5 cm. It has thick walls and is lined by a single-layered columnar epithelium 1, which secrete mucins and resorb water and salt. A thick connective tissue layer 2 with strong collagen fiber bundles, copious elastic fibers and smooth muscle cells underlies the loose subepithelial connective tissue. There is no continuous, closed muscle layer, except at the duodenal end, immediately before the common bile duct reaches the duodenum. Branched or unbranched tubular *biliary glands* 3 are found in the loosely arranged outer wall layers. The glands secrete mucins into the lumen of the bile duct. Mucin probably provides a protective epithelial film and is added to the bile.

1 Bile duct epithelium
2 Connective tissue sheath
3 Tubular glands in the bile duct
Stain: iron hematoxylin—Weigert's picrofuchsin; magnification: × 300

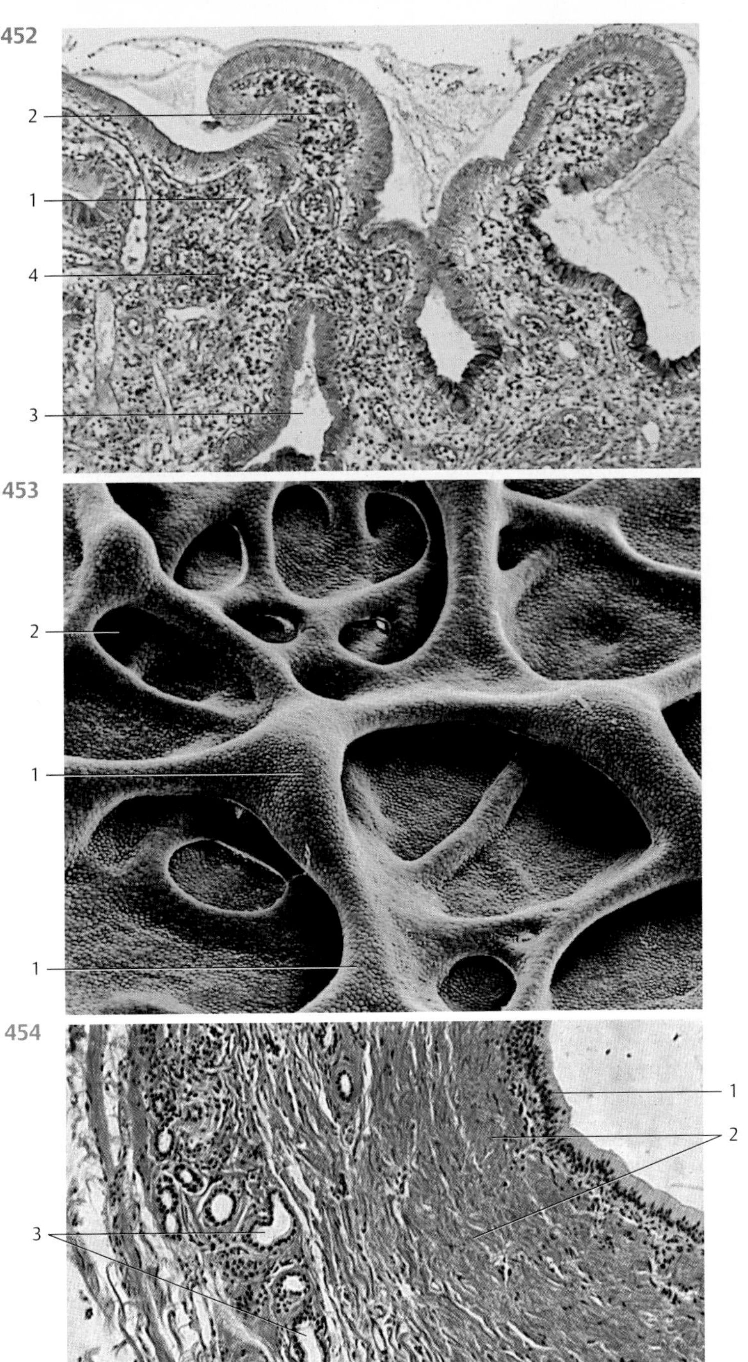

Digestive System

455 Pancreas

There are exocrine and endocrine glands in the pancreas. The endocrine glands are the Langerhans islets, or simply islets (see Figs. 365–369). The exocrine pancreas consists of purely serous glands. It consists of several thousand loosely connected lobes. The diameter of a lobe is about 3 mm. The lobes are separated by thin connective tissue septa. Each lobe contains a group of branched ducts with their acini. Acini may have a multitude of shapes and sizes. There are long, club-shaped 160 µm long acini with humped surfaces, as well as single round acini with a diameter of about 30 µm (cf. Figs. 18, 457, 459). 3–5 acini assemble to a cluster. Their individual ducts combine to a common duct (see 459, 460).

Several acini of different shapes are shown in this figure. The columnar cells of the secretory acini contain basal nuclei. The supranuclear and apical cytoplasmic spaces are densely packed with secretory granules (cf. 18, 456, 457). The secretory granules (zymogen granules) have a diameter of 0.5–1 µm. The almost homogeneous, intensely blue stained basal cytoplasmic regions (basal basophilia) correspond to the ergastoplasm of protein biosynthesizing gland cells (cf. Figs. 18, 19, 22, 23, 456–458).

The lightly stained large nuclei of the centroacinar cells 1 are clearly visible (cf. 18, 455). There are numerous capillaries 2 in the interstitial connective tissue.

1 Centroacinar cells
2 Capillaries
Semi-thin section; stain: methylene blue-azure II; magnification: × 400

456 Pancreas

Section of an acinus from a rat pancreas. The six pyramid-shaped acinar cells have a wide base. Their small apical cell poles are grouped around the gland lumen 1. Like typical serous glands, the acinar cells show round nuclei with diameters of 5–7 µm and an elaborate rough endoplasmic reticulum 2 in the basal two thirds of the cells (*basal basophilia* in light microscopy, cf. Figs. 18, 455). The secretory granules (diameter = 0.5–1 µm) are located in the central and apical parts of the cytoplasm. The granules appear homogeneous and dark in electron microscopy because they bind a lot of osmium tetroxide. Note the gland lumen 1. It is filled with secretory product. There are small, often elongated mitochondria in the interstitial connective tissue.

1 Acinar lumen
2 Granular (rough) endoplasmic reticulum, rER, ergastoplasm)
3 Capillaries
Electron microscopy; magnification: × 2200

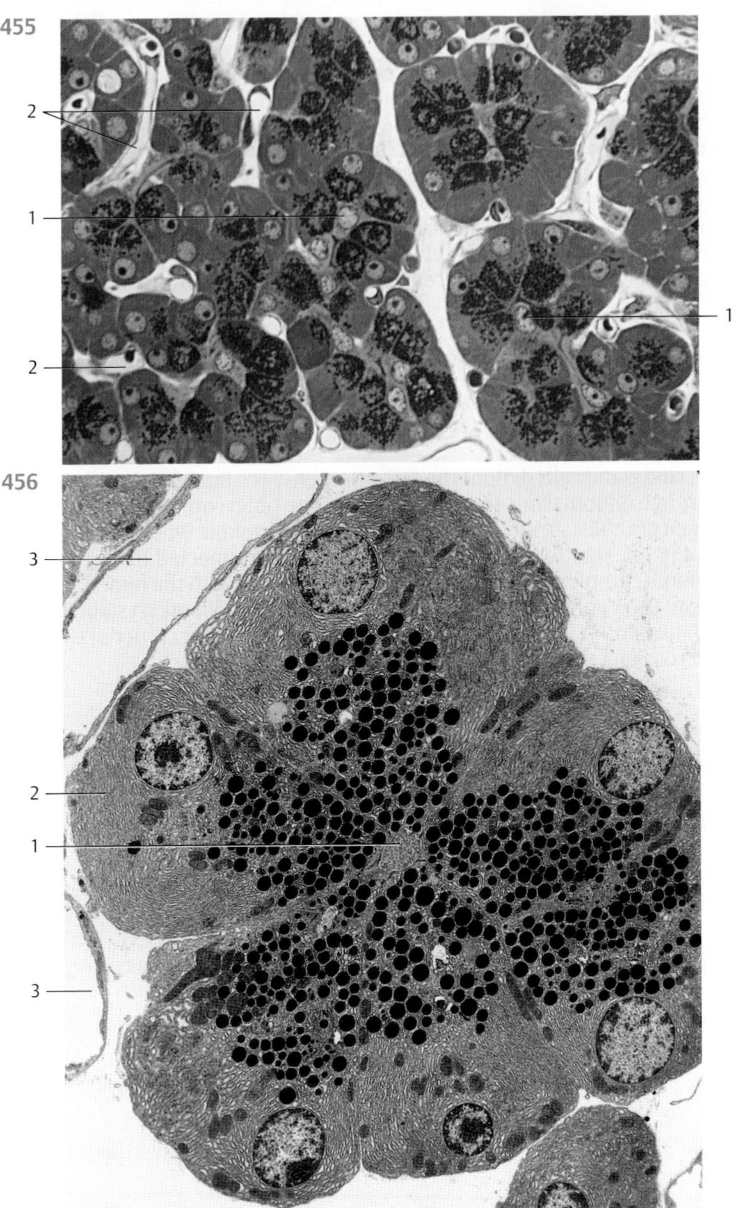
455
2
1
2
1
456
3
2
1
3

457 Pancreas

Paraffin section of a human pancreas with abundant acini.
Many blood-filled vessels [2] are found between acini in the spaces between connective tissue strands (cf. Figs. 455, 456, 459). The basal regions of the gland cells are stained blue-violet (*basal basophilia*, cf. Fig 18). The round cell nuclei are localized in the same area as the rough endoplasmic reticulum. The two compartments are close neighbors. The central and apical cell regions are lightly stained, almost unstained. However, their honeycomb structure is visible. The pattern is due to densely packed zymogen granules (see Figs. 366, 455, 456). Note the centroacinar cells [1] and compare with Fig. 455.

1 Centroacinar cells
2 Capillaries
Stain: hematoxylin-eosin; magnification: × 400

458 Pancreas

Exocrine gland cells delimit the acinar lumen [1] (cf. Fig. 456). Note the elaborate rough endoplasmic reticulum [2] (rER), the Golgi complexes [3] and the zymogen granules [4], which are only weakly osmiophilic when compared with Fig. 456 (cf. Fig. 455). The gland cells are tightly connected to each other via terminal complexes in the apical part of the cell close to the lumen. The cytoplasm also contains long crista-type mitochondria [5] and crystalloid bodies [6]. A nucleus [7] is visible in the left upper and left lower corner of the figure. Pancreas of a mature mouse.

1 Acinar clearance (lumen)
2 Rough endoplasmic reticulum, rER, ergastoplasm
3 Golgi complexes
4 Zymogen granules
5 Crista-type mitochondria
6 Crystalloid bodies
7 Cell nuclei
Electron microscopy; magnification: × 9600

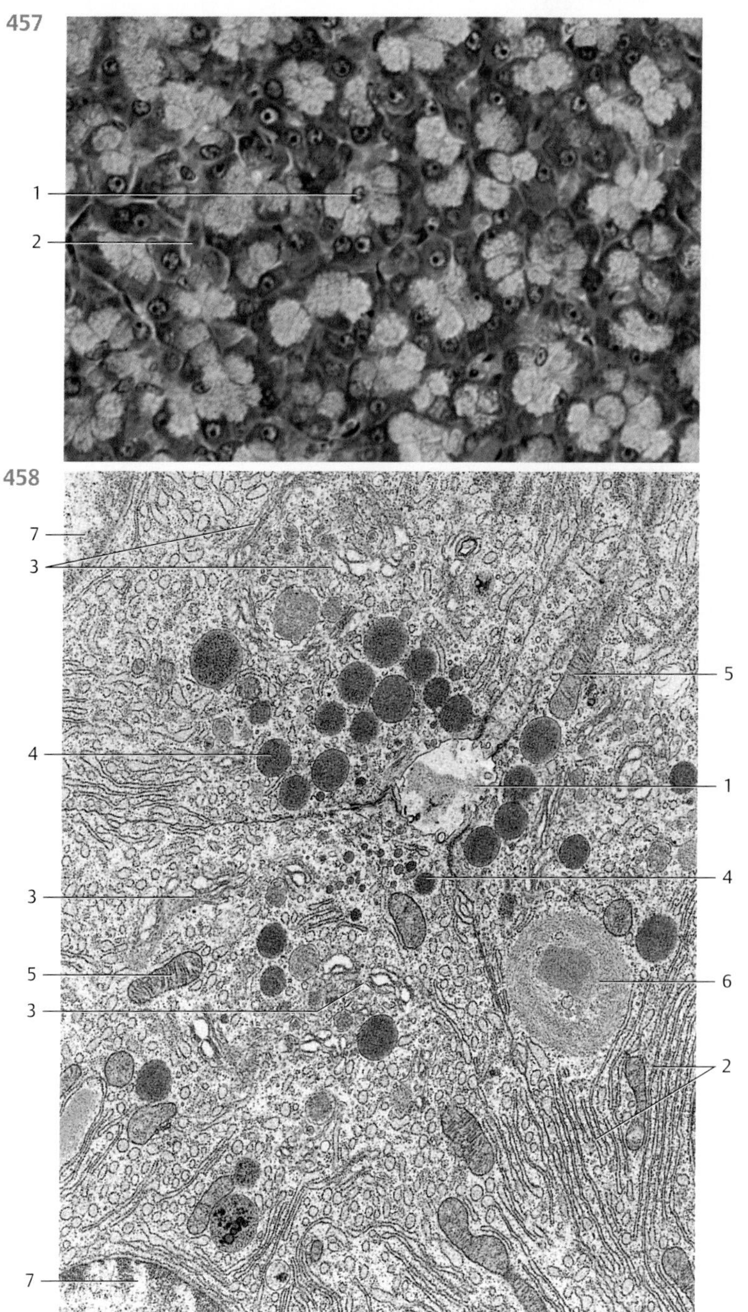

Digestive System

459 Pancreas

The pancreas contains exocrine and endocrine glands. The entire endocrine portion of the pancreas consists of Langerhans islet cells (see Figs. 365–369). The exocrine pancreas consists of purely serous glands. The organ contains many thousand small lobes. The acini are the terminal parts of intralobular and interlobular ducts. Interlobular ducts end in the minor or major pancreatic duct, respectively (see Fig. 461). The pyramid-shaped acinar cells have basal nuclei (cf. 456). The basal cytoplasm is basophilic because of its ergastoplasm (see Figs. 18, 457). Secretory granules are seen in the apical cell portion (cf. Fig. 455, 457). The cells of the intercalated ducts extend into the acinar lumen. Therefore, there are lighter centroacinar cells 1 visible toward the lumen of the acini. They are part of the epithelium 2 that lines the intralobular ducts. An intercalated duct is cut longitudinally 2. Note the different shapes for acini. Acini occur in close vicinity of each other. Human pancreas. This preparation shows intensive staining with eosin.

1 Centroacinar cells
2 Intercalated duct
Stain: alum hematoxylin-eosin; magnification: × 400

460 Pancreas

Cross-section of the intercalated duct from the exocrine pancreas (cf. Fig. 459). Some of the epithelial cells are flat, others are isoprismatic (cuboid). They are layered on a continuous basal membrane. The epithelial cells contain nuclei of all shapes. Elaborately developed Golgi complexes are clearly visible 1. Neighboring epithelial cells connect via apicolateral desmosomes. The intercalated duct contains the granular secretory product.

1 Golgi apparatus
2 Collagen fibrils of the connective tissue layer
3 Fibrocyte processes
Electron microscopy; magnification: × 6500

461 Pancreas

Every pancreatic lobule contains a group of branched intercalated ducts and their acini (cf. Fig. 459). The intercalated ducts continue in small, still intralobular, ducts, which are lined by a cuboid epithelium. In the interlobular connective tissue septa, the ducts turn into interlobular ducts. These are enveloped by a fiber-rich connective tissue sheath 1. Interlobular ducts are covered by a single-layered columnar epithelium 2. The epithelial cells secrete mucins.
Interlobular intercalated duct from a human pancreas.

1 Connective tissue sheath
2 Columnar epithelium
Stain: hematoxylin-eosin; magnification: × 80

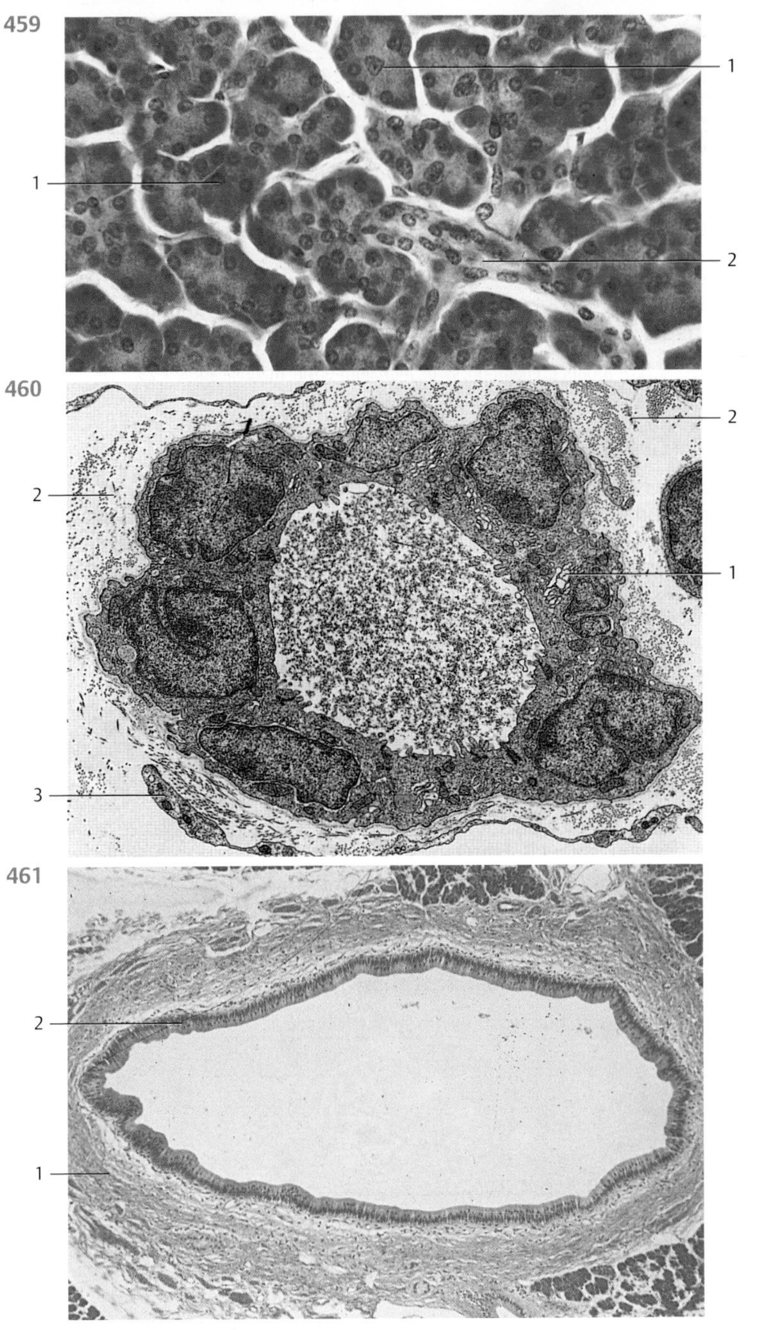
459
1
1
2
460
2
2
1
3
461
2
1

462 Greater Omentum

The connective tissue layer of the omenta and the mesenteries are seen as specialized forms of loose connective tissue. During fetal development, the greater omentum is a continuous cellulous connective tissue membrane, which is covered on both sides with *mesothelium* (*peritoneal epithelium*). After parturition, this layer of tissue becomes perforated, turning into a "net" (net-like *connective tissue*). The connective tissue network of this perforated tissue consists of strong, partially undulating collagen fibers, as well as elastic and reticular fibers. Fibrocytes and free cells are found insides this fiber meshwork. Blood vessels are also clearly visible. They run parallel with the collagen fibers. Note the large perivascular adipocytes and the mesh of the fibrous skeleton.

Whole-mount preparation; stain: hemalum-eosin; magnification: × 25

463 Greater Omentum—Indian Ink Injection

Layer of the canine greater omentum.
The blood vessels are filled with Indian ink. Blood vessels run parallel with the strands of collagen and elastic fibers. They are joined by extended complexes of reticular connective tissue with an underlying dense network of capillaries. The tissue layer also contains fat lobules. The capillary networks are particularly prominent on the right side of the figure. The greater omentum also contains a complex network of lymph vessels. Whole-mount preparation; cells and connective tissue are not stained.

Indian ink injection; magnification: × 40

464 Greater Omentum

This scanning electron micrograph shows the net-like structure of the omentum particularly well. Fibrocytes with long processes are visible in the left part of the figure and on the upper right part. The fiber bundles of the connective tissue scaffolding are part of a network. The fibers form flat extensions in some places, which look like the webbed feet of waterfowl. Toward the peritoneal cavity, the meshwork is completely covered by a mesothelial layer (*peritoneal epithelium*) (not shown in this figure).

Scanning electron microscopy; magnification: × 1500

462

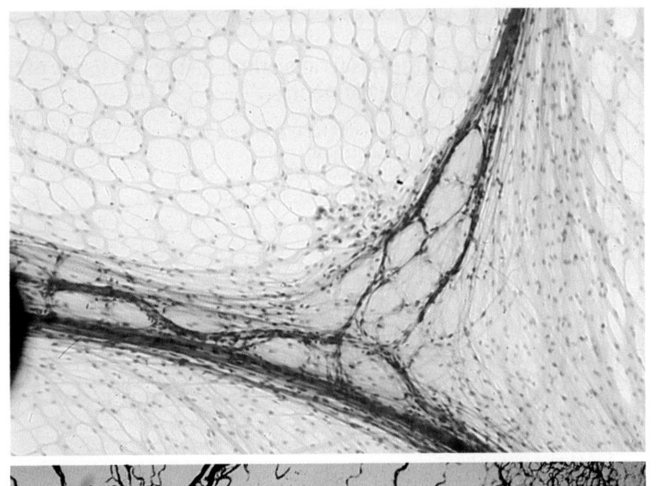

463

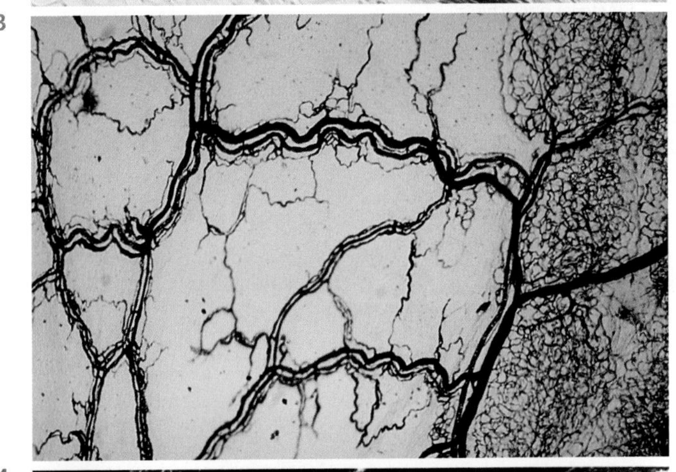

464

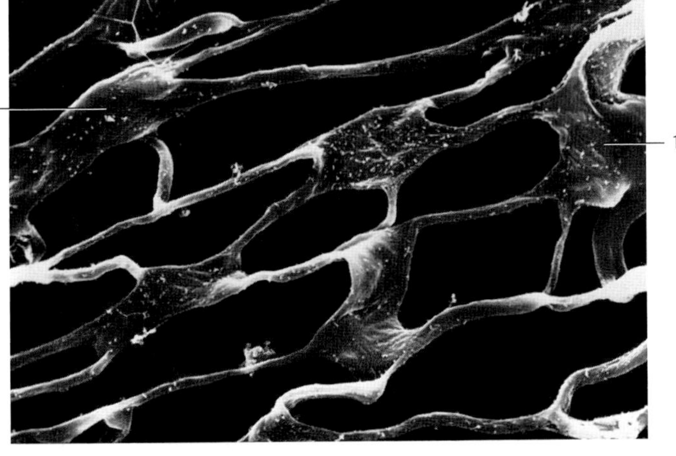

Digestive System

465 Nose

Section, almost parallel to the nasal ridge, through the soft tissue of the outer nose. It contains the following elements:

1 Outer surface, skin, multilayered keratinizing squamous epithelium—epidermis
2 Septum cartilage (cartilago septi nasi)
3 Lower nasal cartilage (cartilago alaris major)
4 Nasal apex
5 Sebaceous gland
6 Hair follicle
7 Dense connective tissue
Stain: iron hematoxylin-picric acid; magnification: × 5

466 Nasal Cavity and Nasal Sinuses

Frontal section through one half of the visceral cranium. It shows the nasal cavity and the nasal sinuses.

1 Anterior cranial fossa
2 Crista galli
3 Nasal septum with respiratory mucosa
4 Nasal cavity
5 Inferior nasal concha
6 Inferior nasal meatus
7 Middle nasal concha
8 Middle nasal meatus
9 Ethmoidal cells
10 Orbital cavity
11 Maxillary sinus
12 Maxilla, upper jaw bone
13 Soft palate
14 Oral cavity
15 Ethmoid bone, lamina perpendicularis
16 Ethmoid bone, lamina orbitalis
17 Maxillary bone
18 Levator palpebrae superioris muscle and superior rectus muscle
19 Superior oblique muscle
20 Medial rectus muscle
21 Retrobulbar fat (corpus adiposum orbitae)

The nasal conchae enlarge the surface of the respiratory region. They are covered with a ciliated multilayered columnar epithelium, which contains numerous goblet cells (cf. Fig. 111, 112). The voluminous corpus cavernosum in the mucosa of the nasal cavity stands out. It reaches a considerable width, especially in the lower and middle concha.

Stain: iron hematoxylin; magnification: × 6

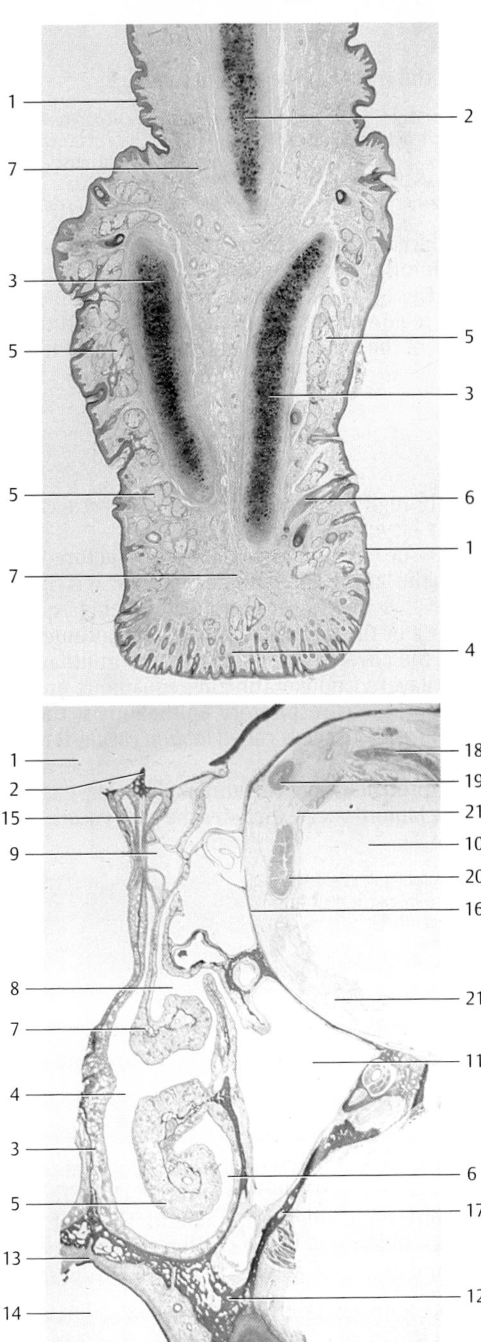
465
1
2
7
3
5
5
3
5
6
1
7
4
466
1
2
15
9
8
7
4
3
5
13
14
18
19
21
10
20
16
21
11
6
17
12

467 Larynx

Cross-section of the throat at the cricoid cartilage.

1 Cricoid cartilage
2 Inferior horn of the thyroid cartilage
3 Esophagus
4 Thyroid gland
5 Adipose tissue
6 Posterior cricoarytenoid muscle
7 Oblique part of the cricothyroid muscle
8 Sternothyroid muscle
9 Laryngeal mucosa
10 Cricothyroid muscle, straight part

The mucosa (*tunica mucosa respiratoria*) of the airways is covered with a multilayered columnar ciliated epithelium that contains mucin-producing goblet cells (cf. Figs. 111, 112). Exceptions: regio cutanea of the nasal vestibule, olfactory region of the upper nasal concha and the upper nasal septum, the mucosa of the vocal cords and the mucosa of the small bronchia.

Stain: azan; magnification: × 12

468 Larynx

Frontal section through the *plica ventricularis* 1, *vocal cord* 2 and *laryngeal ventricle* 3 of the larynx from an infant.
The connective tissue of the mucosa is loosely structured at the beginning of the larynx and in the laryngeal vestibule. However, it is rigidly attached at the vocal fold edge 4. A multilayered nonkeratinizing squamous epithelium covers the mucosa of the laryngeal cavity and continues into the *laryngeal vestibule*. There, the cover changes to a ciliated multilayered stratified epithelium. A multilayered nonkeratinizing squamous epithelium interrupts the otherwise continuous respiratory epithelium at the edge of the vocal cord. This 4–5-nm wide tissue is called *labium vocale*. It allows the firm closing of the glottis.
The vocal fold 2 protrudes into the lumen of the larynx. It delimits the phonation space. The labium vocale includes the *plica vocalis* 2, *vocal ligament* 4 and *vocal muscle* 5.

1 Ventricular fold (plica ventricularis)
2 Vocal chord (plica vocalis)
3 Laryngeal ventricle
4 Vocal ligament
5 Thyroarytenoid muscle with vocal muscle
6 Elastic cone
7 Vestibular fold (plica vestibularis)
8 Seromucous tubuloalveolar glands, laryngeal glands

Stain: azan; magnification: × 8

469 Larynx

The infraglottic cavity is situated under the vocal cords. It continues underneath the ring muscle into the lumen of the trachea. The infraglottic part is covered by a multilayered ciliated epithelium. This epithelium lines the entire lower airways all the way to the small bronchioles.
Ciliated epithelium of the infraglottic tissue from a 76-year-old man.

Scanning electron microscopy; magnification: × 2,500

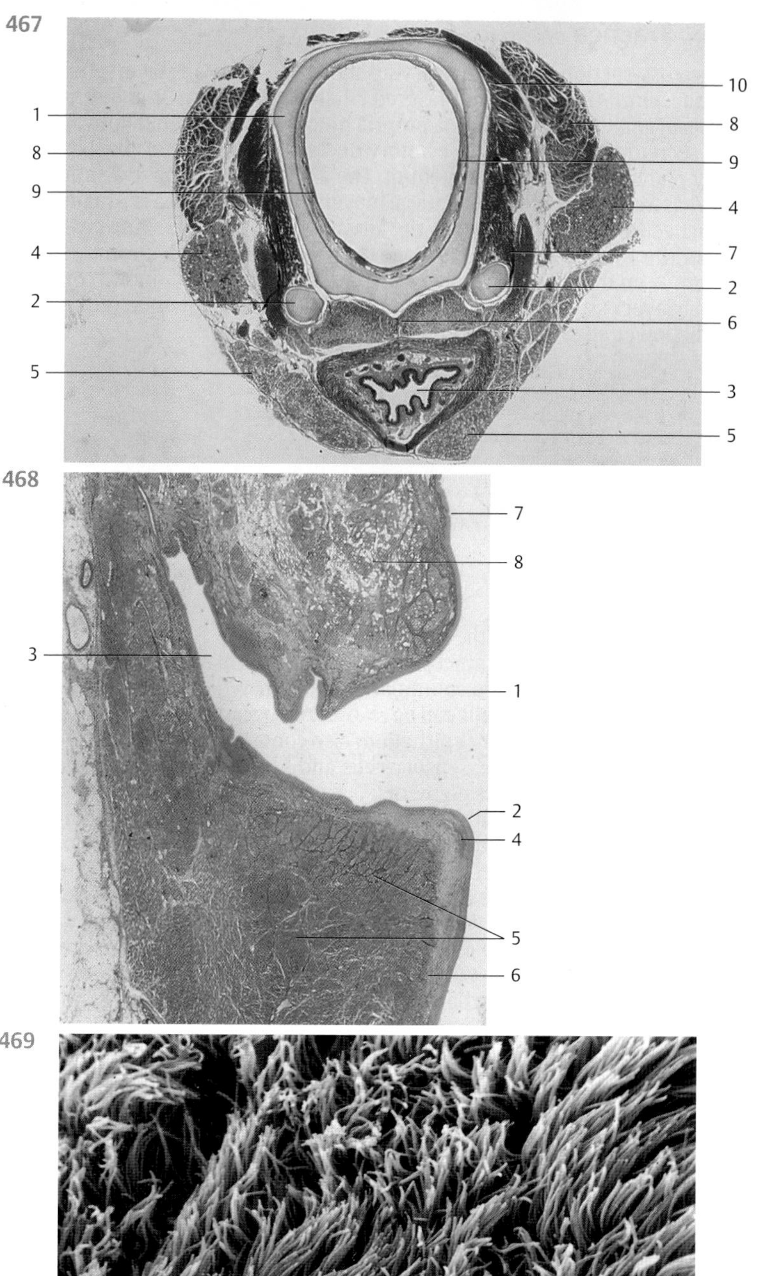

Respiratory System

470 Trachea

This cross-section of the tracheal wall shows the following layers: *tunica mucosa respiratoria* with a multilayered ciliated epithelium 1 and *seromucous tracheal glands* 2 in the lamina propria mucosae 4. The tubular invagination is a secretory duct 3. Many secretory ducts widen to funnel-like bays when they end on the surface epithelium. The airways do not have a submucosal layer as a cushion to dampen lateral movement. The mucosa is usually tightly attached to its base. This keeps the airways open. The following layer represents the hyaline tracheal cartilage 5. It is covered by a strong perichondrium 6 on the side of the mucosa. The very strong perichondral connective tissue layer is stained orange. The tunica adventitia 7 (stained red) is shown at the lower edge of the figure.

1 Respiratory epithelium of the tunica mucosa
2 Tracheal glands
3 Secretory duct
4 Lamina propria mucosae
5 Tracheal cartilage
6 Perichondrium
7 Tunica adventitia
Stain: alum hematoxylin-eosin; magnification: × 20

471 Trachea

Vertical section through the tracheal wall.
The surface of the tunica mucosa consists of a typical respiratory epithelium. It is a ciliated multilayered columnar epithelium, which contains goblet cells (cf. Fig. 112). The goblet cells can be recognized because they appear lighter in this figure. The respiratory epithelium also contains cells, which are covered with microvilli, as well as sensory cells and APUD cells. It requires electron microscopy to show these elements. The epithelium is layered over a strong basal membrane. The epithelial layer is followed by the wide, highly vascularized lamina propria mucosae 2, which contains collagen fibers, longitudinally oriented elastic fiber meshwork and many seromucous tracheal glands 3 Occasionally, there are also lymph follicles. Note the blood vessels in the lamina propria mucosae. The tracheal glands release their secretory product (mucin) directly onto the epithelial surface, thus covering the entire epithelium, including kinocilia, with a film of mucus. The lower parts of the figure show the hyaline ring cartilage of the trachea 5 with the perichondrium 4. Note the blood vessels 6 in the lamina propria mucosae 2.

1 Ciliated, multilayered stratified columnar epithelium with goblet cells (cf. Figs. 111, 112)
2 Lamina propria mucosae with blood vessels and tracheal glands
3 Tracheal glands
4 Perichondrium
5 Tracheal hyaline cartilage
6 Blood vessels
Stain: Masson-Goldner trichrome; magnification: × 200

470

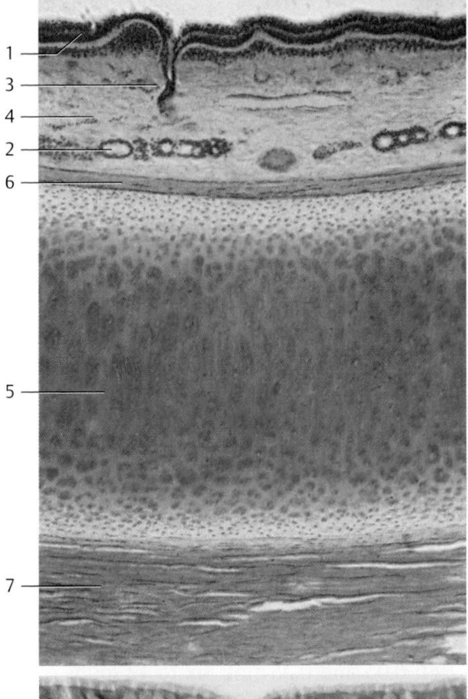

471

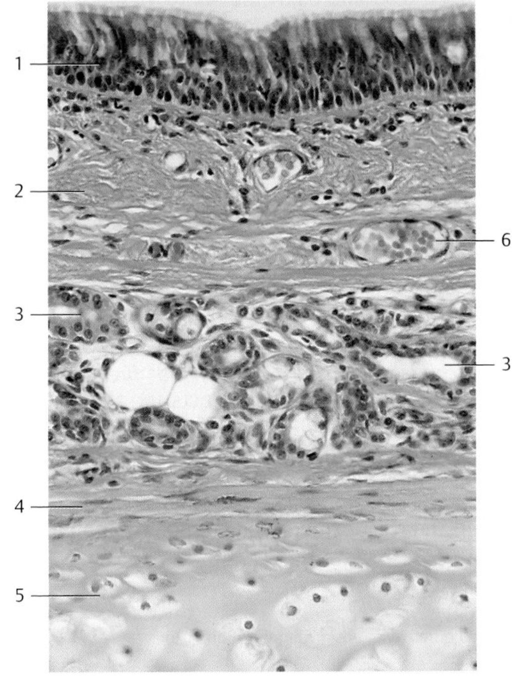

Respiratory System

472 Lung

Section of a human lung, including a small bronchus 1. The mucosa, which lines the bronchus, is folded. This is an artifact. It is caused by the contraction of the smooth muscles during tissue fixation (star-shaped clearance). The mucosa in this figure is covered only by a ciliated, single-layered columnar epithelium. This epithelium contains sporadic goblet cells. The lamina propria (stained blue) is followed by a thin layer of circular muscle cells 2, which are sheathed by elastic fibers. The bronchial glands 3 are situated outside the tunica muscularis 2 in the peribronchial connective tissue. The seromucous glands release a thin or not so thin mucous film of the mucosa surface. Parts of the bronchial cartilage 4 are visible at the upper edge of the figure on the right and in the lower part of the figure to the left of the bronchus. The left part of the figure shows lung alveoli 5 and alveolar ducts 6.

1 Bronchus with folded mucosa
2 Tunica muscularis
3 Bronchial glands
4 Cartilage
5 Alveoli
6 Alveolar ducts
Stain: azan; magnification: × 40

473 Lung

Perspective view of the lung tissue from an adult human. It shows *alveolar ducts* 1 and *alveoli*, which facilitate the gas exchange 2. The alveoli have diameters between 0.05 and 0.25 mm. Six to 12 loops of capillaries weave around each alveolus. The *interalveolar septum* is the common wall between adjacent alveoli. The interalveolar partitions are called alveolar septa. Rings of smooth muscles, which appear knob-like in cross-sections, partition the peripheral septa. This ring of smooth muscles is covered with cuboid epithelium. The upper right of the figure shows a pulmonary vessel (cf. Figs 474–476).

1 Alveolar duct
2 Alveoli,
3 Alveolar sac
Stain: hematoxylin-eosin; magnification: × 80

474 Lung

Respiratory bronchioles divide into wide *alveolar ducts* 1. Alveoli and alveolar sacs are arranged alongside the alveolar ducts and are continuous with them. They open into the long alveolar duct. The walls of the alveolar ducts ↗ widen at the end. There are muscle cells in that end region (see. Figs. 473, 475–477). A thin connective tissue septum (*alveolar wall*) is shared between the epithelia of two adjacent alveoli. The connective tissue consists of a network of collagen and elastic fibers. The pulmonary capillaries are part of this meshwork.

1 Alveolar duct
2 Alveoli
Stain: alum hematoxylin-eosin; magnification: × 200

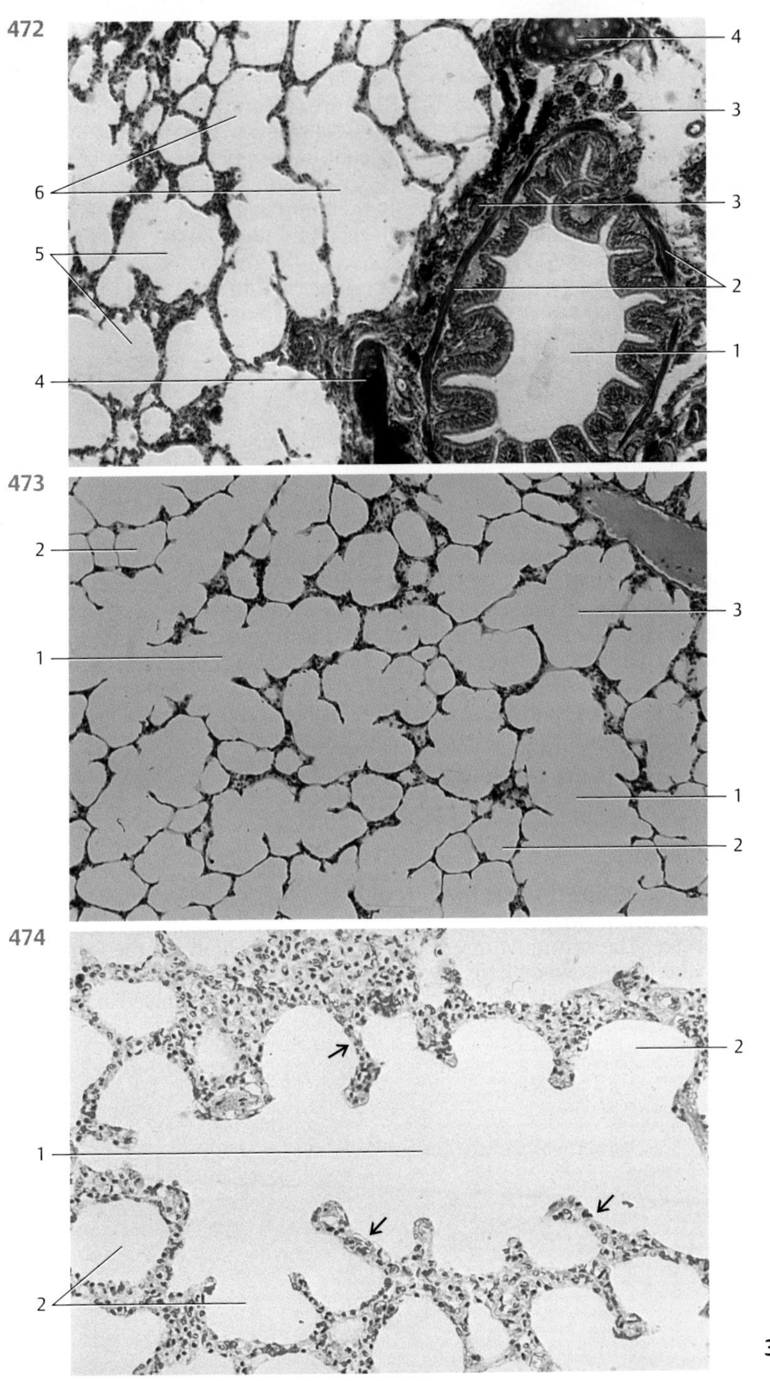

Respiratory System

475 Lung

This is a semi-thin section of lung tissue from a rat. The rich capillarization of the *alveolar septa* is clearly visible. There are still erythrocytes in the lung capillaries ②. Note the extremely thin blood-air barrier. It consists of nonfenestrated capillary endothelium and the continuous epithelial layer of the pulmonary alveoli (alveolar epithelium). Two basal membranes separate both layers (see Fig. 478). The alveolar epithelium consists of two different cell types, the flat *alveolar epithelial* cells or type I pneumocytes, and the large type II pneumocytes. *Type I pneumocytes* contribute about 93% of the alveolar surface cells. The *type II pneumocytes* produce a thin surfactant lipoid covering. Due to their numerous inclusion bodies (*lysosomes*), type II alveolar epithelial cells are also called *granulated pneumocytes.*

1 Alveoli
2 Capillaries with erythrocytes
3 Alveolar duct
Semi-thin section; stain: methylene blue-azure II; magnification: × 400

476 Lung

Vibratome section of a feline lung. Adjacent alveoli are separated only by *interalveolar septa* (cf. Figs. 473, 475). The viewer looks through the septa onto the cut surfaces of the section. On both sides, the septa are covered by a flat *alveolar epithelium*, which consists of type I and type II pneumocytes. A dense capillary network pervades the septa. The septa also contain elastic, reticular and collagenous fibers as well as apart from fibrocytes, leukocytes, macrophages, mast cells and nerve fibers (not visible in this figure). The surface of the alveolar epithelium is recognizable in a few places only.

Scanning electron microscopy; magnification: × 560

477 Lung

This razor section through the lung of a rat shows the branches of a *bronchiolus* ①. The terminal bronchioli ② constitute the ends of the conductive bronchial tree. The continuations of the terminal bronchioli are the respiratory bronchioles, followed by the alveolar ducts ③ and the alveoli ④. The section shows the epithelial lining of many alveoli and the interalveolar septa (cf. Figs. 475, 476, 478).

1 Bronchiolus
2 Terminal bronchioli
3 Alveolar duct
4 Alveoli
Scanning electron microscopy; magnification: × 90

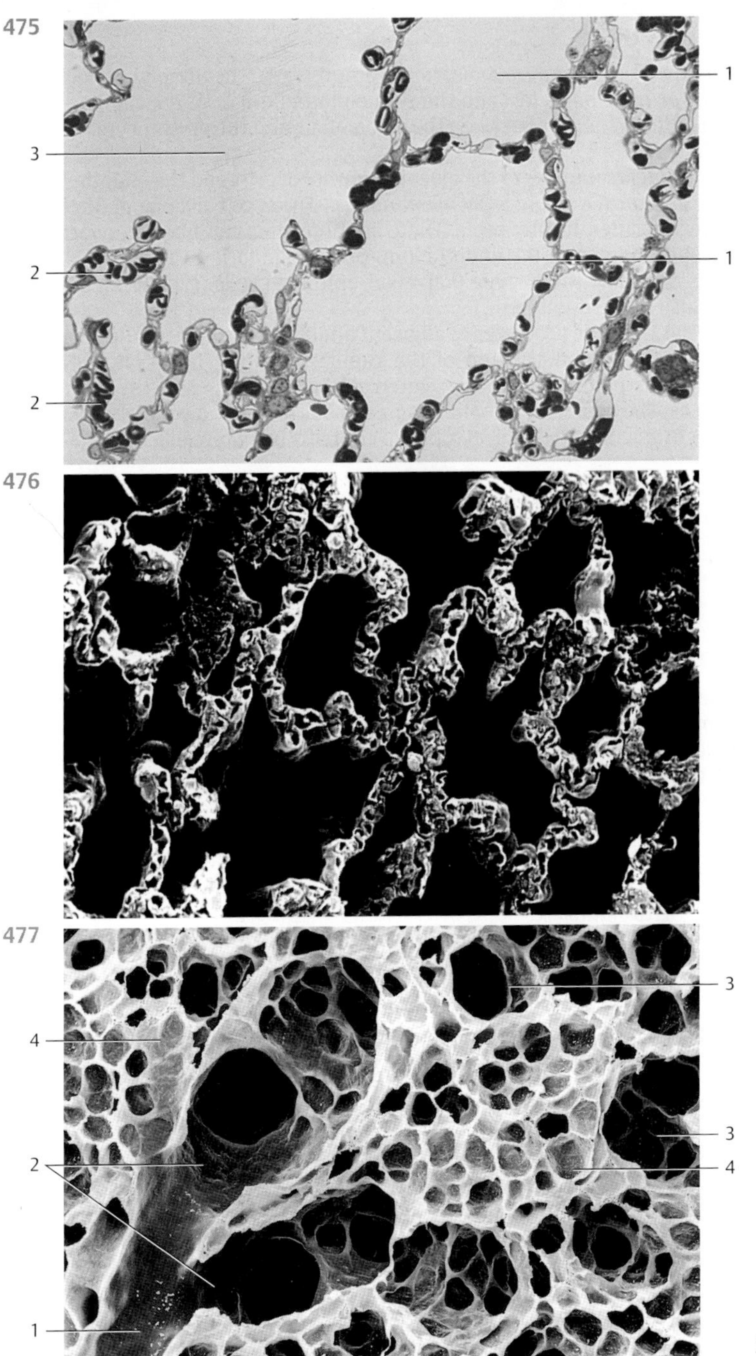
475
1
3
1
2
2
476
477
3
4
3
2
4
1

478 Lung

Section of an *interalveolar septum* (compressed). The *alveolar epithelial cells* 1 (*type I pneumocytes*) and the thin endothelium 2 of the capillaries form the *diffusion barrier* between the alveolar air and the erythrocytes in the capillaries.

The *basal membranes* of the alveolar epithelial cells and the endothelial cells fuse and form a single *basal membrane* 3. The type I alveolar epithelial cells cover the interalveolar septa. There are fibrocytes and fibers between alveolar epithelium and the endothelium of the capillaries. However, this figure does not show them. Type II alveolar epithelial cells (type II pneumocytes) are also not present here.

The cytoplasmic processes of adjacent endothelial cells partially overlap like shingles. The endothelium of the capillaries is not fenestrated. Note the numerous *pinocytotic vesicles*. Intercellular junctions seal the intercellular spaces. The alveolar epithelium spreads out in a thin layer ("anuclear layer" of light microscopy). The cytoplasm contains few organelles.

1 Type I alveolar epithelial cells
2 Capillary endothelium
3 Combined basal membranes
4 Alveolus
5 Capillary lumen
Electron microscopy; magnification: × 30 000

479 Fetal Lung

The epithelial bronchi of the entodermal pulmonary germ layer grow by *dichotomous* (equal) *division* to form the branched bronchial tree. This bronchial tree keeps on branching in the mesenchyme 1. The mesenchyme in the vicinity of the bronchi is conspicuously dense. Its building unit consists of a tube of columnar epithelium 2.

At this developmental stage, the first cell aggregation that intimates the forming lung organ resembles a branched tubuloacinar gland.

1 Mesenchymal interstitial connective tissue
2 Epithelial bronchi
Stain: hemalum-eosin; magnification: × 5

478

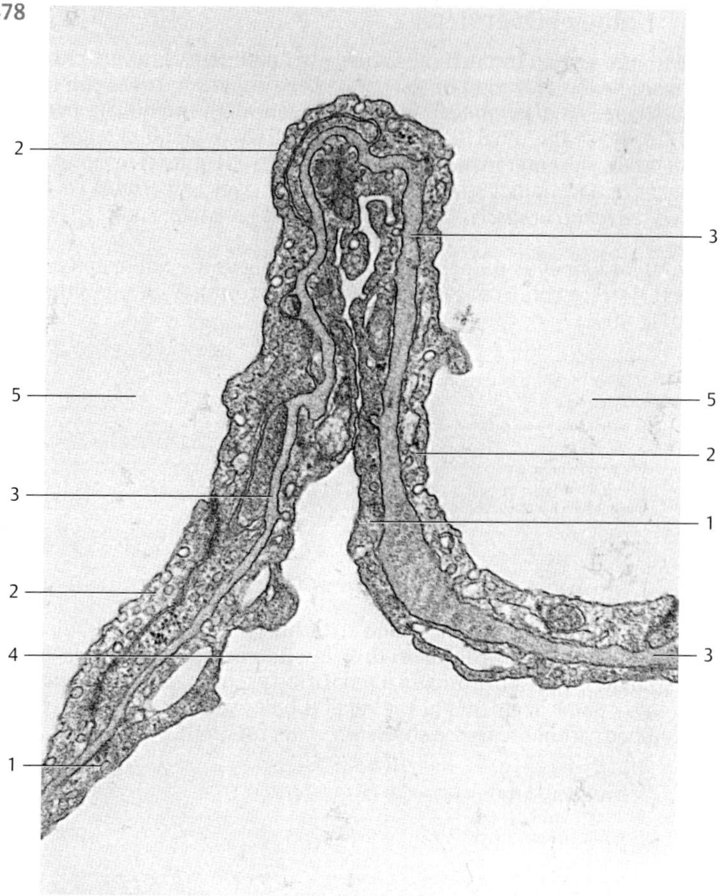

2

3

5

5

2

3

1

2

4

3

1

479

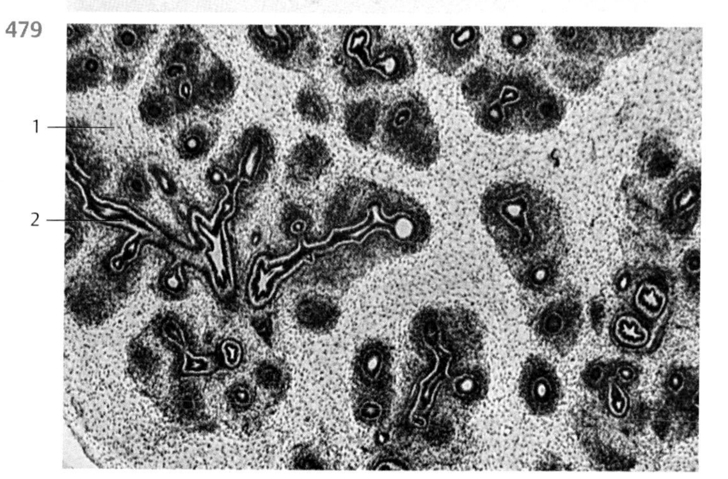

480 Kidney—Overview

This frontal section through the kidney of a rabbit renders a very clear image of the radial organization of the organ. Long collecting tubes run from the cone-shaped *renal pyramid* [1] to the inner zone of the medullary pyramid [2] and finally, to the renal surface. The medullary pyramid extends into the *renal pelvis*. The outer medullary pyramid [4] tissue contains *renal tubules* and appears to have radial stripes. The following layer is the *renal cortex* [5]. It shows the *renal corpuscles* (*Malpighi corpuscles*) as darker spots (cf. Figs. 481–485).
The rabbit kidney is unipapillary; human kidneys are *multipapillary* (8–18 lobes). A strong connective tissue capsule (*renal capsule*) envelops the kidney (see Fig. 499).

1 Pyramid
2 Renal medulla, inner zone
3 Renal pelvis
4 Renal medulla, outer zone
5 Renal cortex
6 Renal papilla
7 Renal sinus
Stain: alum hematoxylin-eosin; magnification: × 2

481 Kidney—Cortical Labyrinth

The renal corpuscles and the coiled distal and proximal renal tubules (*tubuli contorti*) form the *cortical labyrinth* [1], i.e., the cortical components between the straight limbs of the proximal renal tubules (*medullary segments, medullary rays*). Some segments of the renal tubules continue into the cortex [2]. The upper part of the figure shows the *renal capsule* [3].

1 Cortical labyrinth
2 Straight medullary renal tubules (medullary rays)
3 Renal capsule
Stain: alum hematoxylin-eosin; magnification: × 6

482 Kidney—Intrarenal Vascularization

This figure shows the *renal cortex* from a rabbit kidney. Carmine gelatin was injected into the vascular system to demonstrate the organization of the vessels. There is an *interlobular artery* in each *renal column* [1]. It changes direction at the border between cortex and medulla and then continues as the *arcuate artery* [2] along the base of the renal pyramid (right lower corner of the image). The arcuate artery branches into radial *interlobular arteries* (*arteriae corticales radiatae*), which continue as thinner arterioles (*arteriolae rectae*) [3] in the renal medulla (bundle of vessels at the lower edge of the figure). The *afferent glomerular arterioles* branch from the interlobular arteries. They supply the *glomeruli* [4]. The glomeruli appear as black berry-shaped shapes (cf. Figs. 483–485).

1 Interlobular artery
2 Arcuate artery
3 Arterial and venous vasa recta
4 Renal corpuscles
Vascular injection with carmine gelatin; magnification: × 15

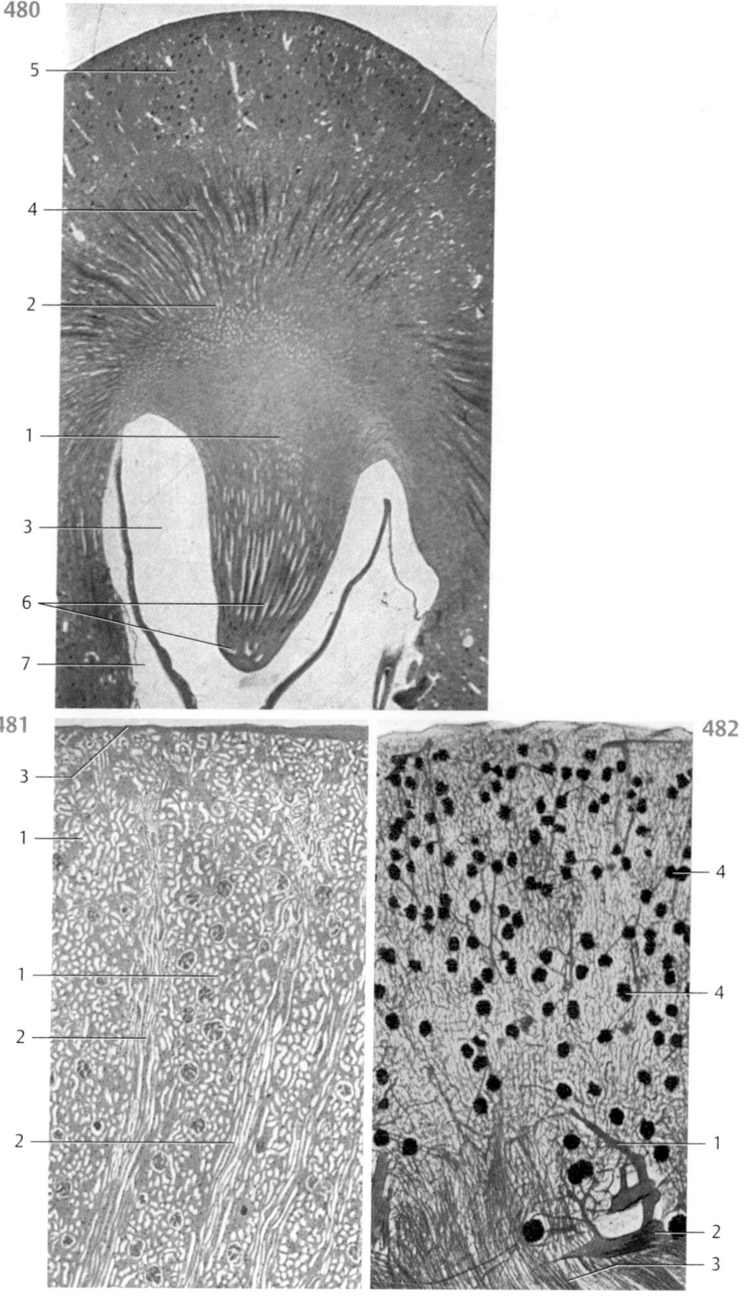
480
5
4
2
1
3
6
7
481
3
1
1
2
2
482
4
4
1
2
3

483 Kidney—Intrarenal Blood Vessels

This vertical section through a rat kidney shows the renal vascular system. The vessels are filled with Indian ink via the renal artery. The *arcuate arteries* 1 are located at the border between cortex and medulla. The border is clearly visible. The black spots in the cortex 2 are blood-filled *glomerular capillaries.* The bundled vessels that radiate toward the renal papilla are the *arteriolae rectae* 3. The renal papilla 4 protrudes into the renal pelvis 5 (cf. Fig. 480).

1 Arcuate artery
2 Renal cortex
3 Renal medulla
4 Renal papilla
5 Renal pelvis
6 Renal sinus
Indian ink injection; stain: picric acid; magnification: × 15

484 Kidney—Intrarenal Blood Vessels

Enlarged section from Fig. 483. At the medulla-cortex border, interlobular renal arteries branch from the *arcuate artery* and vertically ascend to the renal surface. The *afferent glomerular arterioles*, which supply the glomerular capillaries, arise from the interlobular arteries. The medullary *arteriolae rectae* 3 are visible at the lower edge of the figure (see Fig. 482, lower edge and Figs. 470, 483).

1 Arcuate artery
2 Medulla-cortex border
3 Arteriolae rectae
Indian ink injection; stain: picric acid; magnification: × 40

485 Kidney—Intrarenal Blood Vessels

Section from Fig. 483. The interlobular arterioles (*arteriae corticales radiatae*) in the cortex are clearly visible. The *afferent glomerular arterioles*, which supply the *glomerular capillaries*, arise from the interlobular arterioles. The glomeruli seem to hang from short peduncular connections from the interlobular arterioles, like grapes on a vine. The lower part of the figure shows the first segments of the *arteriolae rectae* 3 (see Figs. 483, 484).
Arcuate artery and *interlobular arterioles* are *terminating arteries*.

1 Cortex-medulla border
2 Interlobular artery
3 Arteriolae rectae
Indian ink injection; stain: picric acid; magnification: × 80

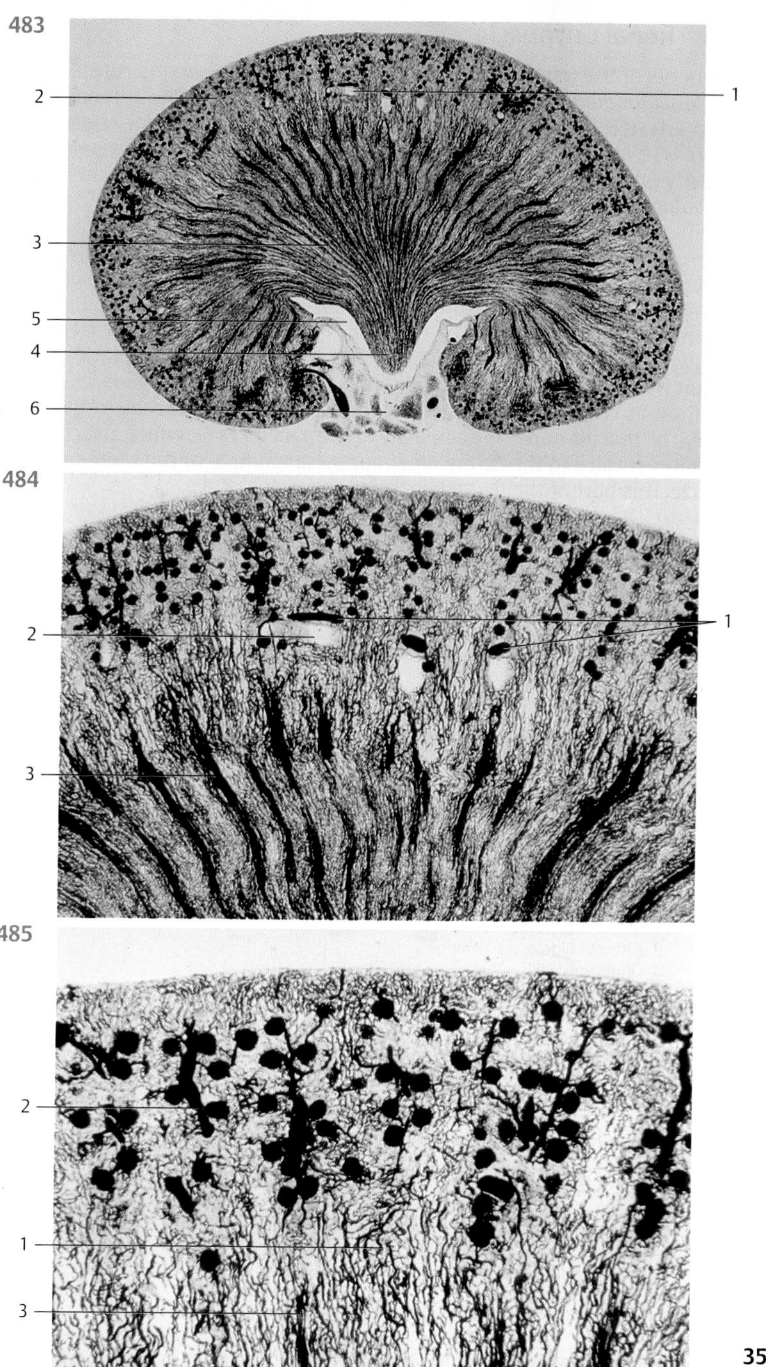
483
2
1
3
5
4
6
484
2
1
3
485
2
1
3

486 Renal Corpuscle

Elements of the *renal corpuscle* are the *glomerulus, Bowman's capsule* [1] and the *vascular pole*. The vascular pole is the point at which the afferent glomerular arteriole enters (*vas afferens*) and the efferent glomerular arteriole (*vas efferens*) exits. The urinary pole is situated opposite the vascular pole. At the urinary pole, the capsule space [2] continues in the proximal tubulus [3] (*pars convoluta*) (see Fig. 488). The parietal lamina of Bowman's capsule [1] consists of a flat single-layered squamous epithelium. At the vessel pole, the single-layered squamous epithelium becomes the visceral lamina (*podocytes*) and covers the capillaries of the glomerulus starting at the capsule space (see Fig. 491). Capillaries arise from the glomerular arterioles. The capillaries anastomose with each other. The efferent capillaries merge and form the *efferent glomerular arteriole*. The walls of the renal glomerular capillaries are different from the walls of other capillaries. A *macula densa* is generated in the location at which the pars recta of the distal tubule attaches to the vessel pole. The macula densa is a cell plate of the pars recta [5], which attaches with its outer surface to the *extraglomerular mesangium* [6] of the same renal corpuscle. It is part of the *juxtaglomerular apparatus* (*JGA*).

1 Bowman's capsule, parietal lamina
2 Bowman's space
3 Proximal tubule
4 Macula densa
5 Distal tubule, pars recta
6 Extraglomerular mesangium cells
Semi-thin section; stain: methylene blue-azure II; magnification: × 400

487 Renal Corpuscle

Renal corpuscle [1] with *afferent glomerular arteriole* [2]. There are granulated cells [3] immediately before the vas afferens [2] enters the renal corpuscle. The granulated cells are the equivalents the smooth muscle cells of the tunica media of this vessel. The granulated (*epithelioid*) cells synthesize the hormone renin. They are part of the *juxtaglomerular apparatus* (*JGA*).

1 Glomerulus, coiled capillaries
2 Afferent glomerular arteriole
3 Granulated cells
4 Bowman's capsule, parietal lamina (lining)
5 Bowman's space
6 Proximal tubule
Semi-thin section; stain: methylene blue-azure II; magnification: × 400

488 Renal Corpuscle

Vibratome section through the cortex of a rabbit kidney (cf. Figs. 486, 487). Scanning electron microscopy renders a three-dimensional image of the renal corpuscle and the adjacent tubules.

1 Bowman's capsule
2 Bowman's space
3 Afferent glomerular arteriole
4 Distal tubule, straight limb
5 Macula densa (dense spot)
6 Urinary pole
7 Proximal tubule, coiled part
8 Proximal tubule
Scanning electron microscopy; magnification: × 510

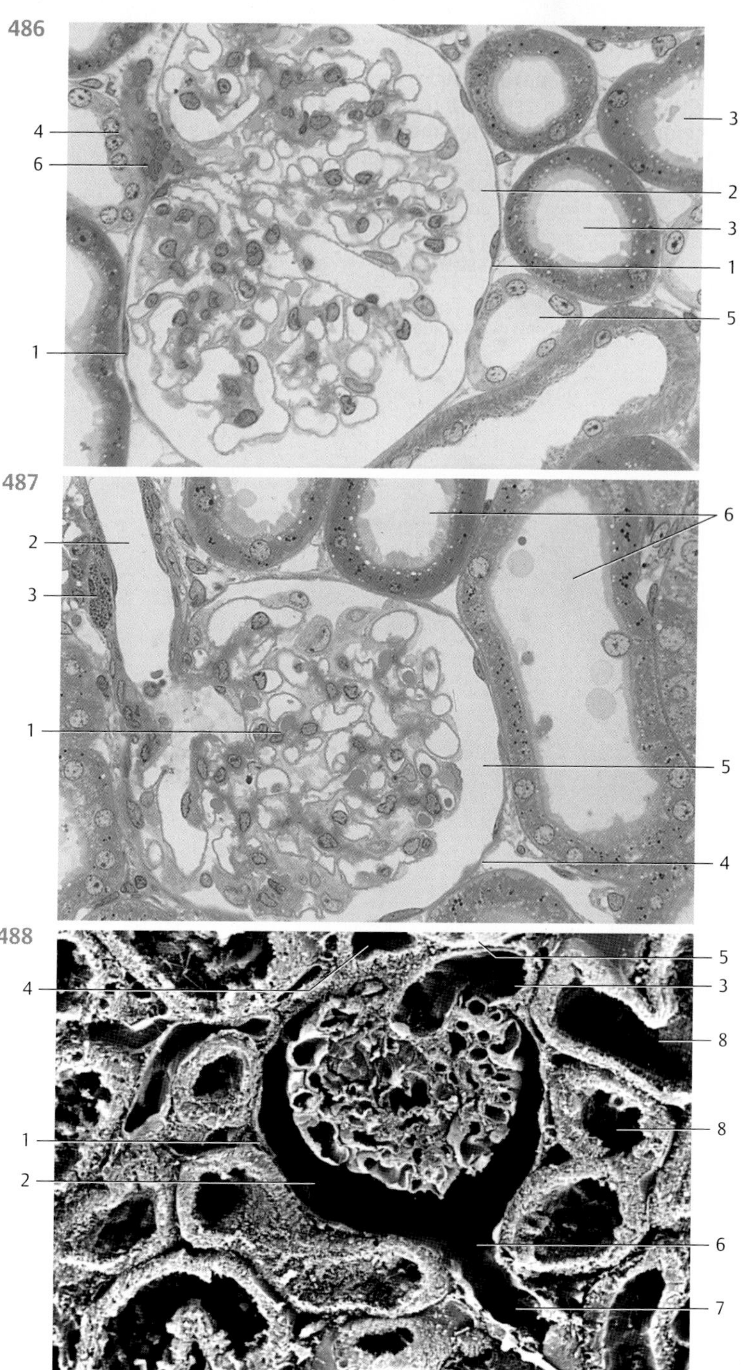

Urinary Organs

489 Renal Glomerulus

General view of a renal corpuscle (section). It shows the glomerular capillary coil ① and Bowman's space ② (cf. Figs. 471–473).
The glomerular basal membrane, the endothelial cells ④, the mesangium cells and the podocytes ⑤ (visceral epithelial cells) are constituents of the glomerular capillary plexus. Details are given in Fig. 491.

1 Capillaries
2 Bowman's space (urinary space)
3 Bowman's capsule, parietal lamina
4 Endothelial cell nuclei
5 Podocyte nuclei
Electron microscopy; magnification: × 2000

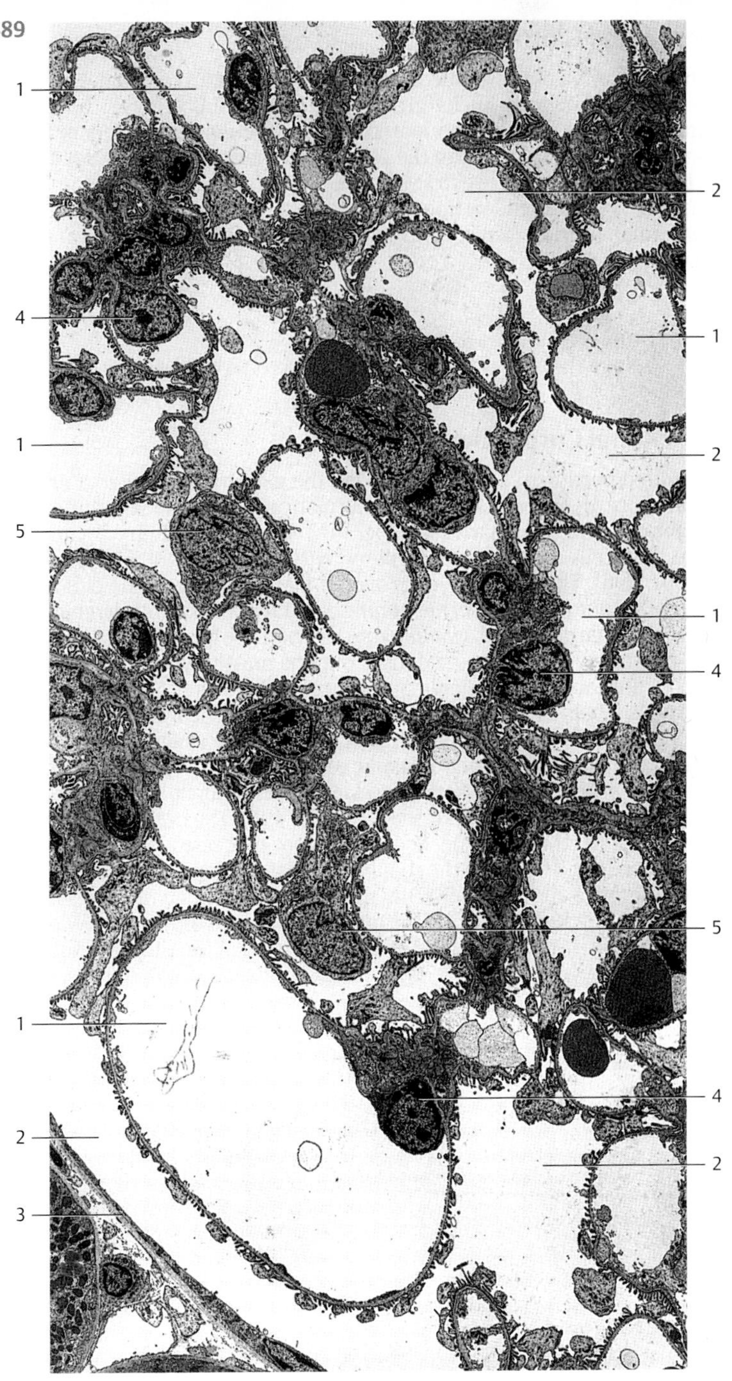
1
2
4
1
1
2
5
1
4
5
1
4
2
2
3

490 Renal Glomerulus

Cast preparation of the glomerular vessels (*glomerulus*) in a renal corpuscle. The renal parenchyma, including the two lamina of Bowman's capsule, was removed by maceration. The view is onto the *vascular pole* 1. Four or five primary capillaries emerge from the afferent glomerular arteriole (*vas afferens*) 2. Each capillary gives rise to a "*lobulus*," which consists of anastomosing capillaries. The efferent portions of the capillaries converge to the efferent glomerular arteriole (*vas efferens*) 3, which exits the capillary coil at the vascular pole 1.

1 Vascular pole
2 Afferent glomerular arteriole
3 Efferent glomerular arteriole
Scanning electron microscopy; corrosion specimen; magnification: × 400

491 Renal Corpuscle

Magnified portion of a section showing the *glomerular capillaries* and *Bowman's space* 2. The walls of the glomerular capillaries are structured differently from other capillaries (cf. Fig. 301). The endothelium 3 consists of large, flat cells, which contain *pores* with diameters of 50–100 nm (see Fig. 301, 496). The pores are not covered by a *diaphragm*. The endothelium covers the glomerular *basal membrane* 4, which consists of a *lamina rara interna, a lamina densa* and a *lamina rara externa*. The basal membrane is about 250–350 nm wide. Its lamina densa contains mostly type IV collagen. *Podocytes* 5 are found facing Bowman's space 2. Podocytes are visceral epithelioid cells. Their large cell bodies (*perikarya*) protrude into Bowman's space 5 (see Figs. 493–495). Podocytes contain elaborate Golgi complexes 6, copious rough and smooth endoplasmic reticulum membranes and lysosomes. There are *primary cytoplasmic processes*, which branch into numerous *secondary processes* 8 (*pedicles*) (see Figs. 494, 495). The branches reach to the glomerular basal membrane. Pedicles or foot processes look like small pistons in sections. They have the shape of interdigitating fingers (see Figs. 493–495). There are about 300–500 nm deep and 35–50 nm wide pores between the pedicles, which are called *filtration slits*. Diaphragms 4 nm wide (only visible at higher magnification) span the bottom of the filtration slit.

1 Capillary lumen
2 Bowman's space
3 Endothelium with pores ↗
4 Glomerular basal membrane
5 Podocyte
6 Golgi apparatus
7 Primary podocyte process
8 Secondary podocyte processes and filtration slits
9 Parietal lamina of Bowman's capsule, single-layered squamous epithelium
10 Subepithelial connective tissue fibers
11 Erythrocyte
Electron microscopy; magnification: × 7200

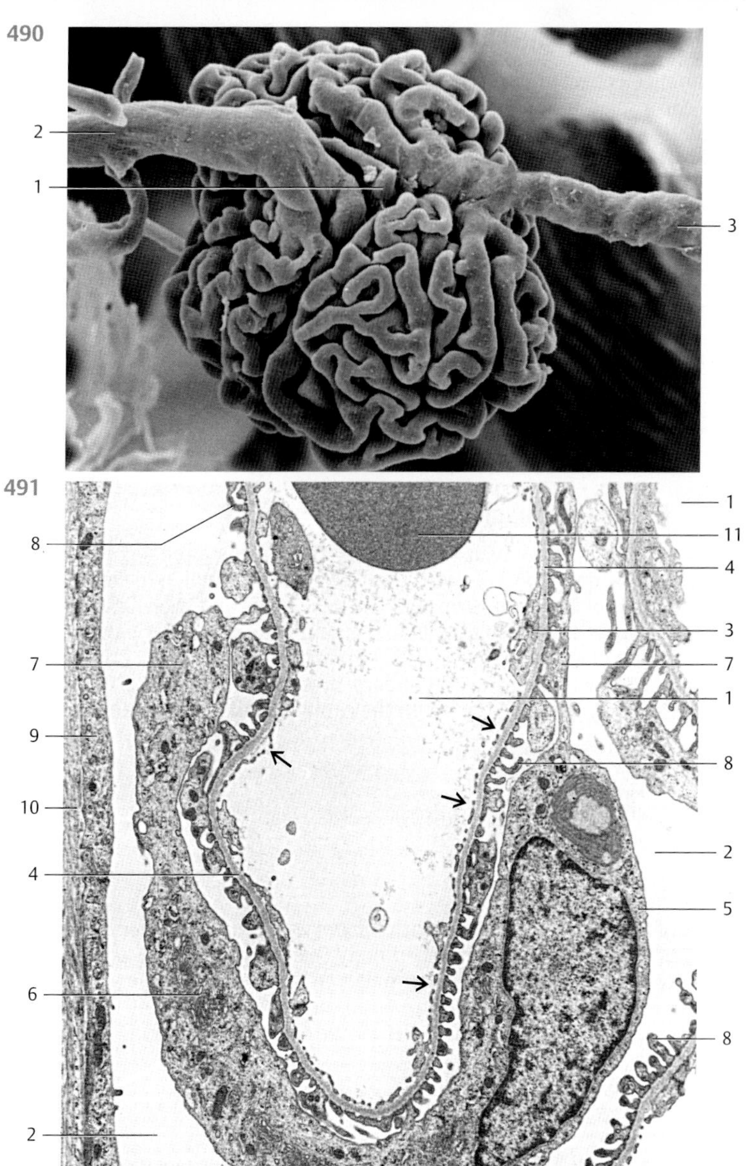
490
2
1
3
491
8
7
9
10
4
6
2
1
11
4
3
7
1
8
2
5
8
6

492 Renal Corpuscle

Scanning electron microscopy of a renal corpuscle and adjacent renal tubule. The corpuscles are opened.
The left side of the figure renders a view into *Bowman's space* 1. The vascular coil is removed. The *vascular pole* 2 is found in the upper part of Bowman's space. The flat epithelial cells of the parietal lamina from Bowman's capsule slightly protrude into Bowman's space. Cell borders are barely recognizable. The capillary coil on the right side of the image is only partially broken apart. This allows a view of the capillary lumina (see Fig. 488). The vascular pole 2 with macula densa 3 is visible in the top part of this corpuscle (cf. Figs. 486, 487).

1 Bowman's space, parietal lamina of Bowman's capsule
2 Vascular pole
3 Macula densa (dense spot)
4 Renal tubules
Scanning electron microscopy; magnification: × 580

493 Renal Corpuscle

Three-dimensional view at the capillary coils inside a renal corpuscle. This figure shows the *podocytes* with their processes 1, which make up the *visceral lamina* of *Bowman's capsule*. The podocytes and their branching processes encircle the capillaries like gripping octopuses. The bulges indicate the location of the podocyte nuclei (*perikaryon*) (cf. Fig. 491). Primary podocyte processes branch into secondary processes (*foot processes*) (see Figs. 491, 494, 495). The space between the capillary coils is Bowman's capsule 3.

1 Podocyte, perikaryon, cell body
2 Primary processes
3 Bowman's space
Scanning electron microscopy; magnification: × 3400

494 Renal Corpuscle

View of a glomerular capillary with a *podocyte* 1 and its primary and secondary *pedicles* 3. Note the large cell body (*perikaryon*), which protrudes into Bowman's space 4. The cell body makes contact only with the primary urine in Bowman's space, not with the basal membrane (cf. Fig. 491). The spaces between pedicles are *filtration slits* 5 (see Figs. 491, 493, 495).

1 Podocyte, perikaryon, cell body
2 Primary pedicles
3 Secondary pedicles (foot processes)
4 Bowman's space
5 Filtration slits
Scanning electron microscopy; magnification: × 7850

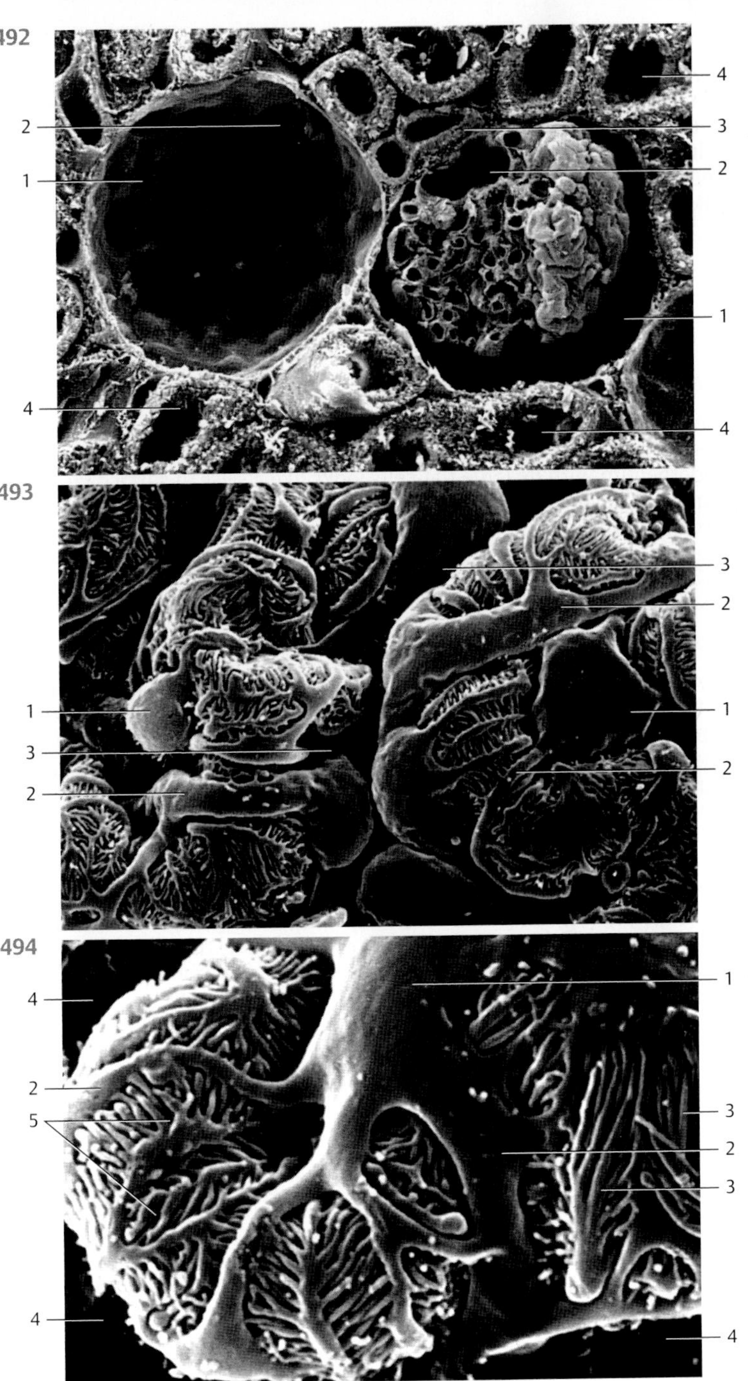
492
4
2
3
1
2
1
4
4
493
3
2
1
1
3
2
2
494
1
4
2
5
3
2
3
4
4

495 Renal Corpuscles

View of the primary and secondary pedicles 2 of podocytes in the glomerulus of a rabbit kidney. The slender pedicles resemble finger-like cytoplasmic processes (see Fig. 491). The primary pedicles interdigitate with adjacent primary pedicles in regular intervals. However, primary and secondary pedicles can also interdigitate. The spaces between pedicles are the filtration slits 3 (see Fig. 491). The slits are 300–500 nm deep and 35–40 nm wide.

1 Primary pedicles
2 Secondary pedicles (foot processes)
3 Filtration slits
Scanning electron microscopy; magnification: × 12 000

496 Renal Corpuscle

View into the inner glomerular capillary and on the endothelium with pores (real holes). Diaphragms to cover the pores are absent (see Fig. 301, 491). The endothelium with its large flat cells looks like a *sieve* in surface view. Their pores have diameters of 50–100 nm. There are thick cytoplasmic ridges between the very thin endothelial processes.

Scanning electron microscopy; magnification: × 23 000

497 Renal Tubules

Parallel cut along the medulla-cortex border (see Figs. 483–485) through the outer layer of the outer zone of the renal medulla. Cross-sections of proximal tubules 1 (pars recta) and of distal tubules 2 (*pars recta, ascending branch*). The cuboidal epithelium of the proximal tubules is covered with a high brush border of dense microvilli (stained green) (cf. Figs. 74, 498). The cell borders of the epithelium in the proximal tubules are not visible. The cytoplasm can be heavily stained using acidic stains. It frequently appears granular, turbid and diffuse. The basal striation of the epithelial cells is also elusive in this preparation. *Distal tubules* (*pars recta, ascending branch*) occur between proximal tubules. Their diameters are considerably smaller than those of proximal tubules, while their clearances are roughly the same. This is due to the flat epithelium of the distal tubules, which is only about 0.5–2.0 μm high. The nuclei of these epithelial cells have the form of disks.

1 Proximal tubules
2 Distal tubules
Stain: Masson-Goldner trichrome; magnification: × 400

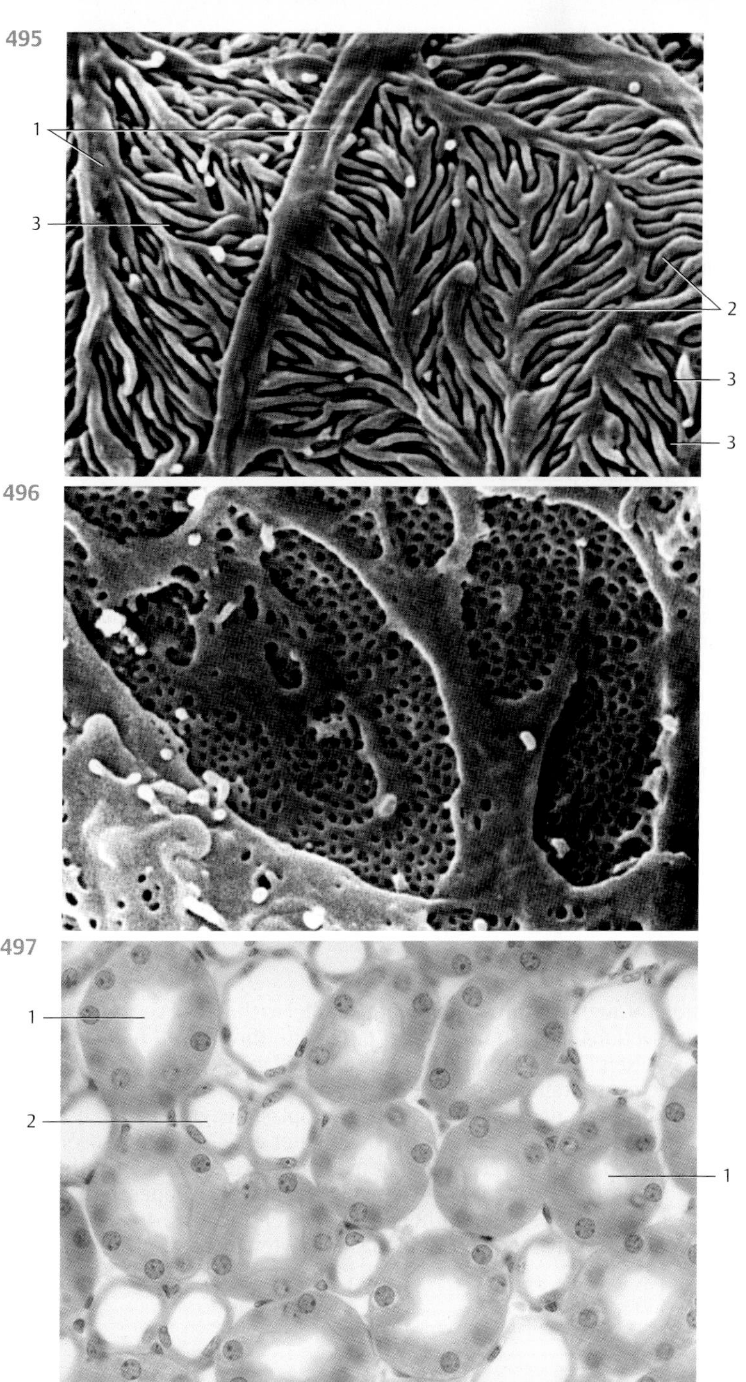
495
1
3
2
3
3
496
497
1
2
1

498 Renal Tubules

Cross-section of the straight parts of a *proximal tubule* 1 and several *distal tubules* 2 (*large ascending limb of Henle's loop*). The cytoplasm of the epithelial cells in the proximal tubules stains intensely with acidic dyes. Staining reveals the granular or striated cytoplasmic structure. The characteristic morphological feature of proximal tubules is the high *brush border* of dense microvilli (stained slightly grayish blue) (see Figs. 497, 500). Note the voluminous nuclei. Cell borders are barely visible. The epithelium of the *distal tubules* (*middle limbs*) 2 from the straight, ascending limbs is considerably lower. There is no brush border or only a very sparse one.

1 Proximal tubules
2 Distal tubules
3 Vessels
Stain: azan; magnification: × 800

499 Renal Tubules

Vertical section of a *cortical labyrinth* and *renal capsule* (*capsula fibrosa* 1 and *subfibrosa* 2). The reticular fibers of the inner capsule layer continue into the center of the kidney where they form a delicate meshwork (cf. Fig. 159). Numerous *proximal tubules* (*pars convoluta*) 3 and two *distal tubules* (*pars convoluta*) 4 are visible in the subfibrous renal capsule. The cuboidal epithelium of the proximal tubules shows its characteristic turbid consistency. A brush border (cf. 495, 498) is absent. Instead, the free epithelial surface shows a diffuse border toward the lumen. The cell borders cannot be recognized here. In contrast, the epithelium of distal tubules 4 (*pars convoluta*) is clearly delimited toward the lumen. The cell nuclei are located closer to each other.

1 Capsula fibrosa
2 Capsula subfibrosa
3 Proximal tubule, pars convoluta
4 Distal tubule, pars convoluta
Stain: van Gieson iron hematoxylin-picrofuchsin; magnification: × 120

500 Renal Tubules

Section through the *cortical labyrinth* parallel to the renal surface. The figure shows sections of several *proximal tubules* 1, three *distal tubules* 2, three larger vessels 3 and capillaries. The epithelial cells of the proximal tubules (*pars recta*) are stained dark blue (cf. Figs. 497, 498). They are covered with a brush border (stained light blue). The cytoplasm is granulated. It contains some lysosomes (stained soft blue) and lighter vesicles. Both lysosomes and vesicles are part of the vesicular system of the proximal tubular epithelium. A straight distal tubule is cut longitudinally (visible in the upper right corner of the figure). Note the different heights of the cells (cf. Figs. 498, 499). The interstitial connective tissue 4 contains fibrocytes and several capillaries.

1 Proximal tubules
2 Distal tubules
3 Vessels
4 Interstitial connective tissue
Semi-thin section; stain: methylene blue-azure II; magnification: × 400

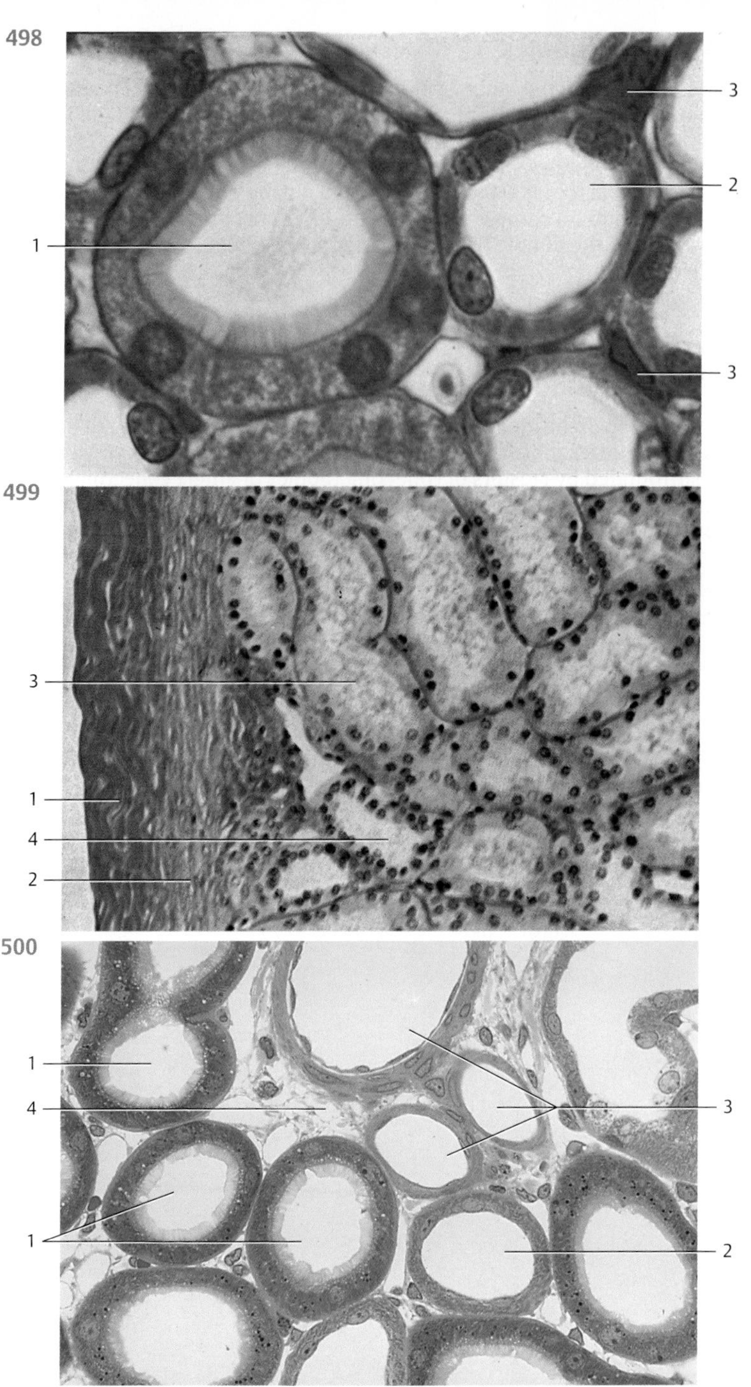
498
3
2
1
3
499
3
1
4
2
500
1
4
3
1
2

501 Renal Tubules

This is a section of the inner layer of the outer zone of the renal medulla. The tissue is cut parallel to the medulla-cortex border (see Figs. 483–485). Intermediary tubules (*descending limb of the thin part of Henle's loop*) surround the vascular bundles (*arteriolae rectae*). The intermediary tubules are followed by distal tubules (middle limbs) and, finally, collecting tubules, which are arranged like a corona that completes the concentric arrangement of tubules around the bundle of vessels (arterial and venous vasa recta).
Rat kidney.

Stain: azan; magnification: × 40

502 Renal Tubules

Cross-section of the inner zone of the renal medulla at the border to the inner layer of the outer zone. The bundles of vessels (*arterial and venous vasa* recta) are surrounded by clusters of collecting tubules or single collecting tubules, which are interspersed with intermediary tubules (*the narrow portion of Henle's loop*). The blood-filled vessels in this cross-section are venous portions of the *vasa recta*. Note the regular structure of the cuboidal epithelium of the collecting tubules.
Rat kidney.

Stain: alum hematoxylin-eosin; magnification: × 80

503 Renal Tubules

Cross-section of the outer layer of the outer medullary zone close to the medulla-cortex border. The renal tubules are arranged in a concentric layer around the bundle of vessels. It is possible to recognize proximal tubules (*pars recta* , main limb) and distal tubules (*pars recta*, middle limb). The epithelium of the proximal tubule is covered with a brush border (cf. Figs. 497–500).

Stain: Masson-Goldner trichrome; magnification: × 200

501

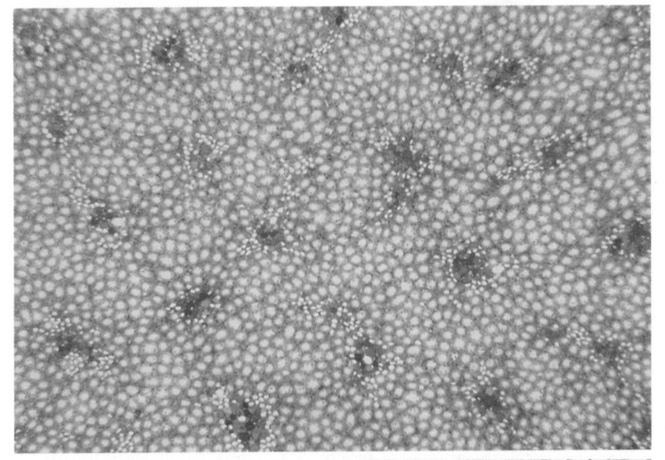

502

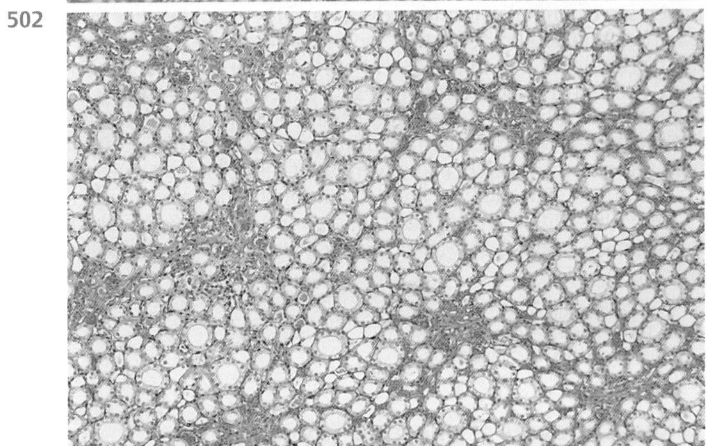

503

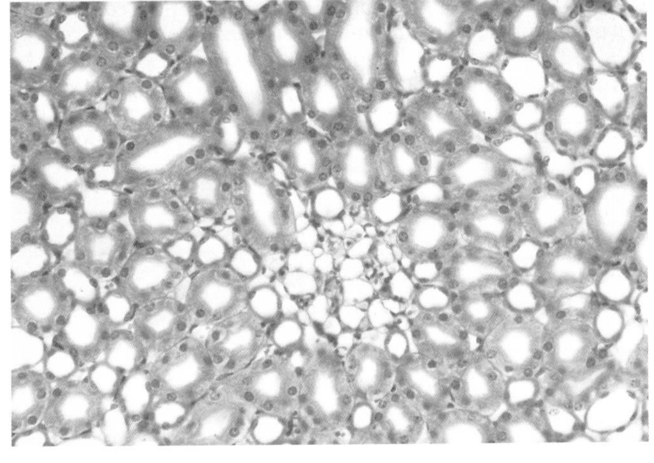

504 Renal Tubules

Cross-section of the inner layer of the outer medullary zone close to the border to the inner zone. Two large collecting tubules [1] with cuboidal epithelial cells (cf. Figs. 106, 107, 505) are presented in the left part of the figure. The remaining cross-sections represent the straight portions of the distal tubules (middle limb) [2] (cf. Figs. 501–503). Two cross-sections of intermediary tubules [3] can be seen in the right part of the image. Capillaries are sporadically found between the tubules. They can be recognized by their narrow lumina and a flat endothelium.

1 Collecting tubules
2 Straight portions of the distal tubules, middle limb
3 Intermediary tubules
Stain: van Gieson iron hematoxylin-picrofuchsin; magnification: × 300

505 Renal Tubules

Cross-section of a renal pyramid in the area of the inner layer of the medulla close to the *renal papilla*. The figure shows numerous cross-sections through collecting tubules [1], the thin segment of Henle's loop [2] and vessels. In contrast to the cortical collecting tubes between the medullary rays (see Fig. 506), the medullary collecting tubules are lined with a single-layered columnar epithelium, which consists of principal cells only (cf. Fig. 107). The columnar epithelium has a light cytoplasm (light cells), distinct cell borders and round cell nuclei. The cuboidal epithelial lining of the cortical collecting tubules (see 506) contains principal cells and intercalate cells, which have a dark cytoplasm (dark cells). Note the numerous arterial and venous vasa recta.

1 Collecting tubules
2 Thin portion of Henle's loop
Stain: azan; magnification: × 200

506 Renal Tubules—Collecting Tubule

Vibratome section through a rabbit kidney. A cortical collecting tubule is broken open and the epithelial lining is visible. The epithelial cells bulge into the lumen. The dark cell in the epithelium is an intercalate cell [1]. Microvilli, which look like pushpins, protrude from its apical plasmalemma. The principal cells [2] often display a single cilium. The large round cell nuclei [3] are prominently exposed in the cut epithelial surfaces at the upper and lower edge of the figure.

1 Intercalate cell
2 Principal cell with cilium
3 Nucleus of a principal cell
Scanning electron microscopy; magnification: × 3000

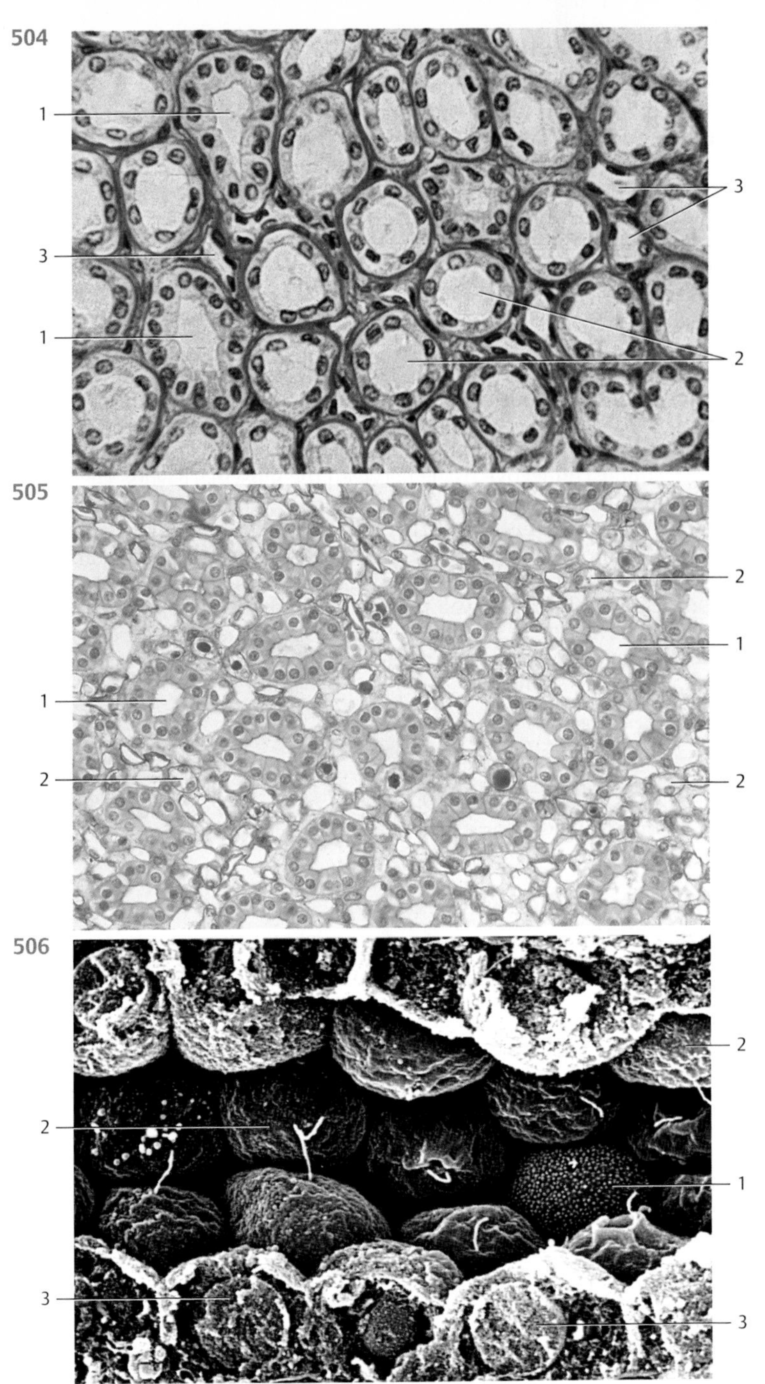
504
1
3
1
3
2
505
2
1
1
2
2
506
2
2
1
3
3

507 Kidney—Renal Papilla

Papilla of a rat kidney. The collecting tubules merge and form 100–200 μm-wide, papillary ducts which end at the tip of the papilla. The openings of the papillary ducts are not round but rather shaped like slits of different sizes. The columnar epithelium of the papillary ducts turn into urothelium at the opening of the papilla. The urothelium covers the outside of the papilla. The renal papilla is perforated. It is named *area cribrosa*.
The renal papilla protrudes into the renal pelvis.

Scanning electron microscopy; magnification: × 160

508 Ureter

The *tunica muscularis* forms the strong muscle coat of the ureter. It has two or three layers. The ureter consists of the internal and external longitudinal muscle bundles [1] with an interleaved layer of circular muscle bundles [2]. There is ample connective tissue between the muscular layers. The mucosa consists of the *urothelium* [3] (cf. Figs. 113–115) and the *lamina propria* [4], which contains copious fibers. The mucosa forms six to eight longitudinal folds when the wall musculature contracts. This explains the star-shaped center clearance in the cross-section. There are sloughed off epithelial cells in the clearance. With the wall muscles relaxed, the ureter folds disappear. The *tunica adventitia* is shown at the left edge of the figure. It contains copious collagen fibers and is traversed by many vessels and nerves. The lamina propria is heavily stained.

1 Internal longitudinal muscle bundles
2 Circular muscle layer
3 Urothelium
4 Lamina propria
5 Tunica adventitia
Stain: van Gieson iron hematoxylin-picrofuchsin; magnification: × 16

509 Urinary Bladder

The layered structure of the ureter is also found in the urinary bladder (*vesica urinaria*). The urothelium is found in the upper part of the figure (blue line). The underlying *lamina propria* consists of a relatively thick layer of connective tissue. The strong muscle fibers of the *tunica muscularis* form a complex network with inner and outer longitudinal muscle bundles, which are intercalated by a layer of circular muscles. The connective tissue strands of the subserosal tissue are visible at the lower edge of the figure.
Urothelium (see Figs. 113–115, 510, 511).
The very strong muscular wall of the urinary bladder forms the detrusor muscle.

Stain: alum hematoxylin-eosin; magnification: × 4

507

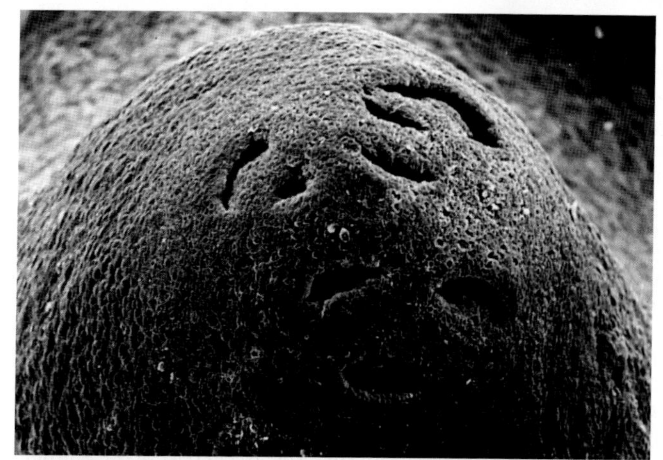

508

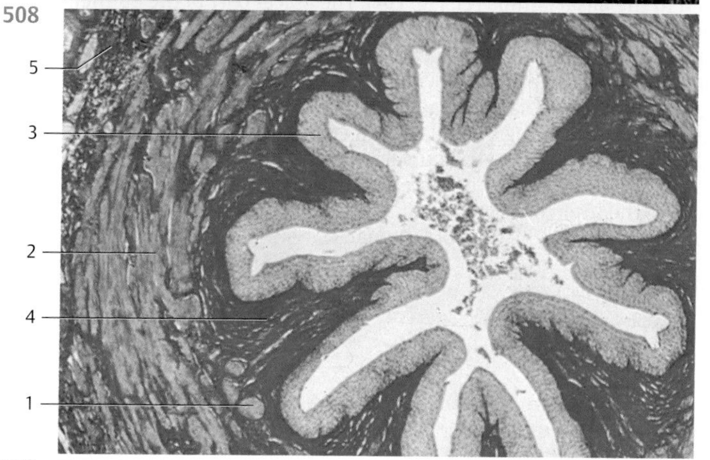

509

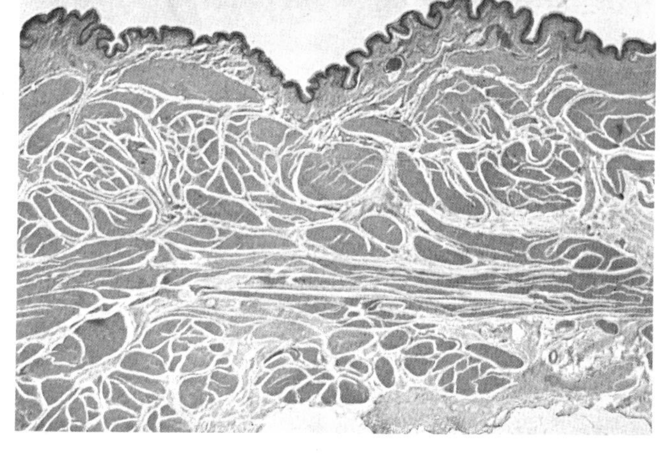

510 Ureter—Urothelium

The urinary collecting system includes *renal calices*, the *renal pelvis*, the *ureter*, the *urinary bladder* and the *urethra*. Save a few portions of the urethra, all parts of the urinary collecting system are lined by a specifically adapted epithelium that can withstand permanent contact with urine. This epithelium appears sometimes multilayered stratified and sometimes multilayered pseudostratified. It was therefore named *transitional epithelium* or *urothelium* (cf. Figs. 113–115). The urothelium is of different heights in different locations in the urinary collecting system. The urothelium in the small renal calices has only two or three layers; the ureter and the urinary bladder display five or six layers. Dependent on the distention of the ureters and the urinary bladder, the epithelium transitions from one form to another (transitional epithelium). In the relaxed state of the ureters and bladder, the epithelium displays the basal 1, intermediary 2 and surface cells 3 of a pseudostratified epithelium. The basal cells are cuboidal, the intermediary cells are polygonal and the superficial cells are columnar. Basal cell processes may reach to the basal lamina (cf. Fig. 114). The apical part of the epithelium protrudes into the lumen. The tall columnar cells of the epithelium are occasionally also called "umbrella cells" (covering cells) (see Fig. 511). The surface cells form the barrier to the urine. Their apical cytoplasm contains a dense network of intermediary and actin filaments, which account for the heavier staining in this cell region. This apical cell region is also called *crusta* 4 (cf. Fig. 113). Intermediary cells and surface cells contain many lysosomes 5 (cf. Fig. 511). Lymphocytes 6 migrate through the urothelium and can often be found in the intercellular space.
Urothelium from a 54-year-old woman.

1 Basal cells
2 Intermediary cells
3 Surface (umbrella) cells
4 Crusta
5 Lysosomes
6 Lymphocytes
Stain: Laczkó-Lévai polychromatic staining of lysosomes; magnification: × 500

511 Ureter—Urothelium

Part of the urothelium in the ureter of a 54-year-old woman. The large surface cells 1 contain many lysosomes 2 mostly in the supranuclear cell region. Intermediary cells 3 may also contain lysosomes (cf. Fig. 510). Some of the surface cells contain two nuclei. The light apical cytoplasmic seam represents the crusta. It contains a dense network of microfilaments, which can be intensely stained. The cytoplasm contains many other vesicles, which are pushed into the apical cell region when the ureter or the urinary bladder expands. As seen before (cf. Fig. 510), the urothelium contains lymphocytes 5.

1 Surface cells with crusta
2 Lysosomes
3 Intermediary cells
4 Basal cells
5 Lymphocytes
Electron microscopy; magnification: × 1800

510

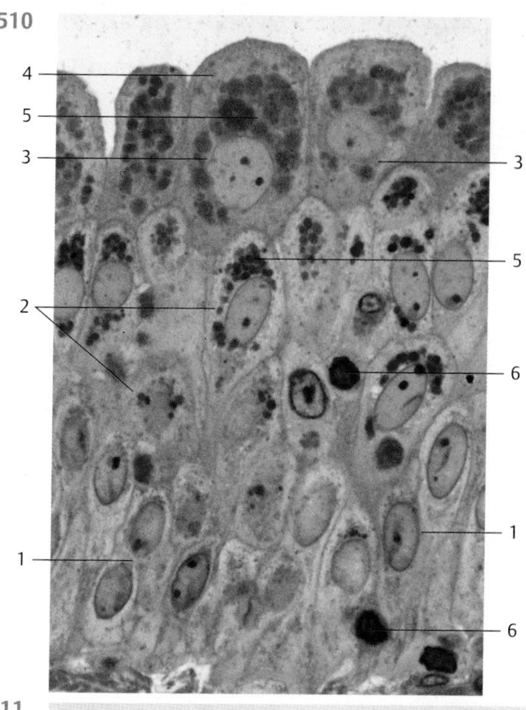

511

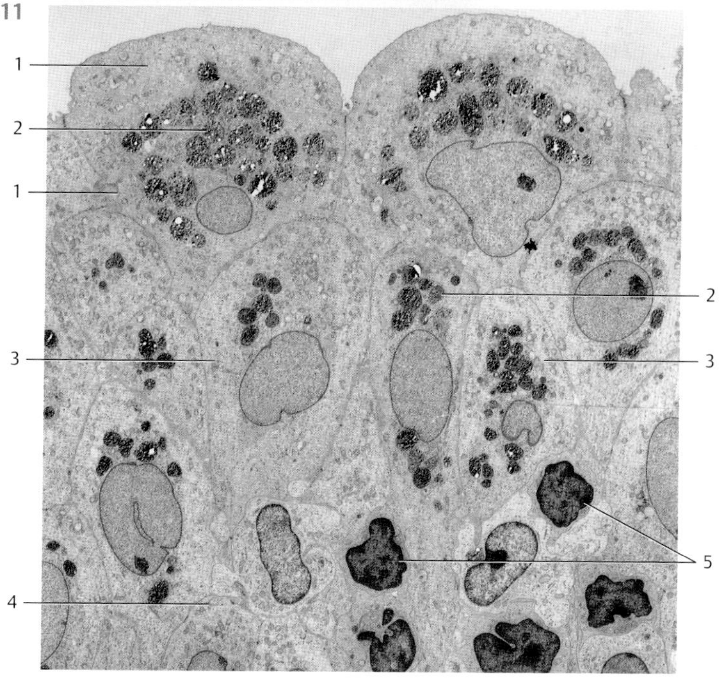

1
2
1
2
3
3
5
4

512 Testis

Cross-section of the testis with *rete testis* 1 of a 19-year-old man. The epididymis is shown in the lower right of the figure.

1 Tunica albuginea
2 Septula testis
3 Lobulus testis
4 Rete testis
5 Epididymis
Stain: azan; magnification: × 2.5

513 Rete Testis

Cross-section of the *rete testis* 1 with *lobuli testis* 2 and *septula testis* 3. The *rete (net) testis* attaches on the dorsal side of the testes to the inside of the tunica albuginea 4. It consists of a network of communicating slits and spaces, which are enclosed in the mediastinum of the testis (*corpus highmori*). The elongated mediastinum consists of connective tissue with lymph and blood vessels as well as muscle cells and nerve fibers. The slit-shaped spaces are lined by a single-layered cuboidal epithelium. However, there are also columnar epithelial cells. Fine cords of connective tissue, which are covered by epithelium, traverse the intercellular spaces of the rete testis. The tortuous seminiferous tubules end either directly in the rete testis or via a short straight tubule (tubuli seminiferi recti). The rete testis continues in the *efferent tubules* (see Figs. 525, 526).

1 Rete testis with blood vessels
2 Lobulus testis with seminiferous tubule
3 Septulum testis
4 Tunica albuginea
Stain: Masson-Goldner trichrome; magnification: × 12

514 Rete Testis

Detail magnification of the rete testis (cf. Fig. 513). The septum of the testis 2 is an elongated body of connective tissue with irregularly shaped slits 1. The slits are lined by a single-layered cuboidal epithelium, which also contains ciliated columnar cells. There are smooth muscle cells underneath the epithelium. The rete testis penetrates the tunica albuginea and continues in the efferent tubules of the caput epididymidis.
The epithelial lining of the rete testis creates a large surface. It regulates the composition of the rete fluid through the processes of secretion and resorption.

1 Rete crevices
2 Septum of the testis, connective tissue
Stain: alum hematoxylin-eosin; magnification: × 20

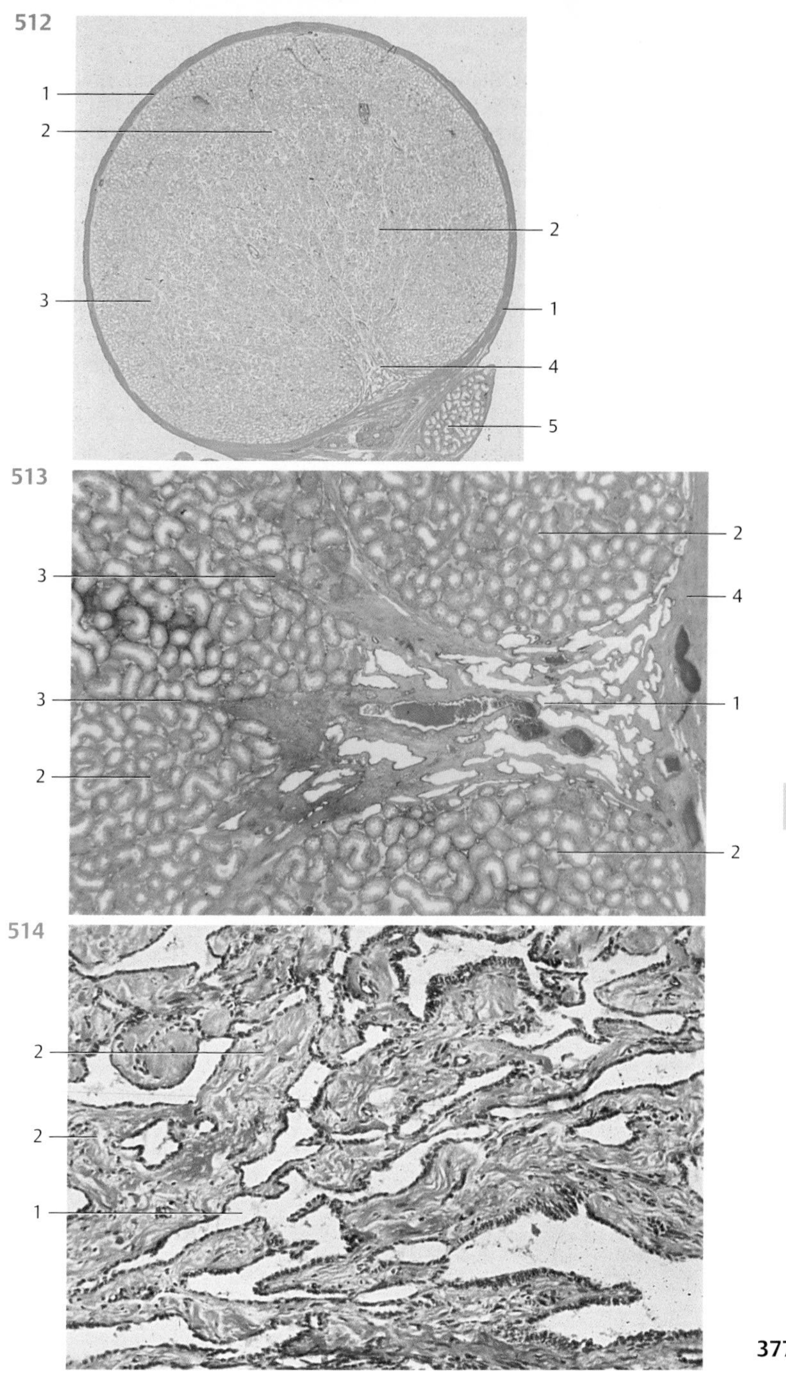
512
1
2
2
3
1
4
5
513
3
2
4
3
1
2
2
514
2
2
1

515 Testis

The *seminiferous tubules* (diameter 180–300 µm) are coiled in the *lobuli testis*. The *septulae testes* (see Fig. 512) intersect the lobuli. The interstitial connective tissue contains fibrocytes and histiocytes as well as the *interstitial Leydig cells* 1. The secretory Leydig cells (see Fig. 522) biosynthesize the male hormone *testosterone*. The tortuous seminiferous tubules have a sheath of muscular connective tissue (lamina propria). Their lining consists of the 60–80 µm high germinal epithelium. It consists of cells in different stages of *spermatogenesis* and of supportive *Sertoli cells*. The spermatogonia are attached to the basal membrane. These are round cells with chromatin-rich nuclei. The layers of cells over the spermatogonia contain the slightly larger primary *spermatocytes*. Primary and secondary spermatocytes (prespermatocytes) are hard to distinguish in this figure. The small dark elements close to the lumen are sperm cells. Compare with Figs. 516–521.

1 Interstitial Leydig cells
Stain: hematoxylin-eosin; magnification: × 250

516 Testis

Male Sexual Organs

Seminiferous tubules of a 42-year-old man. The myofibrous lamina propria limitans or boundary tissue 1 of the tubular wall is visible in the lower part of the figure. This connective tissue sheath consists of a basal membrane, fibrocytes, myofibroblasts and collagen fibers (cf. Figs. 519, 520). The basal membrane (*hyaloid membrane*) is located between lamina propria and parenchyme. The spermatogonia 2 are found at the basal membrane and numerous primary spermatocytes 3 (pachytene stage) are located above it. The spermatocytes can be recognized by their large nuclei with distinct chromatin structure (see Figs. 518, 519). Spermatids 4 with dense round nuclei are present close to the lumen. The darker stained acrosomal caps of the spermatid nuclei are clearly discernible.

1 Lamina propria limitans, boundary tissue
2 Spermatogonia
3 Primary spermatocyte
4 Spermatids
Semi-thin section; stain: toluidine blue-pyronine; magnification: × 800

517 Testes

Section of the wall from a tortuous seminiferous tubule. The *lamina propria limitans* 1 can be seen in the right part of the figure. A *Sertoli cell* 2 is present at the inner basal membrane. The Sertoli cell body narrows as it spans the germinal epithelium. Note the darker stained small spermatids. Three spermatids appear to be located in the Sertoli cell cytoplasm.

1 Lamina propria limitans
2 Sertoli cell with mature spermatids
3 Tubular lumen
Semi-thin section; stain: toluidine blue-pyronine; magnification: × 800

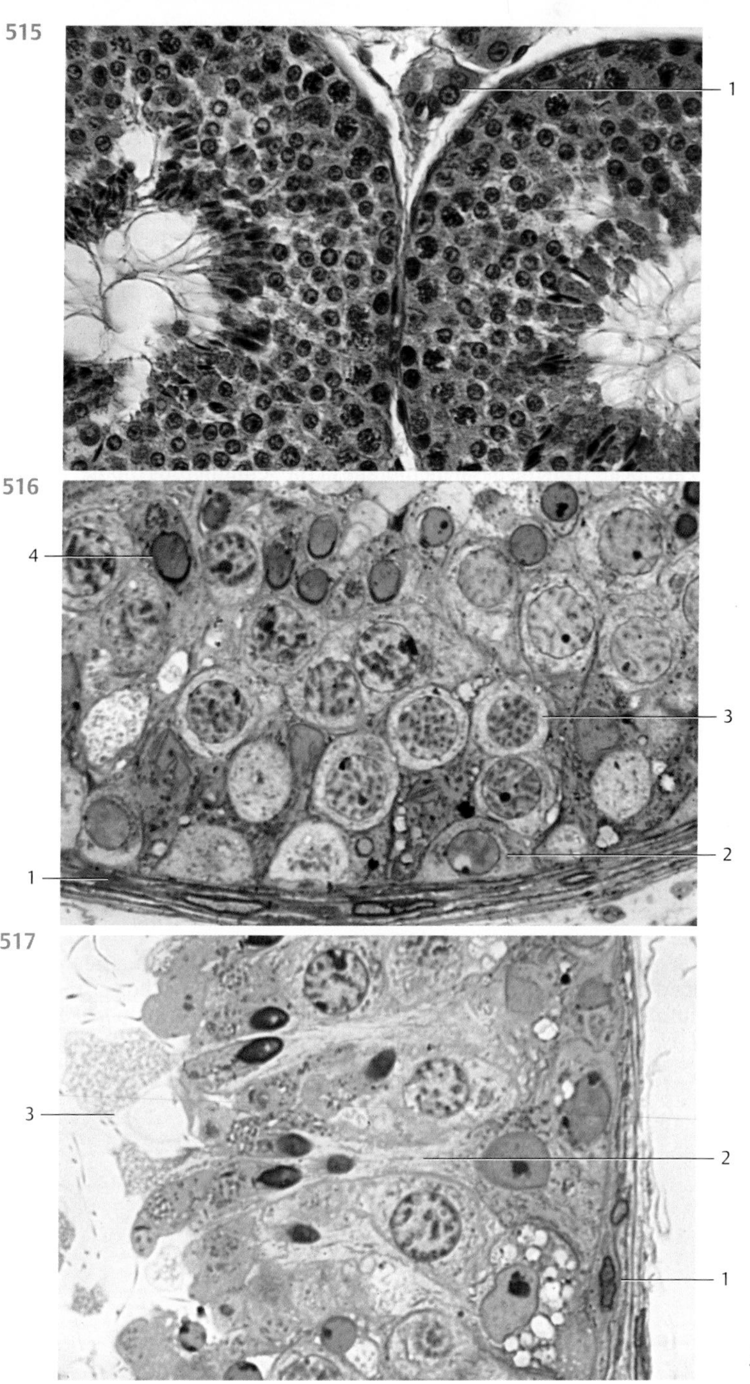
515
1
516
4
3
2
1
517
3
2
1

Testes

Section of a *seminiferous tubule* from a 25-year-old man with intact *spermatogenesis*. The germ cells proliferate in the germinal epithelium and differentiate into sperm cells.

The development starts with the *spermatogonia*. They form the basal layer of the germinal epithelium. There are *spermatogonia of type A* 1 with rounded nuclei and *spermatogonia type B* with nuclei, which contain several nucleoli. Spermatogonia of different types stain differently. Most type A spermatogonia have nuclei, which bind only small amounts of dye. They are *type A pale* cells, in contrast to the *type A dark* cells, which bind more dye and show a cytocenter.

The germinal epithelium in this figure also contains *spermatocytes type I* 2, *spermatids* 3 and *Sertoli cells* 4. The spermatids are the smallest cells of the germinal epithelium. They are usually found near the tubular lumen. Early spermatids are rounded cells with rounded nuclei. Mature spermatids can be identified by their condensed nuclei. Sertoli cells have a columnar shape. They are located on the basal membrane of the seminiferous tubule. The apical poles of the Sertoli cells bulge into the tubular lumen (cf. Fig. 517). Their lobed nuclei are a characteristic feature. Several residual bodies 5 are visible in the left upper part of the figure. They contain parts of the spermatid cell body and consequently organelles of the spermatid cytoplasm (cf. Fig. 519). The figure shows the lamina propria limitans 6 at the lower right corner.

1 Spermatogonia type A, pale
2 Spermatocyte type I
3 Mature spermatid
4 Sertoli cell
5 Residual body
6 Lamina propria limitans
Electron microscopy; magnification: × 900

519

Testes

Section of a seminiferous tubule from a 25-year-old man with intact spermatogenesis (cf. Fig. 518). Spermatogenesis is a continuous process in the mature testes. It involves several stages.

The seminiferous tubules have a diameter of 180–300 µm. They are enveloped by the *myofibrous lamina propria* 6 (cf. Fig. 520). The germinal epithelium is 60–80 µm high and consists of germ cells and supportive Sertoli cells (cf. Fig. 521).

1 Residual body
2 Dividing spermatocyte
3 Spermatocyte type I
4 Sertoli cells
5 Spermatogonia type A, pale
6 Lamina propria limitans
Electron microscopy; magnification: × 1500

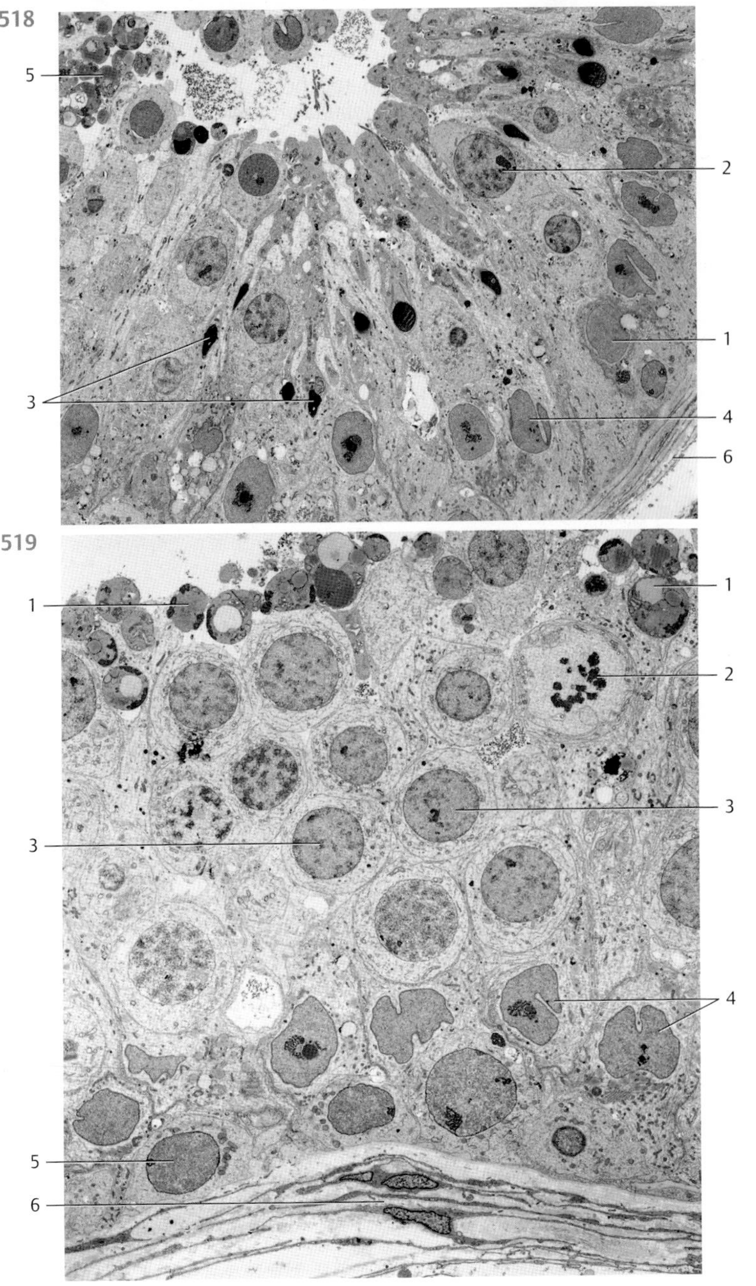

Male Sexual Organs

520 Testis

Lamina propria (boundary tissue) of a seminiferous tubule from the testis of a 30-year-old man with intact spermatogenesis.

The left part of this figure shows the *lamina propria* of a seminiferous tubule. The germinal epithelium is located on the basal membrane 1, which can be clearly recognized. Collagen fibrils 2, fibroblasts 3 and myofibroblasts 4 form the following 8–10 μm wide outer layer. These cells are elongated and so are their nuclei. The myofibroblasts are contractile and account for the peristaltic movements of the seminiferous tubules. The newly generated spermatozoa by themselves are not yet motile. The peristaltic movements transport them from the germinal layer to the rete testis. Note that the collagen fibrils between the spindle-shaped fibroblasts and myofibroblasts are cross-sectioned or cut longitudinally. A pale, type A spermatogonium 5 is visible in the right upper part of the figure.

Compare this figure with the light micrographs 516 and 517 and with the electron micrographs in Figs. 518 and 519.

1 Basal lamina
2 Collagen fibrils
3 Fibroblasts
4 Myofibroblasts
5 Spermatogonium type A, pale
Electron microscopy; magnification: × 4800

521 Testis

Basal section of a seminiferous tubule from a 37-year-old man with intact spermatogenesis.

The spermatogonia 1 are located next to the basal lamina 2 (left lower corner of the figure). The basal lamina is followed by the lamina propria limitans 3 (cf. Figs. 516, 517, 520). The spermatogonia 5 divide repeatedly and give rise to spermatocytes 4. *Sertoli cells* 6 are named after the histologist Enrico Sertoli (1842–1910). They are support cells and line the seminiferous tubules. With the exception of spermatogonia, Sertoli cells surround practically all germ cells. Their wider basal part borders on the basal membrane. From the basal membrane, Sertoli cells pervade the entire germinal epithelium. As their cell bodies extend toward the lumen, they get thinner and often form finger-like processes at their apical cell region. In light microscopy, the calling card for Sertoli cells is their slender cell body and their light oval or pear-shaped nuclei 6. The nucleus is frequently lobed or notched (cf. Fig. 517). Sertoli cells usually have prominent nucleoli.

1 Spermatogonium
2 Basal lamina
3 Lamina propria limitans
4 Spermatocyte type I
5 Spermatogonium type A, pale
6 Sertoli cell nucleus with nucleolus
Electron microscopy; magnification: × 4000

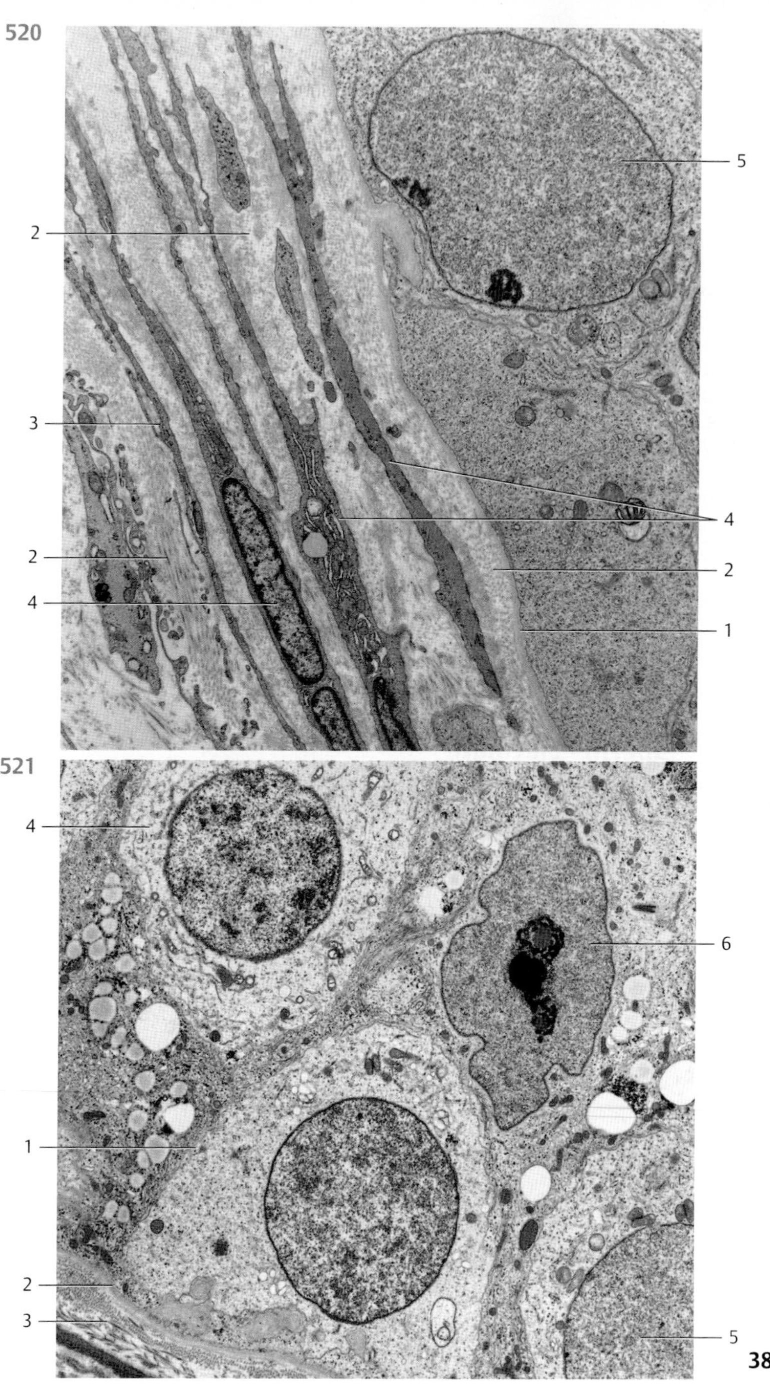

Male Sexual Organs

522 Leydig Cells

The *interstitial* Leydig cells occur in the loose intertubular (interstitial) connective tissue of the testis (see Fig. 515) and occasionally also inside the tunica albuginea testis and in the spermatic cord. With a diameter of 15–20 µm, Leydig cells are conspicuous due to their size. They are found as single cells or as clusters. Larger groups of Leydig cells give the appearance of an epithelial complex. Leydig cells have round nuclei ① and a polygonal cell body. Their cytoplasm is rich in smooth endoplasmic reticulum membranes ②, which are seen as vesicles and tubules. There are also tubular type mitochondria ③ and numerous lysosomes, often also lipofuscin granules. Beginning at puberty, many Leydig cells display rod-shaped or wedge-shaped rectangular or diamond-shaped protein crystals in different numbers and sizes. These protein crystals are named *Reinke crystals* ④. Electron microscopy reveals a grid-like organization of proteins for the Reinke crystals (see inset; cf. Fig. 69).

Leydig cells closely adhere to the winding capillaries. Copious fiber meshworks and nerve fibers are found between them. The Leydig cells synthesize mostly male hormones; the most important one is *testosterone*.

(Franz von Leydig, anatomist, 1821–1910; Friedrich B. Reinke, anatomist, 1862–1919).

1 Cell nucleus
2 Smooth endoplasmic reticulum
3 Mitochondria
4 Reinke crystals
Electron microscopy; magnifications: × 13 000; inset: × 31 500

523 Sperm—Ejaculate

Sperm has a corpuscular and a liquid component. The corpuscular components are spermatozoa, immature germ cells, sloughed-off epithelial cells from the seminiferous tubules, *spermatophages, cytoplasmic droplets* and sporadically leukocytes. Cells of the testes, epididymis and the accessory glands secrete the liquid components of the seminal plasma. The seminal plasma also contains proteolytic enzyme, which stem mostly from the prostate gland.

This figure shows the corpuscular components of sperm in the lumen of the ductulus efferentes from a healthy 27-year-old man.

Electron microscopy; magnification: × 1300

522

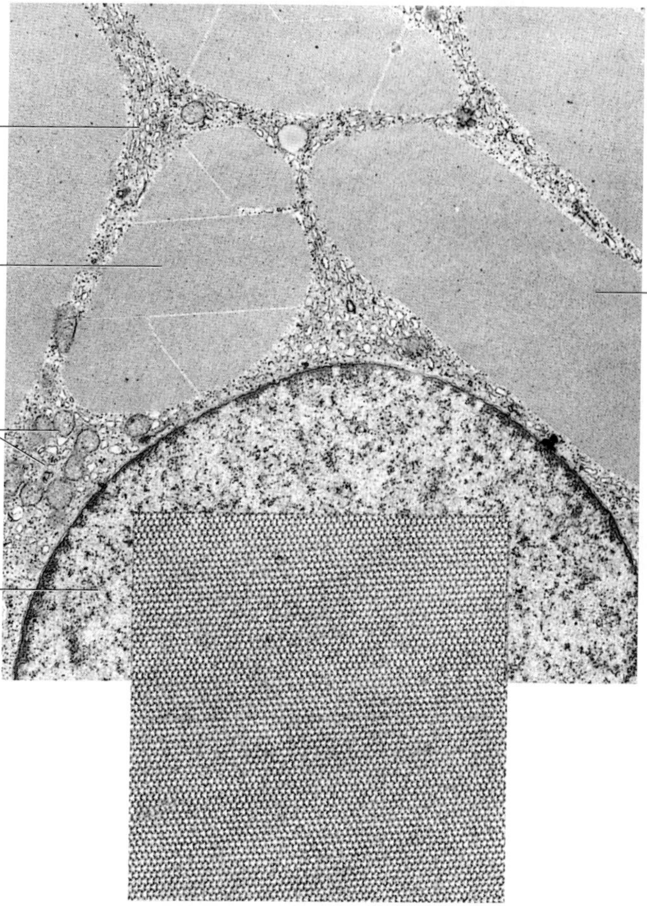

2

4

4

3

1

523

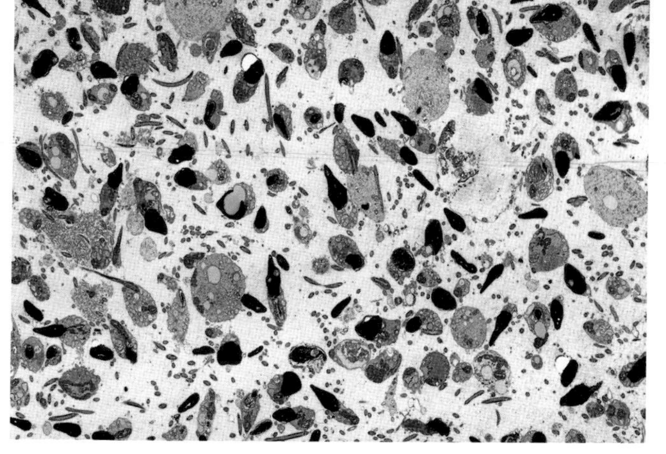

524 Spermatozoon

Spermatozoon from the ejaculate of a 48-year-old man.

I = Spermatozoon, head region
1 Nuclear vesicle
2 Acrosome
3 Nucleus
4 Post-acrosomal region
II = Spermatozoon, neck region
5 Cytoplasmic droplet
6 Connecting piece, striated column
III = Spermatozoon, middle piece
7 Mitochondrial sheath
8 Annulus
IV = Spermatozoon, principal piece
9 Fibrous sheath
10 Axonema

The principal piece continues in the spermatozoon tail.
The entire spermatozoon is enveloped by the plasmalemma. The acrosome is derived from the Golgi apparatus of the spermatid. It contains the acrosomal proteinase acrosin, which plays an important role in fertilization.
The axis of the middle piece forms the flagellum, which emerges from the distal centriole. The flagellum consists of nine peripheral double tubules and two central tubules (9 × 2 + 2 structure).

Electron microscopy; magnification: × 17 000

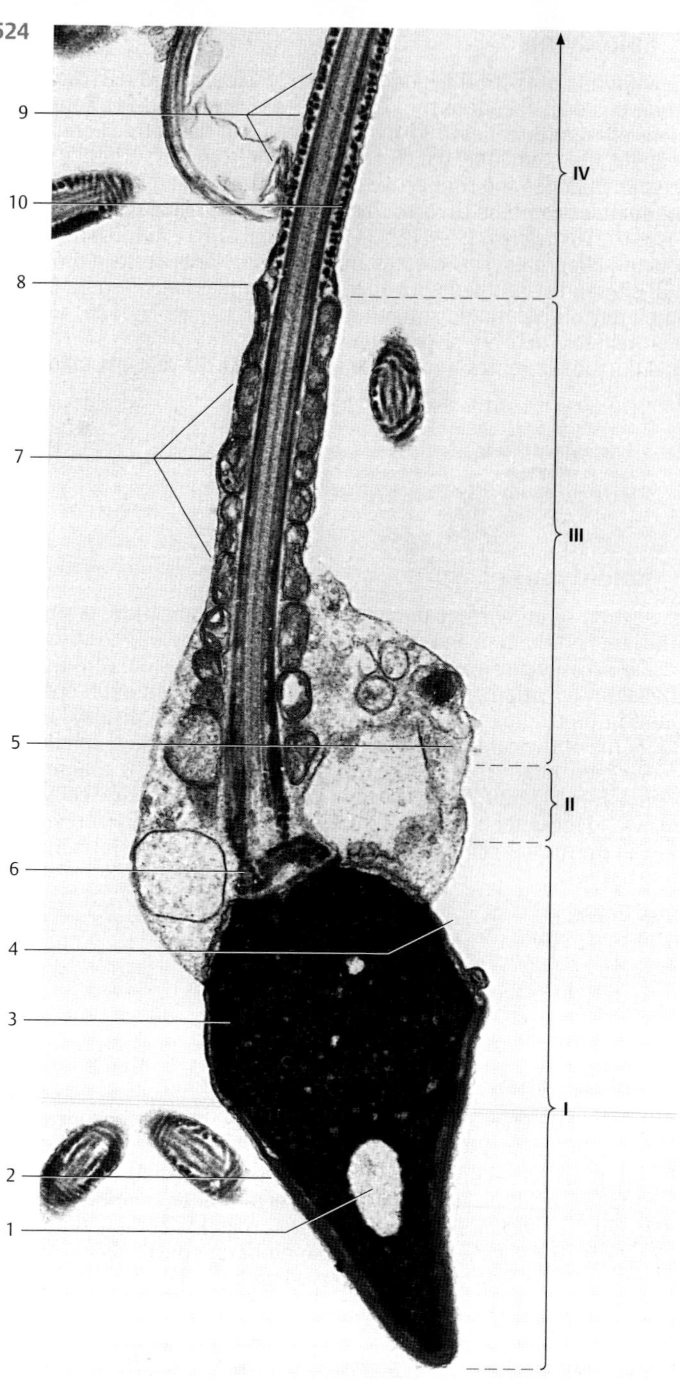
9
10
8
7
5
6
4
3
2
1
IV
III
II
I

525 Epididymis

The epididymis consists of head (*caput*), body (*corpus*) and tail (*cauda*). The seminiferous ducts begin in the rete testis (see Figs. 513, 514). Some 10–16 tortuous efferent ductules 1 form the next part of the path. These are ductules about 10–12 cm long, which are separated from each other by connective tissue. Ductules and connective tissue form the *epididymal head*. The efferent ductules combine to form the winding epididymal duct, which continues as the *vas deferens* (see Fig. 534). Epithelial cells of different height line the ductuli efferentes. This creates an undulating inner surface profile. The ductuli efferentes are filled with sperm and seminal fluid. Several layers of incompletely differentiated smooth muscle cells 3 (see Fig. 526) are under the epithelium. There are also lymph vessels 4.
Several ductuli efferentes from the epididymis of a 50-year-old man.

1 Efferent ductules of the testis
2 Interstitial connective tissue
3 Smooth muscle cells
4 Lymph vessels
Stain: alum hematoxylin-eosin; magnification: × 20

526 Epididymis

Cross-section of an *efferent ductule* at higher magnification. It shows the multilayered epithelium and its irregular height (cf. Fig. 525).
There are occasionally areas with only one layer of cuboidal cells inside the epithelial invaginations, while multilayered stratified columnar epithelium is found in protruding areas. The protruding epithelium displays irregular forms. Some of the columnar cells may have kinocilia, others microvilli (cf. Fig. 528). The supranuclear cytoplasm of the columnar cells contains many lysosomes (see Fig. 528). A thin layer of circular smooth muscle cells 2 is located next to the outer basal membrane. Adrenergic nerve fibers regulate the activity of the muscle cells. Lymph vessels 4 are found in the interstitial connective tissue 3.

1 Kinocilia
2 Smooth muscle cells
3 Interstitial connective tissue
4 Lymph vessels
Stain: alum hematoxylin-eosin; magnification: × 500

527 Epididymis

The tortuous epididymal duct is cut in all planes when cross-sectioned. Its total length in humans is 5–6 m.
The *epididymal duct* is lined by a high two-layered pseudostratified columnar epithelium (cf. Figs. 110, 529, 530). The high columnar epithelial cells are covered with *stereocilia*. The latter often stick together at their ends (cf. Figs, 86, 87, 529, 530). As is the case for other seminiferous ducts, a layer of smooth muscles 1 (cf. Figs. 529, 530) envelops the epididymal duct. The lumina contain spermatozoa 2 (cf. Fig. 523).

1 Smooth muscle cells
2 Interstitial connective tissue
Stain: hematoxylin-eosin; magnification: × 80

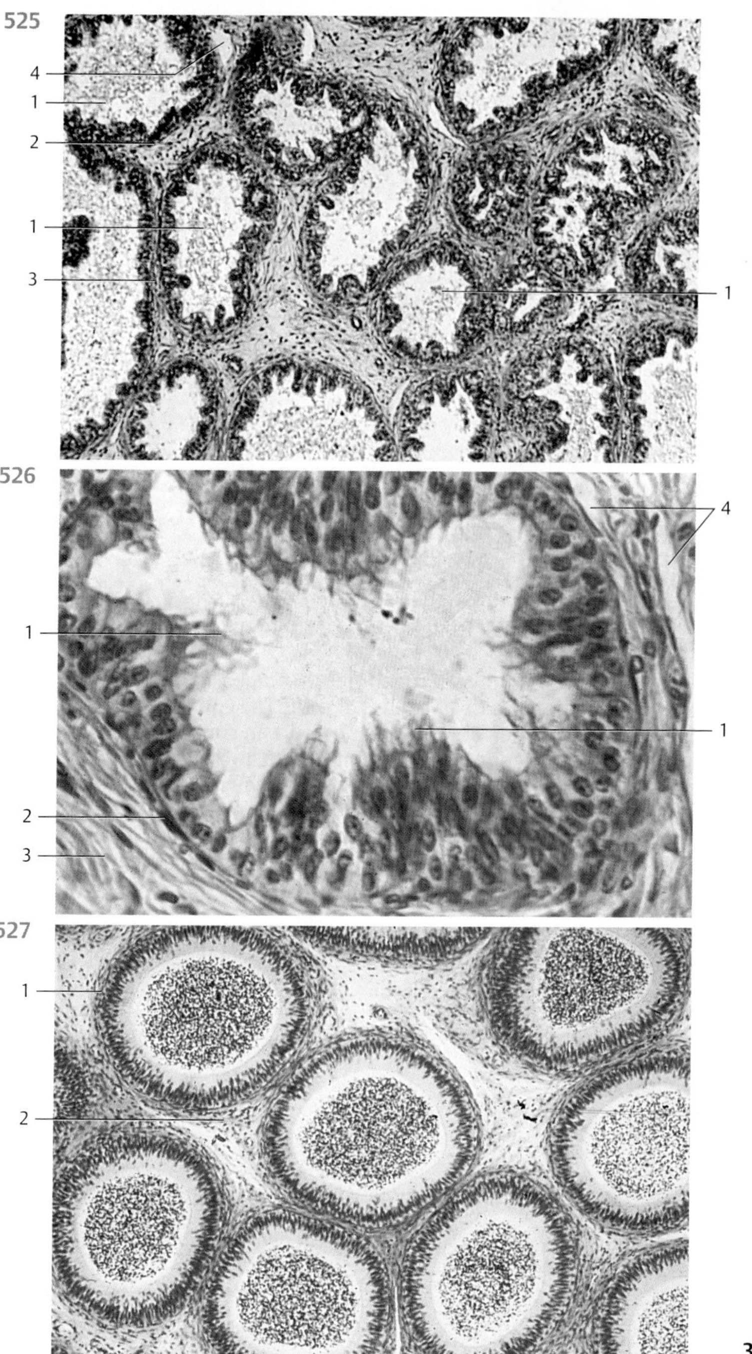

Male Sexual Organs

528 Epididymis

Vertical section through the wall of an *efferent ductule* with columnar epithelium and smooth muscle cells [1]. Darker cells with kinocilia [2] are found in the epithelium. The directional movement of the kinocilia causes semen and seminal fluid to stream through the ductulus. The microvilli at the surface of the lighter cell in the right part of the figure partake in absorption with resorption.

The ciliated cells contain lobed nuclei [3] and elaborate ergastoplasm in the perinuclear region, as well as many lysosomes [4] in the supranuclear cytoplasm. Elongated mitochondria and numerous small Golgi complexes occur in the apical cell region. Circular smooth muscle cells [1] surround the epithelium of the duct. They are shown in the lower part of the figure.

Compare this image with those in Figs. 525 and 526.

1 Smooth muscle cells
2 Kinocilia, cross-sectioned or cut in other planes
3 Lobed nuclei
4 Lysosomes
Electron microscopy; magnification: × 3000

529 Epididymis

This cross-section shows part of the *epididymal duct* from a 65-year-old man, with its high two-layered pseudostratified columnar epithelium (cf. Figs. 86, 87, 530).

The basal cells are round with round nuclei [1]. A basal membrane supports them. Basal cells replace dead columnar cells. The columnar surface cells [2] contain oval nuclei. Their supranuclear cytoplasm contains large Golgi complexes, many rough endoplasmic reticulum membranes, numerous mitochondria and other cell organelles, such as vacuoles, lysosomes and secretory granules. The columnar epithelial cells (height = 40–70 μm) in the epididymal duct show stereocilia [3]. These are not motile and their ends usually stick together (cf. Figs. 86, 87, 530). The lamina propria contains circular *myofibroblasts* [4].

1 Basal epithelial cells
2 Columnar epithelial cells
3 Stereocilia
4 Myofibroblasts in the lamina propria
Semi-thin section; stain: methylene blue-azure II; magnification: × 400

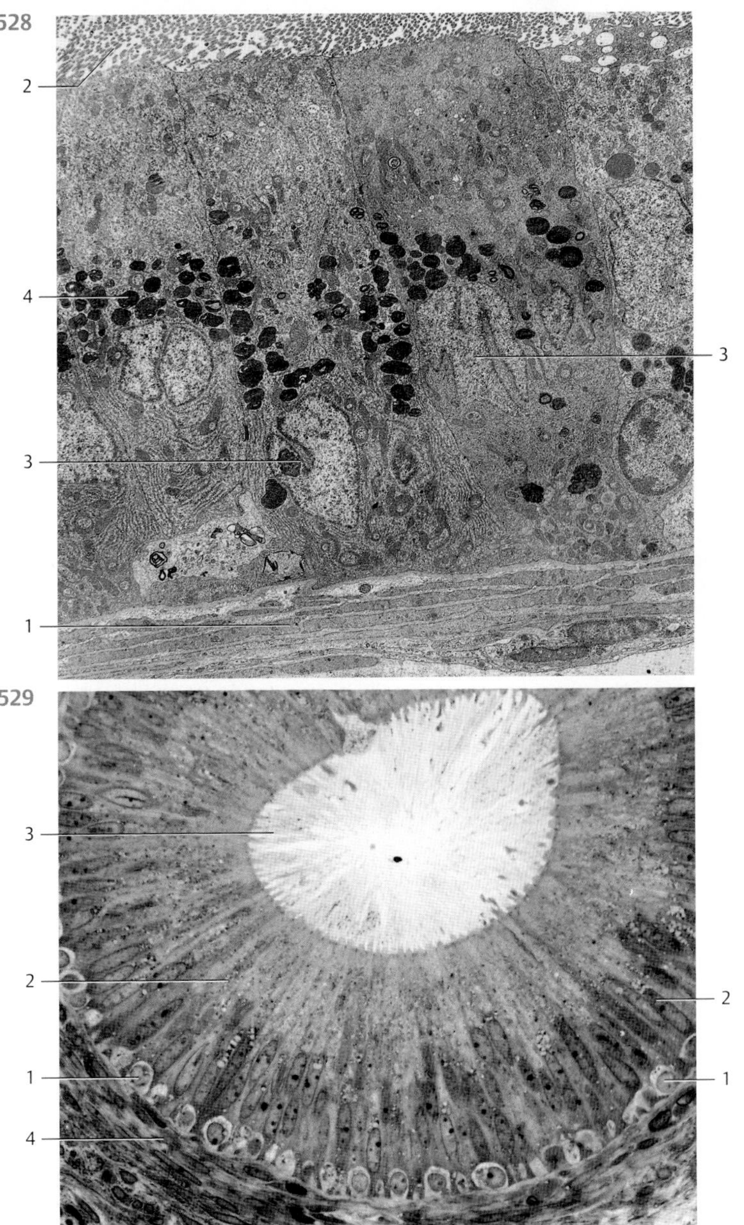

Male Sexual Organs

530 Epididymis

Cross-section of the *epididymal duct* (cf. Fig. 529). Note the two-layered pseudostratified columnar epithelium with stereocilia 1, which often stick to each other (cf. Figs. 86, 87). The basal membrane (cf. Fig. 529) supports the round basal cells. The lamina propria 2, which consists of circular smooth muscle cells, myofibroblasts, and fibrocytes, is a part of the epididymal duct as well. The lumen of the duct contains sperm cells 3. A sectioned vein 4 is present in the left part of the figure.

1 Stereocilia
2 Lamina propria with smooth muscle cells
3 Sperm cells
4 Vein
5 Interstitial connective tissue
Stain: alum hematoxylin-eosin; magnification: × 300

531 Ampulla of the Ductus Deferens

Immediately before entering the prostate gland, the ductus deferens widens and forms the *ampulla of the ductus deferens*. The muscular layer is thinner in this ampulla than in the vas deferens. The typical three-layer structure is replaced by a meshwork of muscles 1. The smooth muscles are predominantly circular. Copious connective tissue 2 exists between the smooth muscles. The structure of the mucosa is especially remarkable. It reminds of the seminal gland structure (cf. Figs. 536, 537). The mucous membrane forms many shallow, sometimes branched invaginations. They appear as isolated alveolar glands in cross-sections. Occasionally, they extend into the muscular layer. The epithelium is two-layered and shows secretory activity.
Human ampulla of the ductus deferens.

1 Tunica muscularis, meshwork of muscle cells
2 Loose connective tissue
3 Glands of the mucosa
Stain: azan; magnification: × 8

532 Ampulla of the Ductus Deferens

This scanning electron micrograph shows the ampulla from a rabbit vas deferens in more detail. It better reveals the *segmentation of its mucous membrane*. Several segments of variable size 2 surround the central lumen 1 of the vas deferens. Involutions and invaginations from the central mucosa form these segments. The segments communicate with the central lumen. Lumen and segments are lined by a two-layered pseudostratified epithelium with basal and surface cells. The height of the epithelium varies. The left edge of the micrograph shows the tunica muscularis 3.

1 Central lumen
2 Gland segments (chambers)
3 Tunica muscularis
Scanning electron microscopy; magnification: × 100

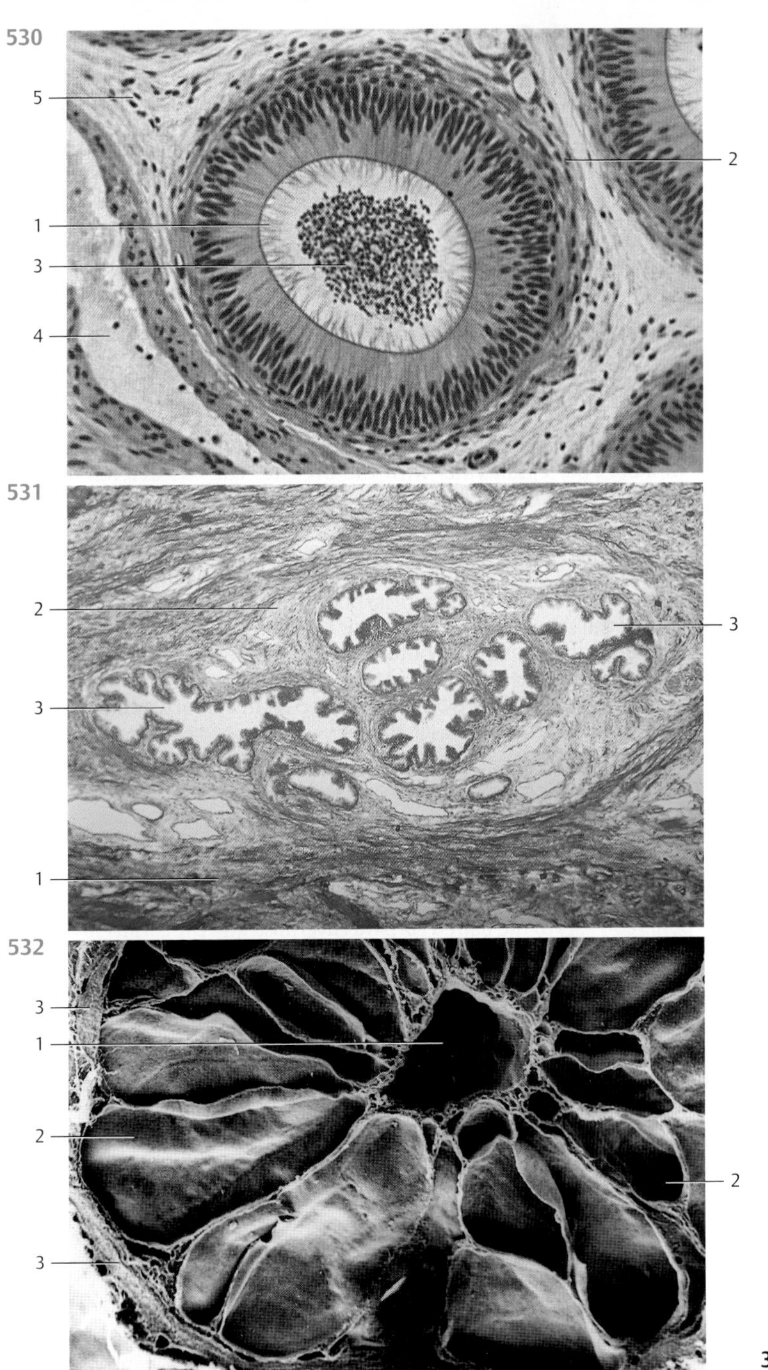
530
5
2
1
3
4
531
2
3
3
1
532
3
1
2
2
3

533 Spermatic Cord

Embedded in loose connective tissue, the *spermatic cord* (*funiculus spermaticus*) contains the strongly muscular ductus deferens 1, numerous veins of the *pampiniform plexus* 2, branches of the *testicular artery* 3, lymph vessels and nerves. The ductus deferens is sheathed by the *internal spermatic fascia* 5, followed by the fibers of the striated *cremaster muscle* 6 (left part of the micrograph). Branches of the ductus deferentis artery 7 are also visible.

1 Vas deferens
2 Veins of the pampiniform plexus
3 Testicular artery
4 Lymph vessels
5 Internal spermatic fascia
6 Cremaster muscle
7 Branches of the artery of the ductus deferentis

Stain: alum hematoxylin-eosin; magnification: × 4

534 Ductus Deferens

The *ductus deferens* is about 3 mm wide. It arises from the epididymal ductus and connects the epididymis with the urethra. The vas deferens is about 35–40 cm long and features strong muscles. It is lined by a mucosa and surrounded by the connective tissue of the tunica adventitia. Submucosal tissue is not found. The folds of the mucosa are covered by a two-layered pseudostratified columnar epithelium with short *stereocilia*. The mucosal connective tissue (*lamina propria mucosae*) is poorly developed. The three-layered structure of the strong *tunica muscularis* can be recognized in this cross-section. There are the inner and outer longitudinal muscle layers 1 3 and a middle circular muscle layer 2. The tunica adventitia contains many muscular vessels. These vessels are branches of the testicular artery and the artery of the ductus deferens 4.

1 Inner longitudinal muscle layer
2 Middle circular muscle layer
3 Outer longitudinal muscle layer
4 Arteries

Stain: azan; magnification: × 20

535 Penis

The penis consists of the paired *corpora cavernosa* and the *corpus spongiosum* of the *urethra-seminal duct*. It terminates with the *glans penis*. The corpora cavernosa of the penis are covered by the *tunica albuginea* 5, which is a tough sheath of connective tissue. The penile pectiniform septum 4 is located between the corpora spongiosa. The urethral corpus spongiosum is encased by a thin *tunica albuginea* 10. The *penile fascia* envelops *corpus cavernosa* and *corpus spongiosum*.
Cross-section of the anterior third of the penis.

1 Penile corpora cavernosa
2 Urethral corpus spongiosum
3 Urethra
4 Pectiniform septum
5 Penile tunica albuginea and fascia
6 Outer membrane
7 Penile dorsal vein (here paired)
8 Penile dorsal artery
9 Arteria profunda penis
10 Thin tunica albuginea of the urethral corpus spongiosum

Stain: hematoxylin-eosin; × 4

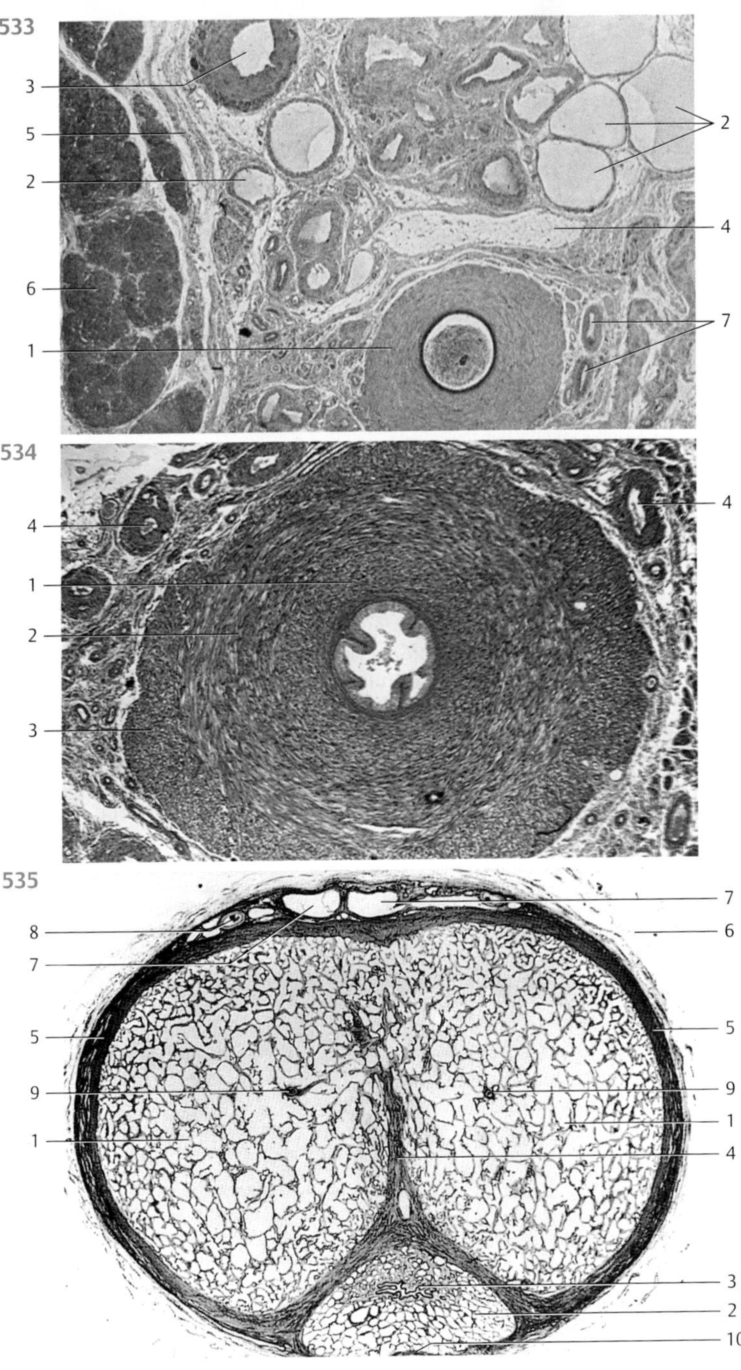
533
3
5
2
6
1
2
4
7
534
4
1
2
3
4
535
8
7
5
9
1
7
6
5
9
1
4
3
2
10

536 Seminal Gland—Seminal Vesicles

The seminal gland is often erroneously called *seminal vesicle*. It consists of a coiled, unbranched tubule, 15–20 cm long. Usually, it is cut several times in cross-sections. The wall of the duct is built of strong smooth muscle cells [1], which form both right-handed or left-handed helices. A connective tissue capsule encases the duct. The mucosa consists of the elastic fibers of the lamina propria, which forms high, narrow folds [2] with complex structures. There are primary, secondary and tertiary folds. Tubuloalveolar glands are located between the folds. Both the folds and the invaginations of the glands are lined by a single- or two-layered columnar epithelium. Note the bizarre folds (cf. Fig. 537). The wide lumen of this duct contains irregularly condensed secretory products, pigment inclusions and sloughed off epithelial cells [3].

1 Tunica muscularis
2 Surface folds (plicae)
3 Secretory products in the lumen
Stain: alum hematoxylin-eosin; magnification: × 5

537 Seminal Gland—Seminal Vesicles

This section shows the seminal gland with its typical relief of mucous membrane plicae and the complex system of *gland segments* [1]. They are separated by thin septa. Mucosal folds (mucosa plicae) often fold over the surface opening of the ducts. The cuboidal epithelium is single-layered and, at the ends of the folds, two-layered or multilayered. The strong *muscular tunica* [3] is shown at the left edge of the micrograph (cf. Fig. 536). Its smooth muscle cells are arranged in counter-directional helices. The muscular wall is interspersed with strong collagen fibers (stained blue). The wall of the seminal gland is richly vascularized and innervated. Frequently, there are also sympathetic ganglia. The lumen of the gland contains secretory product.

1 Gland segment
2 Mucosal folds (mucosa plicae)
3 Tunica muscularis
Stain: azan; magnification: × 800

538 Prostate Gland

Transverse section of the human *prostate gland* and the *pars prostatica* of the urethra [1] in the area of the *seminal colliculus* [2]. Some 30–50 tubuloalveolar glands reside in the fibromuscular stroma (see Figs. 539–541).

1 Urethra
2 Seminal colliculus
3 Prostatic ducts
4 Prostatic ducts, tubuloalveolar glands
5 Inner zone
6 Periurethral sheath
Stain: azan; magnification: × 8

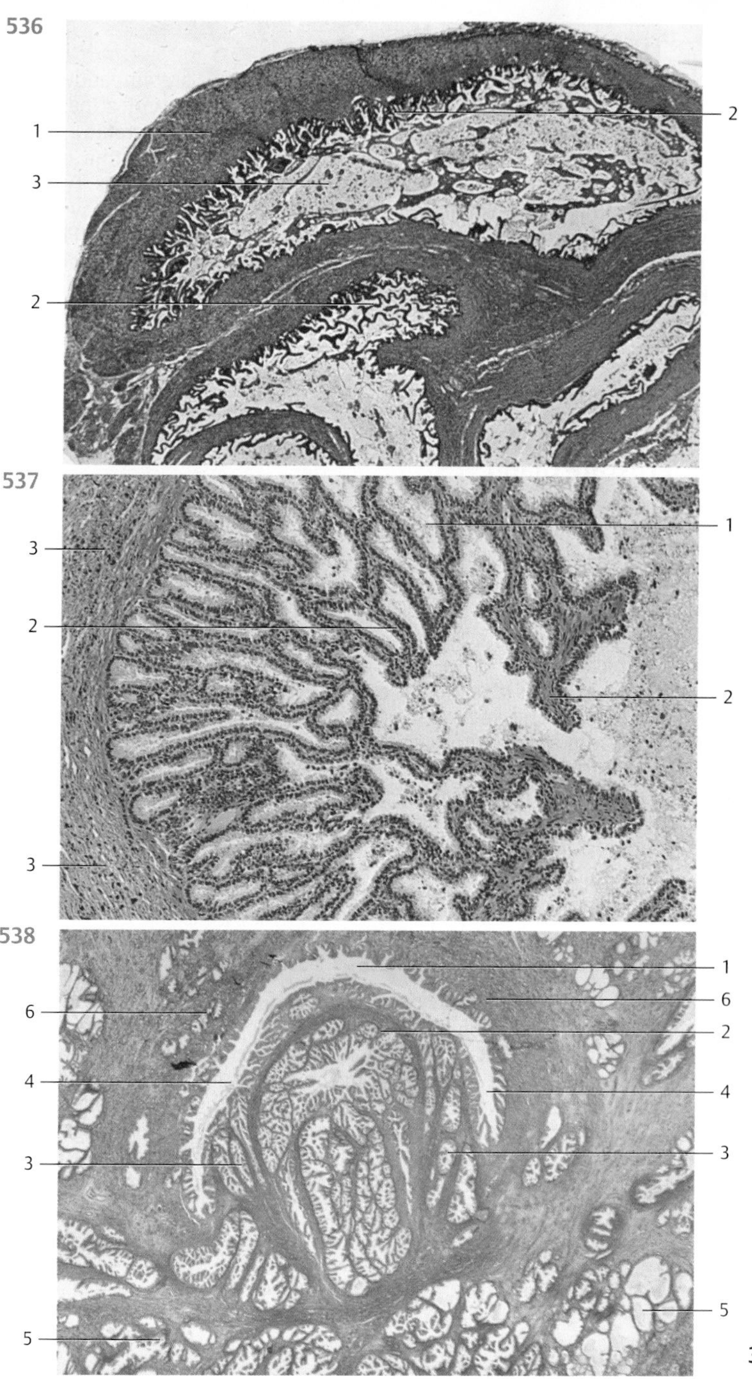

Male Sexual Organs

539 Prostate Gland

About 30–50 branched single tubuloalveolar glands [1] are embedded in fibrous collagenous connective tissue, which is interwoven with a meshwork of smooth muscle cells (stained bright red) [2] (*fibromuscular stroma*). Epithelial plicae [3] protrude into the lumen of the gland ducts. The lumina are lined by a cuboidal epithelium. The nuclei are found at different heights. The cytoplasmic secretory vesicles bind different amounts of stain and may remain very light and without visible structure in routine preparations (see Fig. 540). Each gland has 15–30 secretory ducts, which end around the seminal colliculus in the *prostatic sinus* of the urethra (see Fig. 538).

1 Tubuloalveolar single gland
2 Smooth muscle cells
3 Epithelial plicae
Stain: alum hematoxylin-eosin; magnification: × 80

540 Prostate Gland

This figure shows the epithelium of the prostate gland at higher magnification. The lining of the branched *tubuloalveolar glands* consists in part of single-layered, in part of two-layered or multilayered epithelium. The shapes of the epithelial cells range from flat to cuboidal to columnar. Dependent on the secretory activity and the presence of hormones, epithelial cells appear in different configurations. Age also influences the appearance of the epithelium. The apical regions of the gland cells contain secretory granules, which bind variable amounts of stain. The apical regions also contain lipid granules, glycogen granules and vacuoles. Occasionally, cytoplasmic protrusions are pinched off from the secretory cell and sequestered into the lumen. Undifferentiated, flattened basal cells are found between the secretory epithelium and the basal membrane. They are considered progenitor cells of the gland cells. The connective tissue fibers are stained red and the muscle tissue appears yellow (cf. Figs. 539, 541).

Stain: van Gieson iron hematoxylin-picrofuchsin; magnification: × 400

541 Prostate Gland

The capsule around the gland contains numerous veins. Its components include a muscular layer, which is connected to the interstitial tissue.
This figure shows a prostate gland area close to the capsule from an adult human. A secretory duct is depicted in the center. It shows a rounded corpuscle with concentric layers in the lumen. This is a *prostatic concretion* [1], which consists of condensed secretory products from the prostate gland. Occasionally, it is found in a calcified form in older men. The strong muscle fiber bundles [2] are stained yellow. Connective tissue fibers appear red (cf. Fig. 539).

1 Prostatic concretion
2 Smooth muscle cells
3 Collagen fibers
Stain: van Gieson iron hematoxylin-picrofuchsin; magnification: × 200

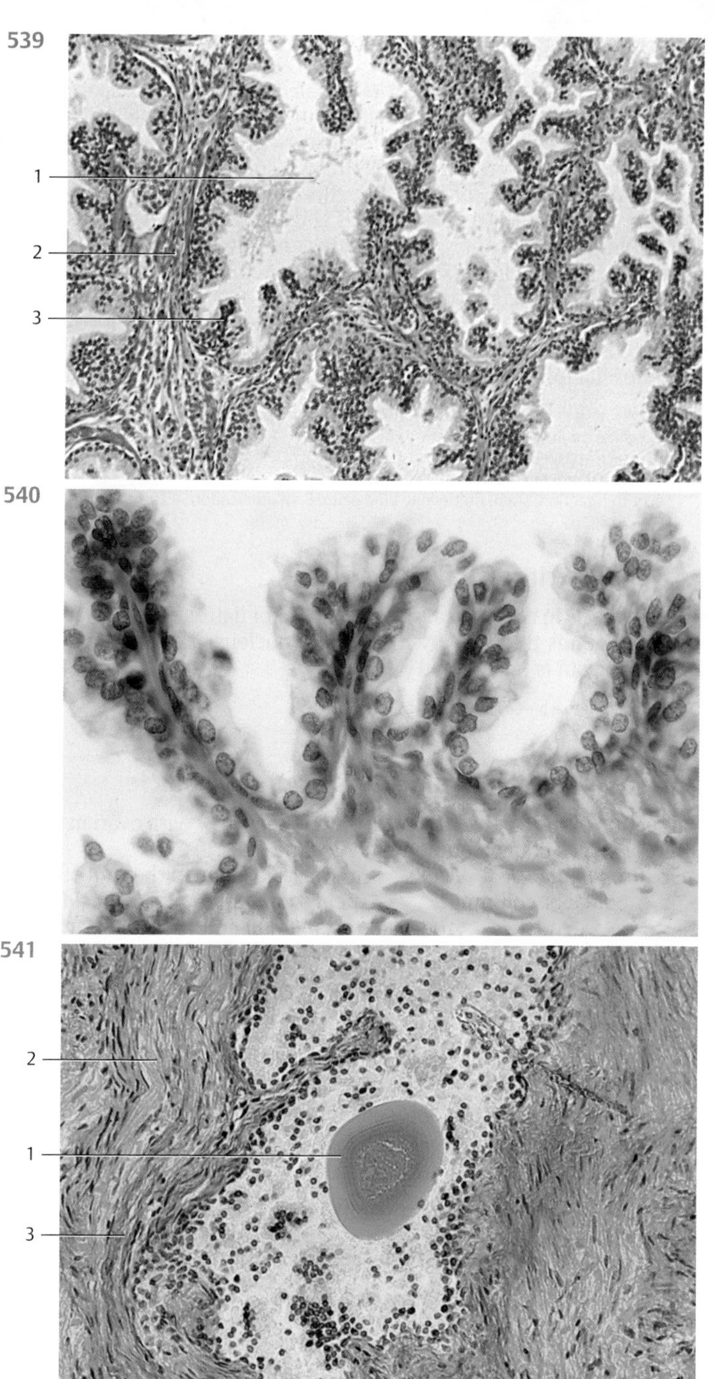
539
1
2
3
540
541
2
1
3

542 Ovary—Primordial Follicle

The ovary consists of an *outer cortex* 1 and an *inner medulla* (*zona vasculosa*) 2. The medulla contains connective tissue, muscle cells, elastic and reticular fibers and vessels. Follicles are not present.
This figure shows the cortex of a feline ovary. It consists of the *surface epithelium* (also called *germinal epithelium*) 3, the tunica *albuginea* 4 and the *cortical stroma* 1. The surface epithelium is single-layered, and its cells are cuboidal or columnar. At the *mesovarium*, it becomes continuous with the squamous peritoneal epithelium. The layer of cells and fibers of the *tunica albuginea* 4 underneath the surface epithelium does not contain follicles. This layer is followed by the cortical stroma (*zona parenchymatosa*). It consists of connective tissue cells, myofibroblasts and interstitial gland cells and contains primordial follicles and primary follicles.

1 Cortical stroma with many primordial and primary follicles
2 Ovarian medulla (zona vasculosa)
3 Surface epithelium
4 Tunica albuginea
Semi-thin section; stain: methylene blue-azure II; magnification: × 200

543 Ovary—Primordial Follicle

Primordial follicle in the cortical stroma. A layer of flattened follicular epithelial cells surrounds the *oocyte* with its large nucleus and prominent nucleolus. The ooplasm is not stained (cf. Fig. 542).

Stain: hematoxylin-eosin; magnification: × 500

544 Ovary—Primary Follicle—Secondary Follicle

Partial section of the cortical stroma from a feline ovary with ovarian follicles in different stages of development and decline.
a) and b) *Primary follicle.* The cells of the single-layered epithelium of the follicle are cuboidal or columnar. A basement membrane (*zona pellucida*) is interleaved between the oocyte *plasma membrane* and the follicular epithelium. A basal membrane and a connective tissue sheath (*theca folliculi*) encase the primary follicle. The connective tissue of the theca folliculi is poorly developed at this developmental stage.
c) A multilayered epithelium is formed in the course of the *maturation of the follicle*:
Secondary follicle (*preantral follicle*). The surface epithelium (*follicular epithelium, stratum granulosum*) is also called granular epithelium. The zona pellucida is well defined as a homogeneous glycoprotein layer. The connective tissue sheath (theca folliculi) follows it. The sheath shows a concentric arrangement of cells.
d) *Atresia of a secondary follicle.* The follicle shows remnants of the follicular epithelium. The oocyte is completely resorbed. The folded reddish band is the now hyaline zona pellucida.

a) and b) stain: alum hematoxylin-eosin; c) and d) alum hematoxylin-chromotrope 2R (acid red 29); magnification (all): × 240

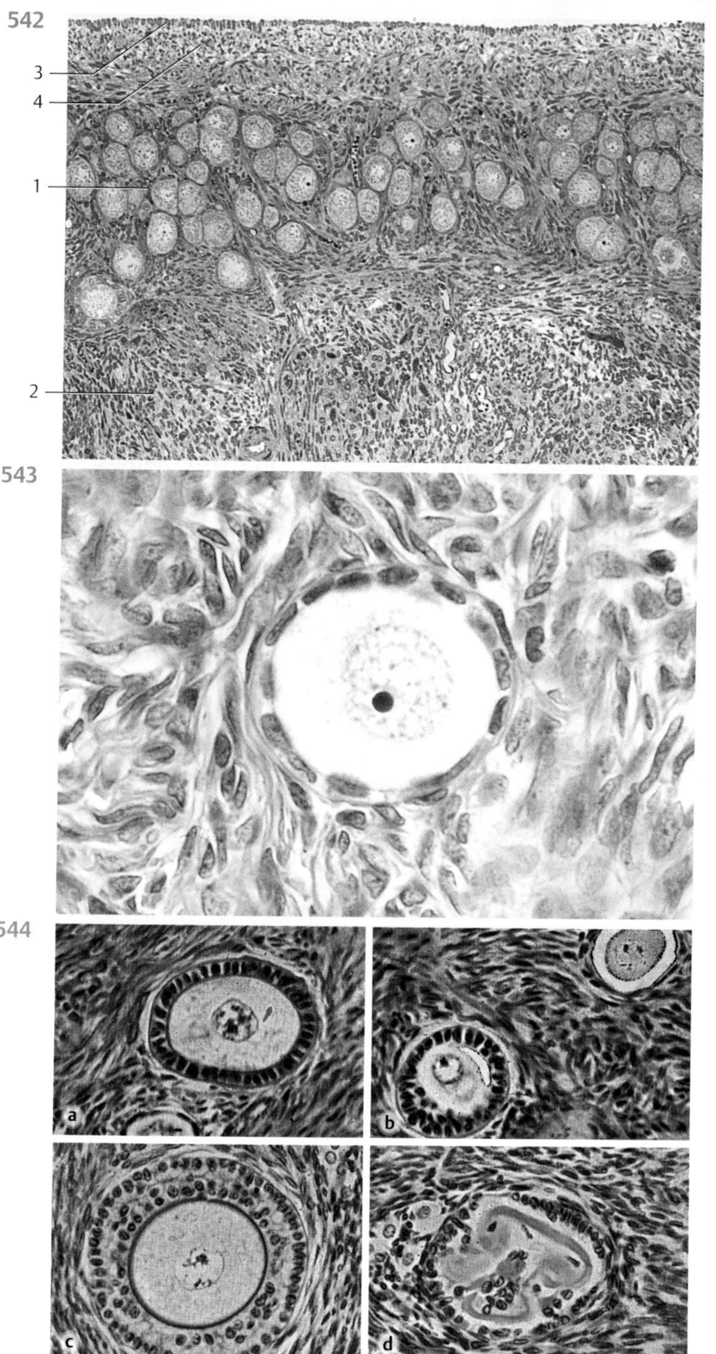
542
3
4
1
2
543
544
a
b
c
d

545 Ovary—Secondary Follicle or Preantral Follicle

Secondary follicle or *preantral follicle* from the ovary of a 30-year-old woman. The follicular epithelium 1 is now multilayered (*granulosa epithelium, stratum granulosum*). Secondary follicles can become up to 400 µm thick. Note the *zona pellucida* 2 between oocyte plasma membrane and granulosa epithelium as well as the basal membrane 3 between granulosa epithelium and the theca folliculi (the connective tissue sheath of the cortical stroma) (cf. Fig. 543, 544c, 546–549). The ovarian cytoplasm is sparsely granulated. The large nucleus contains a prominent nucleolus (cf. Fig. 543).

1 Follicular epithelium
2 Zona pellucida
3 Basal membrane
4 Theca folliculi
Stain: hematoxylin-eosin; magnification: × 300

546 Ovary—Secondary Follicle or Preantral Follicle

Large secondary follicle with beginning development of the *antrum*. The oocyte is situated in the *zona pellucida*. It shows a nucleus with a prominent nucleolus. The granulosa cells of the developing follicle are pushed apart by the secretory product of the *liquor folliculi*. This creates liquid-filled crevices, which finally combine to larger cisternae 1. The secondary follicle in this figure has already developed a larger cistern 1 with eosinophilic content. This content consists of filtered serum and the secretory products from granulosa cells. At this stage, the theca folliculi displays two layers, a cellular, vascularized inner layer (*theca folliculi interna*) 2 and a fiber-enriched outer layer (*theca folliculi externa*) 3.
Four primordial follicles in the cortical stroma are visible in the right half of the figure (cf. Figs. 542, 543).

1 Beginnings of a follicular antrum
2 Theca folliculi interna
3 Theca folliculi externa
4 Cortical stroma
5 Primordial follicle
Stain: alum hematoxylin-chromotrope 2R (acid red 29); magnification: × 120

547 Ovary—Secondary Follicle or Preantral Follicle

Large secondary follicle with advanced antrum development. Transition to a tertiary follicle (*mature follicle, antral follicle*) from a rabbit ovary.
Call-Exner corpuscles 1 have the form of vesicles. They are found between epithelial granulosa cells. Their consistency and staining attributes are similar to those of cells in the zona pellucida. The theca folliculi interna 2 and externa 3 can also be recognized (cf. Fig. 546).

1 Call-Exner corpuscles
2 Theca folliculi interna
3 Theca folliculi externa
Stain: hematoxylin-orange G-phosphomolybdic acid-aniline blue; magnification: × 100

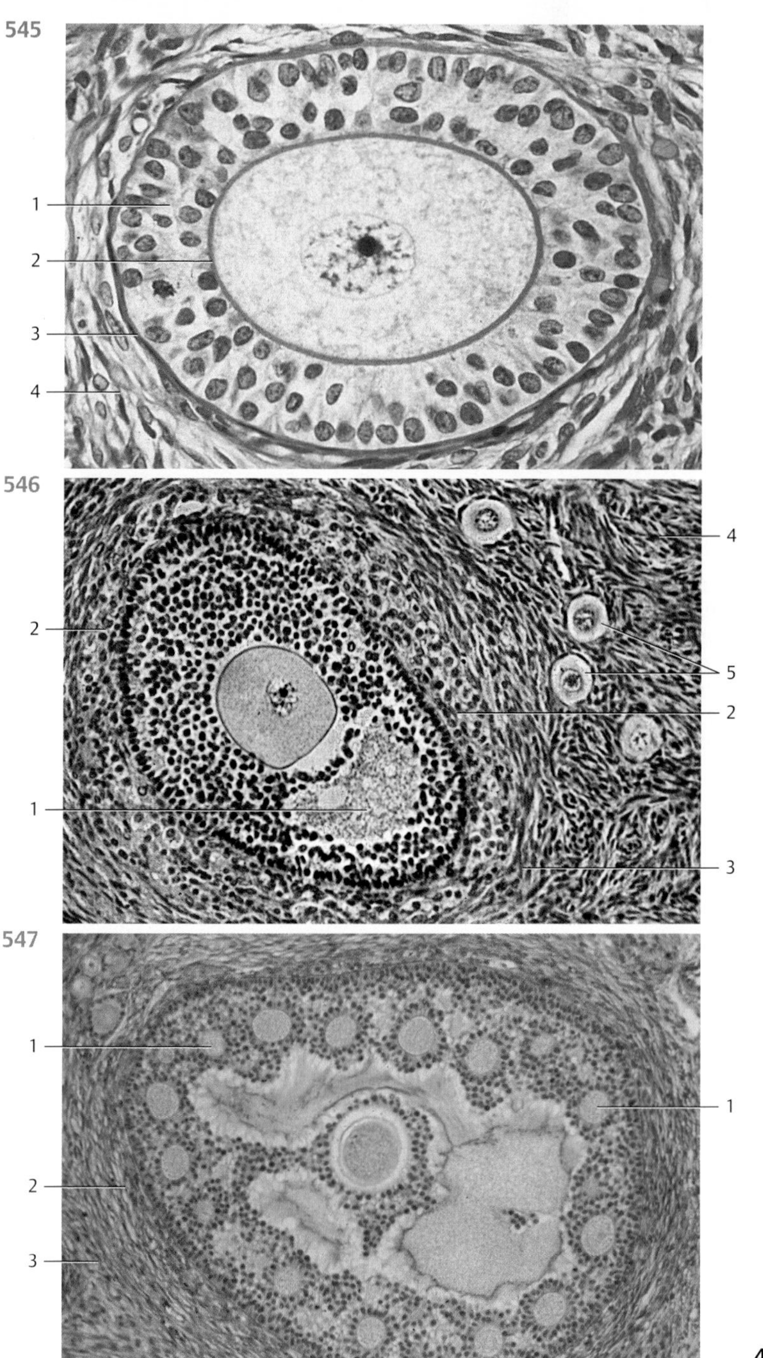
545
1
2
3
4
546
4
2
5
2
1
3
547
1
1
2
3

548 Ovary—Secondary Follicle or Preantral Follicle

Secondary follicle (*preantral follicle*) in the ovary of a rabbit. The cytoplasm of the ovum 1 contains small vacuoles and yolk particles. The nucleus is not shown in this section. The oocyte is enveloped by a thick *membrana* (*zona*) *pellucida* 2. Short cytoplasmic processes of the oocyte as well as processes of the follicular epithelium extend into the membrana pellucida (cf. Fig. 558). The following layer is the multilayered *granulosa cell epithelium* 3, which already has larger irregular cisternae that are filled with follicular liquid (*beginning antrum formation, transition to a tertiary follicle*). The secondary follicle is encased by a richly vascularized *theca folliculi* 4. Note the interstitial gland cells 5 with lipid content (see Fig. 551).

1 Oocyte
2 Membrana (zona) pellucida
3 Multilayered granulosa cell epithelium
4 Theca folliculi interna
5 Interstitial gland cells
Semi-thin section; stain: methylene blue-azure II; magnification: × 200

549 Ovary—Tertiary Follicle or Antral Follicle

Ovarian follicles with a developed antrum are called *tertiary follicles* (*antral follicles* or *Graafian follicles*). The completely vessel-free, multilayered *granulosa cell epithelium* lines the *antrum folliculi* 1. It forms a dome-like protrusion in one spot called *cumulus oophorus* 2 that protrudes into the follicular cavity. The cumulus oophorus contains the oocyte. The oocyte is encased by the strong *zona pellucida*. The whole follicle is enveloped by stroma cells, which form the *theca folliculi* 3.

1 Antrum folliculi
2 Cumulus oophorus with oocyte
3 Theca folliculi
Stain: hematoxylin-eosin; magnification: × 220

550 Ovary—Graafian Follicle

Human follicles reach a diameter of 20–25 mm shortly before ovulation. The preovulatory follicles are called *Graafian follicles*. This section shows the *cumulus oophorus* 2 with the oocyte, the multilayered *granulosa epithelium* 3 and the *theca folliculi* 4 of a Graafian follicle. The granulosa epithelial cells in the immediate vicinity of the oocyte are arranged in radial order. This dense corona granulosa consists of the *corona radiata cells* 5. The next layer of cells contains the loosely arranged *cumulus cells*. The wide nonvascularized granulosa cell epithelium 3 lies underneath the cumulus oophorus. The following underlying layer is the *theca folliculi* 4, which runs parallel with the lower edge of the figure. The multilayered follicular epithelium appears granulated because of the dense row of cell nuclei, especially at lower magnification. This explains the name granulosa cells or granulosa epithelium. Human ovary.

1 Antrum folliculi
2 Cumulus oophorus
3 Granulosa epithelial cells
4 Theca folliculi
5 Radial corona cells
Stain: alum hematoxylin-eosin; magnification: × 25

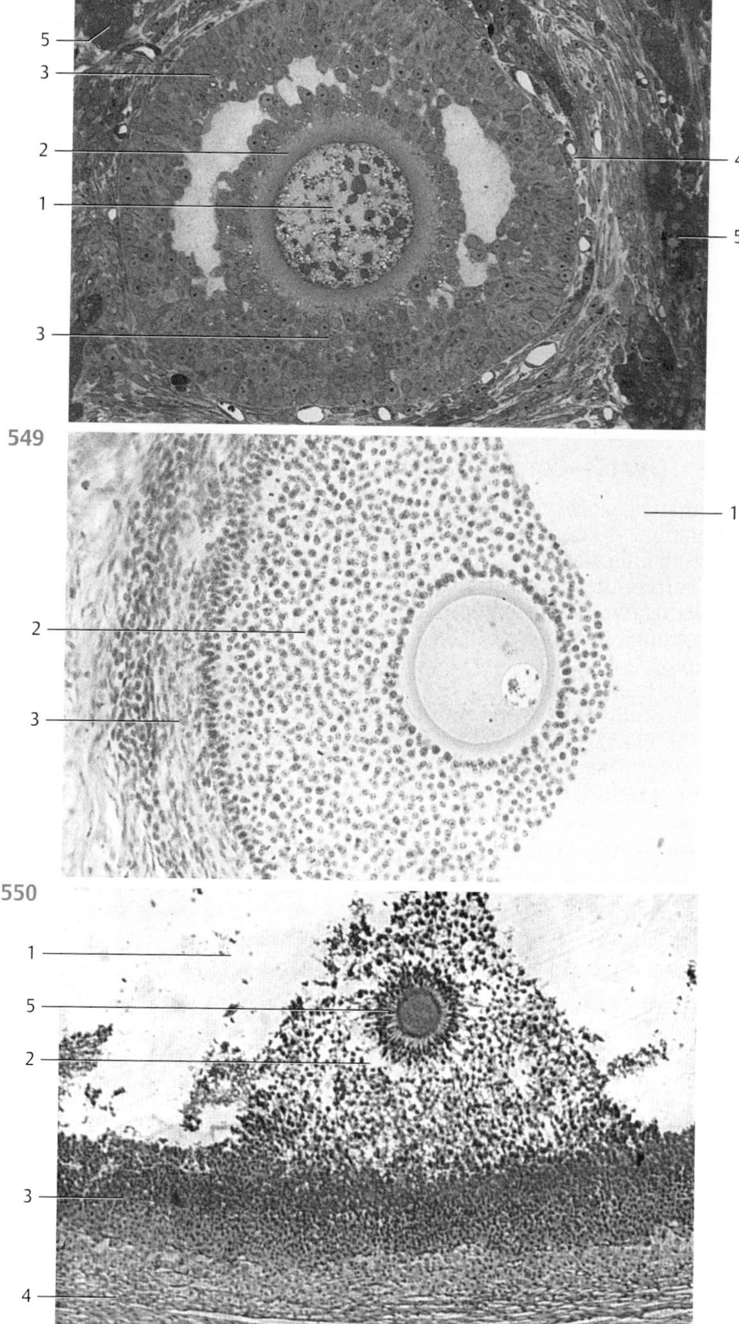
548
5
3
2
1
3
4
5
549
1
2
3
550
1
5
2
3
4

551 Ovary—Interstitial Cells

Partial section of the ovarian cortex from a rabbit. It shows the interstitial cells, which are derived from the theca folliculi interna. All interstitial cells form the *interstitial endocrine gland* of the ovary or *theca organ*. They are epithelioid cells, which contain lipid droplets as stored starting material for the biosynthesis of androgens. These cells have an elaborate honeycomb structure, which is similar to that of theca lutein cells. The highly vascularized spinocellular connective tissue with its delicate fibers is located between the interstitial cell complexes (cf. Fig. 180). Interstitial and theca cells biosynthesize androgens, which are taken up by the granulosa cells. Theca cells contain an aromatase, which turns androgens into estrogens. Outside pregnancy, the interstitial cells in humans are less active than the interstitial cells of the rabbit ovary. The interstitial glands of the human ovary look more like fibroblasts.

Semi-thin section; stain: methylene blue-azure II; magnification: × 400

552 Ovary—Corpus Luteum

Dramatic changes ensue in the follicles after the oocyte is released during ovulation. A complicated restructuring process occurs in the remaining ovarian follicular sheath during the first 2–3 days. The sheath is turned into the corpus luteum, which is an endocrine gland. The zona granulosa is folded upward, and its cells become hypertrophied. They store lipids and develop into *granulosa lutein cells* 1 (cf. Figs. 553, 554). At this stage, the cells have all the morphological criteria of hormone producing cells. Capillaries and larger vessels from the theca layers grow into this transformed tissue and form a dense capillary network. A histological section shows an undulating band that is 15–20 cellular layers wide. The genesis of the corpus luteum is now complete. The upper part of the figure shows a follicular cavity 3 with remnants of a clotted fibrin body. New connective tissue from the theca folliculi is found immediate underneath it. The wide, undulating, already vascularized band of granulosa lutein cells is enveloped by the theca folliculi 2.

1 Granulosa lutein cells
2 Theca folliculi
3 Former follicle cavity

Stain: azan; magnification: × 10

553 Ovary—Corpus Luteum

Lipid droplets are present in the *granulosa lutein cells* 1 at the peak of corpus luteum development. At this stage, the outer cells of the theca interna grow in size and proliferate. They also store lipid droplets and turn into *theca lutein cells* 2. These cells will finally fill all spaces and crevices. This generates cords and islets in the granulosa lutein cell population. The large light cell clusters of the theca lutein cells can be clearly recognized. They are interspersed with vascularized connective tissue 3, which pervades the corpus luteum as well. Lutein is a yellow carotene pigment.

1 Granulosa lutein cells
2 Theca lutein cells
3 Connective tissue of the theca folliculi

Stain: azan; magnification: × 90

551

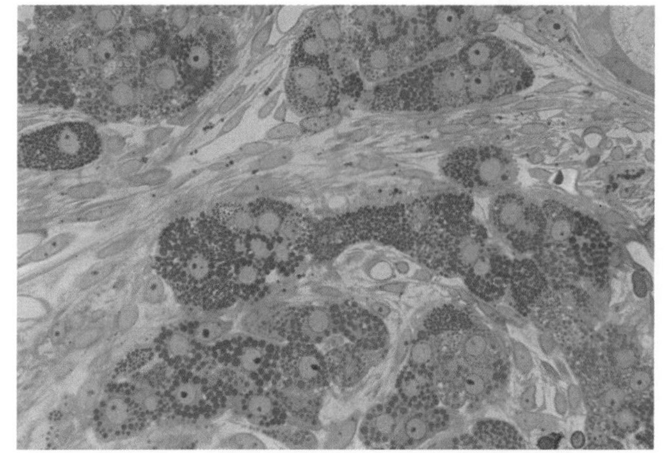

552

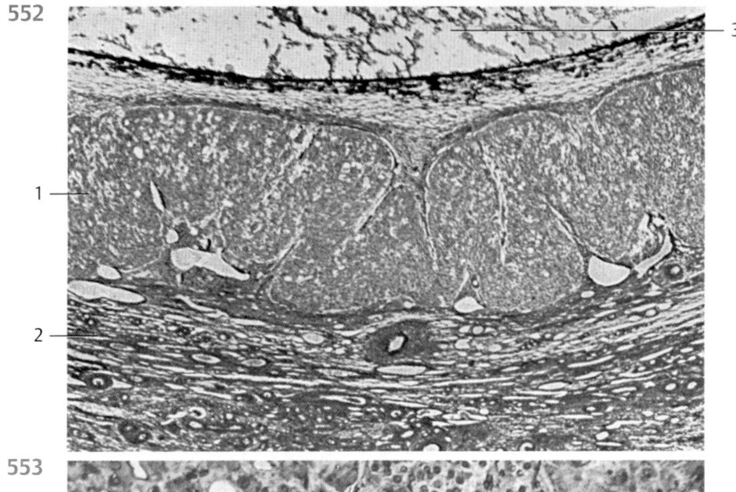

553

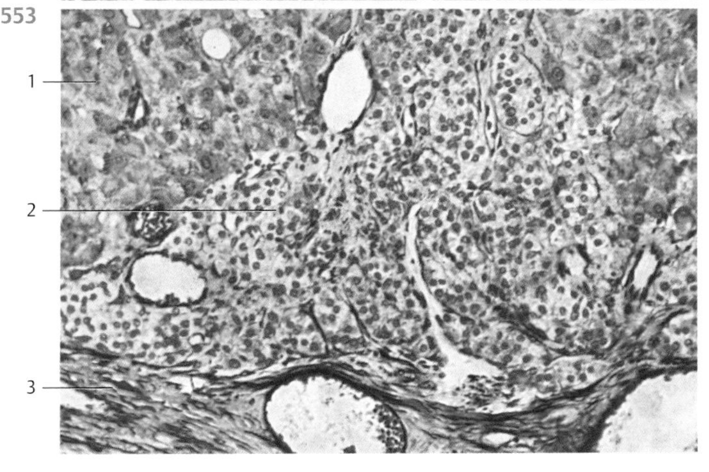

Female Sexual Organs

554 Ovary—Corpus Luteum

Segment of a *corpus luteum* at its developmental high point. Hormones of the anterior lobe of the pituitary gland regulate its secretory activities. The sizes of the polyhedral *granulosa cells* have increased two- or threefold. Their diameters may be up to 30 µm. After lipid droplets and the yellow lipochrome pigments have been formed, they are now called granulosa lutein cells (*corpus luteum*). In histological preparations, lipophilic solvents are used to remove water from the tissue. The same solvents also remove the lipid droplets of the cells. The removal of the lipid droplets gives the cell a perforated or honeycomb-like appearance. Numerous spindle-shaped or elongated endothelial cells occur between the granulosa lutein cells. In case the oocyte is not fertilized, the corpus luteum remains potent for 8–10 days (*luteal phase*). It has been transformed to a cyclical endocrine gland (*corpus luteum cyclicum sive menstruationis*). The granulosa lutein cells secrete mostly progesterone.

Stain: hematoxylin-eosin; magnification: × 120

555 Ovary—Corpus Luteum

When a fertilized egg implants itself in the endometrium, the corpus luteum develops into the *corpus luteum graviditatis*. However, if fertilization does not occur, the *corpus luteum menstruationis sive cyclicum* will quickly regress. During the phase of regression, fibrocytes and macrophages pervade the corpus luteum, and *apoptoses* occur. Later stages of regression involve shrinkage of the granulosa lutein cells and the increasing presence of lipoid bodies (*luteolysis*). Connective tissue increasingly invades the wall of the regressing corpus luteum from the outside. The theca lutein cells also show a high degree of lipoid content.

The adjacent figure shows a regressing corpus luteum. The granulosa lutein cells have become considerably smaller. Debris of fibrocytes and macrophages are now found in the extended intercellular spaces (cf. Fig. 554). In this phase, a hematoma may be caused by the flow of blood into the regressing corpus luteum.

Stain: hematoxylin-eosin; magnification: × 120

556 Ovary—Corpus Albicans

The granulosa lutein cells as well as the theca lutein cells of the *corpus luteum cyclicum* are degraded and the debris is cleared during regression (see Fig. 555). Invading connective tissue will take over. This creates a shiny white corpuscle (*corpus albicans sive fibrosum*) 1. The corpus albicans looks like a hefty, knotted connective tissue scar. Degradation is slow, and the corpus albicans may exist for several months. The tissue has a shiny surface like tendons. Hemosiderin inclusions are often found in the regressing corpus albicans.

1 Corpus albicans
2 Ovarian medulla
Stain: alum hematoxylin-eosin; magnification: × 14

554

555

556

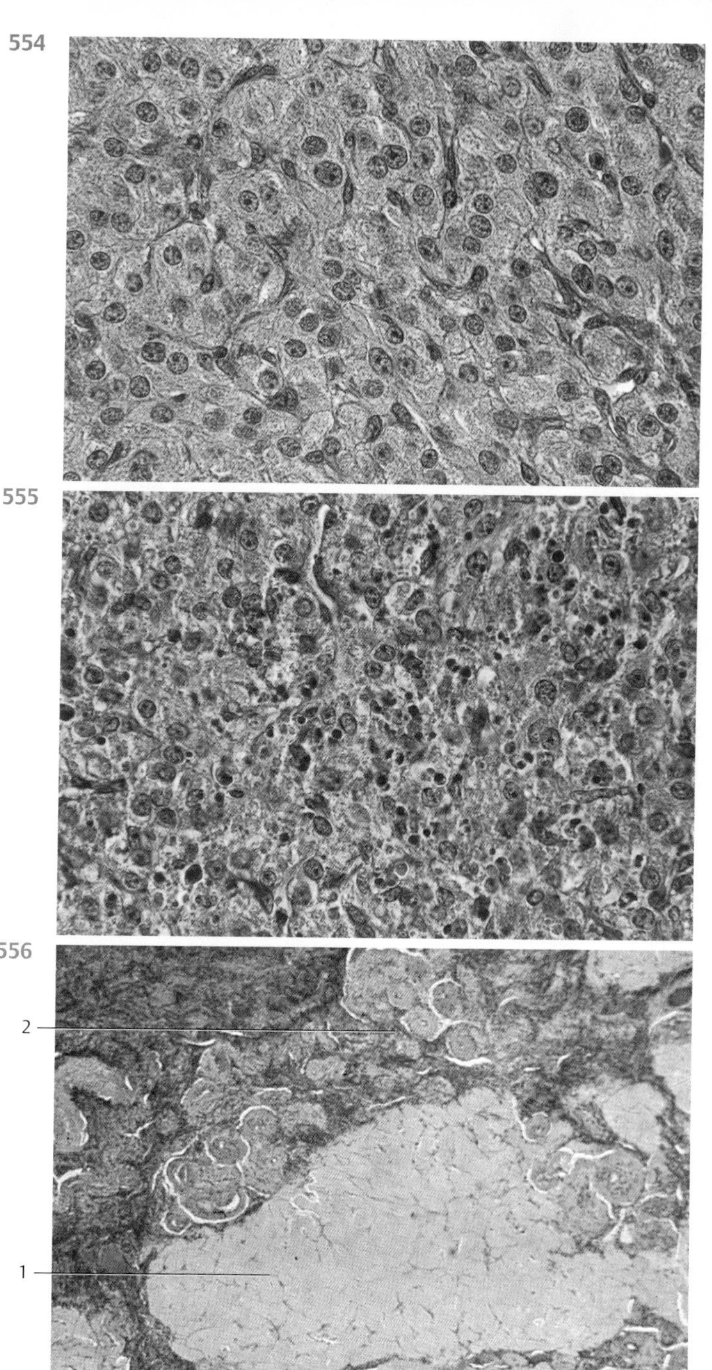

Female Sexual Organs

557 Oocyte

Human oocyte after assisted (in vitro) fertilization by intracytoplasmic sperm injection (ICSI), which negotiates the oocyte plasmalemma as the last barrier between sperm and oocyte cytoplasm. Using a light microscope, a single sperm cell is directly injected into the oocyte.
This electron micrograph shows the head region 1 of the spermatozoon in the center 1. Electron-dense granules are scattered through the cytoplasm of the oocyte. Small vesicles 2 occur mostly in the cell center. The cell nucleus is not part of this section. The oocyte is enveloped by the *zona pellucida* 3, which is formed by the glycoproteins of the extracellular matrix. In this case, the follicular epithelial cells of the *cumulus oophorus* have already been lost (cf. Fig. 558). The light space between zona pellucida and oocyte surface is the *perivitelline space* 4.
At the time of ovulation, the oocyte has a diameter of 120–130 μm. This makes it one of the largest cells in the human body.

1 Head region of the spermatozoon
2 Vesicle
3 Zona pellucida
4 Perivitelline space
Electron microscopy; magnification: × 1000

558 Oocyte

Section of a *preantral* follicle. The band in the lower part of the figure represents the outer region of an oocyte 1 (cf. Fig. 559). The cytoplasm in that region contains vesicles and vacuoles with content of variable density. Short, stump-like microvilli extend from the oocyte plasma membrane. They reach into the fine granular material of the *zona pellucida* 2. Toward the outer border (top of the micrograph), follow the *follicular epithelial cells* 3 and their cytoplasmic processes. The latter extend through the zona pellucida and form contacts with the oocyte plasmalemma (not seen in this figure). Follicular epithelial cells have large nuclei. Their cytoplasm contains elongated mitochondria, short fragments of rough endoplasmic reticulum membranes (rER) and vesicles.

1 Oocyte
2 Zona pellucida
3 Follicular epithelium
Electron microscopy; magnification: × 6400

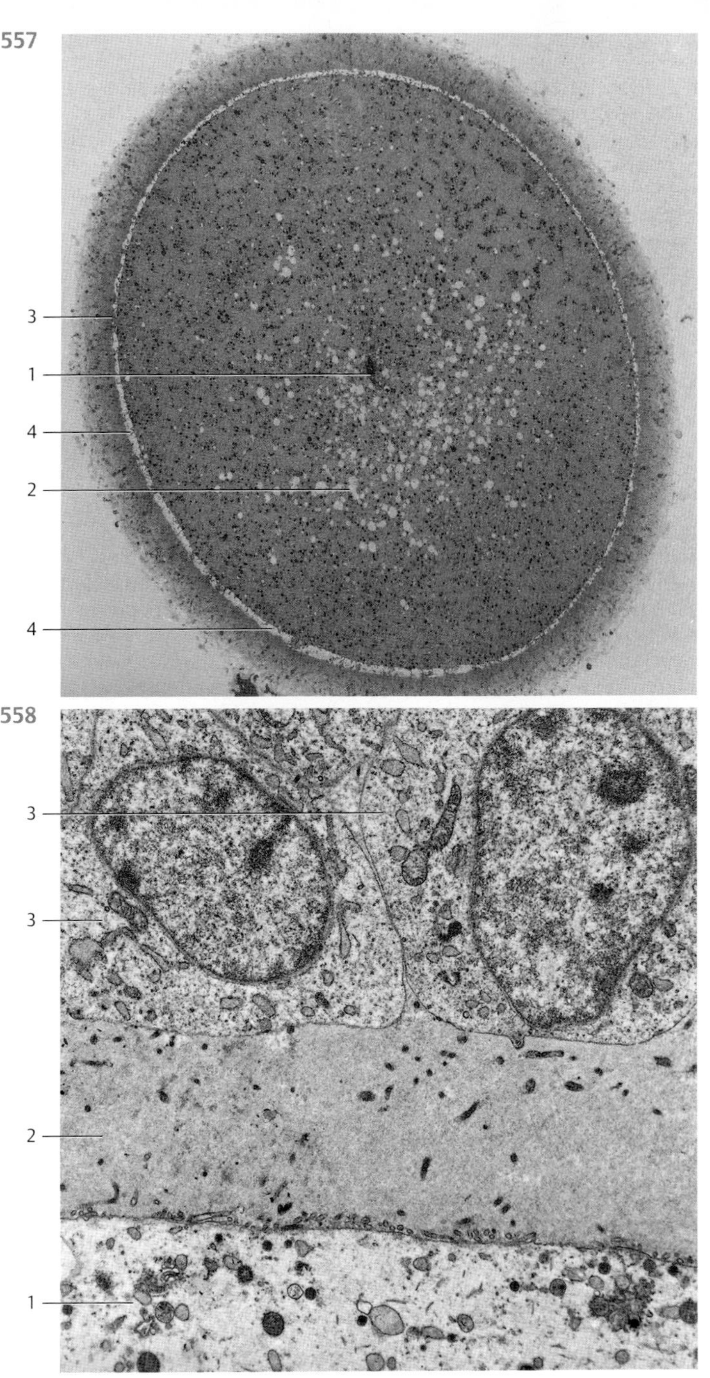
557
3
1
4
2
4
558
3
3
2
1

559 Oocyte

With a diameter of 120–130 μm, the human oocyte is considerably larger than the spermatozoon. The loosely structured round nucleus 1 of the oocyte has a diameter of about 25 μm. It was formerly called *blastosphere.* The cytoplasm appears fine granular in light microscopy. Electron microscopy reveals that these granules consist of osmiophilic granules, Golgi complexes, vacuoles, small mitochondria and short rough endoplasmic reticulum membranes (rER).
Ovulated oocyte, partial section.

1 Nucleus
2 Cytoplasm
Electron microscopy; magnification: × 8000

560 Oviduct—Ampulla Tubae Uterinae

The human oviduct (*tuba uterina, Fallopian tube*) is about 10–15 cm long. It consists of *tunica mucosa, tunica muscularis*, the vascularized *tela subserosa* and the *tunicaserosa*. All layers are shown in this section. The mucosa of the ampulla of the Fallopian tube rises to high longitudinal folds 1. The folds subdivide into elaborately branched *secondary* and *tertiary folds* . This considerably reduces the lumen of the oviduct. The tunica muscularis (*tuba uterinae musculature*) consists of three layers. These layers are helical and show very irregular configurations. The inner and outer layers are *longitudinal muscle bundles*, and the muscle bundles in the middle layer have a *circular* structure. The wide subserosal tissue layer contains numerous vessels 3 4. There are also cords of smooth muscle cells of variable density in the *subperitoneal muscle layer*, which connects with the *uterus*, the *mesosalpinx* 5 and the *mesovarium*. The muscles enable changes in the positioning of the oviduct. The single-layered peritoneal epithelium is very shiny and flat. The *tunica serosa* 6 covers the *subserosal tissue.*

1 Mucosa fold (plica)
2 Oviduct musculature
3 Artery
4 Vein
5 Mesosalpinx
6 Tunica serosa
Stain: iron hematoxylin-eosin; magnification: × 10

561 Oviduct—Isthmus Tubae Uterinae

The diameter of the oviduct decreases steadily toward the *opening of the uterine tube*. The width of the tunica muscularis 1 increases. The relatively wide mucosa plicae 2 with copious connective tissue rarely branch and completely disappear at the beginning of the *uterine part of the oviduct* (*pars intramuralis, inner uterine wall*) (cf. Fig. 562). The *tunica serosa* 3 is visible in the lower left corner of the figure. Compare this cross-section with the cross-section of the labyrinth-like ampulla of the uterine tube. Blood vessels 5 are found in the *subserosal tissue* 4.

1 Smooth musculature
2 Mucosa plicae
3 Tunica serosa
4 Subserosal tissue
5 Artery
Stain: alum hematoxylin-eosin; magnification: × 40

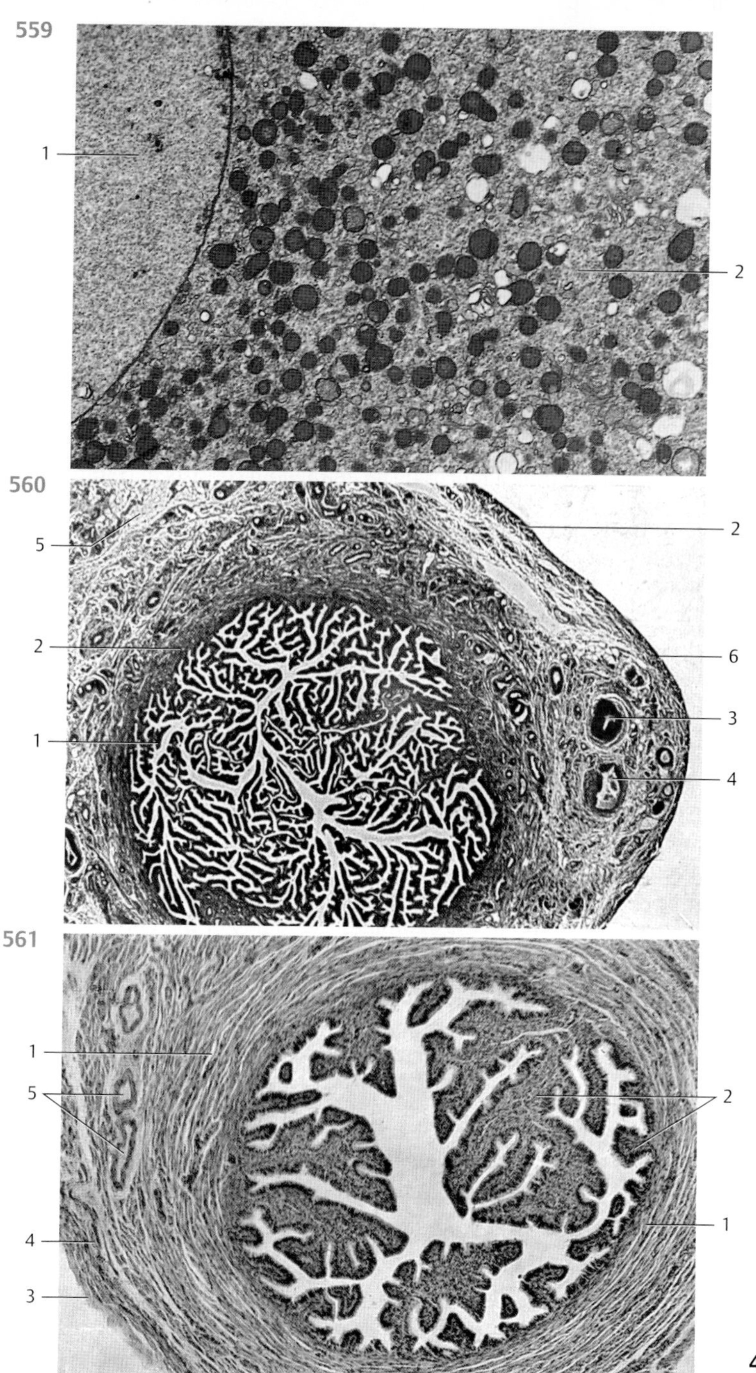

Female Sexual Organs

562 Oviduct—Uterine Part of the Oviduct

The *pars uterina tubae* (*pars intramuralis*) starts at the *isthmus of the uterine tube* and extends through the uterine wall. It ends at the uterine fundus (*cavum uteri*) with a very narrow clearance (*ostium uterinum*). A thick circular muscular layer 1 encases the narrow lumen of the duct (*sphincter mechanism*?). Note the complete lack of mucosa plicae. The outer musculature of the tube is already part of the uterine wall 2. Note the blood-filled vessels 3.

1 Muscular layers
2 Myometrium
3 Blood vessels
Stain: hematoxylin-eosin; magnification: × 25

563 Oviduct—Ampulla Tubae Uterinae

This semi-thin section of the mucosa plicae of the ampulla was stained with methylene blue-azure II. It shows the single-layered cuboidal to columnar epithelium of the tunica mucosa. The epithelium consists of columnar cells with *kinocilia* 1 (see Fig. 82–85) and *secretory cells* (nonciliated cells) 2. The secretory cells show a slender basal portion and an expanded apical portion. Secretory granules are predominantly found in the apical cytoplasmic protrusions. Numerous blood vessels 4 are present in the thin, loosely structured lamina propria 3 immediately underneath the epithelium.

1 Ciliated cells
2 Gland cells
3 Lamina propria mucosae
4 Blood vessels
Semi-thin section; stain: methylene blue-azure II; magnification: × 400

564 Oviduct—Isthmus Tubae Uterinae

Mucosa plicae from the *isthmus of the uterine tube* from a rabbit. The mucosa of this segment of the oviduct epithelium contains more secretory cells 1, which are only sporadically interspersed with ciliated cells 2. The secretory cells bulge in a dome-like fashion into the lumen of the duct (cf. Fig. 563). They are loaded with secretory granules in the supranuclear cell region. The secreted product provides nourishment for the fertilized egg on its path through the oviduct. The oviduct also contains a neutral or weakly acidic mucus, as well as different ions, sugars, amino acids and enzymes, along with globulins and albumin from circulating blood. There are strong cyclical fluctuations in the composition of the secretory products and components in the oviduct. Small, rod-like cells are found among the cells. These are probably exhausted secretory cells. The secretory cells contain dark, elongated nuclei in the basal part of the cell. Note the numerous capillaries 4 in the lamina propria mucosae 3.

1 Secretory cells
2 Ciliated cells
3 Lamina propria mucosae
4 Capillaries
Semi-thin section; stain: methylene blue-azure II; magnification: × 400

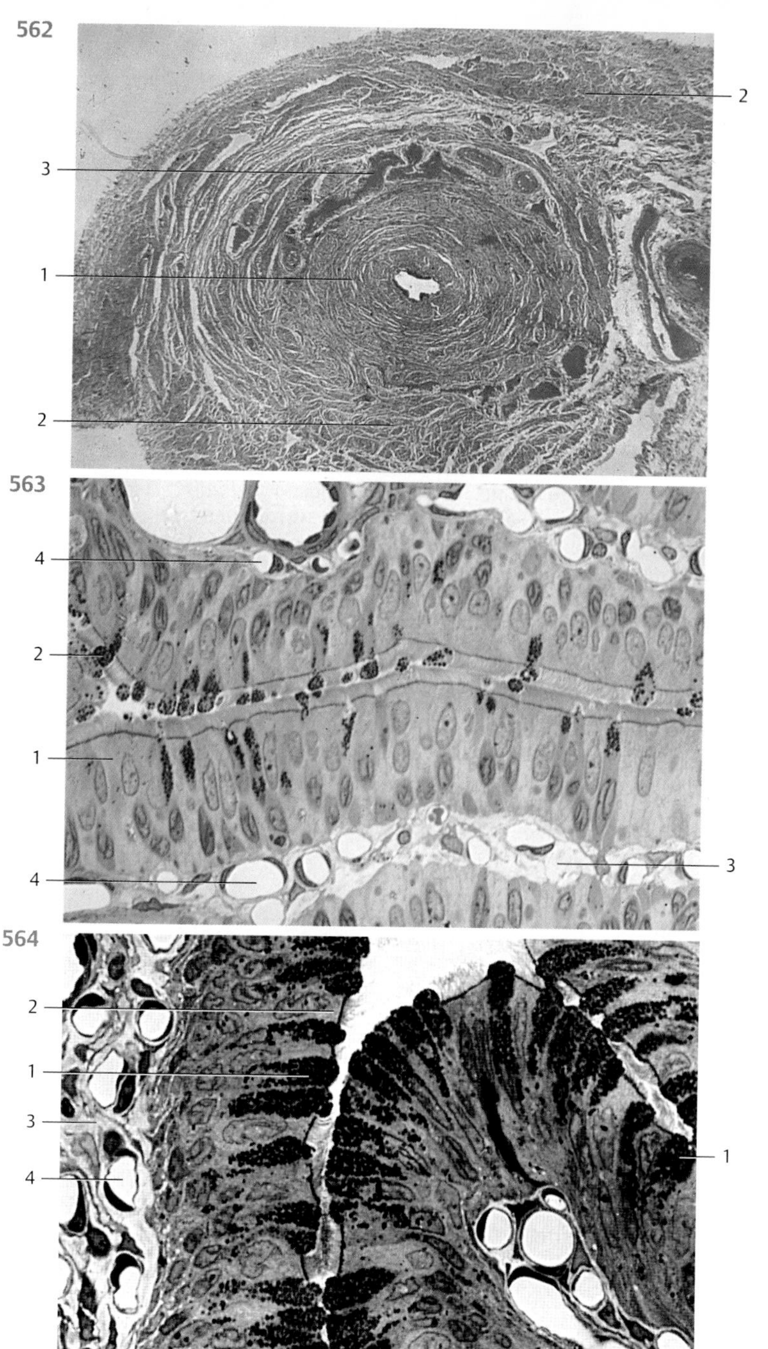
562
2
3
1
2
563
4
2
1
4
3
564
2
1
3
4
1

565 Oviduct—Ampulla Tubae Uterinae

The mucosa plicae of the ampulla are densely lined with *ciliated cells* and interspersed *secretory cells* 1 (see Fig. 563). The 7–15 μm long kinocilia are by far the tallest structures on the cell surface, far taller than the secretory cells. The figure clearly shows short, thick microvilli on the apical surfaces of secretory cells. Two cilia are distended at their ends like clubs. Compare with Figs. 82–85.
The ciliated cells generate a streaming motion of liquid toward the uterus, which supports the movement of the oocyte.

1 Gland cells
Scanning electron microscopy; magnification: × 4800

566 Uterus—Uterine Cervix

Central sagittal section through the *vagina* and *uterine cervix*. The uterine cervix or *collum uteri* is the narrow caudal third of the uterus. The uterine cervix has the shape of a cone. Its cusp is the *portio vaginalis cervicis*, which protrudes freely into the vagina 1. The cusp is surrounded by the fornices of the vagina 2. The center of the cusp displays a small indentation, which is the outer mouth of the uterus (*ostium externum uteri*) 3. It lies between the anterior 4 and posterior 5 labia of the vaginal mouth (*labium anterius et posterius*). The single-layered cuboidal epithelium of the cervical mucosa continues in the nonkeratinizing multilayered squamous epithelium of the *portio vaginalis*, which also covers the vagina 1 (see Fig. 567). The cervical canal is spindle-shaped and forms mucosa plicae (*plicae palmatae*) 6 (see Fig, 567). They remind of tubular glands. Submucosal tissue does not exist. The mucous membrane directly covers the musculature 7.

1 Vagina
2 Posterior fornix of the vagina
3 Outer vaginal mouth
4 Anterior labia of the vaginal mouth
5 Posterior labia of the vaginal mouth
6 Cervical canal with plicae palmatae
7 Smooth musculature of the uterine cervix
Stain: hematoxylin-eosin; magnification: × 12

567 Uterus—Uterine Cervix

The structures of the mucosa in the uterine cervix and the uterine corpus show considerable differences. The tunica mucosa of the uterine cervix is 2–5 mm thick. The plicae of the mucosa (plicae palmatae) 1 create a ragged surface relief (cf. Fig. 566). Numerous ciliated cells occur in the columnar epithelium, which continues in the irregularly branched glands. The glands secrete mucins. The lamina propria 2 of the cervical mucosa is richer in fibers and stronger than the tunica propria of the endometrium. It borders directly on the musculature.
This sagittal section of the cervical canal shows a magnified portion of Fig. 566.

1 Plicae palmatae
2 Lamina propria
Stain: hematoxylin-eosin; magnification: × 40

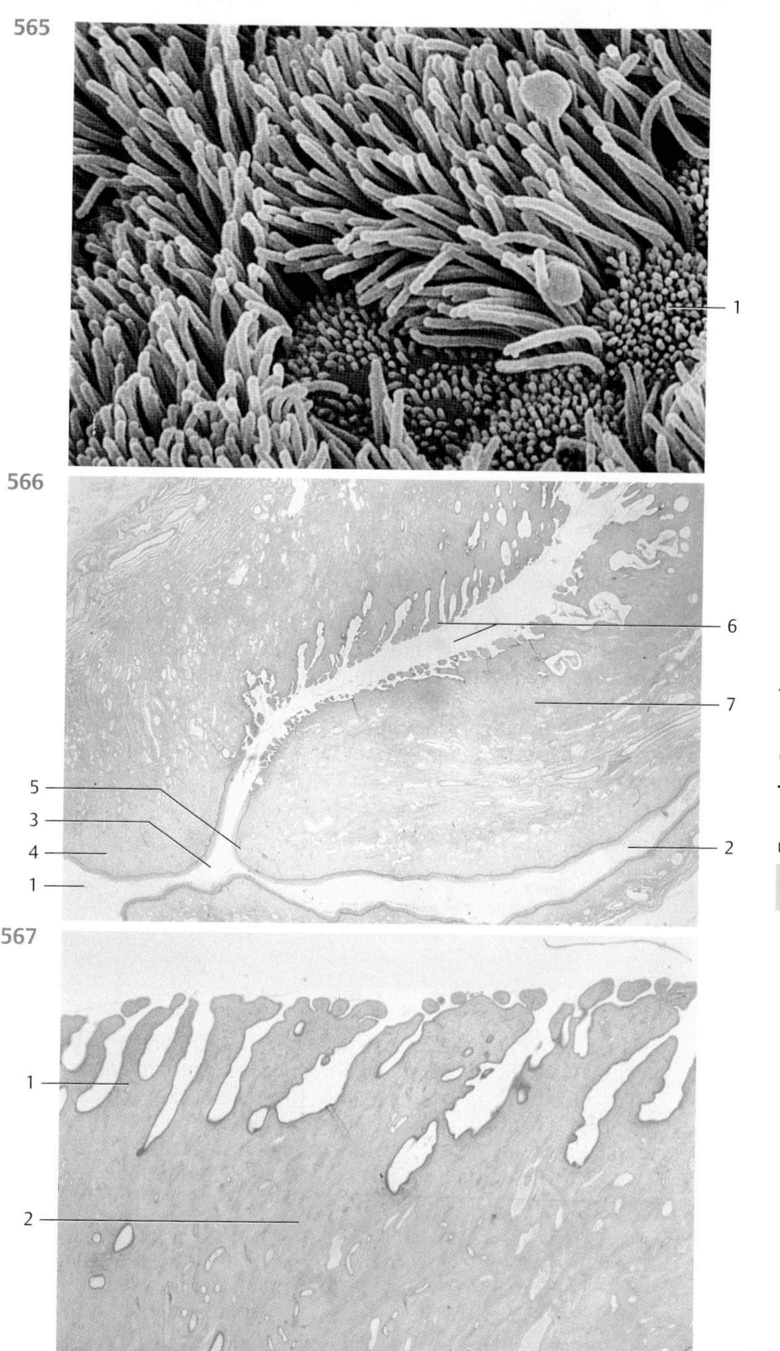

Female Sexual Organs

568 Uterus

The uterus is a pear-shaped hollow organ. It is about 7–9 cm long, 3–4 cm wide, 2–3 cm thick and weighs 100–120 g. The uterus is located in the *plica lata uteri*. The structural parts of the uterus are the body of the uterus with its upper uterine fundus and the cylindrical cervix. A portion of the uterine cervix protrudes into the vagina where it forms the vaginal part of the cervix (*portio vaginalis*) (cf. Fig. 566). The uterine cavity (*cavum uteri*) has the shape of a slit. In frontal view, it appears triangular. The uterine wall is 1.5 to 2 cm thick. Starting at the outer limit, there are the following layers: *perimetrium* [2] or tunica serosa (*peritoneal epithelium*), *myometrium* [3] or tunica muscularis with four layers (*stratum submucosum sive subvasculare, stratum vasculosum, stratum supravasculosum, stratum subserosum*) and the *endometrium* [4] or tunica mucosa.
The almost central sagittal section shows all layers.

1 Uterine cavity
2 Perimetrium
3 Myometrium
4 Endometrium
Stain: hematoxylin-eosin; magnification: × 5

569 Uterus

Section from the wall of a human uterus with *myometrium* [1] and *endometrium* [2]. Note the tubular glands in the endometrium (*late proliferation phase*). The basal cell layer of the endometrium is stained blue-violet [3]. The myometrium is about 1 cm thick. Its vascularized meshwork of smooth muscle fibers is interspersed with connective tissue (cf. Fig. 568). The myometrium consists of four layers: the submucosal layer, the vascular layer, the supravascular layer, and the subserosal layer.
Detail from Fig. 568.

1 Myometrium with submucosal and vascular layers
2 Endometrium
3 Basal cell layer
4 Uterine cavity (cavum uteri)
Stain: hematoxylin-eosin; magnification: × 15

570 Uterus

Section from a human uterine wall with *endometrium* [1] and *myometrium* [2] (cf. Figs. 569, 571b). The mucosa is in the late phase of *proliferation* (*follicular phase*). Following the *desquamation phase*, the endometrial glands grow into elongated tubules. The tubules have an undulating path in the late follicular phase, as shown in this figure. The gland tubules in the basal cell layer are cross-sectioned. The epithelium in the uterine cavity is single-layered and columnar. The bottom part in this figure shows the myometrium [2].

1 Endometrium
2 Myometrium
Stain: hematoxylin-eosin; magnification: × 25

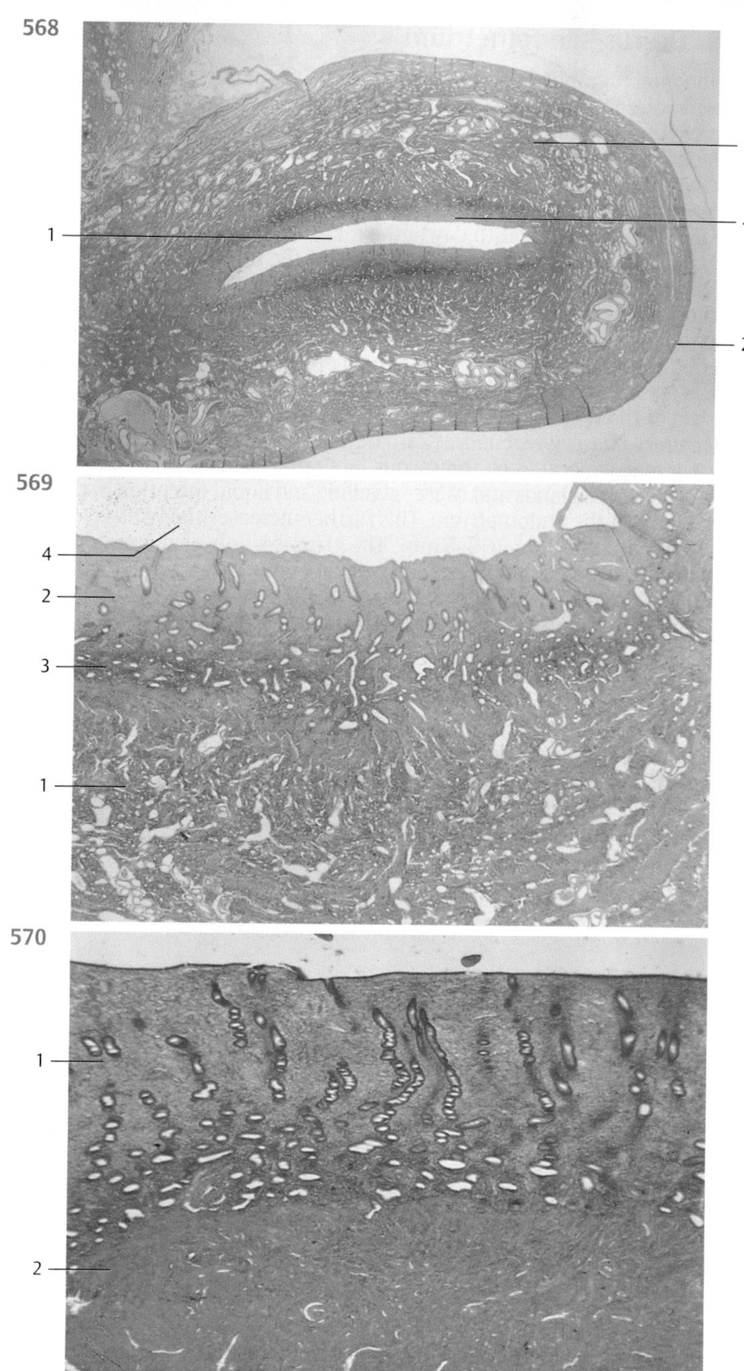
568
3
4
1
2
569
4
2
3
1
570
1
2

571 Uterus—Endometrium

All four micrographs have been done at the same magnification. The specimens were mounted in such a way that the borders between *endometrium* (tunica mucosa) and *myometrium* (tunica muscularis) can be viewed side-by-side. The sequence of micrographs shows the cyclical changes of the uterine mucosa.

a) *Early follicular phase* (9th day of the menstrual cycle).

b) *Late folliculin phase* (16th day of the menstrual cycle).

Both figures show the division into zones of the uterine mucosa. The basal cell layer of the endometrium 1 (*basalis*, deep layer of the endometrium next to the myometrium) contains irregularly distributed tubular glands. The functional layer of the endometrium (*functionalis*) shows an increased density of the connective tissue in the lamina propria. Another obvious morphological feature is the presence of long tubular uterine glands. The tubules run vertical to the tissue surface.

c) *Secretory phase, luteal phase* (23rd day of the menstrual cycle).

Progesterone generated by the corpus luteum initiates very active secretion from the uterine glands and causes swelling and liquid retention in the functional layer of the endometrium. This further increases the width of the mucous membrane to about 6–8 mm. The cross-section of the endometrium now displays a dense population of strongly undulating, winding gland tubules with saw-like acini. The tubules are particularly prominent in the tissue next to the basal cell layer (*zona spongiosa*) 2. The layer close to the lumen has a denser structure because the connective tissue cells in the tunica propria have increased in size and push the tubular glands away from each other (*zona compacta*) 3.

d) *Desquamation phase*, menstruation (1st day of menstrual cycle).

The entire functional layer of the endometrium is sloughed off (menstruation). The desquamation creates a wound. It consists of the basal cell layer with ruptured tubular glands, which initiate the building of an epithelium and wound healing (regeneration phase).

1 Basal cell layer of the endometrium, basalis
2 Zona spongiosa
3 Zona compacta
Stain: van Gieson iron hematoxylin-picrofuchsin; magnification: × 5

572 Uterus—Endometrium

Parallel section through the endometrium. The tissue has been cut at the level of the *zona compacta* in the functional layer of the endometrium. The *tubular uterine glands* have been cross-sectioned. The tubules are lined by a columnar epithelium. Many epithelial cells are about to divide. The *lamina propria mucosae* 1 consists of reticular connective tissue. Its cells are arranged like a school of fish. Lymphocytes and granulocytes are present between branched reticulum cells.

1 Endometrial lamina propria mucosae
Stain: alum hematoxylin-eosin; magnification: × 240

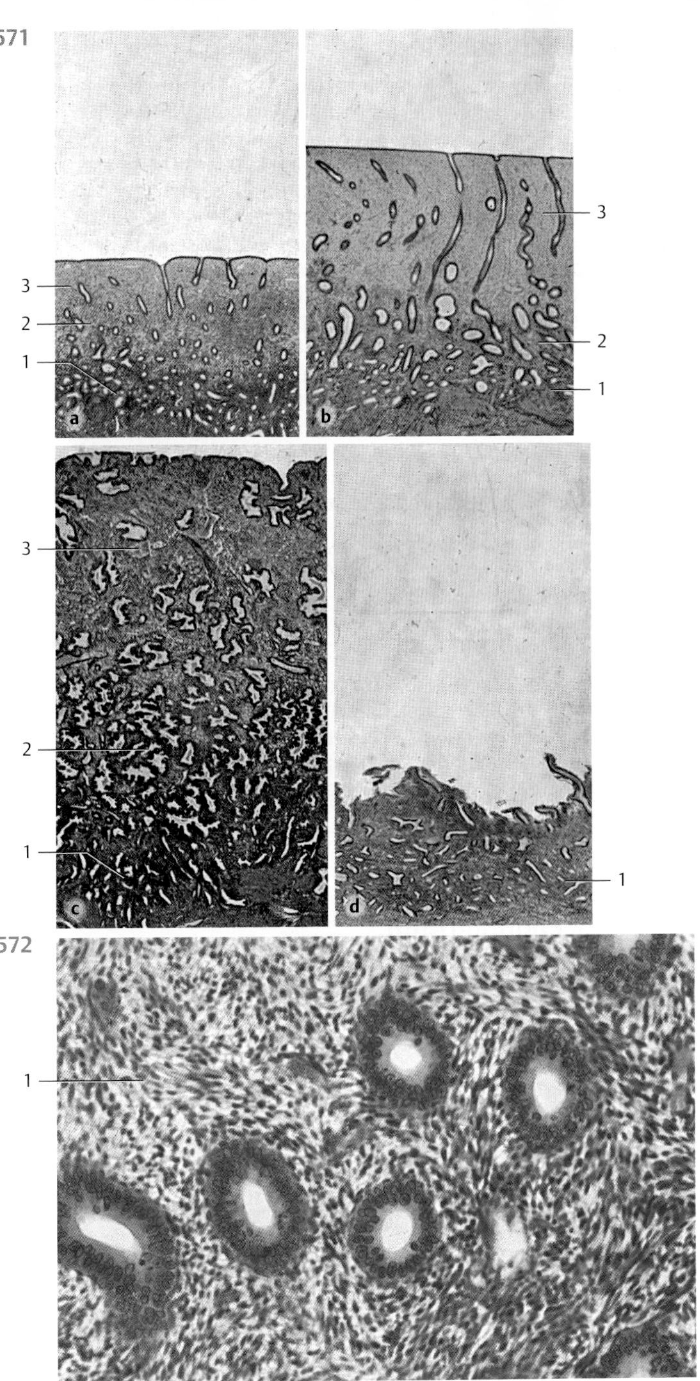
571
3
2
1
a
b
3
2
1
3
2
1
c
d
1
572
1

573 Uterus—Endometrium

The endometrium consists of the lining of the *uterine cavity* (right edge of the figure), the *functional endometrial layer* and the *basal cell layer of the endometrium* (cf. Fig. 570, 571). Single-layered columnar cells form the parietal epithelium of the uterine cavity, some of them are ciliated. The functional layer of the endometrium undergoes the most pronounced changes during the menstrual cycle. It is sloughed off during *menstruation* at the end of the *desquamation phase*. This figure shows endometrial tissue in the late follicular (proliferation) phase. The functional layer of the endometrium consists of cellulous connective tissue with only a few fibers (*stroma endometrii*). It contains a tubular gland. Its duct starts in the epithelial cavum lining (right part of the figure). The uterine glands are covered with a columnar epithelium, which is thicker than the parietal epithelium of the uterine cavity. The high columnar epithelium of the glands has elongated basal nuclei. The endometrial stroma resembles mesenchymal tissue. It is often called *lamina propria mucosae* and contains nerves and many vessels, such as the undulating arteries (*spiral arteries*). The arterioles feed the capillary network on the endometrial surface. Many dividing cells are found during the early follicular phase.

Stain: alum hematoxylin-eosin; magnification: × 130

574 Uterus—Endometrium

In the early follicular phase, the tubular uterine glands in the deeper, approximately 5-mm thick functional layer of the endometrium show a *corkscrew configuration*. Consequently, they are cut several times in vertical sections (cf. Fig. 570). The secretory ducts are empty because secretion has not yet started. The increased density of the connective tissue gives the stroma a compact appearance.

Stain: alum hematoxylin-eosin; magnification: × 130

575 Uterus—Endometrium

This figure shows the *endometrial basal layer* of the *uterine mucosa* on the 25th day of the menstrual cycle in the final part of the *secretion phase*. It is not lost during menstruation. The basal cell layer is about 1.5 mm high and borders on the myometrium (*stratum submucosum*) 1. The endometrial basal cell layer consists of fiber-rich connective tissue with embedded segments of tubular glands 3. The glands often extend into the *myometrium*. The *regeneration* of the mucosa, which has been sloughed off during menstruation, starts at the basal cell layer (cf. Fig. 571 d).

1 Myometrium
2 Fibrous connective tissue
3 Sectioned tubular glands
Stain: hematoxylin-eosin; magnification: × 80

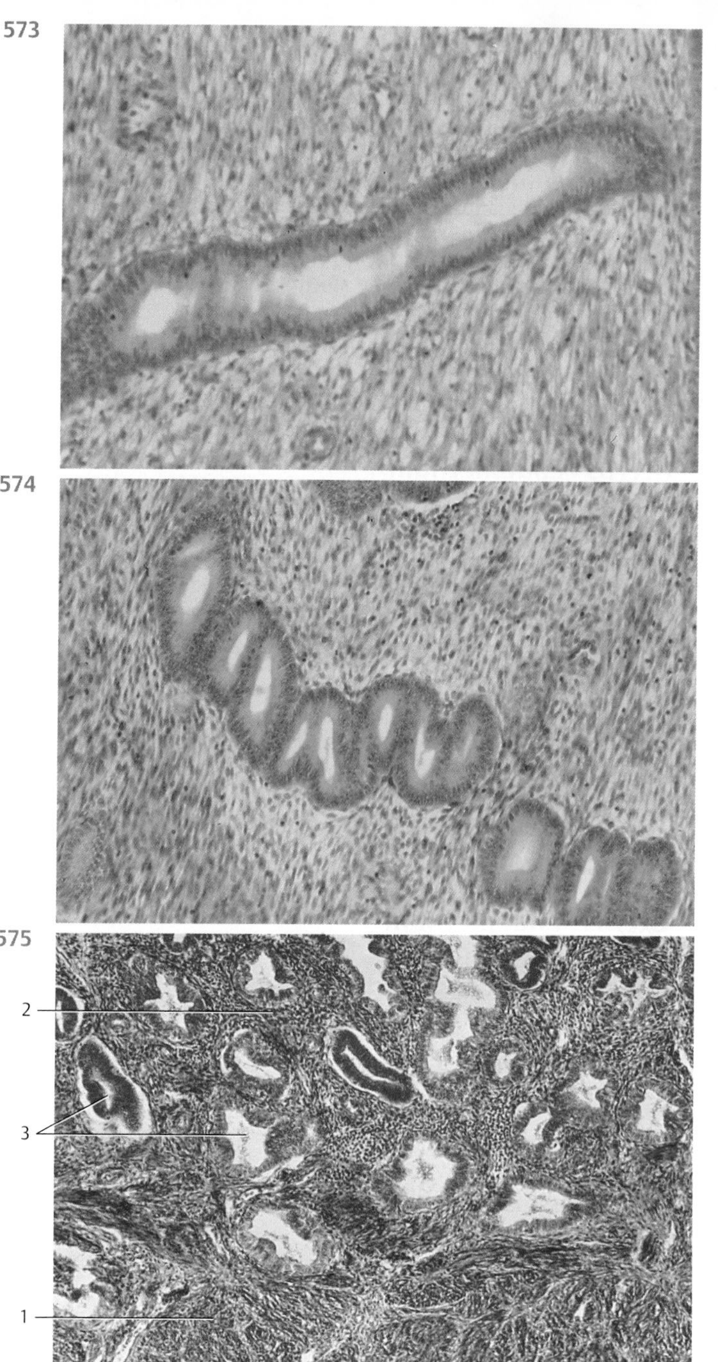
573
574
575
2
3
1

576 Uterus—Endometrium

This figure shows a detail of endometrium on the 25th day of the menstrual cycle in the final part of the *secretion phase*. The *uterine glands* 1 have become more voluminous and often undulate. The tubules that branch from the gland have a characteristic ragged form. The resulting surface structure is therefore often said to have a saw-blade profile 1 or show an accordion folding. The lumina of the glands contain secretions, which are rich in glycogen. Glycogen synthesis in the uterine glands is stimulated by progesterone. The connective tissue cells in the lamina propria mucosae 2 of the endometrial functional layer also grow lager while storing glycogen and lipids (cf. Figs. 571, 572, 576, 578).

1 Tubular gland with accordion folds
2 Lamina propria mucosae
Stain: hematoxylin-eosin; magnification: × 40

577 Uterus—Endometrium

Detail from the functional layer of the human endometrium in the human uterine mucous membrane on the 25th day of the menstrual cycle at the end of the secretion phase (same preparation as Fig. 576 at greater magnification). The micrograph shows the bellies of the distended tubular glands 1 with their irregularly structured epithelium. The supranuclear cytoplasm often bulges like a dome into the uterus. The cytoplasm has a foamy structure. When secretory product is released, apical cytoplasmic membranes may also be pinched off and become part of the uterine secretory product. Note the loose structure of the lamina propria mucosae 2 (cf. Figs. 571, 576, 578). A typical spiral artery 3 is visible in the upper center.

1 Lumen of a uterine gland
2 Lamina propria mucosae
3 Spiral artery
Stain: hematoxylin-eosin; magnification: × 200

578 Uterus—Endometrium

Detail from the functional layer of the human endometrium on the 25th day of the menstrual cycle (cf. Figs. 571c, 576). The micrograph shows that the tubular volumes of the uterine glands have increased (toothed blade structure, accordion folds) 1. The height of the epithelium varies, the epithelial cells are swollen and the structure appears to be in flux. The whole endometrial stroma appears edematous. The secretory tubules contain secretory products.

Endometrium in the secretory phase (cf. Figs. 571c, 576, 577).

1 Gland tubules
2 Endometrial stroma
Stain: hematoxylin-eosin; magnification: × 200

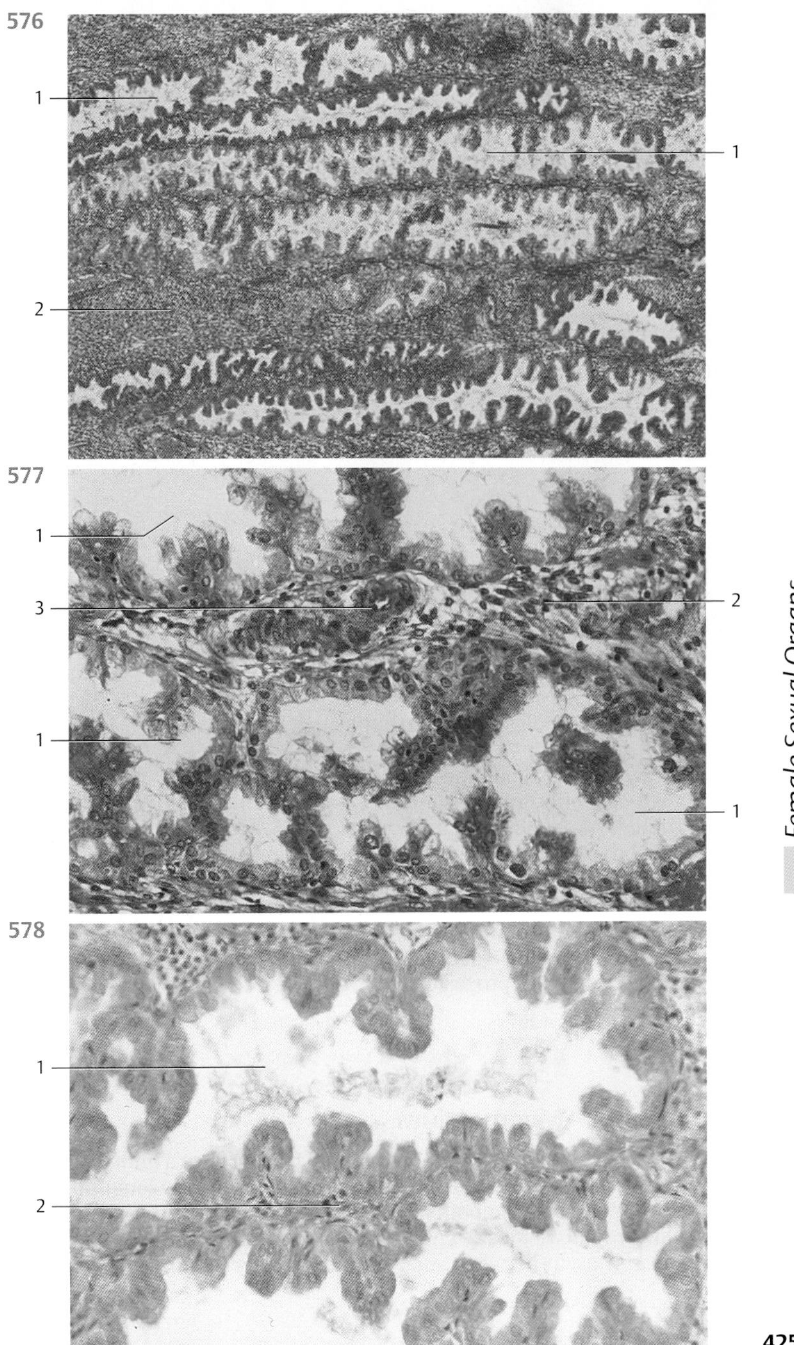
576
1
1
2
577
1
3
2
1
1
578
1
2

579 Uterus—Endometrium

During menstruation in the *desquamation phase*, the functional layer of the endometrium is sloughed off (*withdrawal bleeding*). Only the 1.5-mm thick *endometrial basal cell layer* 1 stays intact. It will be the basis for the generation of the new functional layer in the *regeneration phase*. The fibrous basal cell layer contains the branched, winding final segments of the uterine glands. The basal layer continues in the myometrial tissue 2 without demarcation (shown in the lower part of the figure). The epithelium of the uterine cavity is absent in the state of desquamation. This creates an open *wound bed*. The endometrium is regenerated immediately after menstruation. The wound is covered with epithelial and connective tissue cells. This *epithelialization* of the basal layer begins on day three or four of the menstrual cycle at the residual gland bodies.
Uterine cavity in the upper part of the figure (cf. Fig. 571d).

1 Endometrial basal layer, basalis
2 Myometrium
Stain: hematoxylin-eosin; magnification: × 80

580 Uterus—Endometrium

a) Curettage material obtained on day 17 of the menstrual cycle.
The presence of storage vesicles with glycogen or glycoproteins causes the apparent basal vacuolization of the uterine gland epithelium and pushes the nuclei into a more apical position. This type of epithelium is transitional and is seen on the 3rd and 4th day following ovulation, i.e., in the *early secretory (luteal) phase*. This characteristic cell transformation is an *early effect* of *progesterone*. The vacuoles underneath the nuclei are also known as *subnuclear vacuoles*.
b) Curettage material obtained on day 27 of the menstrual cycle.
In the late secretion phase, the uterine glands undulate considerably, and their tubules have wider lumina (cf. Figs. 574, 576–578). Copious specific secretory product is released into the tubules, along with pinched off plasmalemma vesicles. Concomitantly, glycogen and lipids are stored in the lamina propria connective tissue cells of the endometrial functional layer. This causes extensive swelling of the connective tissue cells, which are now rounded and called *endometrial decidual cells*. The *decidual reaction* is considered a late effect of progesterone.

Stain: Tonutti alum hematoxylin-orange G-phosphomolybdic acid-aniline blue (HOPA); magnification: × 160

581 Uterus—Myometrium

Section of the myometrial *stratum supravasculosum* from a human uterus (cf. Fig. 582). The upper part of the micrograph shows mostly longitudinally or tangentially sectioned smooth muscle cells. The smooth muscle cells shown in the lower half are mostly cut across their long axis. Note the vasculature. Blood vessels occur between adjacent muscle fiber bundles (cf. Fig. 221).

Stain: hematoxylin-eosin; magnification: × 400

579

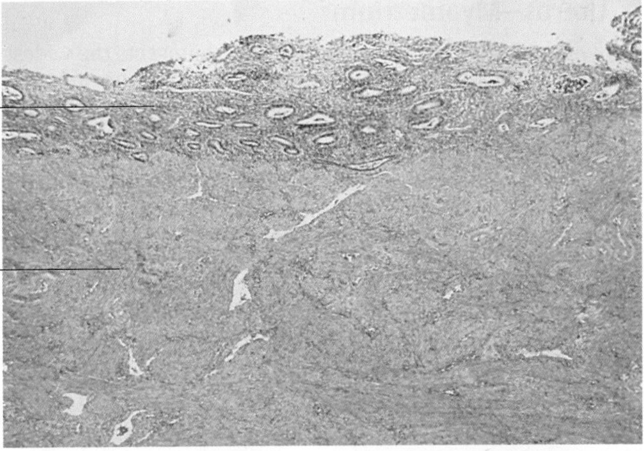

1

2

580

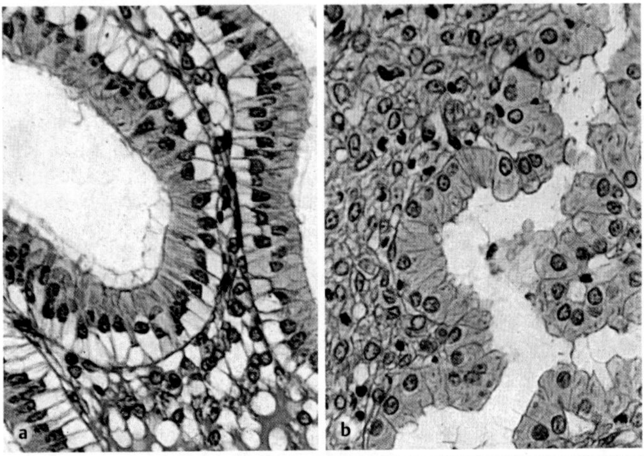

a

b

581

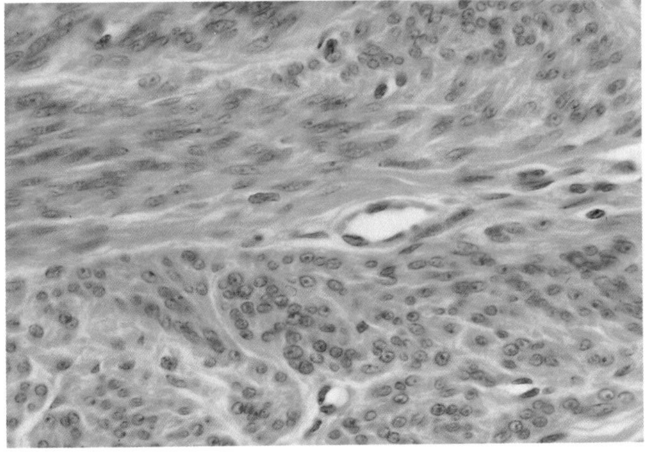

582 Uterus—Myometrium

With a width of 1.5–2.0 cm, the *myometrium* represents the widest layer of the uterine wall. It is built as a dense interwoven structure of smooth muscle bundles with interspersed vascularized connective tissue strands. The muscle bundles in this preparation have been cut in all planes (cf. Figs. 221, 568–570, 581). During pregnancy, the ordinarily 50-μm long and 5-μm thick smooth muscle cells become hypertrophied and can grow to be 800 μm long and 12–18 μm thick. Four myometrial layers with diffuse borders are discernible. The thickest layer in the center contains mostly circular muscle fibers as well as lymph and blood vessels. The presence of blood vessels explains the name *stratum vasculosum*. The inner thin layer is the submucosal layer. It lies underneath the endometrium and is called *stratum subvasculosum*. The outer thin layer is named *stratum supravasculosum*. It consists of several smooth muscle lamellae. The layer underneath it is the thin *subserosal* layer.

Stain: hematoxylin-eosin; magnification: × 200

583 Vagina

The wall of the vagina consists of the *tunica mucosa, tunica muscularis* and *tunica adventitia*. The tunica mucosa does not contain glands. It is covered by a multilayered nonkeratinizing squamous epithelium with surface plicae. The epithelial cells are rich in glycogen. The lamina propria 2 with elastic fibers and a venous plexus borders on the epithelium. The epithelium interlocks via papilla with the connective tissue of the vagina wall. The epithelium consists of *basal cells, parabasal cells, intermediary cells* and *surface cells*. It can be influenced by hormones and shows cyclical changes. Numerous free cells, especially lymphocytes, are found immediately underneath the epithelium in the lamina propria.

1 Multilayered nonkeratinized squamous epithelium (stratified)
2 Lamina propria
Stain: van Gieson iron hematoxylin-picric acid; magnification: × 90

584 Labia Minora—Labia Minora Pudendi

The labia minor are skin folds, which are homologous to the penis. They are covered by a multilayered squamous epithelium 1. The *labia majora pudendi* cover the labia minor partially or completely. The surface shows keratinization of the multilayered squamous epithelium. The subepithelial basal cell layer is frequently heavily pigmented. The loose connective tissue 2 of the labia contains collagen fibers as well as elastic fibers. It forms high papilla. There are hardly any adipocytes. Due to abundant blood vessels, the tissue appears red. Hair is not present. However, there are many sebaceous glands 3. This micrograph shows the vestibular face of the *labium minus pudendi* from an adult woman.

1 Multilayered stratified keratinizing squamous epithelium
2 Loose connective tissue
3 Sebaceous glands
Stain: azan; magnification: × 40

582

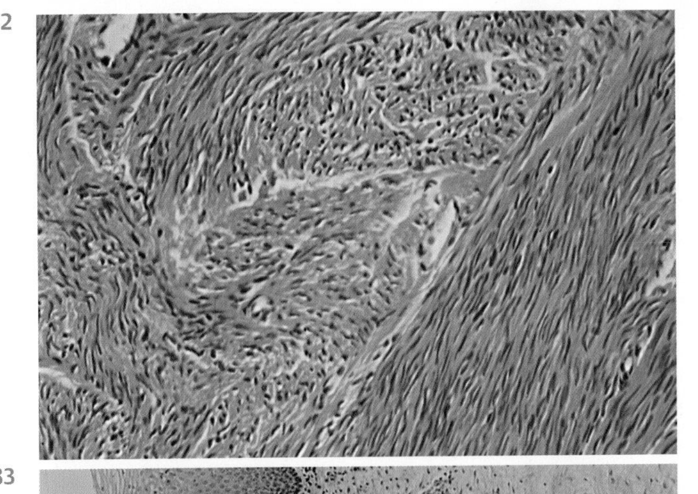

583

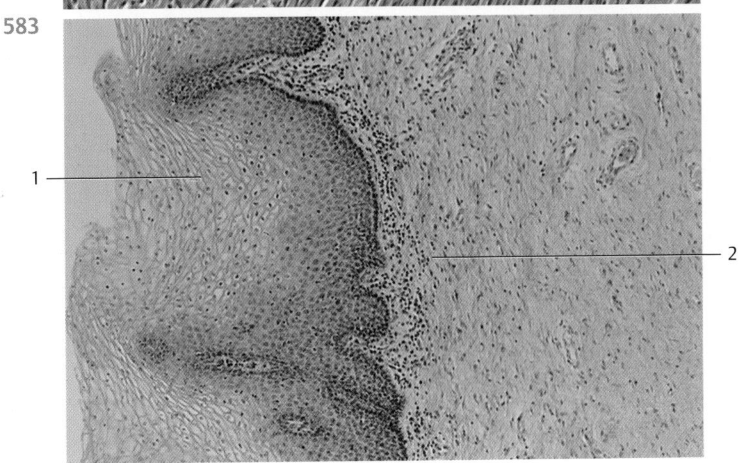

584

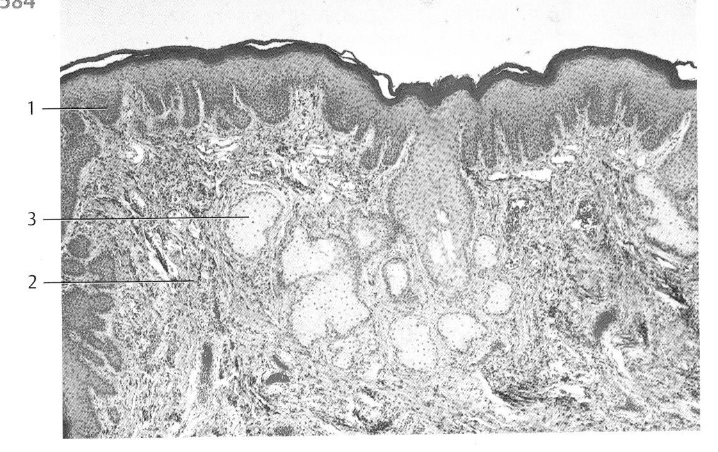

585 Placenta

Vertical section through a mature *placenta*. It consists of the *chorionic plate* (*membrana chorii*) 1, the *branched microvilli* and the *basal plate* (not shown here). The *intervillous space* 2 with the maternal stream of blood is located between the villi. This micrograph shows the chorionic plate 1 (upper part of the figure), which is covered by a single-layered cuboidal to columnar *amnion epithelium* 3 (see Fig. 590). *Syncytiotrophoblasts* cover the chorionic plate at the intervillous space. Many termini of villi 4 and branches of villi underneath the chorionic plate are sectioned. They are covered with syncytiotrophoblasts as well (see Fig. 587). *Fibrinoid* (Langhans) is present between villi and subchorionic tissue. Fibroid material is acidophilic.

1 Chorionic plate, membrana chorii
2 Intervillous space
3 Amnion epithelium, fetal side of the placenta
4 Placental villi
5 Subchorionic fibrinoid
Stain: alum hematoxylin-eosin; magnification: × 40

586 Placenta

Detail of the *labyrinth* from a human placenta (39 weeks of gestation) with multiple villi (overview). With the exception of a few sporadic cells, the *cytotrophoblast* layer has degenerated. Therefore, the villi 1 are only surrounded by the *syncytiotrophoblast*. Darker *proliferation nodes* are seen in some places on the surface. The center part of the villi consists of loose chorionic mesodermal tissue and erythrocyte-filled capillaries. There are maternal blood cells in the intervillous space 2 (*maternal milieu*).

1 Placental villi
2 Intervillous space
Stain: Masson-Goldner trichrome; magnification: × 65

587 Placenta

Cross-section of the chorionic villi from a human placenta in the 4th gestational month. The chorionic villi consist of loosely structured chorionic mesoderm 1 and a cover of ectodermal trophoblasts. Capillaries 2 and rounded, eosinophilic cells with granules or vacuoles (*Hofbauer cells*) are found in the chorionic mesoderm. Up to the end of the 4th gestational month, the trophoblast covering is two-layered. The inner epithelium with *cytotrophoblasts* (*Langhans layer*) 3 clearly shows the borders of the cuboidal cells. The outer layer consists of polynucleated cells with undefined borders. The intervillous space contains sporadic maternal blood cells and fibrin clots (cf. Figs. 585, 586, 588).

1 Mesenchymal villi stroma
2 Capillaries
3 Cytotrophoblast
4 Syncytiotrophoblast
Stain: azan; magnification: × 210

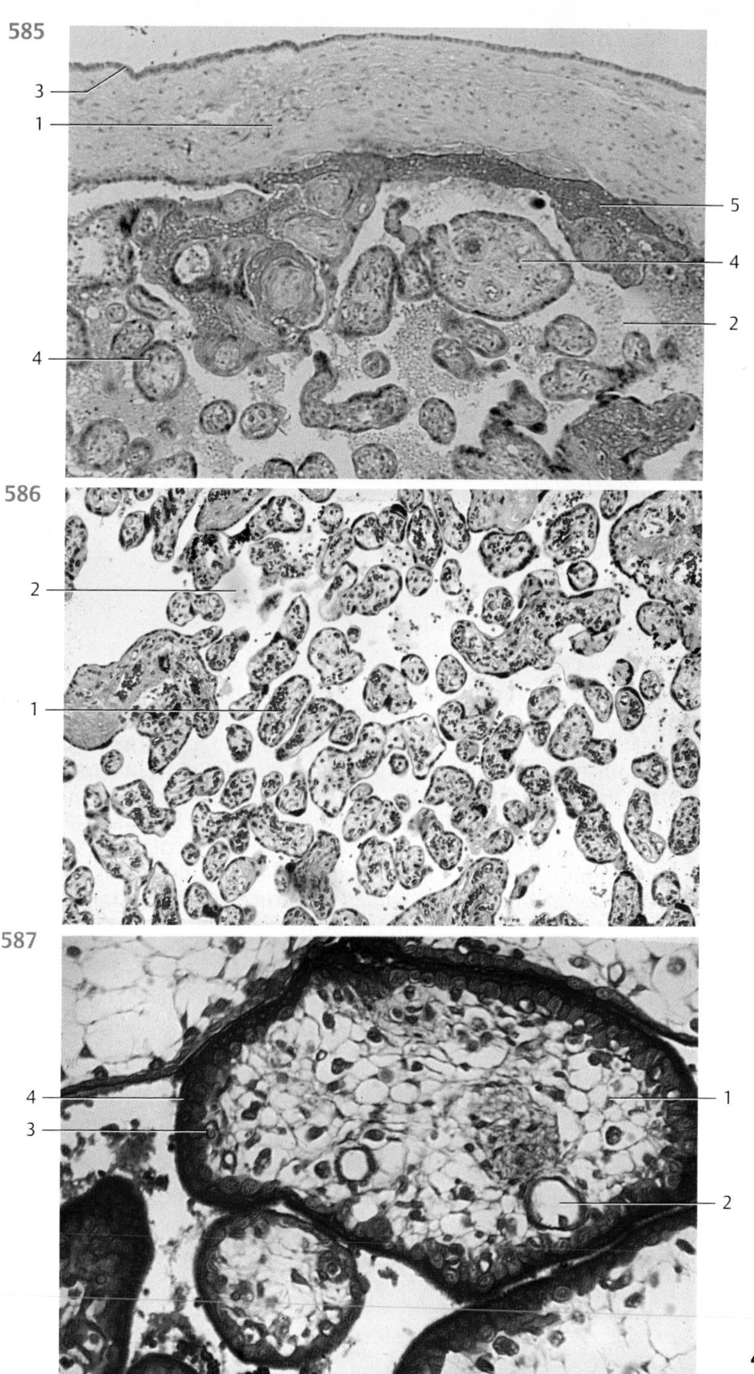
585
3
1
5
4
2
4
586
2
1
587
4
3
1
2

588 Placenta

Cross-section of a terminal villus from the mature placenta (cf. Figs. 585–587) with four fetal capillaries, which have dilated and formed sinusoids. They bulge into the intervillous space. Their trophoblast cover is extremely thin. That decreases the *maternal-fetal diffusion zone* considerably. On the left and in the upper left part, the figure shows two nondilated capillaries 2. All fetal capillaries contain erythrocytes. The loosely structured chorionic mesoderm contains macrophages (*Hofbauer cells*) 3 and fibroblasts 4. The syncytiotrophoblast 5 covers the outer villi. It is directly bathed in maternal blood in the intervillous space. Villi of different length protrude from the syncytiotrophoblast. A cytotrophoblast cell 6 (*Langhans giant cell*) is still present. It is shown in the upper left of the figure. A syncytial node 7 is also shown.

1 Fetal sinusoids
2 Fetal capillaries
3 Macrophage, Hofbauer cell
4 Fibroblast
5 Syncytiotrophoblast
6 Cytotrophoblast, Langhans cell
7 Syncytial node
Electron microscopy; magnification: × 1200

589 Placenta

After a fertilized egg is implanted, the maternal uterine mucosa (now called *decidua*) and the germ cell chorion establish a unique relationship, which creates the very complex placenta. There are clearly discernible structural changes of the endometrium, even before egg implantation. The changes encompass both uterine glands and the endometrial connective tissue. The connective tissue cells grow larger and appear epithelioid with polygonal geometry. These cells are the *decidual cells* 1. They store lipids and glycogen. This figure shows the basal cell plate (*decidua basalis*) of a placenta in the 5th gestational month. The densely stacked, swollen decidual cells 1 can be clearly recognized. They are surrounded by fibrin deposits 2 (stained bright red). A uterine gland 3 is visible in the right part of the micrograph.

1 Decidual cells
2 Fibrin
3 Uterine gland
Stain: alum hematoxylin-chromotrope 2R (acid red 29); magnification: × 90

590 Placenta—Amnion Epithelium

The chorionic plate (membrana chorii) forms the fetal side of the placenta. It is covered by a single layered columnar epithelium (cf. Fig. 585). Note the round apical nuclei. The connective tissue of the chorionic plate is shown in the lower half of the figure.

Stain: hematoxylin-eosin; magnification: × 400

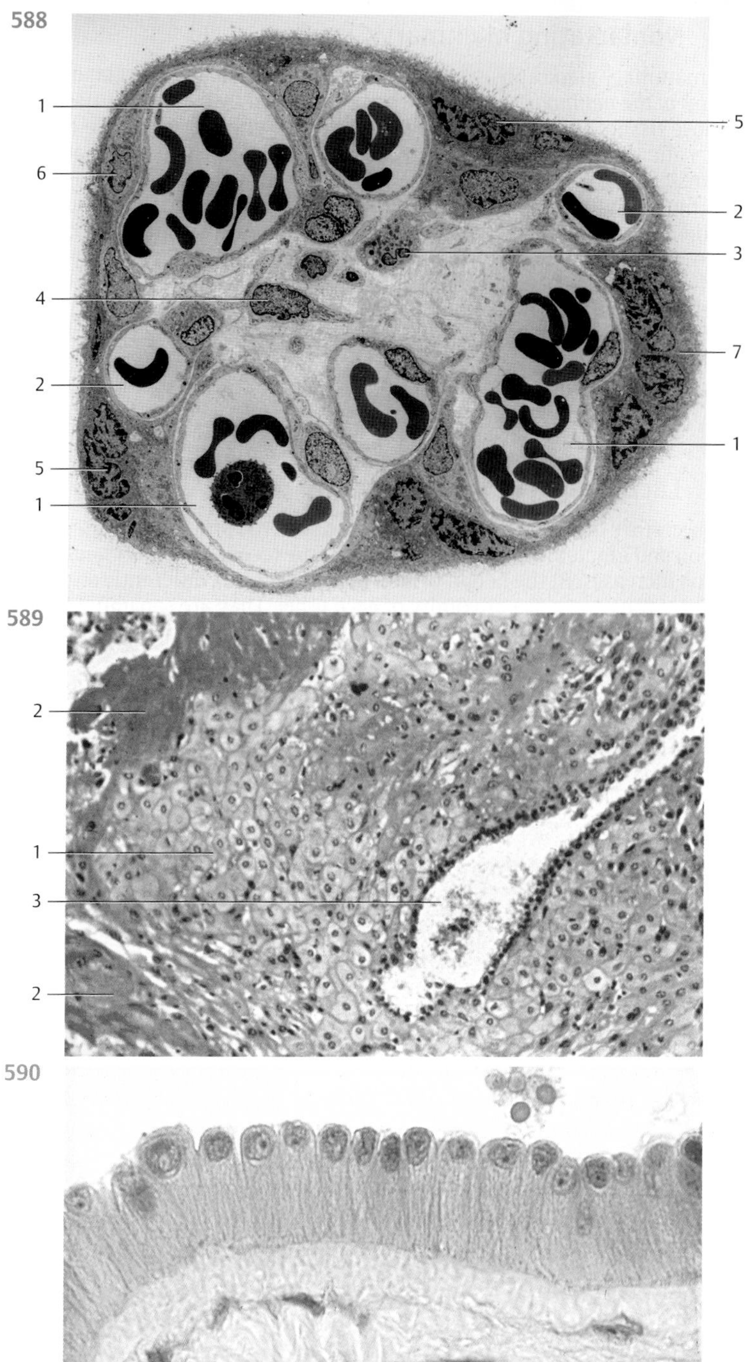

Female Sexual Organs

591 Nonlactating Mammary Gland

The mammary gland consists of 15–25 separate tubuloalveolar glands in the *lobules of the mammary gland*, which are separated by connective tissue and adipose tissue. Their alveoli are fully developed only in the course of pregnancy and lactation. Alveoli are rarely present in quiescent glands that do not lactate, especially in nulliparous women.
This figure shows the central secretory duct (*sinus lactiferi*) 1. Tubuli with blind ends and incompletely developed ducts (*ductus lactiferi*) branch from it. Note the loose sheath of cellular connective tissue 2. It is clearly distinguished from the coarse fibrous connective tissue stroma 3.
Quiescent, nonlactating human mammary gland.

1 Sinus lactiferi
2 Connective tissue sheath
3 Coarse fibrous collagenous connective tissue
Stain: alum hematoxylin-eosin; magnification: × 80

592 Lactating Mammary Gland

The secretory ducts of the mammary gland start to sprout during pregnancy. Alveoli and lobules form. The connective tissue recedes and the gland parenchyma increases. At the height of *lactation* (the figure), differently shaped alveoli are found in close proximity of each other. They are separated by delicate connective tissue fibers. The gland epithelium 1 has different heights, dependent on its secretory state.
Lactating mammary gland. Secretory products are visible in some of the gland lumina (cf. Fig. 593).

1 Alveoli
2 Connective tissue septa
Stain: azan; magnification: × 80

593 Lactating Mammary Gland

In the active, lactating mammary gland, the epithelium of the alveoli features a rich ergastoplasm and apical fat droplets. It shows different heights. The usual preparations display round empty spaces 1 where fat droplets have been (cf. Figs. 594, 595). The apical cell membrane may rupture or, in other places, bulge dome-like into the lumen. These attributes are characteristic of apocrine glands (see Fig. 133). There are patches with secretory product 2 and occasionally sloughed-off epithelial cells (upper figure). Elaborately branched myoepithelial cells 3 form an incomplete layer around the alveolar wall.

1 Secretory product in gland cells (vacuoles)
2 Secretory product
3 Myoepithelial cells
Stain: alum hematoxylin-eosin; magnification: × 160

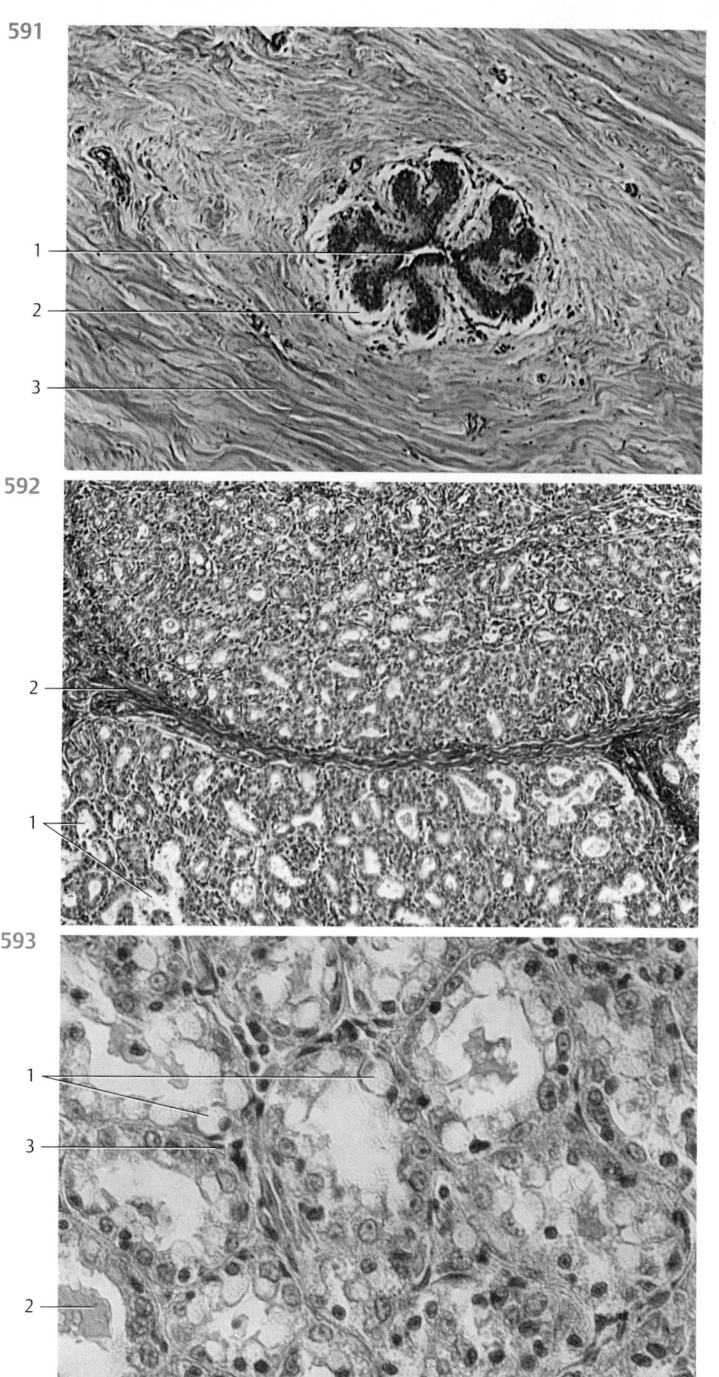
591
1
2
3
592
2
1
593
1
3
2

594 Lactating Mammary Gland

The fat droplets of the milk are blackened with osmium tetroxide in this section of a lactating mammary gland. They correspond to the vacuoles, which are seen in Fig. 593. Note that small droplets combine to larger spheres in some places. The gland cells and the connective tissue are stained yellowish brown.

Stain: osmium tetroxide; magnification: × 160

595 Lactating Mammary Gland

The lactating mammary gland concomitantly synthesizes several different substances, which are released into the alveoli. During periods of lactation, the secretory cells produce fat droplets (see Fig. 594). They combine to larger droplets and are moved to the apical cell region. Finally, they become part of vesicular formations at the plasmalemma (*apical protrusions*) and are pinched off as milk droplets.

The figure displays two membrane encased fat droplets 1 in the alveolar lumen. The large central, membrane encased fat droplet is still connected to the plasmalemma. It will obviously be pinched off shortly. At the same time, the ergastoplasm 2 of the gland cells in conjunction with the Golgi apparatus biosynthesize proteins, in particular casein and α-*lactalbumin* and packaged as secretory vesicles. The small *casein granules* 4 have a dense structure. They are osmiophil and can therefore easily be found. Casein granules fuse with the plasmalemma and are released by *exocytosis*. Four gland cells with many protein vesicles 4 are visible in this section. The gland cells have an elaborate endoplasmic reticulum 2 (*ergastoplasm*), Golgi complexes 3 and mitochondria. Sporadically, casein granules are already present in the lumen of the alveoli 5.

Lactating mammary gland from a guinea pig.

1 Membrane-encased fat droplet
2 Ergastoplasm
3 Golgi apparatus
4 Vacuole with casein granule
5 Casein granule in the alveolar lumen
Electron microscopy; magnification: × 6000

596 Nonlactating Mammary Gland

Whole-mount preparation of a nonlactating mammary gland from a rat. The branched secretory ducts (*ductus lactiferi*) are shown. Their ends are distended in a bud-like fashion. These ends contain the germ tissue for the alveoli which are fully developed only during pregnancy. Adipose mammary gland tissue is present in the light, unstained spaces between the branched secretory ducts. Its mass decreases with the growth of the mammary gland secretory tissue.

Stain: hematoxylin; magnification: × 25

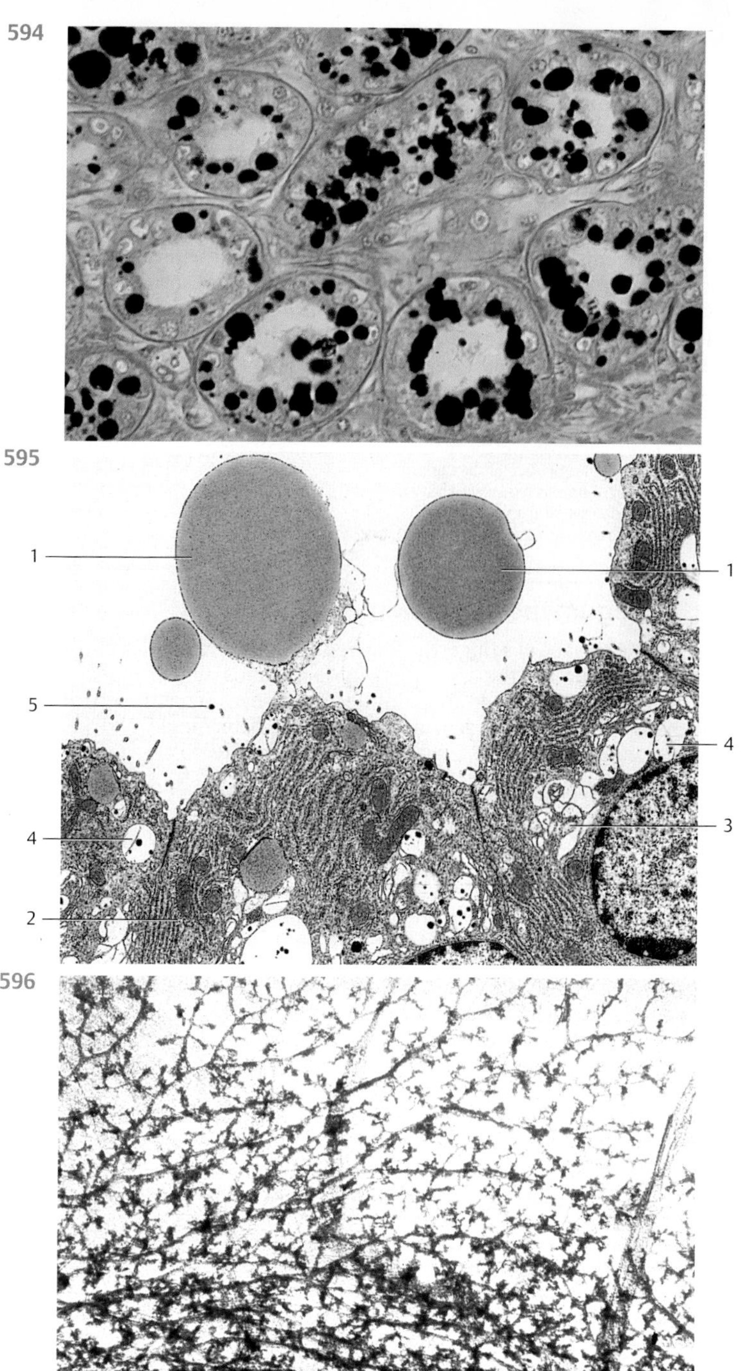
594
595
1
1
5
4
4
3
2
596

597 Integument—Thick Skin

Skin (*cutis*) consists of the epithelial *epidermis* 1 and the connective tissue of the *dermis* (*corium*) 2 3. Subcutaneous tissue 4 is found underneath the dermis (*subcutis*). The epidermis is a multilayered keratinizing squamous epithelium (cf. Figs. 119–121, 598–601). The corium is built of connective tissue elastic fibers. The epidermal surface displays grooves, which delimit patches or fields (see Fig. 602). However, the epidermis of the palms of the hands and soles of the feet (thick skin) have parallel grooves that create ridges (ridged skin) (cf. Fig. 598). This figure shows the layered structure of the skin from a fingertip. The connective tissue of the corium (*dermis*) consists of the *stratum papillare* 2 and the *stratum reticulare* 3. These layers are followed by the *subcutaneous tissue* 4. Most of the skin's glands 5 are located between dermis and subcutaneous tissue. Subcutaneous tissue is rich in adipose tissue.

1 Epidermis with friction ridges
2 Stratum papillare of the corium
3 Stratum reticulare of the corium
4 Subcutaneous tissue with fatty tissue
5 Eccrine sweat glands
Stain: benzopurpurin (diamine red); magnification: × 16

598 Integument- Thick Skin

View of the surface of a fingertip. The figure shows a resin cast. It displays the *ridged epidermis* and the apertures of sweat glands, which appear to sprout on the surface. The ridges are delimited by grooves (cf. Figs. 597, 599, 600). The patterns on ridged skin are genetically determined and permanent through life (fingerprint).

Scanning electron microscopy; magnification: × 50

599 Integument—Thick Skin

Vertical section through the skin of the fingertip. The micrograph displays the epidermis and the stratum papillare 5 of the dermis (cf. Figs. 597, 598, 600). The four layers of the epidermis are clearly defined: the *stratum corneum* 1 with keratinocytes, the *stratum lucidum* 2, the *stratum granulosum* 3 with the basophilic *keratohyaline granules* as the precursor of the keratinous matrix and the *stratum germinativum* 4 (cf. Figs. 600, 601). Some parts of the epidermis protrude like deep cutaneous spikes (rete lamellae) into the dermis. They extend between dermal papilla (*corium papilla*) 5. This figure shows two cutaneous rete lamellae, which are traversed by the corkscrew-shaped secretory ducts of sweat glands (cf. Fig. 600).

1 Stratum corneum
2 Stratum lucidum (absent in thin skin)
3 Stratum granulosum
4 Stratum germinativum
5 Stratum papillare of the corium (dermal papillary layer)
Stain: hematoxylin-eosin; magnification: × 40

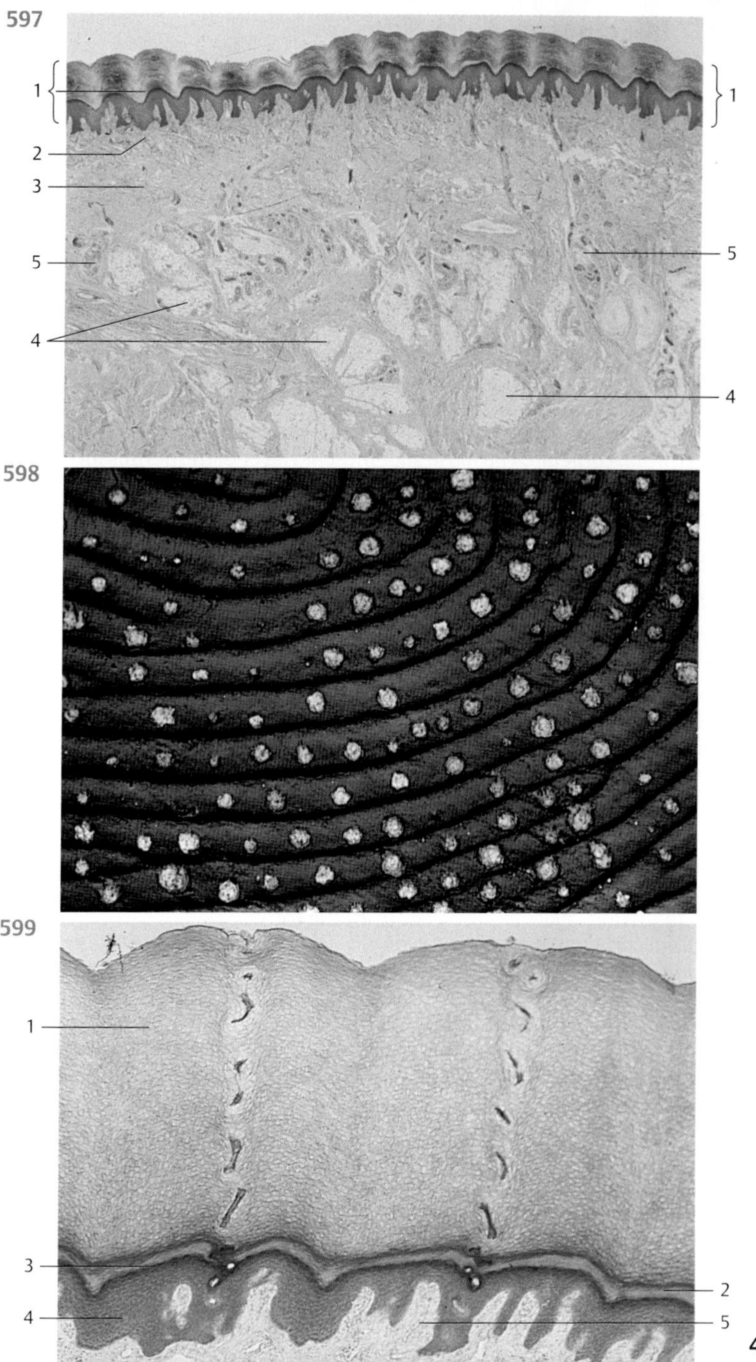

Integumentary System, Skin

600 Integument—Thick Skin

This vertical section shows the skin of the sole of a human foot. The wide *subcutaneous* layer is not shown. The epidermis consists of a multilayered keratinizing squamous epithelium. The outer, *cornified layer* (*stratum corneum*) is particularly thick at the sole of the foot (0.75–1.5 mm) (cf. Fig. 599, fingertip). It is composed of anuclear dead *corneocytes* that are filled with the filamentous protein *keratin*. The basal layer is the stratum germinativum 2. It forms rete lamellae 3, which interlock with the dermal papillae 4 (cf. Figs. 597, 599, 601). The germinal layer (*stratum germinativum*) 2 consists of the *stratum basale* (see Fig. 93, 118) and the *stratum spinosum* (see Figs. 93, 94, 601). The thin, granulated *stratum granulosum* 5 (stained dark blue) underlies the upper keratinized layer of the epidermis. Cell nuclei in this layer already show structural changes. The cytoplasm contains basophilic keratohyaline granules. Immediately over the granular layer lies the shiny stratum lucidum (not clearly recognizable in this image, see Fig. 599, 601). A helical secretory duct 6 longitudinally traverses the left dermal lamella in the lower half of the *stratum corneum*. The loose subepithelial layer of the dermis forms papillae. It is therefore called papillary layer (*stratum papillare*) (cf. Figs. 597, 599). The epidermis also contains melanocytes, Langerhans cells, tactile disks (Merkel's disks) and Meissner's corpuscles (not shown here, see Figs. 614, 615).

1 Stratum corneum
2 Stratum germinativum
3 Epithelial spine
4 Dermal papillae
5 Stratum granulosum
6 Intraepidermal secretory duct of a sweat gland
7 Stratum papillare of the dermis (corium)
Stain: alum hematoxylin-eosin; magnification: × 12

601 Integument—Thick Skin

Epidermis of the finger and dermal stratum papillare at higher magnification (cf. Figs. 597, 600).
The following layers are present (from the top):
Stratum corneum 1, *stratum lucidum* 2, *stratum granulosum* 3, *stratum spinosum* 4 (cf. Figs. 93–95, 120, 603) and the *stratum basale* 5. Stratum spinosum and *stratum basale* form the *stratum germinativum*. The following layers are the *stratum papillare* 6 and the stratum reticulare 7 of the dermis (corium). Note: the corneocytes of the stratum corneum do not have nuclei. The stratum granulosum consists of only two or three layers.

1 Stratum corneum
2 Stratum lucidum
3 Stratum granulosum
4 Stratum spinosum
5 Stratum basale sive cylindricum
6 Stratum papillare
7 Stratum reticulare
Stain: alum hematoxylin-eosin; magnification: × 300

600

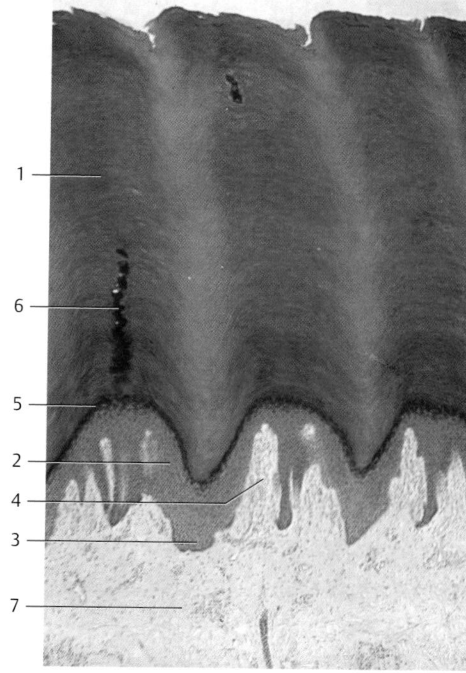

601

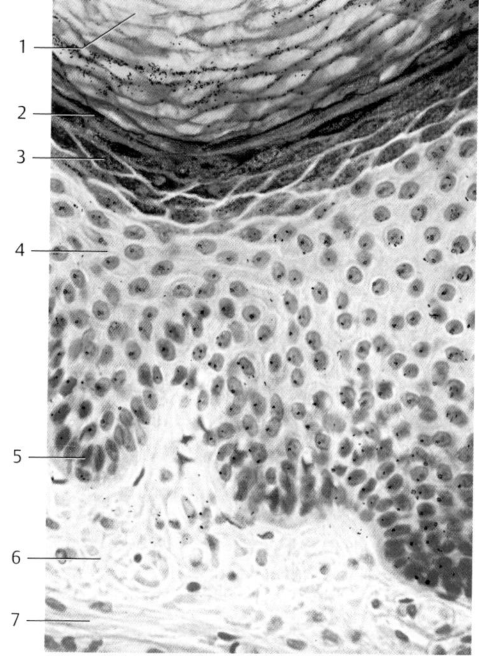

602 Integument—Thin Skin

In contrast to *thick skin* (see Figs. 597–602), the grooves on the surface of *thin skin* subdivide the surface into patches or fields. The hair is located in the grooves, mostly at intersecting grooves. Deep grooves diagonally traverse the image shown here. There are also finer grooves, which define the irregularly shaped areas (patches, fields). Skin from the human face.

Scanning electron microscopy; magnification: × 30

603 Integument—Thin Skin

Vertical section through the skin of the lateral thoracic wall. Note the thin *stratum corneum* 1 (cf. Figs. 597, 599, 600) and the *stratum granulosum* 2 with only one layer. The prickle cell layer (*stratum spinosum*) 3 with its intercellular bridges is clearly defined (cf. Figs. 93, 118, 601). It is part of the *stratum germinativum*. The lowest cell layer is the *stratum basale* 4. It forms fine basal cytoplasmic processes (rootstocks) (see Fig. 93). This creates an enlarged connecting layer between dermis and epidermis. The dermal papillae are interlocked via epidermal rete lamellae. The stratum papillare 6 forms a dense fiber meshwork at the border to the epidermis. It sporadically contains fibroblasts.
Axillary skin (cf. Fig. 120).

1 Stratum corneum
2 Stratum granulosum
3 Stratum spinosum
4 Stratum basale
5 Dermal papilla
6 Stratum papillare of the corium
Semi-thin section; stain: methylene blue-azure II; magnification: × 400

604 Integument—Scalp

The skin of the scalp consists of epidermis, dermis (corium) and subcutaneous tissue, which continues in the *aponeurosis epicranialis* (*galea aponeurotica*) 5. This vertical section of the scalp reveals that the hair roots sit vertically in funnel-shaped epidermal invaginations. The hair shafts (*scapus pili*) usually extend over the epithelium. They have broken off. The *hair follicles* 1 are found in the *subcutaneous layer* 2 (see Fig. 605). Note the smooth arrector muscle bundles (*arrector muscles of the hair*) 3, which originate with the papillary layer of the dermis and extend to the connective tissue sheaths of the hair follicles (*goose flesh*). Each hair follicle has one or more sebaceous glands 4. (Histology of the hair: see Figs. 605 and 606). The tendon fiber bundles of the galea aponeurotica (*aponeurosis epicranialis*) 5 are shown in the band that runs parallel to the lower edge of the figure.

1 Hair follicle (bulbus)
2 Subcutaneous adipose tissue
3 Musculus arrector pili
4 Sebaceous glands
5 Galea aponeurotica
Stain: benzopurpurin (diamine red); magnification: × 15

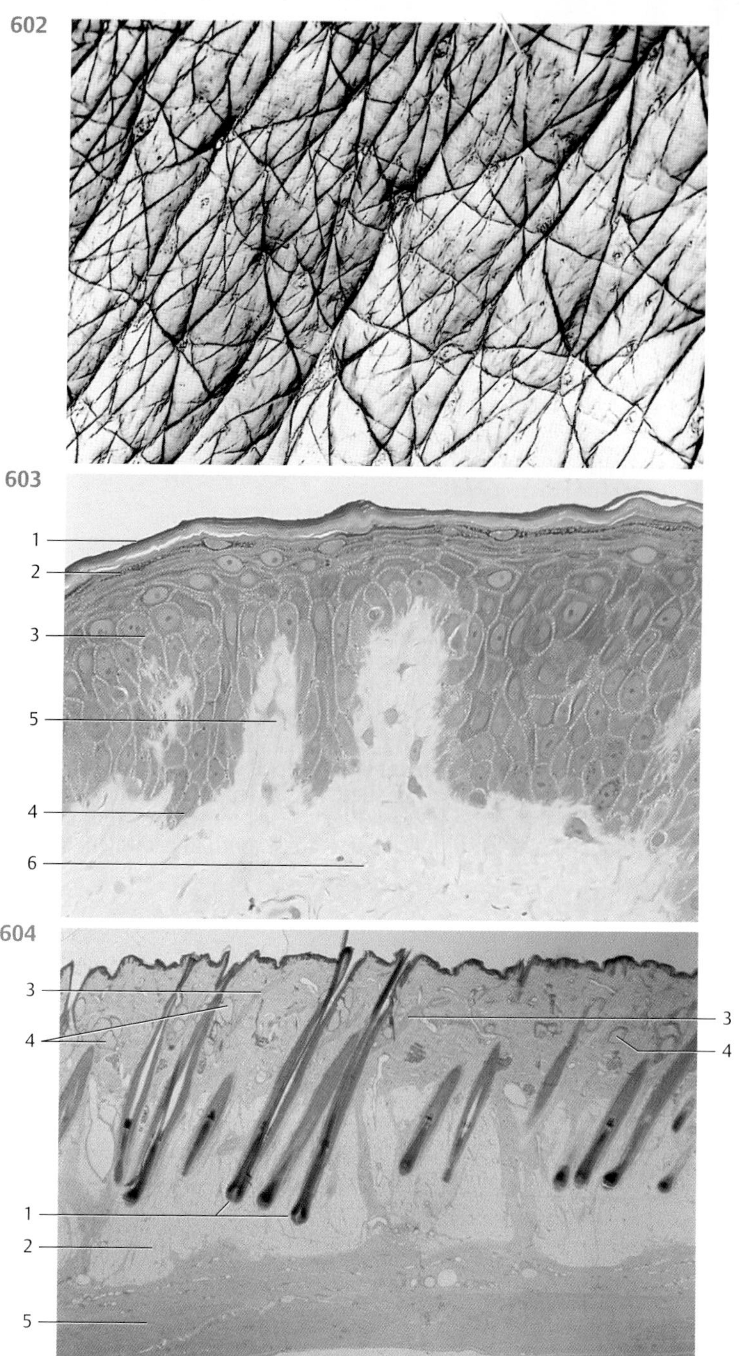
602
603
1
2
3
5
4
6
604
3
4
1
2
5
3
4

605 Hair—Pili

Hair, like nails, consists of the protein keratin. The keratin strands are flexible. Hair originates with the epidermis. There are *terminal hairs* and *vellus hairs*. Thickness and distribution of hair depends on hair growth and body part. Maximum hair density is observed on the scalp where the total number of hairs can reach 100 000. The lifespan of a human hair is 3–5 years.
This image is a montage of longitudinal sections through the hair root of a *terminal hair* (see also Fig. 604).

1 Adipose tissue
2 Hair follicle (bulbus pili) with hair matrix
3 Hair cortex
4 External root sheath
5 Unmyelinated nerve fiber
6 Basement membrane
7 Hair shaft (connective tissue root sheath)
8 Arrector pili muscle
9 Sebaceous gland
10 Hair shaft (scapus pili)
11 End of the inner root sheath
12 Internal root sheath
13 Hair medulla
14 Vessel
15 Henle's layer of the inner root sheath
16 Huxley's layer of the inner root sheath
17 Sheath cuticle and hair cuticle
18 Connective tissue hair papilla (Papilla pili)
Stain: hematoxylin-eosin; magnification: × 64

606 Hair—Pili

Detail section of a hair shaft (*scapus pili*) of a blond scalp hair. The *cuticula pili* form the external sheath of the hair shaft. Its surface consists of hard keratin. The keratin scales are arranged like shingles. Their free edges point in the direction of the follicular ostium. The edges are smooth in healthy hair.

Scanning electron microscopy; magnification: × 1900

607 Nail—Unguis

The nails (*ungues*) of the fingers and toes are arcuate, about 0.5 mm thick, epidermal keratinous horny plates 1. They are located in the nail bed (*hyponychium*) 2. The nail wall surrounds the lateral and proximal edges. The lateral nail wall is embedded in the nail fold (*eponychium*) 3. This vertical section through the nail and fingertip of a human finger shows the sponge-like bone structure of the end phalanx 4 underneath the arcuate nail. Note the eccrine sweat glands 5, the adipose tissue patches 6 and the toothed contour of the fingertip 7 (thick skin) (see Figs. 597–600).

1 Nail plate
2 Nail bed
3 Nail fold
4 Bones of the end phalanx of the finger
5 Eccrine sweat glands
6 Adipose tissue patches
7 Skin of the fingertip
Stain: alum hematoxylin-eosin; magnification: × 10

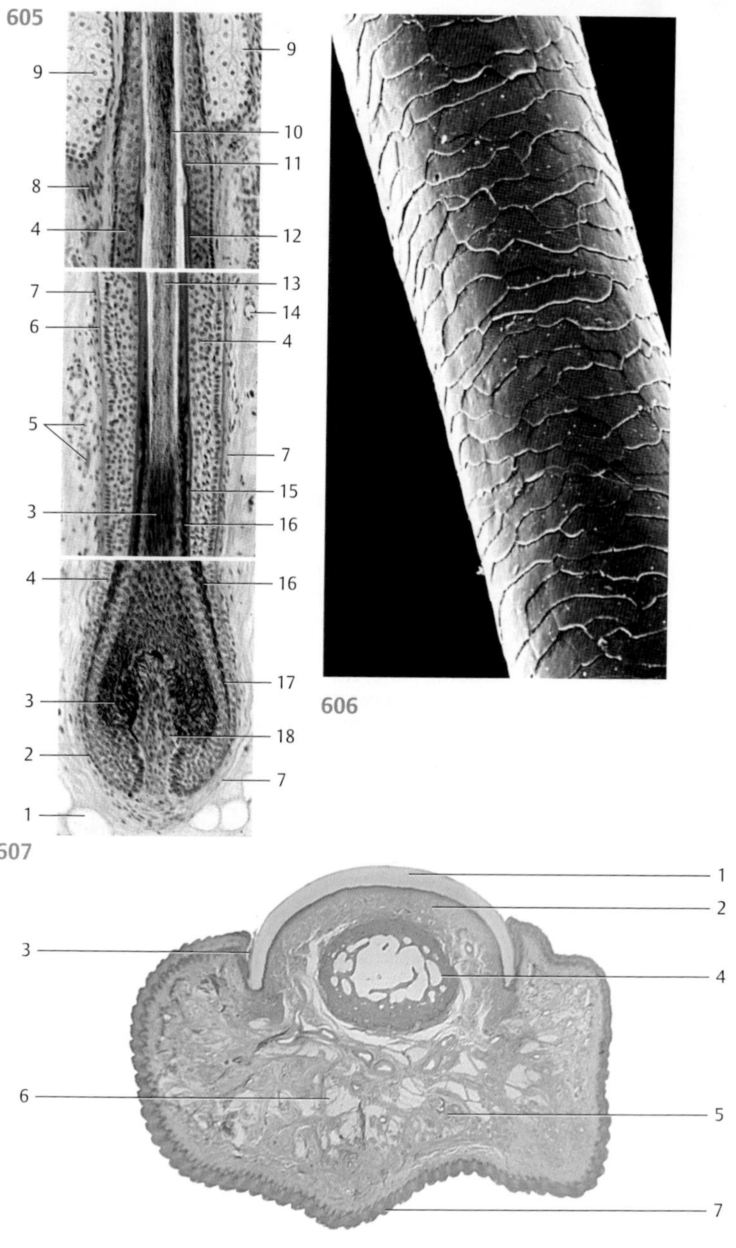
605
9
9
10
11
8
4
12
7
13
14
6
4
5
7
15
3
16
4
16
17
3
18
2
7
1
606
607
1
2
3
4
6
5
7

608 Eccrine Sweat Glands—Glandulae Sudoriferae Eccrinae

The eccrine (*merocrine*) sweat glands are long unbranched tubular glands. The final parts of the tubules form a 0.5 mm large coil at the interface between the dermis and the subcutaneous tissue (*coiled gland*). The secretory ducts 1 undulate strongly and end on the summits of the skin lamellae (see Figs. 598, 600). The wall of the secretory segment of the tubules 2 consists of a single-layered (simple) cuboidal to columnar epithelium. It always appears lighter than that of the secretory ducts in stained preparations. The ducts are clearly visible as short tubules. These are lined by a two-layered epithelium. Note the large adipocytes 3 and the apocrine sweat glands 4 in the lower left corner.

1 Secretory duct
2 Secretory tubule
3 Adipocytes
4 Apocrine sweat gland
Stain: Masson-Goldner trichrome; magnification: × 130

609 Apocrine Sweat Gland—Glandulae Sudoriferae Apocrinae—Scent Glands

Scent glands only occur in specialized parts of the human skin. In line with their development, they end in the hair follicles. Like the eccrine sweat glands, the tubuloalveolar terminal portions of the apocrine sweat glands are coiled. They have wide lumina and are lined by a single-layered epithelium. Dependent on their functional state, the secreting epithelial cells show different shapes. This figure shows several tubuli with a flattened epithelium: *exhausted gland cells* 1. The center of the image depicts gland segments with a high epithelium and dome-like cytoplasmic protrusions 2, which bulge into the lumen. The protrusions are finally pinched off as vesicles: *apocrine extrusion, apocytosis* (cf. Fig. 133). Spindle-shaped myoepithelial cells 3 occur between epithelium and basal membrane. Parallel sections are used to evaluate their morphology (see Fig. 610).

1 Tubules with exhausted secretory cells
2 Tubules with columnar secretory cells and cytoplasmic domes
3 Myoepithelium
Stain: Masson-Goldner trichrome; magnification: × 130

610 Apocrine Sweat Gland—Glandulae Sudoriferae Apocrinae—Scent Glands

Myoepithelial cells are particularly abundant and easy to find in the tubules of the *apocrine scent glands* (cf. Fig. 611). The rod-shaped *myoepithelial cells* occur between epithelium and basal membrane. They are usually arranged longitudinally in the direction of the gland tubules. Therefore, cross-sections only show spot-like structures at the basis of the cell. Only parallel sections can reveal their structure. Myoepithelial cells contain actin and myosin filaments.

1 Myoepithelial cells
2 Cytoplasmic dome
Stain: Masson-Goldner trichrome; magnification: × 130

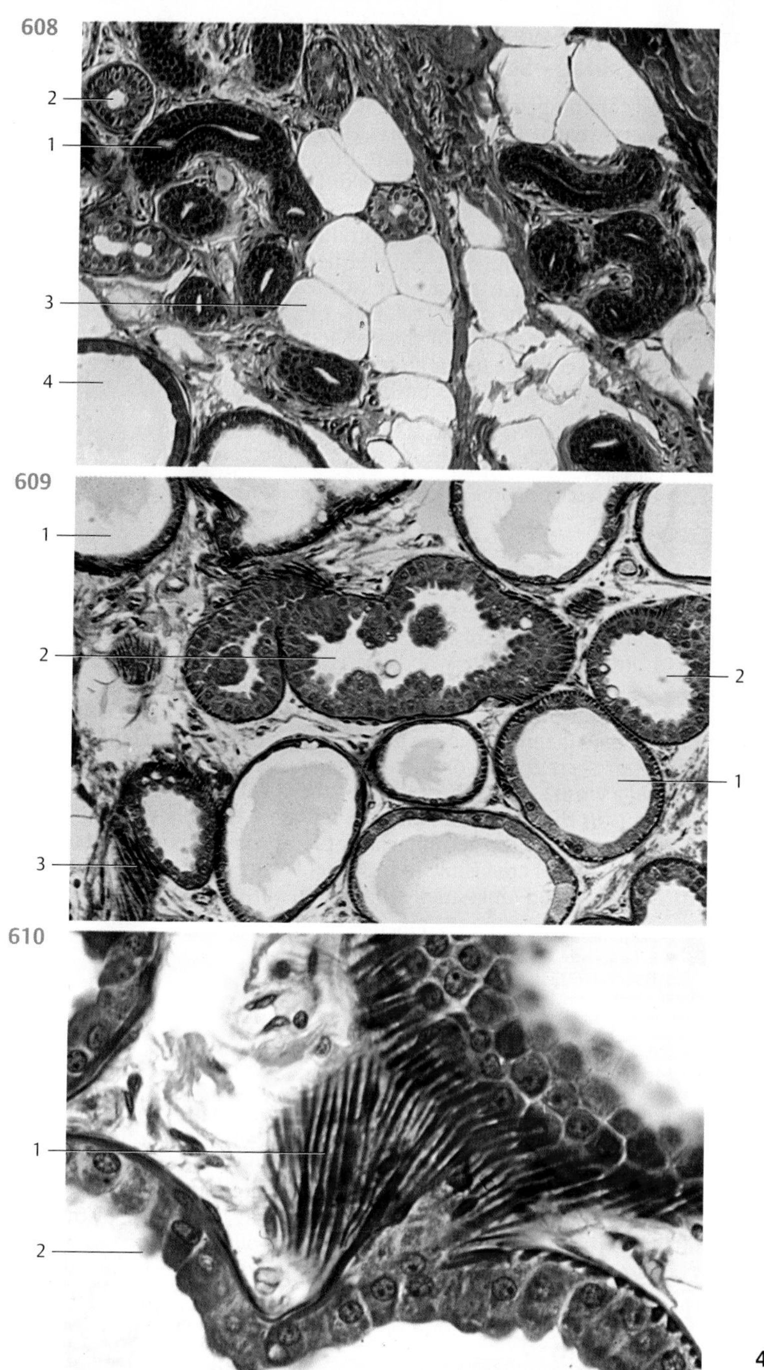

Integumentary System, Skin

611 Apocrine Sweat Gland—Glandulae Sudoriferae Apocrinae—Scent Glands

Scent glands are branched tubuloalveolar glands, which release their products by apocrine extrusion (*apocytosis*). They are located in the subcutaneous tissue close to the hairs and arise from their germ. Their characteristics include wide lumina and epithelial cells of different heights. The epithelium of the gland cells contains several secretory granules. The dome-like plasmalemma protrusions enclose secretory products. The protrusions are pinched off as secretory vesicles into the gland lumen (*apocrine secretion*). Small homogeneous sections of particularly well-developed myoepithelial cells 2 are found at the bases of the glands (cf. Figs. 133, 609, 610). They reside in the basal membrane. The height of the epithelium varies with the functional status. The gland cells are lower after secretory vacuoles have been pinched off (see Fig. 609). Axillary skin from an adult woman.

1 Apical cytoplasmic protrusions
2 Myoepithelial cells
3 Capillaries
Semi-thin section; stain: methylene blue-azure II; magnification: × 400

612 Holocrine Sebaceous Glands

Sebaceous glands (*glandulae sebaceae*) are associated with hair follicles. The alveolar glands have a size of approximately 1 mm. They end in the outer root sheath 2. In the skin of a few body parts also occur free sebaceous glands (not associated with hairs). This figure shows several rounded sacs (alveoli), which are only incompletely separated from each other. Sebaceous glands are multilayered glands without a lumen of their own (cf. Fig. 134). The gland cells die after secretion is completed (*apoptosis*)—i.e., they are turned into sebum (*holocytosis*). The substitution of these cells begins with the outer basal cells 1 in the basal membrane. They are basophilic and their entire population represents the germinal layer of the sebaceous glands. Light cells with pyknotic nuclei are visible in the inner sebaceous acini. The outer root sheath 2 is sectioned tangentially (upper left of the figure).

1 Basal substitute cells (germinal cells)
2 External root sheath
3 Connective tissue
Stain: Masson-Goldner trichrome; magnification: × 80

613 Holocrine Sebaceous Glands

This parallel section of several alveoli of sebaceous glands shows peripheral basal or germinal cells 1. The cells are basophilic and appear homogeneous, although small granules are sporadically found. While accumulating secretory product, the cell size and number of fat droplets increase. This explains the vacuoles in routine preparations. The nuclei become pyknotic and disintegrate. The nuclei in this image are already very deformed. Finally, the cells burst open and become part of the sebum (cf. Figs. 134, 612).

1 Basal germinal cells (matrix cells)
Semi-thin section; stain: methylene blue-azure II; magnification: × 200

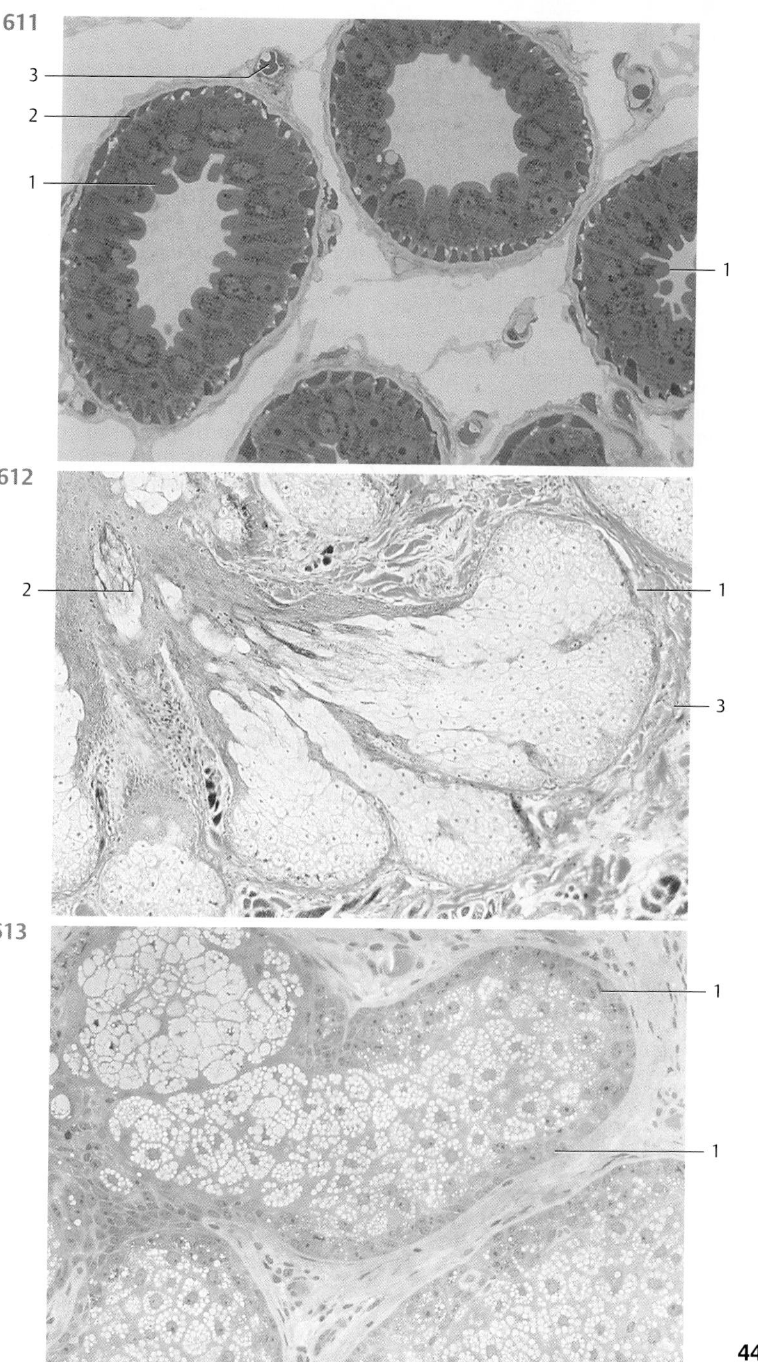
611
3
2
1
1
612
2
1
3
613
1
1

614 Merkel Nerve Endings

Free nerve endings are found in the dermis, the locomotor system and the walls of hollow organs. In addition to these nerve endings, the dermis features *Merkel mechanoreceptors* (Merkel's disks) as specialized nerve endings. They are located in the stratum basale of the epidermis, among other locations. This figure describes Merkel's nerve endings in the epidermis of the nasal planum of a cat. The nerve endings extend from the *ellipsoid Merkel cell* 1. The longitudinal cell axis measures about 9–20 μm. The axon terminates in the *Merkel disk* 2. The Merkel cell nucleus is large and lobed. Merkel cells are connected via desmosomes 4 with the neighboring *keratinocytes* 3 of the epidermal stratum basale. Finger-shaped Merkel cell processes can reach across the intercellular space as far as to the stratum spinosum. The cytoplasm is light. It contains microfilaments and many osmiophilic granules with diameters of 80–120 nm. The granules are mostly found in the cytoplasmic area, which establishes contact with the nerve endings. The *afferent nerve fiber* is initially myelinated (not shown). Shortly before the papillary layer and close to the stratum basale of the epidermis, myelination discontinues and the axon forms a disk-like bulge, which connects to the basal surface of the Merkel cell. There may be synapse-like interactions at this interface.

The right side of this figure represents the basal part of the Merkel nerve ending.

1 Merkel cell
2 Nerve disk with mitochondria
3 Keratinocytes of the epidermal stratum basale
4 Desmosomes
Electron microscopy; magnification: × 10 000

615 Meissner's Corpuscles

Meissner's corpuscles (tactile corpuscles) are part of a group of lamellar bodies. There are lamellar bodies with or without a perineural capsule. Meissner's corpuscles 1 occur singular or in small groups directly underneath the epidermis 2 in the *dermal connective tissue papillae* of the papillary layer. The oval Meissner corpuscles are 100–150 μm long and about 40–70 μm wide bodies. A loosely structured connective tissue capsule envelops them. Up to seven *afferent nerve fibers* 3 approach the tactile Meissner corpuscle, lose their myelin sheath and branch several times inside the corpuscle. The fibers progress as spirals and end as wide *nerve terminals* (see Fig. 616). The nucleated part of the Schwann cells and their stacked cytoplasmic processes (lamellae) cannot be recognized in this figure.

1 Meissner's corpuscle
2 Epidermis
3 Afferent nerve fibers
4 Dermal connective tissue papilla
5 Reticular layer of the dermis
Stain: Bodian silver impregnation; magnification: × 500

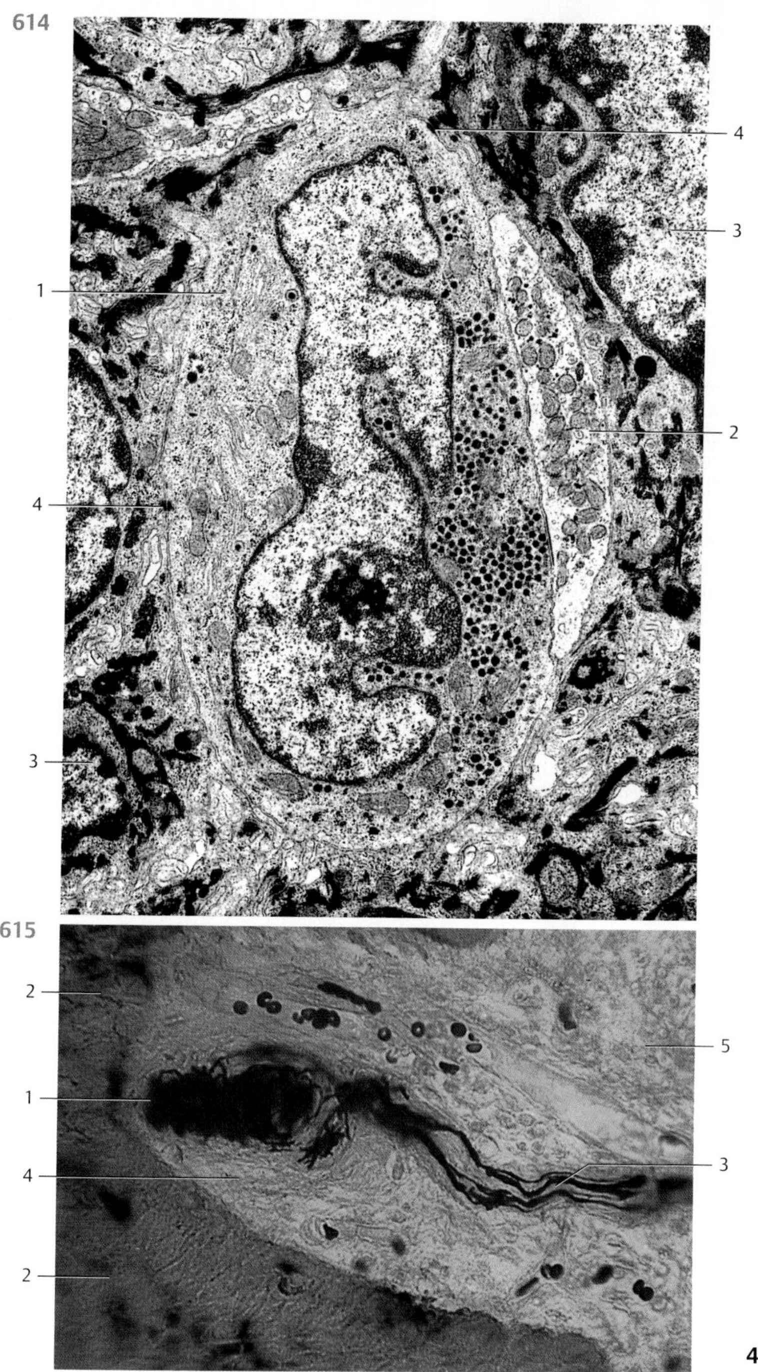
614
4
3
1
2
4
3
615
2
5
1
3
4
2

616 Meissner's Corpuscles

Meissner's tactile corpuscles occur singular or in small groups in the dermal papillae immediately underneath the epidermis. They are long oval and positioned vertical to the skin surface. Meissner's corpuscles are about 40–70 µm wide and 100–150 µm long and consist of myelinated afferent nerve fibers with wide, plate-like *nerve terminals* 1. Apposed cytoplasmic processes of Schwann cells and a connective tissue capsule encase the terminals. Approximately seven myelinated afferent axons are found per corpuscle. The axons lose their myelin sheaths only upon entering the corpuscle. Inside the corpuscle, the individual axons branch several times. The branches form helices and end with wide terminals. The longitudinal axis of these wide, plate-like terminals are arranged parallel to the skin surface. The nuclei of the Schwann cells 3 are found at the periphery of the corpuscle. Schwann cells send narrow, flat cytoplasmic processes (lamellae) toward the center of the corpuscle. The processes envelop the nerve terminals. The sheaths consist of several cytoplasmic processes (*Schwann cell lamellae*) 2. Collagen fibrils occur between the processes and continue in the connective tissue of the dermal papillary layer 5.
The figure shows a Meissner corpuscle from the fingertip of a rhesus monkey. The Meissner tactile corpuscle is located in the dermal papilla next to the basal membrane of the epidermal stratum basale 4 (cf. Fig. 600). Note the cells of the basal layer, which extend delicate cell processes (*root pedicles*, cf. Fig. 93) into the connective tissue of the papillary layer 5. Meissner's tactile corpuscles are *mechanoreceptors*, which react to pressure and *adapt* with medium speed.

1 Nerve terminals
2 Cytoplasmic processes of Schwann cells
3 Nuclei of Schwann cells
4 Cells of the stratum basale with root pedicles
5 Dermal papillary layer
Electron microscopy; magnification: × 3800

617 Vater-Pacini Corpuscles

Vater-Pacini corpuscles (*Pacinian corpuscles, large lamellated corpuscles*) are up to 4 mm long and 2 mm thick. Their giant size makes them easy to detect, e.g., in the subcutaneous tissue of the palms of the hand and the soles of the feet and proximal phalanxes as well as in the vicinity of fasciae, periosteum and tendons, also in mesenteric tissue and the pancreas. The sheaths of these terminal nerve systems are a characteristic attribute. They consist of 40–60 concentric layers of cytoplasmic processes (*perineural lamellae*) in an onion-like arrangement 1. The nerve fiber is found in the center (*inner afferent axon*) 2. The connective tissue capsule around the corpuscle contains a meshwork of elastic fibers.
Human fingertip. Vater-Pacini corpuscles are *pressure* and *vibration receptors.*

1 Lamellae of the perineural capsule
2 Central nerve fiber
3 Dense connective tissue capsule
4 Adipose tissue
Stain: alum hematoxylin-eosin; magnification: × 30

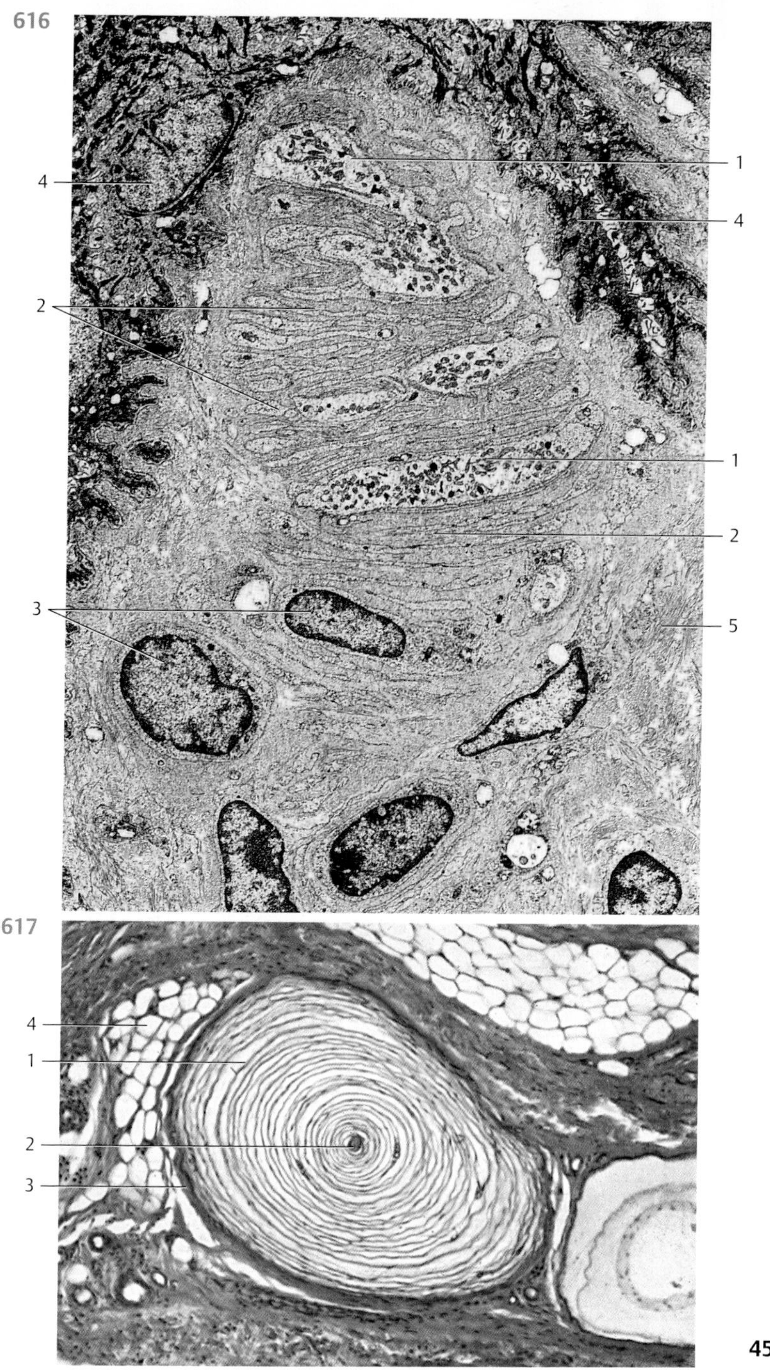
616
1
4
4
2
1
2
3
5
617
4
1
2
3

618 Vater-Pacini Corpuscles

Vater-Pacini lamellated corpuscle from the fingertip of a rhesus monkey. The *afferent axon* is visible in the center. The lamellae of the cytoplasmic Schwann cell processes form the *inner bulb* around the axon (*bulbus internus*). The outer layers are part of the perineural sheath 2 (cf. Fig 617). Very fine connective tissue fibers traverse the lamellar cell processes. The lower right corner of the figure displays a myelinated axon 3, which is attached to the Vater-Pacini corpuscle. An eccrine sweat gland is visible in the right upper corner.
Receptors of the Vater-Pacini corpuscles recognize *vibration.*

1 Inner bulb with afferent axon
2 Layers of the perineural sheath
3 Myelinated axon
4 Capillary
Electron microscopy; magnification: × 350

619 Vater-Pacini Corpuscles

Several oval *Vater-Pacini lamellated corpuscles* from the mesenteric tissue of a cat are shown in this whole-mount preparation (not sectioned). This preparation was stained using methylene blue. It was then bleached. The center consists of axon and *inner bulb*, the surrounding layers form the *perineural sheath*. The thin connective tissue capsule on the surface of the lamellar corpuscle is also visible. All Vater-Pacini corpuscles in this figure are arranged around a mesenteric vessel 1.

1 Mesenteric vessel
Stain: methylene blue; magnification: × 500

620 Golgi-Mazzoni Corpuscles

The sensory corpuscles resemble Vater-Pacini lamellated corpuscles (cf. Figs. 617–619). There are fewer *perineural lamellae* in Golgi-Mazzoni corpuscles. As in Vater-Pacini corpuscles, an afferent axon 1 and *inner bulb* of Schwann cell lamellae are found in the center. However, there are often two or more axons with inner bulbs in one corpuscle. The outer layers build the *perineural sheath* 2.
The figure also shows arterioles 3 and a vein 4 (upper right). Golgi-Mazzoni corpuscles are found in the skin of the fingers, in the nail bed and in the skin of the outer genitals (*genital nerve corpuscles*). They contain tactile mechanoreceptors, which respond to skin movement due to pressure and touch.

1 Central afferent axon and inner bulb
2 Lamellae of the perineural sheath
3 Arterioles
4 Vein
Stain: alum hematoxylin-eosin; magnification: × 300

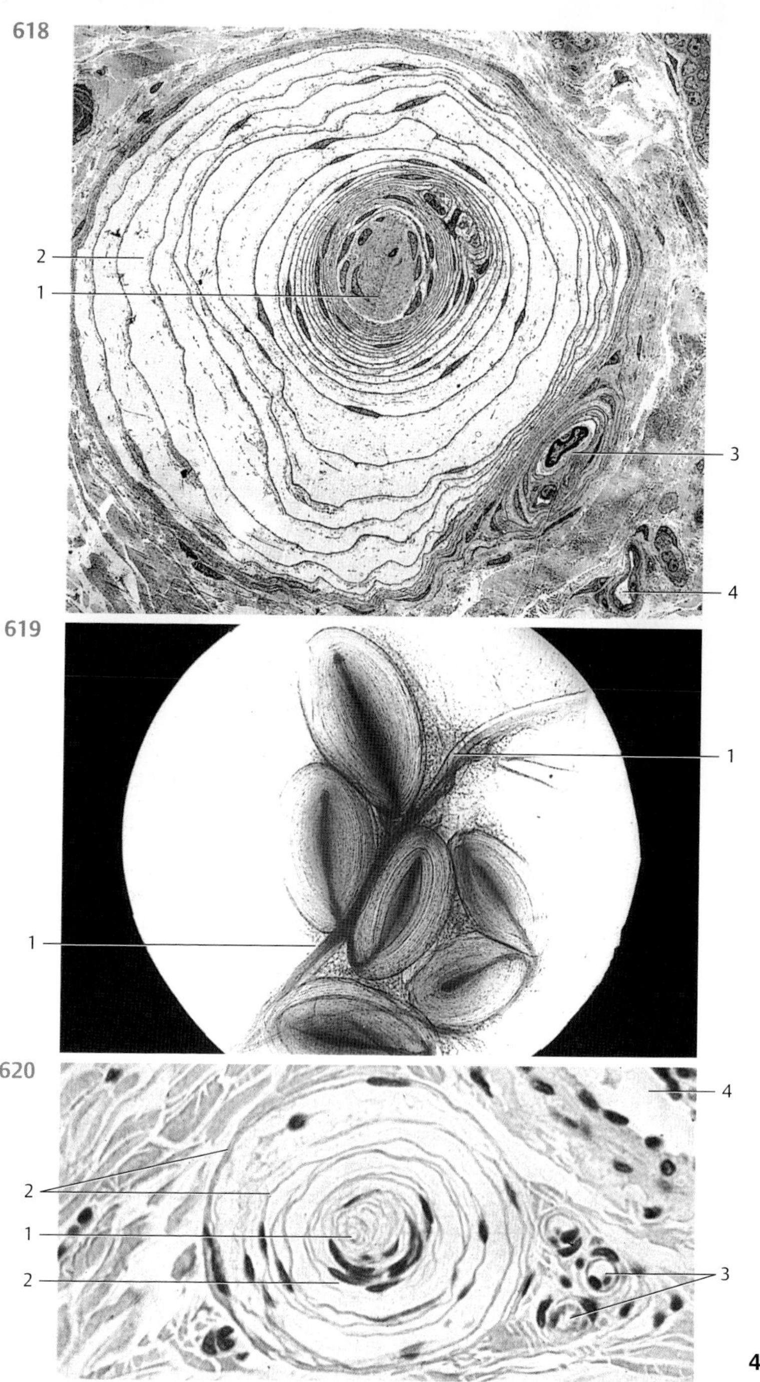
618
2
1
3
4
619
1
1
620
4
2
1
2
3

621 Ruffini's Corpuscles

Ruffini's corpuscles are Stretch receptors. They occur, for example, in the skin, in joint capsules and in the periodontium. The perineural sheath [1] of the corpuscle forms an open cylinder. Both the ends of the cylinder are either rounded or pointed. Dermal collagen fiber bundles traverse the cylinder from end to end. Helical *nerve terminals* are interspersed between the fibers. The *myelinated afferent axon* has a diameter of 5 μm. The collagen fiber bundles [3] in this preparation are stained light brown. The nerve terminals appear black.

1 Perineural sheath
2 Nerve fiber bundle
3 Collagen fiber bundle
4 Connective tissue of the glans penis
Stain: Bodian silver stain; magnification: × 170

622 Ruffini's Corpuscles

Cross-section of the cylinder of *Ruffini's corpuscle* from the knee joint capsule with *perineural sheath* [1]. Several nerve terminals are visible between the collagen fiber bundles inside the cylinder [2]. There are also Schwann cells [4].

1 Perineural sheath
2 Collagen fiber bundles inside the cylinder of Ruffini's corpuscle
3 Nerve terminals
4 Schwann cell
5 Collagen fibril bundle outside the cylinder of Ruffini's corpuscle
Electron microscopy; magnification: × 2000

623 Neuromuscular Spindle—Fusus Neuromuscularis

Neuromuscular spindles (Stretch receptors) are 2–10 mm long and 0.2–0.5 mm thick. They are embedded in *perimysium internum*, which consists of muscular connective tissue. The spindle consists of the *equatorial region* and the tapered *pole regions*. Concentric layers of strong connective tissue fibers (*perineurium*) form the capsule [1]. Five to 10 thin *intrafusal* muscle fibers [2] with a reduced number of fibrils are found in the center. Endomysial cells surround them. There are two groups of intrafusal muscle fibers, dependent on the configuration of their nuclei in the equatorial segment (central segment). The nuclei either form short, thin rows (*nuclear chain fibers)* or occur in piles (*static nuclear bag fibers*). Sensory and vegetative nerves as well as motor nerve fibers penetrate the corpuscular capsule. The helical nerve fibers circumscribe and innervate the central intrafusal muscle fiber. There are *nerve terminals*. Several small rounded cell nuclei are found in the center. They are part of the neurolemma.
Cross-section of a neuromuscular spindle.

1 Perineural sheath
2 Intrafusal nerve fibers
3 Axonal terminals
4 Skeletal muscle fibers
Stain: Heidenhain iron hematoxylin; magnification: × 500

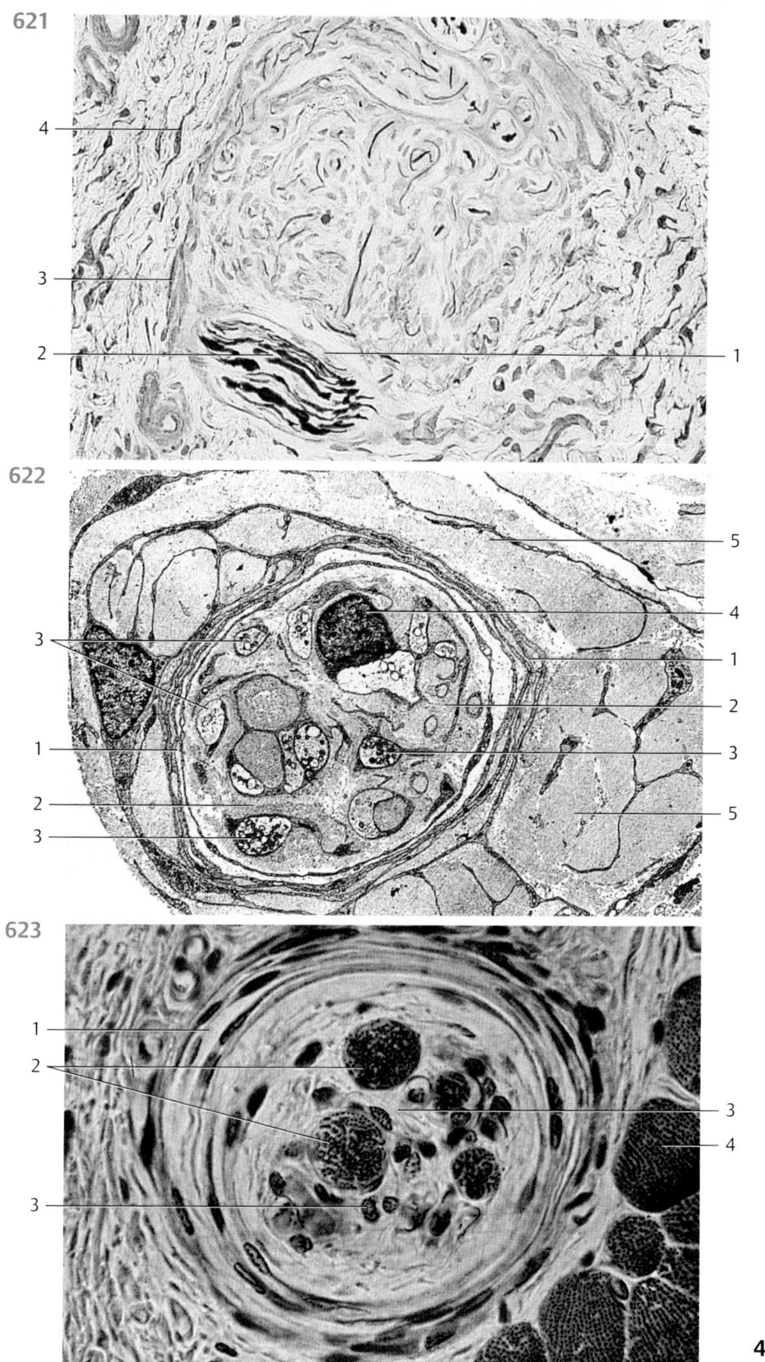
621
4
3
2
1
622
5
4
3
1
2
1
3
2
5
3
623
1
2
3
4
3

624 Eyeball—Bulbus Oculi

Horizontal center section of the left eyeball (*bulbus oculi*).

1 Cornea
2 Anterior camera oculi, anterior chamber of the eye
3 Iris
4 Lens
5 Posterior camera oculi, posterior chamber of the eye
6 Corpus ciliare, ciliary body
7 Sclera, tunica fibrosa bulbi
8 Corpus vitreum, vitreous body
9 Retina
10 Optic nerve
Stain: hematoxylin-eosin; magnifying glass

625 Eyelids—Palpebrae

Eyelids are skin folds, which can be actively moved. They consist of a tough connective tissue skeleton 1 (*tarsus superior* and *tarsus inferior*). Toward the outside, it is covered by the musculus orbicularis oculi (pars palpebralis) 2. The surface covering of the eyelid is a multilayered keratinizing squamous epithelium with only a few velum hairs. The outer lid is about 2 mm wide and consists of a dull anterior 4 and a sharp-edged posterior palpebral limb 5. This tissue continues in the multilayered nonkeratinizing squamous epithelium of the palpebral part of the conjunctiva (*conjunctiva tarsi*) 6. A multilayered columnar epithelium with goblet cells is only found beyond the level of the fornix of the conjunctiva. Long cilia (*eyelashes*) 7 protrude from the anterior rim of the lid. They are rooted in the lid plate (see Fig. 626). The *sebaceous glands* (*Zeis glands*), *apocrine scent glands* and the *sweat glands of the cilia* (*Moll glands*) end in the hair follicle of the eyelashes. The right side of the figure shows numerous tarsal holocrine sebaceous glands (Meibomian glands) 8 with long secretory ducts that end on the anterior edge of the lid (*posterior limbus*). The tight tarsal fiber meshwork envelops the lobed glands. Smooth muscle cells run both before and behind the Meibomian glands at the rim of the lid. The palpebral part of the musculus orbicularis oculi 2 is located in front of the tarsus. The subcutaneous tissue of the lid consists of loosely structured, cell-rich connective tissue 9, which is usually free of adipose tissue. The epithelium on the anterior eyelid is thin. The skin of the lids contains many melanocytes. This explains the dark pigmentation.

1 Tarsus
2 Palpebral part of the orbicularis oculi muscle
3 Skin
4 Anterior palpebral limb
5 Posterior palpebral limb
6 Palpebral part of the conjunctiva
7 Eyelashes
8 Tarsal glands, Meibomian glands
9 Loosely structured subcutaneous connective tissue
10 Deep skin fold of the upper lid
11 Chalazion (infection of the Meibomian gland)
Stain: hematoxylin-eosin; magnifying glass

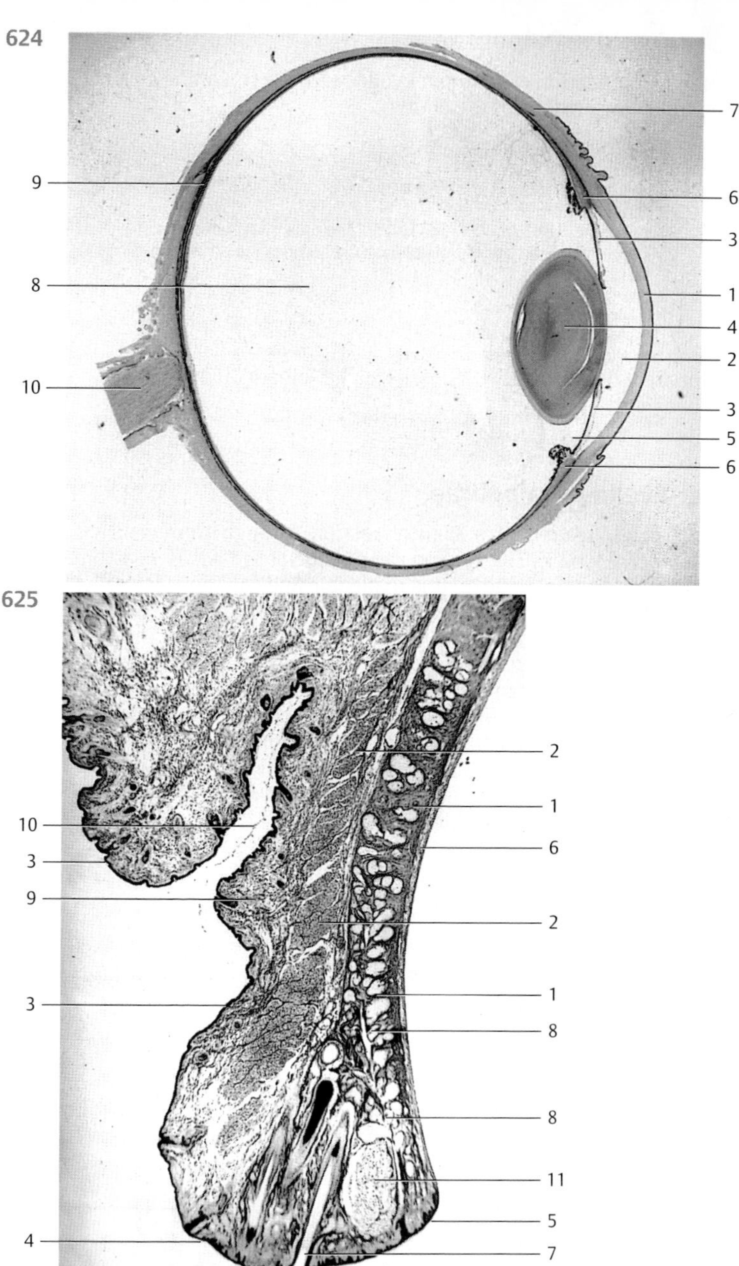
624
9
8
10
7
6
3
1
4
2
3
5
6
625
10
3
9
3
4
2
1
6
2
1
8
8
11
5
7

626 Eyelids—Palpebrae

Detail magnification of an upper eyelid, with the rim of the lid and eyelashes. The following structures are shown:

1 Rim (edge) of the lid
2 Hair funnel
3 Hair shaft, scapus pili of the eyelash
4 Outer root sheath
5 Rim of the eyelid, multilayered keratinizing squamous epithelium
6 The terminal portions of a Meibomian gland end in the hair follicle clearance
8 Tarsus superior
9 Hair bulb
10 Hair papilla
11 Subcutaneous tissue of the lids

Compare with Figs. 625–629. Heinrich J. Meibom (1638–1700).

Stain: alum hematoxylin-eosin; magnification: × 10

627 Eyelids—Palpebrae

Detail magnification of a sagittal section through the eyelid of an adult human (cf. Fig. 625). The skin on the outside of the lids is very thin. There is usually no adipose tissue [1]. It is malleable and can move laterally. Keratinization of the multilayered squamous epithelium of the epidermis is marginal. Dermis and subcutaneous connective tissue are thin. The dermis of the skin on the lid contains branched *chromatophores*. The palpebral part of the striated *musculus orbicularis oculi* [3] is shown in the lower right corner of the microphotograph. Part of the sebaceous follicle of a holocrine Meibomian gland [4] is visible in the upper right of the figure [4].

1 Skin of the eyelid
2 Subcutaneous tissue
3 Palpebral part of the orbicularis oculi muscle
4 Meibomian gland
Stain: alum hematoxylin-eosin; magnification: × 20

628 Eyelids—Palpebrae

The inner face of the eyelids is lined by the moist mucous membrane of the palpebral part of the tunica conjunctiva, which is part of the conjunctival sac. The keratinizing squamous epithelium of the skin of the lid continues in the nonkeratinizing multilayered squamous epithelium of the palpebral part of the conjunctiva at the *posterior palpebral limb* (see Fig. 625). It is only at the *fornix conjunctivae* that a multilayered columnar epithelium is found.
The figure shows a sagittal section of the eyelid close to the fornix conjunctivae with conjunctival epithelium [1] and an underlying accumulation of lymphocytes [2]. The tunica propria [3] contains adipocytes [4].

1 Conjunctival epithelium
2 Accumulation of lymphocytes
3 Lamina propria
4 Adipocytes
Stain: alum hematoxylin-eosin; magnification: × 20

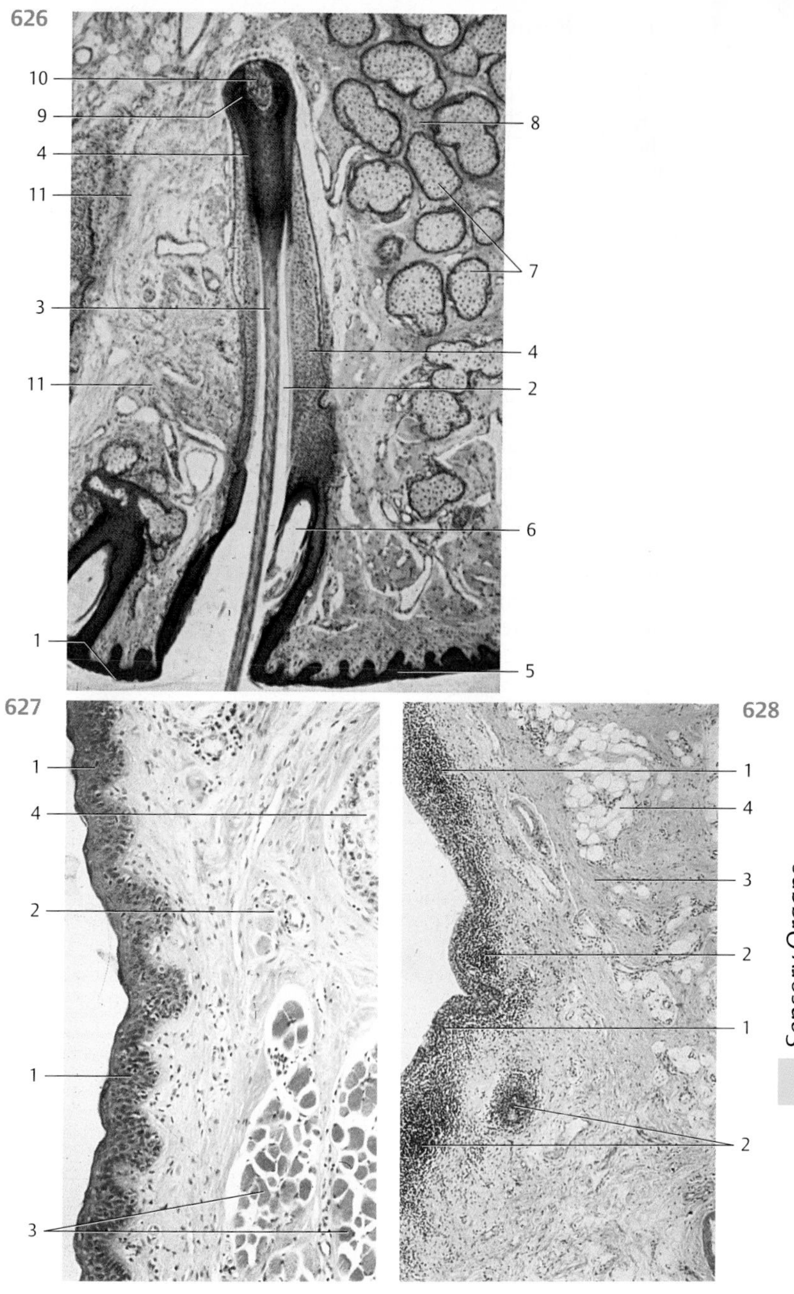
626
10
9
4
11
3
11
1
8
7
4
2
6
5
627
1
4
2
1
3
628
1
4
3
2
1
2

629 Eyelids—Palpebrae

Detail magnification of a sagittal section through the eyelid close to the rim of the lid. It shows the apocrine glands of Moll (*ciliary glands*) 1. They are located in the vicinity of the roots of the eyelashes and end at the rim of the lid or in the hair follicles. The glands of Moll are classified as sweat glands. There are striated muscle fiber bundles of the musculus orbicularis oculi 2 close to the glands. They can pull the rim of the lid to the eyeball (cf. Fig. 625).

1 Glands of Moll, apocrine sweat glands
2 Orbicularis oculi muscle
Stain: alum hematoxylin-eosin; magnification: × 20

630 Lacrimal Gland

The lacrimal gland has approximately the shape of an almond. It consists of lobes that are intersected by connective tissue septae. The lacrimal gland is a tubular, purely *serous gland* without intercalated ducts. The gland tubules end in intralobular ducts 1, which merge to larger ducts. About 8–12 ducts channel the tears to the *fornix conjunctivae*. In cross-sections, the acini of the lacrimal gland resemble those of the parotid glands. They show all the morphological criteria of serous glands (cf. Figs. 129, 379–381). The secretory cells often show a fine cytoplasmic granulation (see Fig. 632). The interstitial connective tissue is sometimes rich in lymphocytes and plasma cells. With increasing age, there are often also adipocytes 2.

1 Intralobular ducts
2 Adipocytes
3 Artery
Stain: azan; magnification: × 80

631 Lacrimal Gland

The tubules of the *lacrimal gland* often have wide lumina. They are therefore often referred to as *tubuloalveolar glands*. The irregularly shaped tubules can be clearly assessed at higher magnification. Note the shape of the gland cells (secretory cells) (cf. Fig. 630). The round nuclei are in basal position. The cytoplasm appears light, and cell borders can be clearly recognized in some places. *Myoepithelial cells* are found between the gland epithelium and the basal membrane. Note the delicate connective tissue between the tubules (here stained blue).
The secretory product of the lacrimal glands (tears) moisturizes the cornea and the conjunctiva of the eyeball as well as the eyelids.

Stain: azan; magnification: × 200

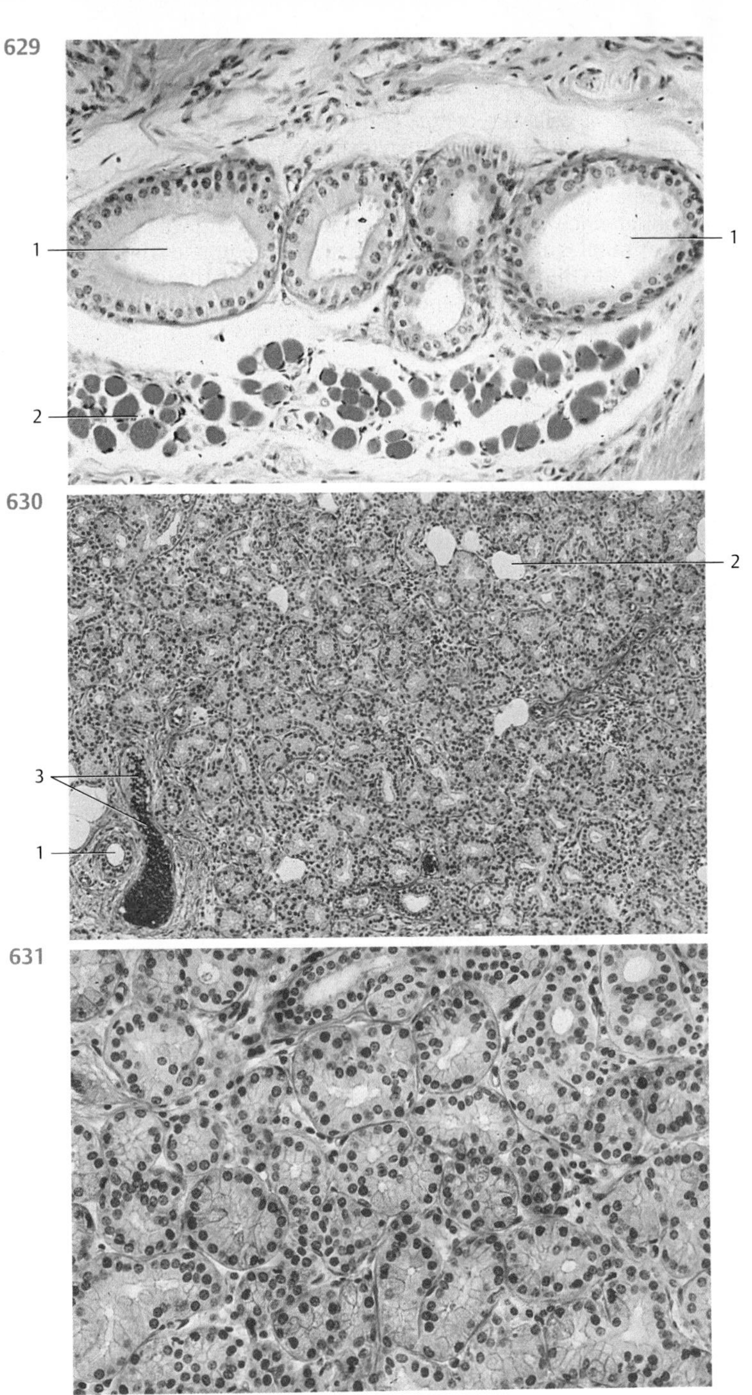

Sensory Organs

632 Lacrimal Gland

The varieties of secretory products of the exocrine and endocrine gland cells are stored in the cells as secretory granules or secretory droplets. Intracellularly stored secretory granules may display a variety of appearances. The figure shows three acinar cells of the lacrimal gland. The secretory granules appear either homogeneous 1 or show low electron microscopic densities. They contain finely dispersed secretory particles. As shown in the figure, the secretory granules are released individually in response to stimuli. Microvilli 3 protrude into the acinar lumen. Note the granule in the lumen 7. It has already lost part of its membrane. The lateral surfaces of the secretory cells show apical junctional complexes (terminal bars) 456 .

1 Secretory granules
2 Mitochondrion
3 Microvilli
4 Zonula occludens
5 Zonula adherens
6 Desmosome
7 Secretory granule in the acinar lumen
Electron microscopy; magnification: × 25 000

633 Cornea

View of the surface of the corneal epithelium (*surface cells, superficial cells*). The polygonal cells are flattened and about 5 µm thick, with diameters up to 50 µm. Their nuclei protrude slightly 1. The surface cells are sloughed off continuously and replaced. The large cell in the center of the figure is about to detach. The cells of the next lower layer contain fine, dense surface plicae 2, which serve the intercellular attachment. Compare the surface view of this tissue with the sections in figures 117, 634–636).
The cornea consists of five layers:

1 Epithelium
2 Lamina limitans anterior (Bowman's membrane)
3 Stroma
4 Lamina limitans posterior (Descemet's membrane)
5 Endothelium (see Figs. 634–636)
Scanning electron microscopy; magnification: × 2000

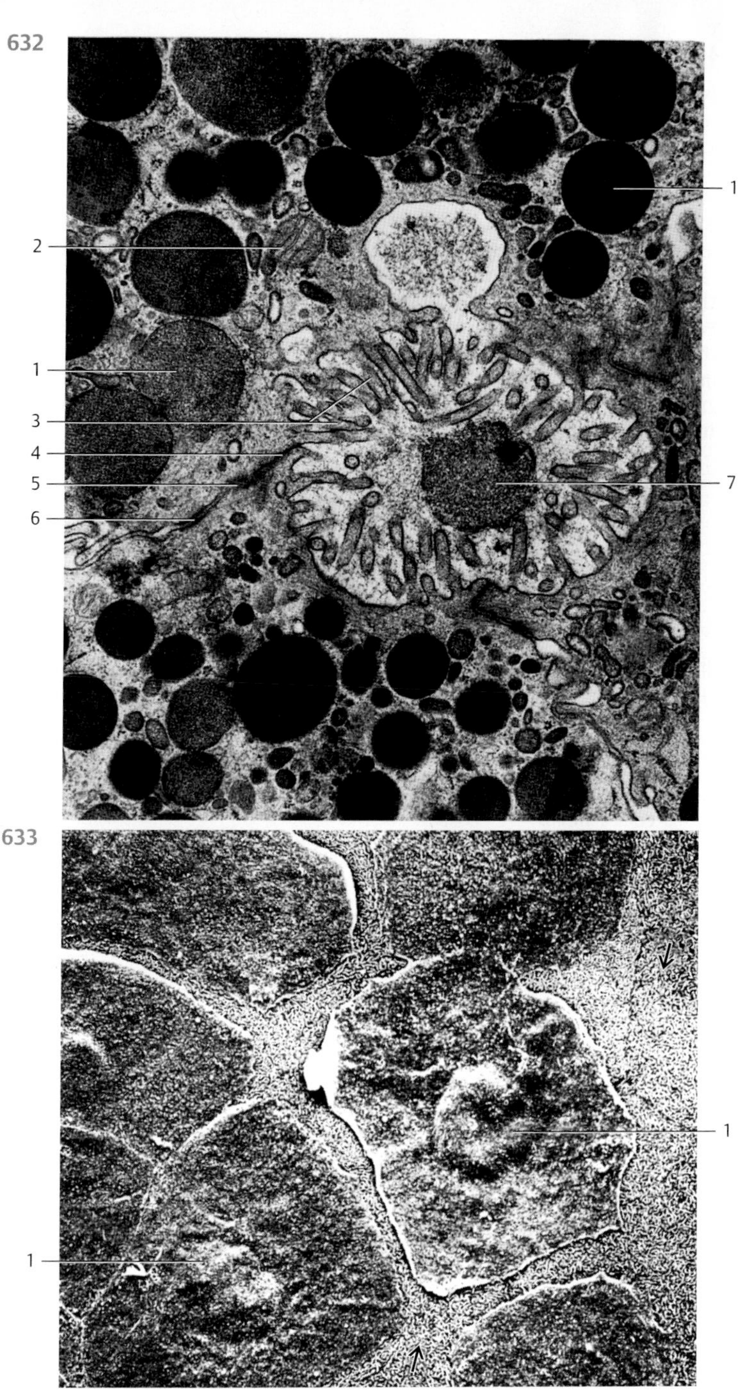

Sensory Organs

634 Cornea

This vertical section through the cornea provides a clear image of the layered structure. The outer covering consists of five or six layers of nonkeratinizing cells (*multilayered nonkeratinizing squamous epithelium*) [1] (cf. Figs. 117, 635, 636). It is about 70 μm high and is supported by a basal membrane. The *limiting lamina* (*Bowman's membrane*) [2] follows as a relatively wide layer (see Figs. 635–637). The thick corneal stroma (*substantia propria corneae*) [3] features 200–250 densely stacked lamellae about 2 μm thick, with interleaved parallel oriented collagen fibrils (see Fig. 638). Fibrocytes (*keratinocytes*) with cytoplasmic processes ("branched fibrocytes"; see Fig. 639) are found between collagen fibrils. The corneal fibrocytes appear spindle-shaped in vertical sections (see Figs. 103, 117, 635, 636). The thinner *posterior limiting lamella* (*Descemet's membrane*) separates the corneal stroma from the about 5 μm thick posterior single-layered corneal epithelium (corneal endothelium) (cf. Figs. 103, 104, 640).

1 Anterior corneal epithelium
2 Anterior limiting lamina, Bowman's membrane
3 Corneal stroma, substantia propria corneae with fibrocytes (keratinocytes)
4 Posterior corneal epithelium (corneal endothelium)
Stain: alum hematoxylin-eosin; magnification: × 50

635 Cornea

Multilayered nonkeratinizing squamous epithelium of the cornea. There are *surface cells* [1], *intermediary cells* [2] and *basal cells* [3]. Compare with Fig. 636.

1 Surface cells
2 Intermediary cells
3 Basal cells
4 Anterior limiting lamina, Bowman's membrane
5 Corneal stroma
6 Keratinocyte
Stain: hematoxylin-eosin; magnification: × 500

636 Cornea

This vertical section of the cornea shows the *corneal epithelium*, *Bowman's membrane* and the *corneal stroma*. Note the different shapes of the basal cells [3] and compare them with those in Fig. 635. An intermediary cell often spans over two basal cells like an umbrella. The two uppermost layers consist of flattened, about 5 μm thick and up to 50 μm long flat surface cells [1] (see Fig. 633). The anterior limiting lamina (*Bowman's membrane*) [4] lies under the epithelium. The lower part of the figure shows the *corneal stroma* [5] with long spindle-shaped fibrocytes (*keratinocytes*) (cf. Fig. 639).

1 Surface cells
2 Intermediary cells
3 Basal cells
4 Bowman's membrane
5 Stroma corneae
Semi-thin section; stain: methylene blue-azure II; magnification: × 80

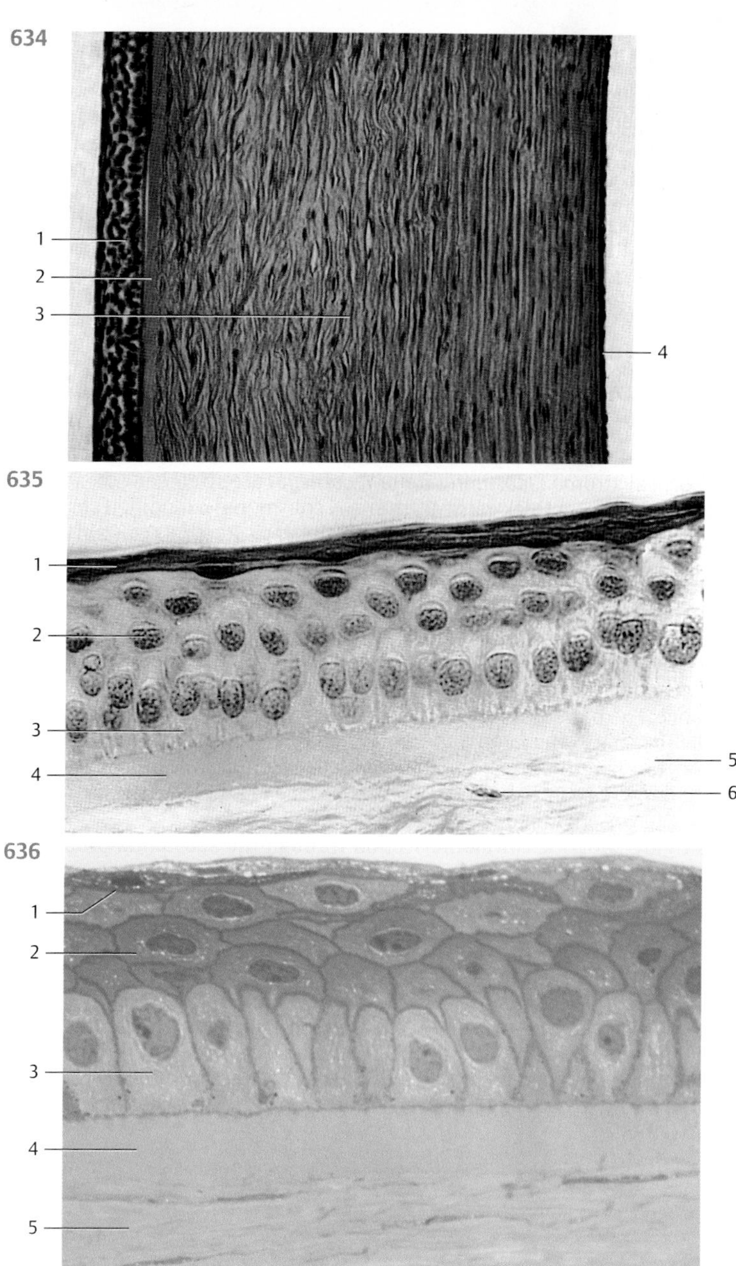

Sensory Organs

637 Cornea—Bowman's Membrane

Bowman's membrane (*anterior limiting lamina*) stretches underneath the subepithelial basal lamina. It appears homogeneous in light microscopic images and is about 8–14 µm thick. Bowman's membrane represents a modified condensed form of the substantia propria corneae. It is free of cells and shows a weakly positive PAS reaction. With 14–17 µm, the collagen fibrils of Bowman's membrane are thinner than the fibrils of the substantia propria. In addition to the collagen fibrils, the lamina contains a proteoglycan-rich basic substance (cf. Figs. 103, 117, 634, 636).

Electron microscopy; magnification: × 42 500

638 Cornea—Corneal Stroma

The sclera consists of a weave of tough undulating collagen fibers, which provide controlled plasticity and tensibility. In contrast, the collagen fibers of the corneal stroma (*substantia propria corneae*) are stretched (see Fig. 634). The about 500-µm thick corneal stroma is considered a modified connective tissue, which ascertains stability and translucency. Its fibrils contain *collagen types I, III, V and VII* and form parallel bundles with a cross-striation periodicity of 21 or 64 nm. The fibers form lamellae, which are layered parallel over the corneal surface. Lamellae are between 1 and 6 µm thick. There are therefore variable numbers of fibrils in each stack of lamellae. There are up to 250 lamellae. The direction of adjacent fibrils may be offset by an angle. However, the fibrils in each lamella are strictly parallel and stacked in equal distance. The basic substance predominantly consists of *glycosaminoglycans.* It fills the spaces between and inside the lamellae (*interfibrillar substance*). Fibrocytes (keratinocytes) and their branched cytoplasmic processes are embedded in the basic substance (not shown; see Figs. 636, 639). Sporadically, macrophages are found.
This figure shows a Vibratome section through the substantia propria corneae with its lamellar structure.

Scanning electron microscopy; magnification: × 700

639 Cornea

This parallel section through the corneal stroma shows the fibrocytes (*keratinocytes*) and their long, branched processes. The processes form a two-dimensional fibrocyte web, which is layered between the collagen lamellae (see Fig. 638). The applied impregnation technique does not stain the collagen lamellae.

Stain: gold chloride impregnation; magnification: × 200

637

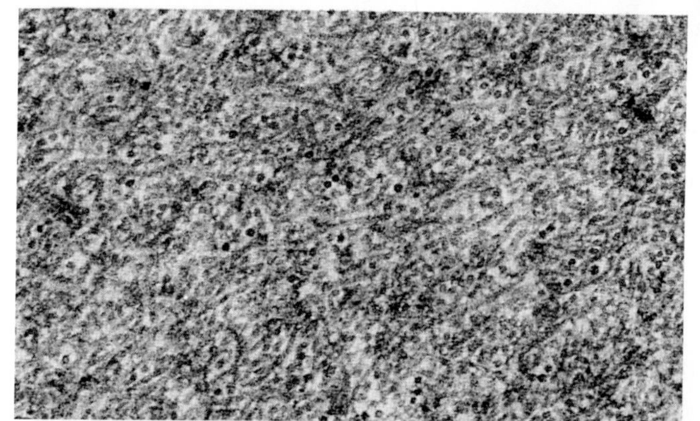

638

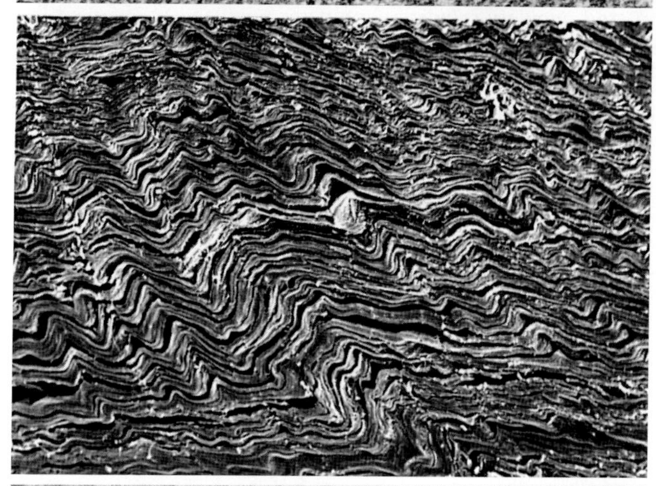

639

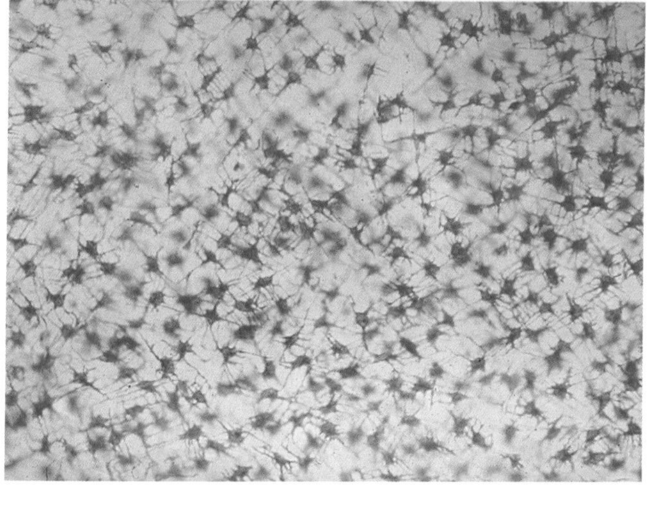

Sensory Organs

640 Cornea

Vertical section through the cornea. It shows the stroma corneae (*substantia propriae corneae*) [1] with spindle-shaped keratinocytes, *Descemet's membrane (posterior limiting lamina)* [2] and posterior corneal epithelium [3] (cf. Figs. 103, 636, 639). Descemet's membrane (basal membrane) is about 10 μm thick and shows a positive PAS reaction.

1 Corneal stroma with keratinocytes
2 Descemet's membrane, posterior limiting lamina
3 Posterior corneal epithelium (corneal endothelium)
Semi-thin section; stain: methylene blue-azure II; magnification: × 800

641 Iris

Section of the *iris* (detail enlargement) with *pigmented epithelium* [1], *iris dilator* [2] and *pupillary sphincter* (sphincter pupillae) [3]. The next layer is the stroma of the iris (*stroma iridis*) [4]. The border between iris and anterior chamber of the eye consists of a discontinuous mesothelium [6].

1 Pigmented epithelium
2 Iris dilator
3 Pupillary sphincter
4 Stroma of the iris
5 Vessels
6 Mesothelium of the anterior face of the iris
7 Crypts of Fuchs
8 Anterior chamber of the eye
Stain: alum hematoxylin-eosin; magnification: × 50

642 Iris and Lens

Section of the pupillary zone of the *iris* and the adjacent *lens* [6] (detail enlargement). The stroma of the iris [4] consists of collagen fiber bundles.

1 Pigmented epithelium
2 Pupillary sphincter
3 Iris dilator
4 Stroma of the iris
5 Ectropion
6 Lens
7 Anterior face of the lens
Stain: alum hematoxylin-eosin; magnification: × 50

643 Eye and Lens

The lens (see Fig. 624) consists of lens capsule (*capsula lentis*), the lens epithelium (*epithelium lentis*), *subcapsular epithelium* and the lens fibers (*fibrae lentis*). The lens fibers arise from the lens epithelium (see textbooks of embryology). Lens fibers are thin cells, 7–10 μm long and about 2-μm thick, containing crystallin. The cells lose their nuclei during development. They form long bands that appear hexagonal in cross-sections. The bands consist of concentric layers of radial lamellae. The lamellae are connected via focal desmosomes (junctional complexes). Interdigitations are present at the corner structures of the hexagonal lamellae. Note the focal desmosomes between intercellular processes. There are about 2300 lamellae in the adult human.

Scanning electron microscopy; magnification: × 4000

640

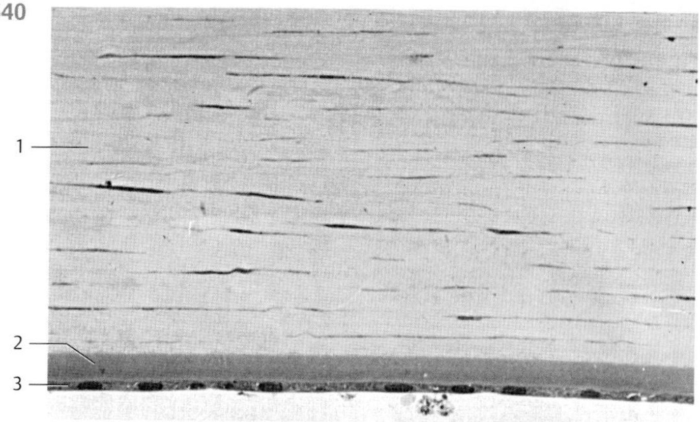

1
2
3

641

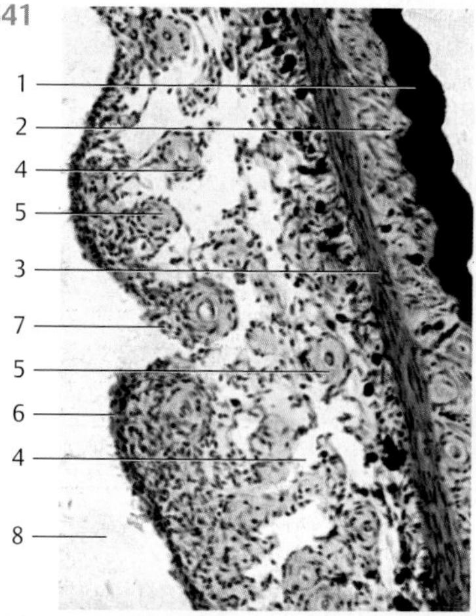

1
2
4
5
3
7
5
6
4
8

642

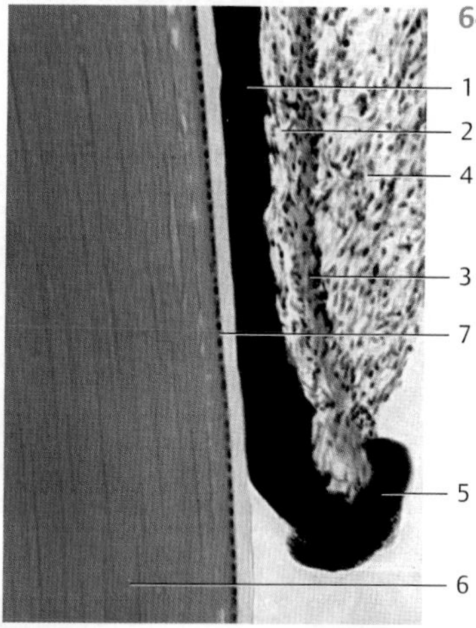

1
2
4
3
7
5
6

643

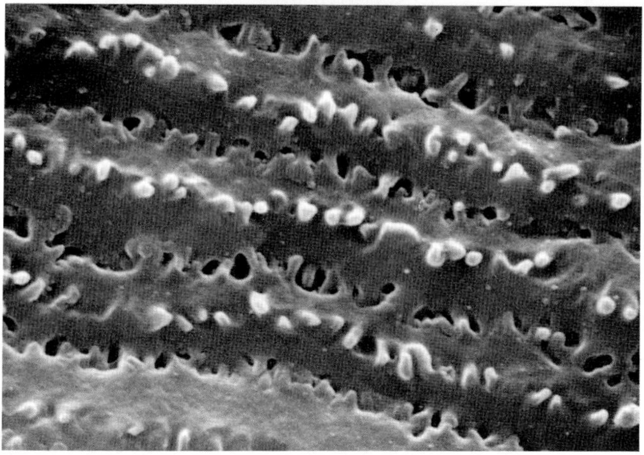

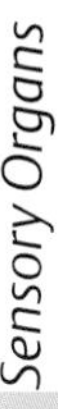

644 Angle of the Eye—Iridocorneal Angle

The upper part of the figure shows the *substantiae propriae sclerae* 1 and the *cornea* 2. The slits in the sclera represent the *canal of Schlemm* (sinus venosus sclerae). The *ciliary body* with the *ciliary muscle* 6 forms lamella-shaped *ciliary processes* with a thin *pars plana* and a *pars plicata*. The processes are covered by a two-layered epithelium, which is thought to produce the intraocular fluid. The pars plicata 8 features about 70 ciliary processes (see Fig. 645).

1 Substantia propria sclerae
2 Substantia propria corneae
3 Angle of the eye (Schwalbe's line)
4 Anterior chamber of the eye
5 Iris
6 Ciliary muscle
7 Pigmented epithelium of the iris
8 Ciliary processus

Stain: hematoxylin-eosin; magnification: × 40

645 Ciliary Processes and Zonula Filaments

The functions of the ciliary body are accommodation and the release of ocular fluid. Both parts of the ciliary body (see Fig. 644) are covered by a two-layered epithelium. The suspensor filaments for the lens (*zonula filaments, zonula lentis, Zinn zonule*) 2 extend from the surface of the ciliary processus 1 to the lens capsule. This establishes the connection between lens and ciliary muscle. There are thick suspensor fibers and thinner tensile fibers. The latter are not anchored in the ciliary epithelium but span the distance between ciliary fold and basal membrane of the nonpigmented epithelium. The thinner fibers may be considered part of the basal membrane.
The figure shows the attachment of the zonula filaments to the walls of the ciliary processus.

1 Ciliary processus
2 Lens zonula, zonula filaments

Scanning electron microscopy; magnification: × 660

646 Angle of the Eye—Corneoscleral Trabeculae

The anterior chamber of the eye is limited in the front by the cornea and the peripheral sclera, in the back by the anterior iris and the pupillary part of the lens. The border between anterior and posterior chamber of the eye is the angle of the eye or Schwalbe's line (*angulus iridocornealis*) (see Fig. 644). At that line, the corneal epithelium continues in the epithelium of the conjunctiva and the lamellae of the corneal stroma interweave with the connective tissue of the sclera. From the corneal epithelium and Descemet's membrane arise the *corneoscleral trabeculae*, which are a loosely arranged sponge-like connective tissue. The ocular fluid flows through the meshwork of this sponge-like tissue to the *canal of Schlemm* . Endothelial cells cover the trabecular surfaces. The intertrabecular space is the *space of Fontana*. It is the connection between Schwalbe's line and the canal of Schlemm. This figure conveys an impression of the trabecular structure. The structure cannot be obtained in this form using light microscopy (cf. Fig. 644).

Scanning electron microscopy; magnification: × 800

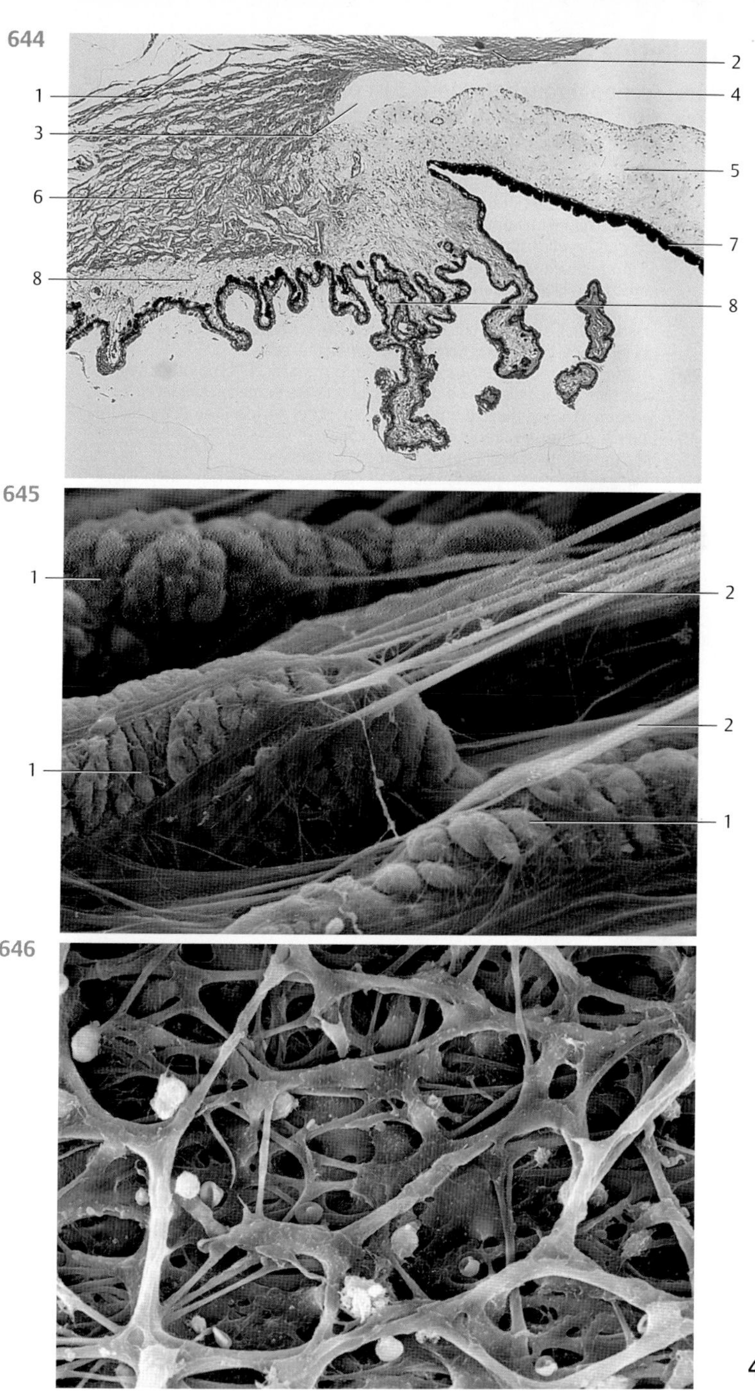
644
1
2
3
4
5
6
7
8
8
645
1
2
2
1
1
646

647 Retina and Choroid

Vertical section through the optic part of the retina and the choroidea. Note: the iris, the choroidea and the ciliary body appear combined as uvea. The choroid is the posterior part of the uvea.

1 Stratum limitans internum (internal limiting lamina)
2 Stratum neurofibrarum, optic nerve fiber layer with anchoring parts of Müller cells
3 Stratum ganglionicum nervi optici (3rd neuron), the ganglion cell layer is single-layered, the multilayered appearance is an artifact due to the thickness of the section
4 Stratum plexiforme internum, inner plexiform layer (IPL) (only lightly stained). The synapses between bipolar and multipolar ganglia cells of the ganglion cell layer are located here
5 Stratum nucleare internum, inner nuclear layer (INL) (2nd neuron) The blue-violet stained nuclei are part of bipolar ganglia cells (amacrine cells)
6 Stratum plexiform externum, outer plexiforme layer (OPL) (lightly stained). Synapses between receptor cells and bipolar ganglia cells are formed in this layer
7 Stratum neuroepitheliale, rods and cones, outer nuclear layer (1st neuron)
8 Inner and outer segments of rods and cones
9 Stratum pigmentosum retinae, pigment epithelium
10 Lamina choroidocapillaris, choroidal capillary layer; its capillaries attach to the lower basal membrane on the pigmented epithelium
11 The lower third of the figure represents the choroidea with the vascular layer and filled veins as well as pigmented epithelial cells (cf. Fig. 648)

Stain: alum hematoxylin-eosin; magnification: × 65

648 Retina

This microphotograph of a retina displays the separate layers particularly well (cf. Fig. 647).

1 External limiting lamina, (junctional complexes)
2 Rods and cones layer
3 Inner nuclear layer
4 Müller cells
5 Nucleus of a neuroglial cell
6 Internal limiting lamina
7 Anchor portion of a Müller cell
8 Ganglia cells of the optic nerve (3rd neuron)
9 Fiber bundle of the optic nerve
10 Inner plexiform layer (IPL)
11 Outer plexiform layer (OPL)
12 Nucleus of a rod cell
13 Nucleus of a cone cell
14 Outer segment of a rod cell
15 Inner segment of a rod cell
16 Inner segment of a cone cell
17 Outer segment of a cone cell

Stain: nuclear fast red-eosin-nigrosin (steel gray); magnification: × 320

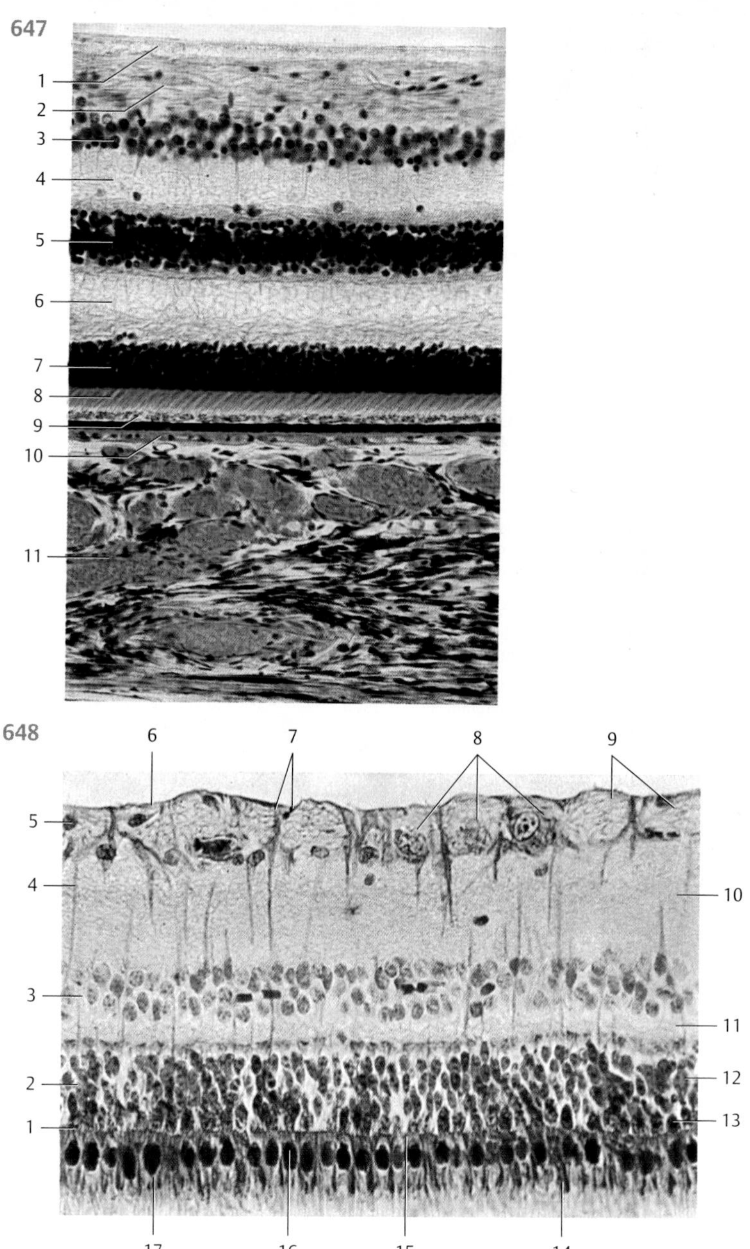
647
1
2
3
4
5
6
7
8
9
10
11
648
6
7
8
9
5
4
10
3
11
2
12
1
13
17
16
15
14

649 Retina

Incomplete section of a human retina. It shows the following layers:

1 External nuclear layer. This layer contains the nuclei of the rods and cones
2 Inner segments of the rods and cones with a distal acidophilic part (ellipsoid) and a proximal basophilic part (myoid). The distal ellipsoid part is filled with mitochondria, the proximal myoid part contains smooth endoplasmic reticulum membranes, Golgi complexes, and free ribosomes
3 Outer segments of the rods and cones. Their structures are in principal similar to the structure of the inner segments. Outer and inner segments of the rods are approximately of equal length. The cylindrical outer segments contain stacks of 600—1000 flat disks, which look like rolls of coins. They are enveloped by a plasma membrane. The outer segments of the cones are cone-shaped and shorter than the outer segments of rods. They are often described as flask-shaped. The membrane stacks of cones consist of equally spaced involutions of the plasma membrane, not of separate disks. The outer third of the outer segments of the cones is surrounded by the microvilli of the pigmented epithelium [7]
4 Pigment epithelium. The single-layered cuboidal epithelium is interwoven with the choroidea. Microvilli protrude from the apical portion of the epithelium. They extend far into outer segments of the rods and cones of the bacillary layer. The basal membrane borders on Bruch's membrane and shows many folds. Pigmented epithelial cells contain large round nuclei [8]. The apical cell region contains many melanosomes and phagosomes
5 Choroidal capillary layer (lamina choroidocapillaris). This layer is found close to the pigment epithelium. It consists of a tight vascular network, which contains capillary lobes. Only one capillary is sectioned longitudinally in this figure. The capillaries contain erythrocytes
6 Lamina vasculosa. The lower right corner of the figure shows an arteriole. There are three layers in the choroidea: the outer layer close to the sclera (Haller's layer), the lamina vasculosa and the lamina choroidocapillaris close to the pigment epithelium. Compare with Figs. 647 and 648

Electron microscopy; magnification: × 3500

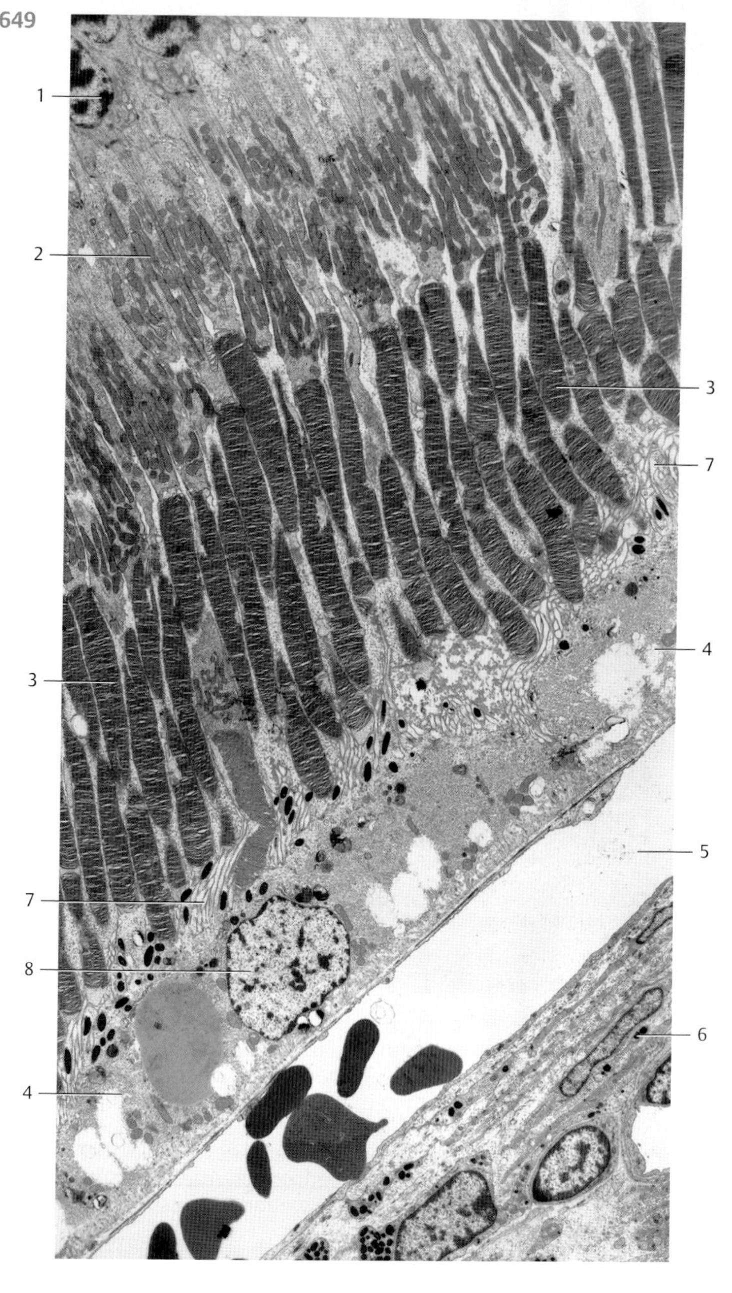
1
2
3
7
4
3
5
7
8
6
4

650 Optic Nerve—Papilla of the Optic Nerve

Exit point of the optic nerve, longitudinal section. The nerve fibers continue as optic nerve at the papilla of the optic nerve (blind spot).

1 External sheath of the optic nerve (dura mater)
2 Subdural space
3 Internal sheath of the optic nerve (pia mater)
4 Arachnoidea
5 Subarachnoidal space
6 Sclera
7 Choroidea
8 Retina
9 Lamina cribrosa sclera (perforated plate of collagen fibrils)
10 Papilla of the optic nerve
11 Unmyelinated nerve fiber bundle before pushing through the lamina cribrosa
12 Myelinated nerve fiber bundle of the optic nerve behind the lamina cribrosa
13 Lamina episcleralis
14 Ciliary nerve

At the eyeball, the dura mater continues in the cornea; the arachnoidea and pia mater continue in the choroid.

Stain: alum hematoxylin-eosin; magnification: × 6

651 Optic Nerve

Section of the optic nerve behind the *lamina cribrosa sclerae* (see Fig. 653).

1 Ciliary nerve
2 Sclera
3 Pigment epithelium of the lamina suprachoroidea
4 Fiber bundles of the optic nerve
5 Central retinal artery
6 Septa of the pia mater
7 Central retinal vein
8 Internal sheath of the optic nerve (pia mater)
9 External sheath of the optic nerve (dura mater)
10 Subdural space
11 Arachnoidea
12 Short posterior ciliary artery
Stain: hematoxylin-eosin; magnification: × 20

652 Optic Nerve

Cross-section of the optic nerve behind the lamina cribrosa sclerae. The axons of the ganglia cells are combined in bundles 1. They are enveloped by a thin *septum of the pia mater* 2. The optic nerve contains a pia mater sheath, an arachnoidea sheath and a dura mater sheath (see Figs. 650, 651). The pia mater sheath attaches directly to the optic nerve. Septa originate with the pia mater and guide blood vessels to the myelinated nerve fibers. The nerve fiber bundles contain astrocytes and oligodendrocytes. *Arteries* 3 and *central retinal veins* 4 are visible in the center of the section. The vessels are sheathed by the loose connective tissue of the pia mater.

1 Nerve fiber bundles
2 Pia mater septa
3 Central retinal artery
4 Central retinal vein
Stain: hematoxylin-eosin; magnification: × 40

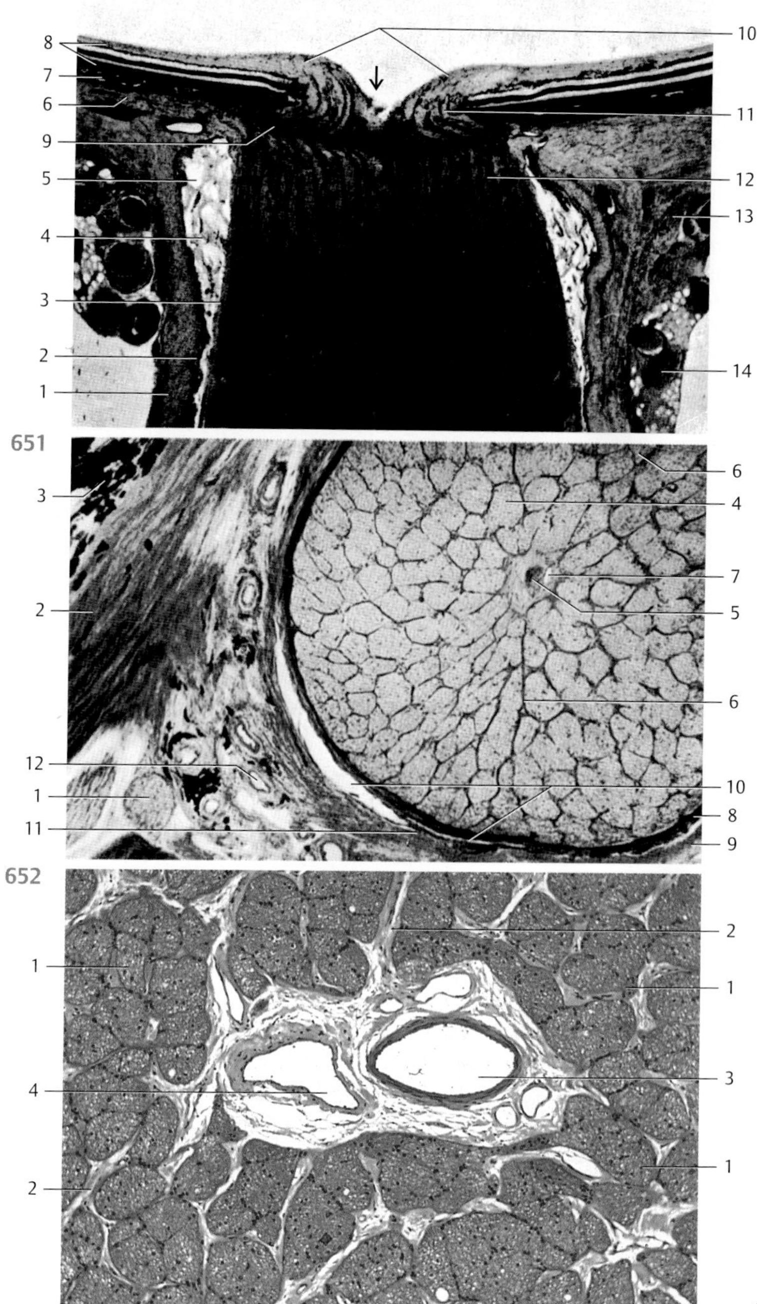

Sensory Organs

653 Optic Nerve—Lamina Cribrosa Sclerae

The optic nerve, a longitudinal fascicle, has an *intraocular, orbital, intracanalicular* and an *intracranial segment*. The about 2-mm long pars intraocularis corresponds to the papilla of the optic nerve (cf. Fig. 650). The nerve fibers in this intraocular segment are unmyelinated. Examination with the ophthalmoscope allows a view of the sieve-like, loosely structured lamina cribrosa sclerae, which shines through the unmyelinated nerve fibers at the point where the optic nerve traverses the lamina cribrosa. The *lamina cribrosa* is a continuation of the sclera. The axons of the optic nerve are myelinated only after traversing the lamina cribrosa.

This figure shows the *lamina cribrosa sclerae*. The viewer looks on the circular arrangements of collagen fibers around each traversing axon. The collagen fibers have been isolated by maceration with a 10% NaOH solution, which disintegrates the axons of the optic nerve. The center represents the space for the artery and the central retinal vein. The collagen fibers around the center are called *scleral ring*.

Lamina cribrosa sclerae of an 89-year-old woman.

Scanning electron microscopy; magnification: × 60

654 Choroid Plexus

The *choroid plexus* consists of a richly vascularized layer of leptomeninges (*pia mater and arachnoidea*), which is covered by a single-layered cuboidal epithelium 1. The plexus structure is tree-like. In the ciliated connective tissue occur fibroblasts as well as plasma cells, mast cells and macrophages. This preparation contains many vessels with erythrocytes 2. The cuboidal epithelium of the choroid plexus stains heavily with Eosin. Note the large, round central nuclei.

1 Epithelium of the choroid plexus
2 Capillaries with erythrocytes
3 Cerebrospinal fluid (CSF) with cells
Stain: alum hematoxylin-eosin; magnification: × 300

655 Axodendritic Synapse

This *axodendritic synapse* consists of the *presynaptic membrane*, the *synaptic gap* and the *postsynaptic membrane* 3. The axolemma region appears denser in the area of the presynaptic membrane. The synaptic bouton of the axon 1 contains several synaptic vesicles 2 with diameters between 20 and 65 nm as well as mitochondria and a few small dense vesicles (*dense bodies*) 4. The synaptic vesicles contain a *transmitter* (chemical synapse).

1 Synaptic bouton of an axon
2 Synaptic vesicle
3 Synaptic membrane complex
4 Dense granule
5 Dendrite
Electron microscopy; magnification: × 35 800

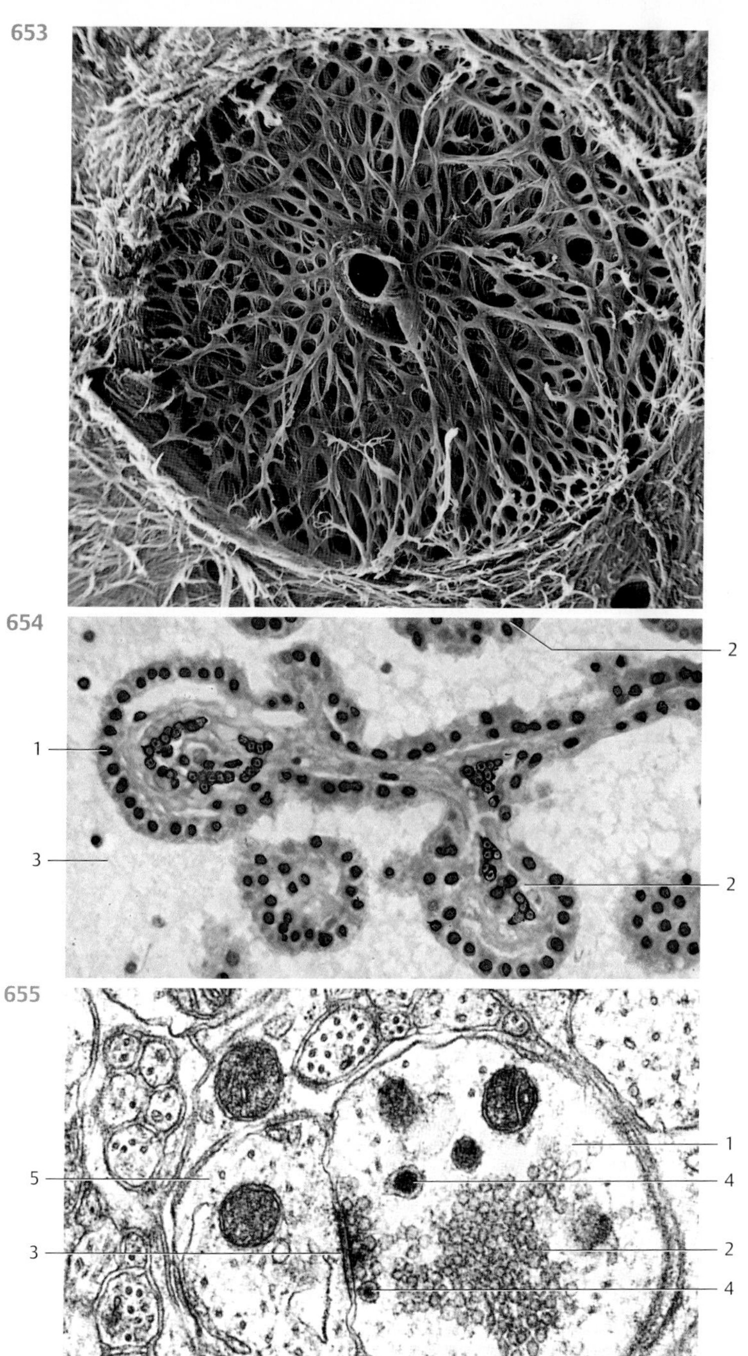
653
654
2
1
3
2
655
1
5
4
3
2
4

656 Inner Ear—Cochlea

Longitudinal section of a human cochlea.

1 Scala tympani (contains perilymph)
2 Cochlear duct (contains endolymph), triangular in cross-sections
3 Scala vestibuli (contains perilymph)
4 Osseous spiral lamina
5 Helicotrema (scala vestibuli and scala tympani join)
6 Cecum cupulare (copular blind sac, caecum cupulare)
7 Modiolus (end of the osseous spiral lamina)
8 Cochlear cupola (azimuth of the apical cochlear turn)
9 Longitudinal canals of the modioli (canales longitudinales modioli), central inner canals of the cochlea
10 Spiral canal of the modioli (canalis spiralis modioli), canal in the outer wall of the osseous spiral lamina
11 Facial nerve in the bony facial canal
12 Vestibular membrane (Reissner's membrane, membrana vestibularis, upper wall of the cochlea)
13 Spiral crest, spiral ligament (ligamentum spirale cochlea)
14 Basilar membrane (connective tissue between cochlear duct and scala tympani)
15 Osseous spiral lamina
16 Area of the facial nerve of the internal acoustic meatus (fundus)
17 Cochlear ganglion (cochlear nerve)
18 Transverse crest
19 Base of the modiolus (base of the cochlea)
20 Cochlear nerve
21 Internal acoustic meatus (fundus)
22 Spiral canal of the modioli (see 10)
Stain: hematoxylin-eosin; magnification: × 10

657 Cochlea—Inner Ear

Middle bend of the cochlea.

1 Cochlear duct (contains endolymph)
2 Spiral ligament, spiral crest
3 Stria vascularis, vascularized tissue over the spiral prominence
4 Reissner's membrane, vestibular membrane
5 Scala vestibuli
6 Osseous spiral lamina
7 Cochlear ganglion
8 Spiral canal of the modioli (bony canal in the outer wall of the osseous spiral lamina)
9 Longitudinal canal of the modioli (central inner canal)
10 Tractus spiralis foraminosus, a few spirally arranged openings around the inner cochlear canal, which permit access of cochlear nerve ganglia to the cochlea
11 Cochlear nerve (branch of the vestibulocochlear nerve for the cochlear audiosensory organ)
12 Internal acoustic meatus (fundus)
13 Scala tympani (contains perilymph)
14 Organ of Corti
15 Basilar membrane (connective tissue layer between cochlear duct and scala tympani)
Stain: hematoxylin-eosin; magnification: × 25

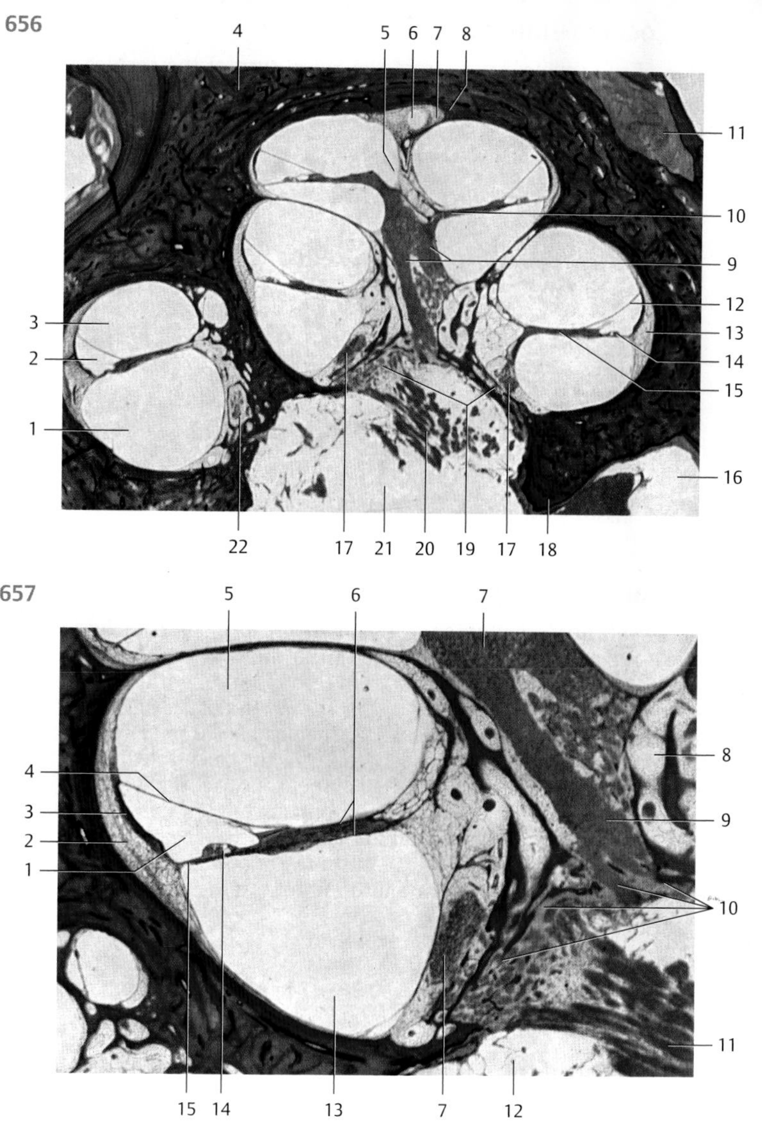
656
4
5 6 7 8
11
10
9
12
13
14
15
3
2
1
16
22
17 21 20 19 17 18
657
5
6
7
8
9
4
3
2
1
10
11
15 14
13
7
12

658 Cochlea—Inner Ear

Section of the cochlear duct from the apical turn of the cochlea with the organ of Corti (*organum spirale*).

1 Spiral ligament, spiral crest
2 External spiral groove of the cochlear duct
3 Spiral prominence (border of the external spiral groove)
4 Stria vascularis
5 Bony wall of the cochlea
6 Cochlear duct
7 Vestibular membrane, Reissner's membrane
8 Scala vestibuli
9 Cochlear nerve
10 Scala tympani
11 Tectorial membrane (located over the organ of Corti and the inner cochlear canal)
12 Inner cochlear canal (canalis spiralis cochleae)
13 Inner hair cells
14 Inner tunnel, contains endolymph
15 Outer hair cells
16 Cells of Henson
17 Cells of Claudius
18 Basilar membrane
Stain: hematoxylin-eosin; magnification: × 80

659 Cochlea—Organ of Corti

The *organ of Corti* (*organum spirale, papilla spiralis*) rests on the *basilar* membrane. It represents the part of the cochlear duct, which has differentiated into a sensory epithelium. There are two groups of cells with different functions in this epithelial layer. 1. The *sensory cells* or *hair cells*. The fibers of the acoustic nerve end at the hair cells. 2. The *phalangeal support cells* 3. Both cell types form rows. A surface view confirms the cell arrangement in rows. This figure shows the singular rows of inner sensory cells (*hair cells*) 1 and the triple or quadruple rows of the outer hair cells 2. The hair consists of stereocilia (*cochlear stereocilia*). Inner and outer hair cells show numerous differences in their morphological attributes, and their functions are different. Both inner and outer hair are directed toward the *endolymph*.

1 Inner hair cells
2 Outer hair cells
3 Phalangeal cells
Scanning electron microscopy; magnification: × 2000

660 Osseous Semicircular Canals—Ampullary Crest

The ampullary crest consists of sensory organs, which extend into the ampullary spaces of the osseous semicircular canals. The laminae of the sensory organs are capped by the gelatinous *cupula ampullaris* 2. A fiber bundle of the *vestibular part* of the ampullary nerve 3 is visible in the center of the figure. The bony capsule of the *ampulla membranaceae* 4 is shown on the right.

1 Sensory epithelium
2 Cupula ampullaris, ampullary dome
3 Ampullary nerve
4 Bony capsule
5 Sensory hair
6 Lamina propria
Stain: hematoxylin-eosin; magnification: × 25

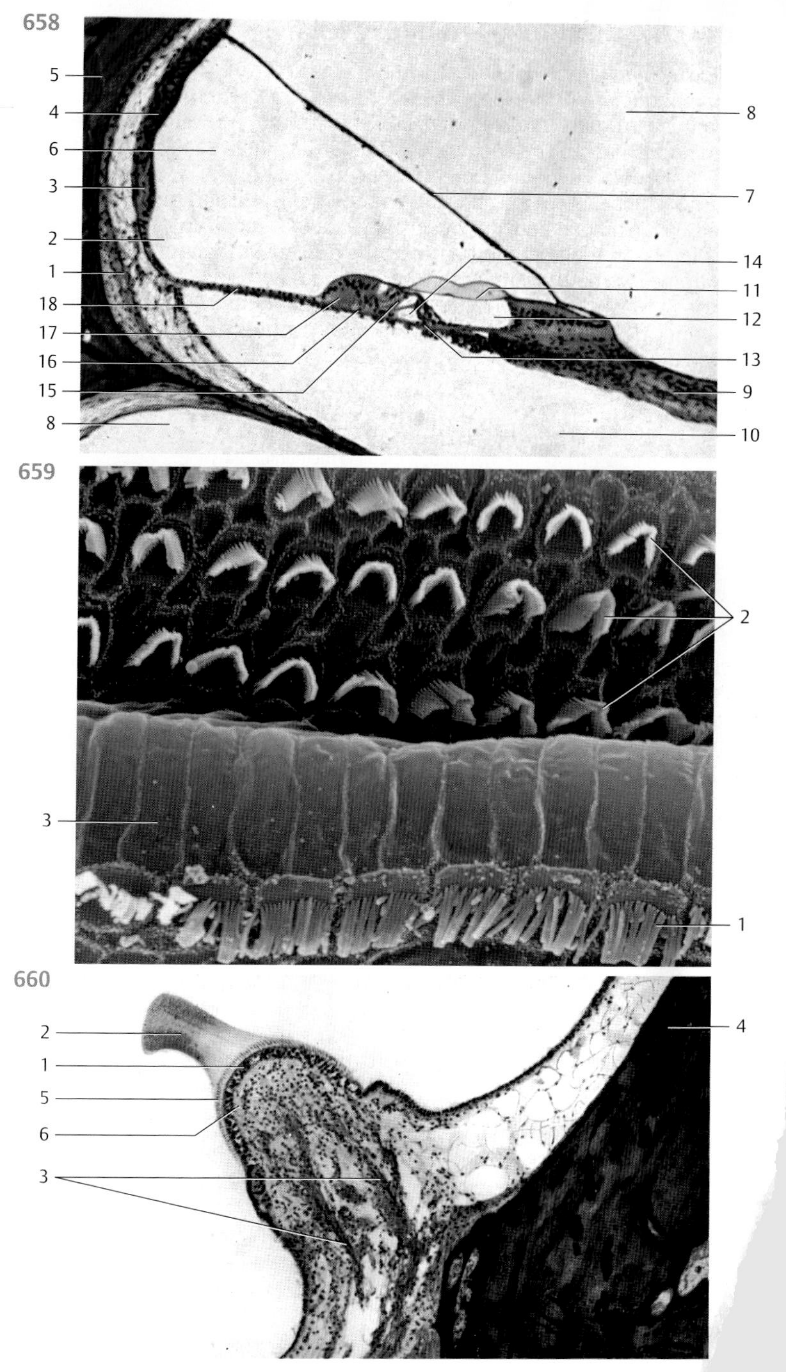
658
5
4
6
3
2
1
18
17
16
15
8
8
7
14
11
12
13
9
10
659
2
3
1
660
2
1
5
6
3
4

661 Eustachian Tube—Auditory Tube

The *Eustachian tube* [1] connects the nasal part of the pharynx and the middle ear. It is about 35–40 mm long. There are a bony part *(pars ossea)* [2] and a cartilaginous part (*pars fibrocartilaginea*) [3] with different wall components. In the medium part of the cochlea, the human hyaline tube cartilage has the form of a hook. The lamina membranacea (basal plate) [4] covers the tube opening which has an oval shape in this segment. The part of the tube that is closed by the hook-shaped tube cartilage (*stapes*) and the basal plate takes the role of a pressure compensating tube [5]. The epithelium of the mucous membrane is a multilayered ciliated epithelium with goblet cells. The lamina propria [6] of the tubular mucous membrane contains *seromucous glands*. It also contains lymphocytes. Cross-section of the *pars fibrocartilaginea* tubae of the guinea pig.

1 Eustachian tube
2 Bone
3 Stapes, hyaline tube cartilage (ossicle)
4 Basal plate (closes the oval window), lamina membranacea
5 Pressure compensation tube with parietal multilayered ciliated epithelium, which contains goblet cells
6 Lamina propria with lymphocytes
Stain: azan; preparation; magnification: × 10

662 Taste Buds

Sections of two neighboring foliate papillae of the rabbit tongue. There are six taste buds in the walls. They consist of *sensory cells* with *taste receptors*, *support cells* and *basal cells*. Taste buds are intraepithelial organs. Cross-sections display their oval shape. Their circumference tapers off at the lamina propria and is even smaller at the epithelial surface. Each taste bud features 40–70 long, longitudinally oriented cells, which are straight in the center, but slightly arcuate, following the overall shape of the taste bud at the ends. The cells have the layered appearance of an onion. The sensory cells reach to the gustatory pores at the epithelial surface. A short duct ends at the epithelial surface. Routine staining leaves the cytoplasm of the sensory cells light.

1 Groove
2 Multilayered nonkeratinizing squamous epithelium
Stain: Heidenhain iron hematoxylin; magnification: × 400

663 Olfactory Epithelium—Olfactory Region

The epithelium of the olfactory mucous lamina is multilayered and contains specific *sensory cells* [1], *support cells* [2] and *basal cells* [3]. The *cones* of the bipolar *olfactory cells* [4] are visible in some areas of the epithelial surface. Olfactory glands [5] are present in the vascularized innervated lamina propria. The serous glands consist of winding tubes. They release mucus to dissolve and remove olfactory materials. Compare with Figs. 664 and 665.

1 Sensory cells
2 Support cells
3 Basal cells
4 Conical olfactory cells
5 Olfactory glands
6 Glimpse of junctional complexes (terminal bars)
7 Plasma cell
8 Capillary
Stain: alum hematoxylin-eosin; magnification: × 100

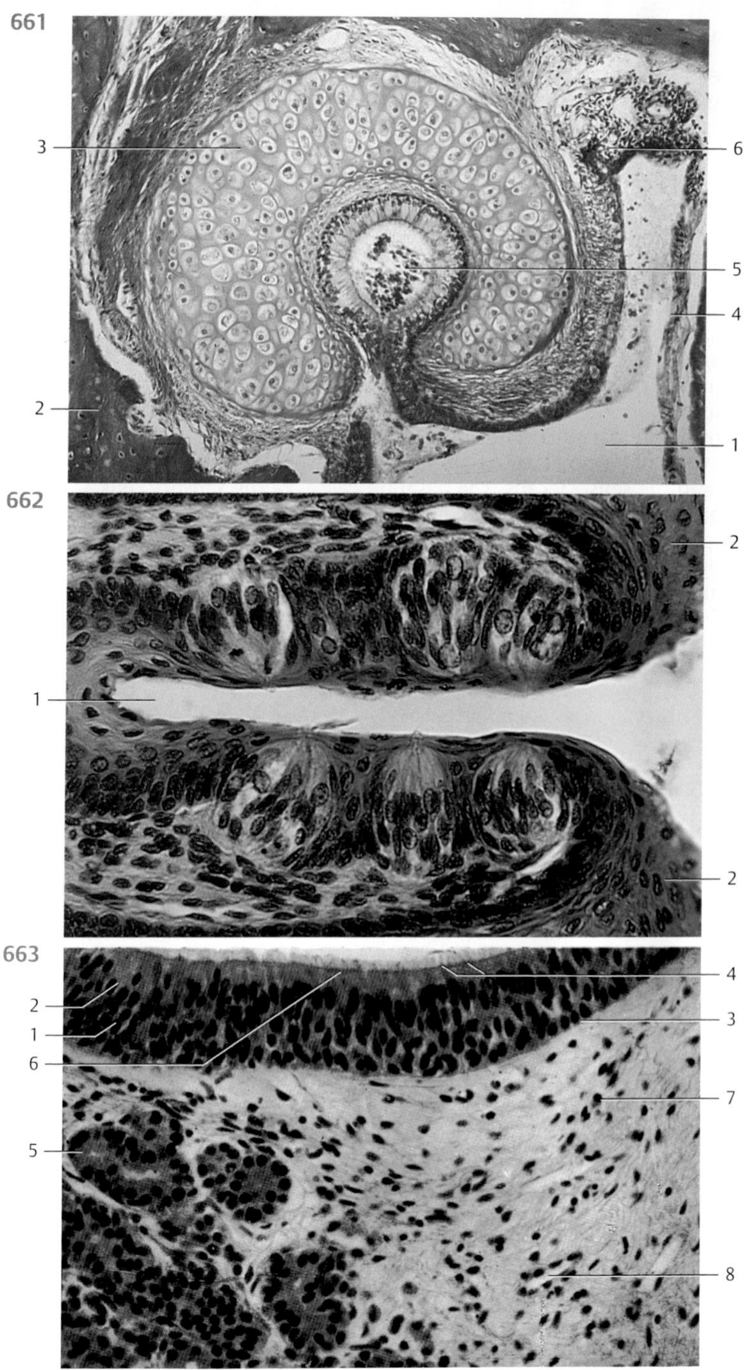
661
3
6
5
4
2
1
662
2
1
2
663
4
2
3
1
6
7
5
8

664 Olfactory Epithelium—Olfactory Region

The multilayered columnar epithelium of the olfactory mucous lamina consists of *basal cells, support cells* and *sensory olfactory cells*. The nuclei of these cells occupy different levels (cf. Fig. 663). The support cells are the most numerous cells. Basal, support and sensory cells originate on the basal lamina, forming a pseudostratified epithelium. This figure shows the apical regions of two support cells and two sensory cells. The support cells are usually wider at their apical surfaces than at their bases. Long microvilli [4] protrude from the free surfaces of support cells. They contain many organelles, a large Golgi apparatus, extended smooth ER and secretory granules. The olfactory sensory cells are bipolar neurons. Their apex is wider than their basal part. Their *olfactory bulbs* extend over the epithelial surface. Six to eight long *cilia* [3] protrude from the olfactory cells, which contain the olfactory receptors. The base of each cilia shows the typical 9 × 2 + 2 microtubule organization. The microtubule continues in a thin nontubular process. The cilia protrude into a mucous film. Olfactory and support cells are connected via a network of terminal bars (tight junctions). Note the abundance of mitochondria in the sensory cells. The basal processes of the sensory cells are axons, which run to the base of the epithelium and traverse the basal membrane. Apposed plasmalemma Schwann cell processes envelop the axons only after they have traversed the basal lamina. The olfactory bulbs with their cilia make up the apical portion of the dendritic processes of these sensory cells.

1 Support cells with microvilli
2 Olfactory bulb with cilia
3 Kinocilia
4 Microvilli
Electron microscopy; magnification: × 24 000

665 Olfactory Epithelium—Olfactory Region

View of an area of the olfactory mucous lamina (cf. Fig. 664). The *olfactory bulbs* extend over the epithelial surface. Long *cilia* protrude from the olfactory bulbs. The sensory cells are interspersed with *support cells* with *microvilli*. The olfactory bulbs are about 4 μm high.

Scanning electron microscopy; magnification: × 17 800

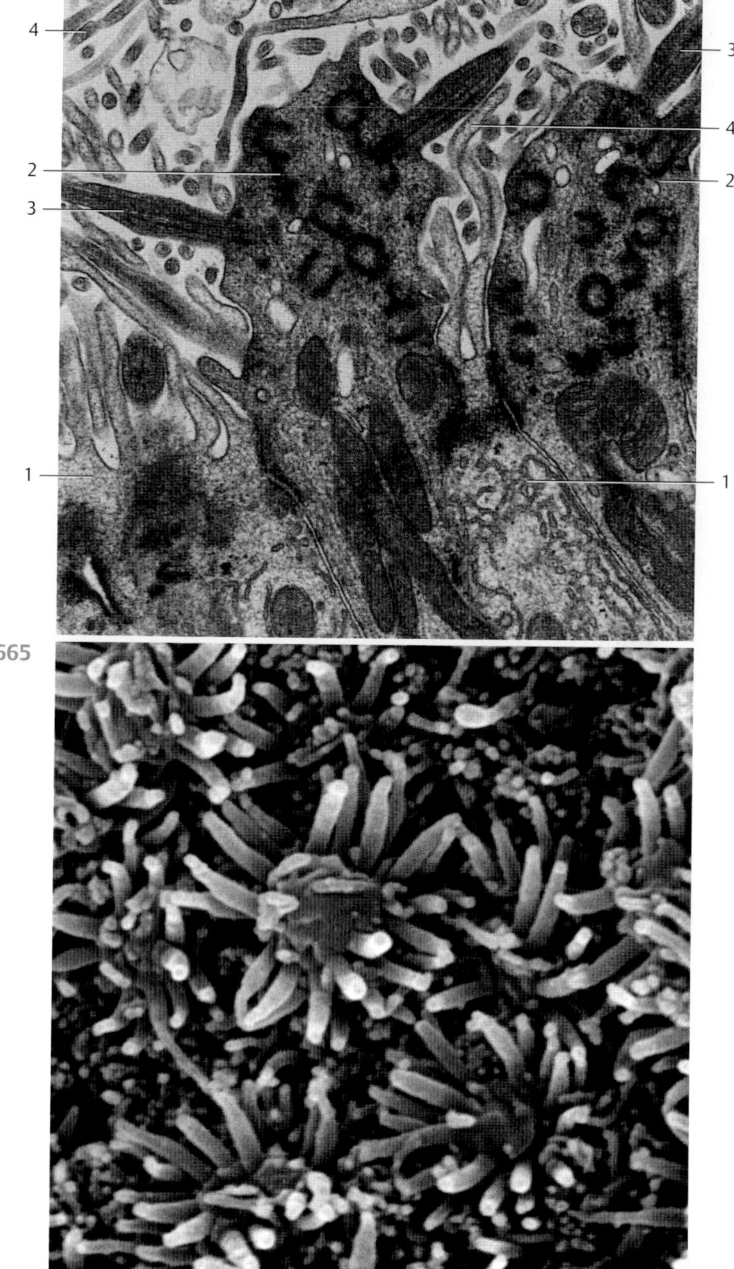
664
4
3
4
2
2
3
1
1
665

666 Spinal Cord—Spinal Medulla

Cross-section of the cervical part (C5)—*cervical intumescence.*
The spinal medulla is traversed lengthwise by the columnar gray matter (*substantia grisea*). It is completely enveloped by the white matter (*substantia alba, medullary sheath*). The columnar gray matter displays a butterfly or H-pattern in cross-sections. There is a deep anterior median fissure (*fissura mediana anterior*), the dorsal median fissure is not as deep (*sulcus medianus posterior*). The gray matter forms extensions, which look like horns in cross-sections. They are therefore named *cornua.* Both halves of the spinal medulla feature a larger anterior horn (*cornu anterius, columna anterior*) and a slender posterior horn (*cornu posterior, columna posterior*). Both sides are connected via the central intermediary matter, which is joined in the center (*commissura grisea*) with the *central canal.* The figure reveals that the posterior horns extend to the surface in the proximity of the posterior root of the spinal nerves. The tissue next to the spinal cord (stained brown) represents the rootlets of the posterior root of the spinal nerves (*fila radicularia*). The darker stained medullary sheath shows a clear substructure. This sheath contains the longitudinal, mostly myelinated nerve fibers of the various afferent and efferent projection tracts.
The surface of the spinal cord is covered by the *spinal pia mater* (stained soft yellow).

Stain: medullary sheath preparation—Weigert carmine; magnification: × 8

667 Spinal Cord—Spinal Medulla

Cross-section of the *thoracic part* (T6). Note the delicate anterior and posterior horns of the gray matter. The gray matter protrudes slightly to the sides (*cornu laterale*).

Stain: medullary sheath preparation—Weigert carmine; magnification: × 8

668 Spinal Cord—Spinal Medulla

Cross-section of the *lumbar part* (L6)—*lumbosacral intumescence.*
The gray matter (anterior and posterior horns) is prominently expressed because the nerves for the extremities exit here.

Stain: medullary sheath preparation—Weigert carmine; magnification: × 8

669 Spinal Cord—Spinal Medulla

Cross-section of the *sacral part* (S3).
Massive posterior horns are characteristic of the sacral spinal medulla. There is a broad interface to the anterior horns. Note the very narrow medullary sheath.

Stain: medullary sheath preparation—Weigert carmine; magnification: × 8

666

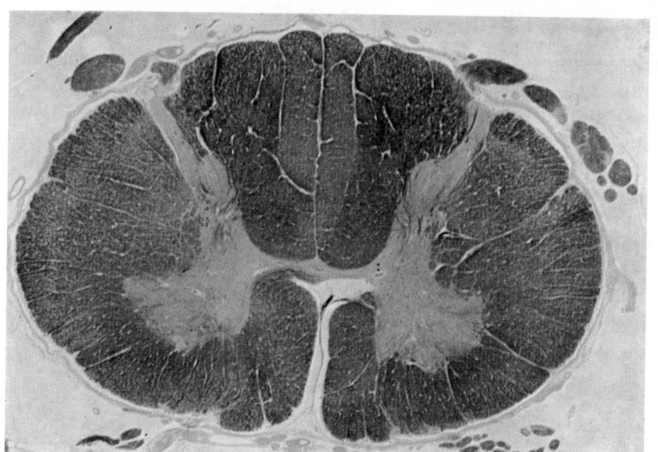

667

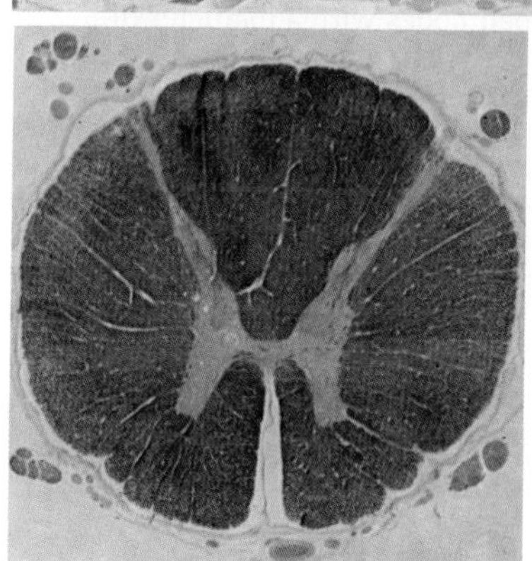

668

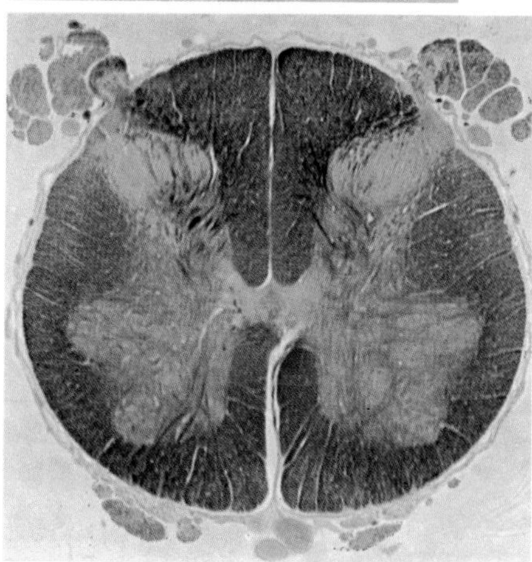

669

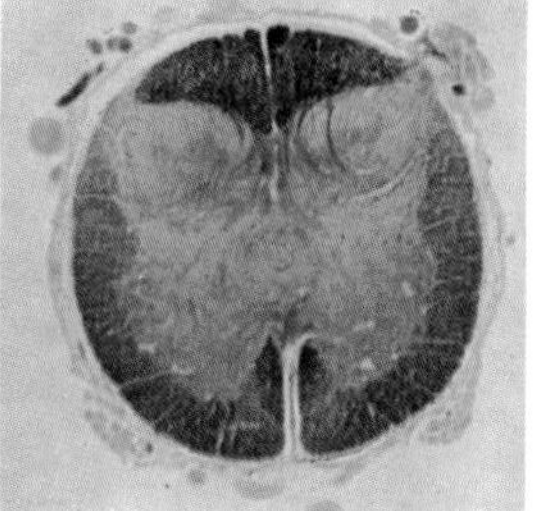

670 Spinal Cord—Spinal Medulla

Cross-section of the white matter (*substantia alba*) of the spinal medulla. The medullary sheath consists predominantly of longitudinal myelinated nerve fibers. Their myelin sheaths [1] are colorless in this preparation and show a wide range of diameters. The dark spots inside the colorless (white) areas are silver impregnated *axons* [2]. Unmyelinated or sparsely myelinated axons occur sporadically. Delicate vascularized connective tissue septa [3] start at the surface and traverse the spinal white matter. This causes a subdivision of the medullary sheath into parcels.

1 Myelin sheaths
2 Axons (neurites)
3 Vascularized connective tissue septa
Stain: Bielschowsky-Gros silver impregnation; magnification: × 500

671 Spinal Ganglion

Spinal ganglia are spindle-shaped nodes with a diameter of 5–8 mm. They are located in the posterior roots of the spinal nerves immediately before posterior and anterior roots merge. Each spinal ganglion is enveloped by a strong collagen fiber capsule [1] (= constituent of the spinal dura mater). Distally, it continues in the *perineurium* of the spinal nerve. Each ganglion is traversed by a delicate vascularized connective tissue (*endoneurium of the spinal nerve*), which is continuous with the connective tissue of the capsule. Embedded in this loose connective tissue are pseudounipolar nerve cell bodies and their satellite cells (= *peripheral glial cells*) as well as the axons of these primary sensory neurons of the spinal nerves (cf. Figs. 256, 672–674).

1 Connective tissue capsule
2 Posterior root of the spinal nerve
Stain: azan; magnification: × 12

672 Spinal Ganglion

Vertical section of a spinal ganglion which is part of the posterior root of the spinal nerve (*radix posterior*) immediately before it merges with the anterior root and forms the spinal nerve. The anterior root of the spinal nerve is not shown. The figure shows fiber tracts, i.e., axon bundles of different sizes, which build the posterior root [1] or the posterior branch of the spinal nerve [2], respectively. The black spots with different diameters represent pseudounipolar ganglia cells [3]. The spinal ganglion is encased by a vascularized connective tissue capsule [4], which is continues with the spinal dura mater (cf. Figs. 66, 256, 671, 673, 674).

1 Posterior root of the spinal nerve
2 Posterior branch of the spinal nerve
3 Group of ganglia cells
4 Connective tissue capsule
Stain: Bielschowsky-Gros silver impregnation; magnification: × 7

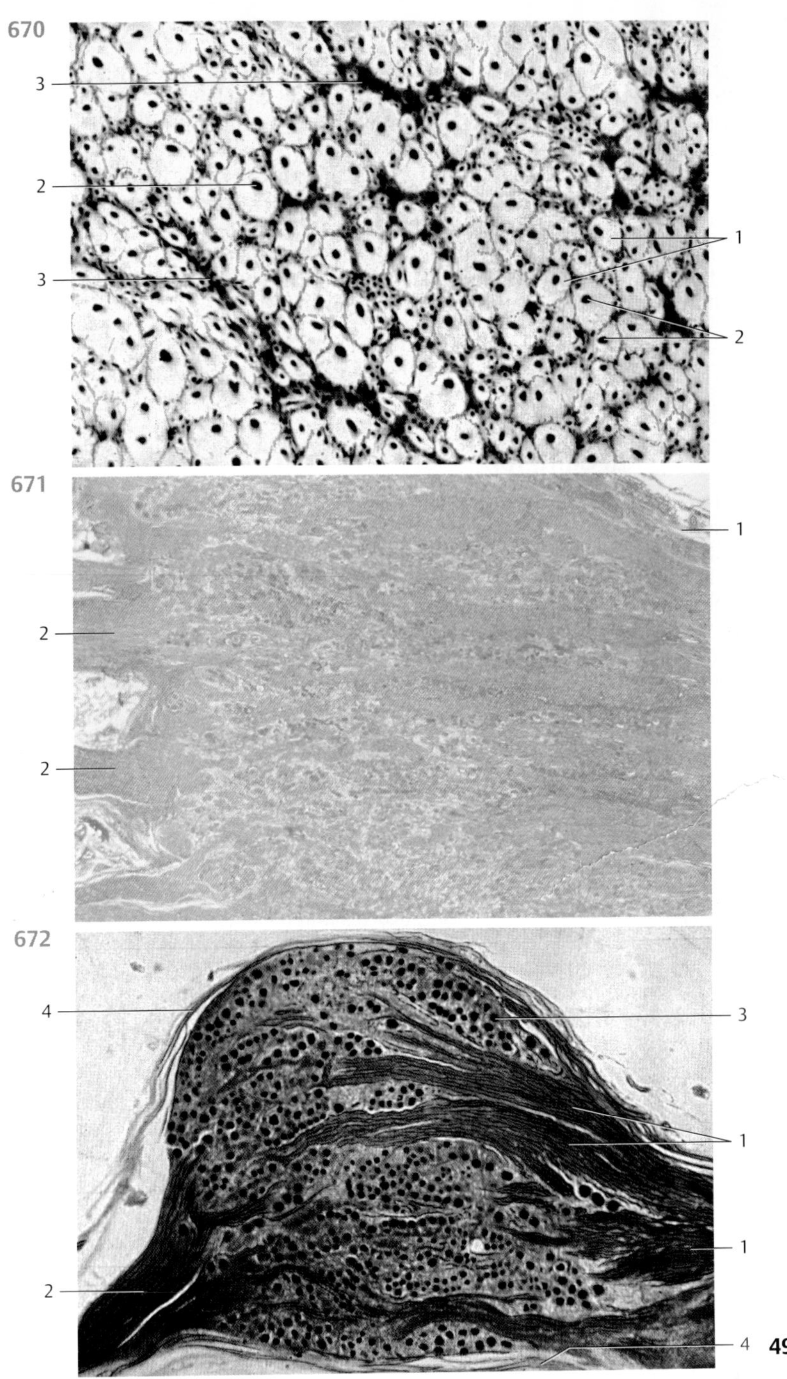
670
3
2
3
1
2
671
1
2
2
672
4
3
1
1
2
4

673 Spinal Ganglion

Detail from Fig. 671. The round or ellipsoid cell bodies [1] are of different sizes, their diameters vary from 20 to 120 µm. Spinal ganglia cells are among the largest cells in the body. They contain large, round nuclei with nucleoli, which show strong affinity to stains (cf. Figs. 1, 66, 256). The cytoplasm contains Nissl bodies. Note the corona of small satellite cells (lemmocytes) and the loose, vascularized connective tissue (*endoneurium*) (stained light blue). The cytoplasmic processes form T-shaped dendritic peripheral branches and a central axon (not seen in this figure). The axon (*radix posterior*, see Fig. 672) ends at the inner cells of the spinal medulla. The center of the figure shows a bundle of myelinated nerve fibers [2] (cf. Figs. 674).

1 Spinal ganglia cells (perikarya of pseudounipolar neurons)
2 Myelinated nerve fibers
Stain: azan; magnification: × 80

674 Spinal Ganglion

Detail from Fig. 656. Vertical section of myelinated nerve fibers from the posterior root of the spinal nerve. The preparation has been treated with lipophilic solvents (alcohol, xylene). This has led to a separation of the myelin sheaths. The lipids have been extracted from the myelin sheath, and only a protein precipitate, the *neurokeratin skeleton*, has remained. Note the delicate loose connective tissue (stained blue), which corresponds to the *endoneurium* of peripheral nerves. The larger nuclei (stained red) are part of Schwann cells. The smaller, spindle-shaped nuclei belong to fibrocytes.

Stain: azan; magnification: × 200

675 Cerebral Cortex

The neurons of the *cerebral cortex* (gray matter) are arranged in horizontal layers (*laminae*). One type of neuron predominates in each layer. The borders of the vertical layers are diffuse. This figure shows the *cytoarchitecture* (*Nissl image*) of the parietal lobe of the *isocortex* and its layers. The preparation depicts only nerve cell perikarya and glial nuclei. The outer layer I (*molecular* or *plexiform layer*) is cell sparse containing only scattered horizontal cells. Layer II, the *external lamina granulosa*, consists of granular cells. The *external pyramidal layer III* contains pyramidal cells of varying sizes together with scattered nonpyramidal neurons (cf. Figs. 676, 677). There are densely packed granular cells in the *internal granular layer*, the *lamina granularis interna IV*. The *internal pyramidal layer V* and spindle layer VI, the *lamina multiformis* , are relatively narrow in the parietal lobe. Apart from vertically running vessels (cut in various planes), there are also smaller vessels, which run in horizontal direction (cut longitudinally).

Stain: cresyl violet; magnification: × 30

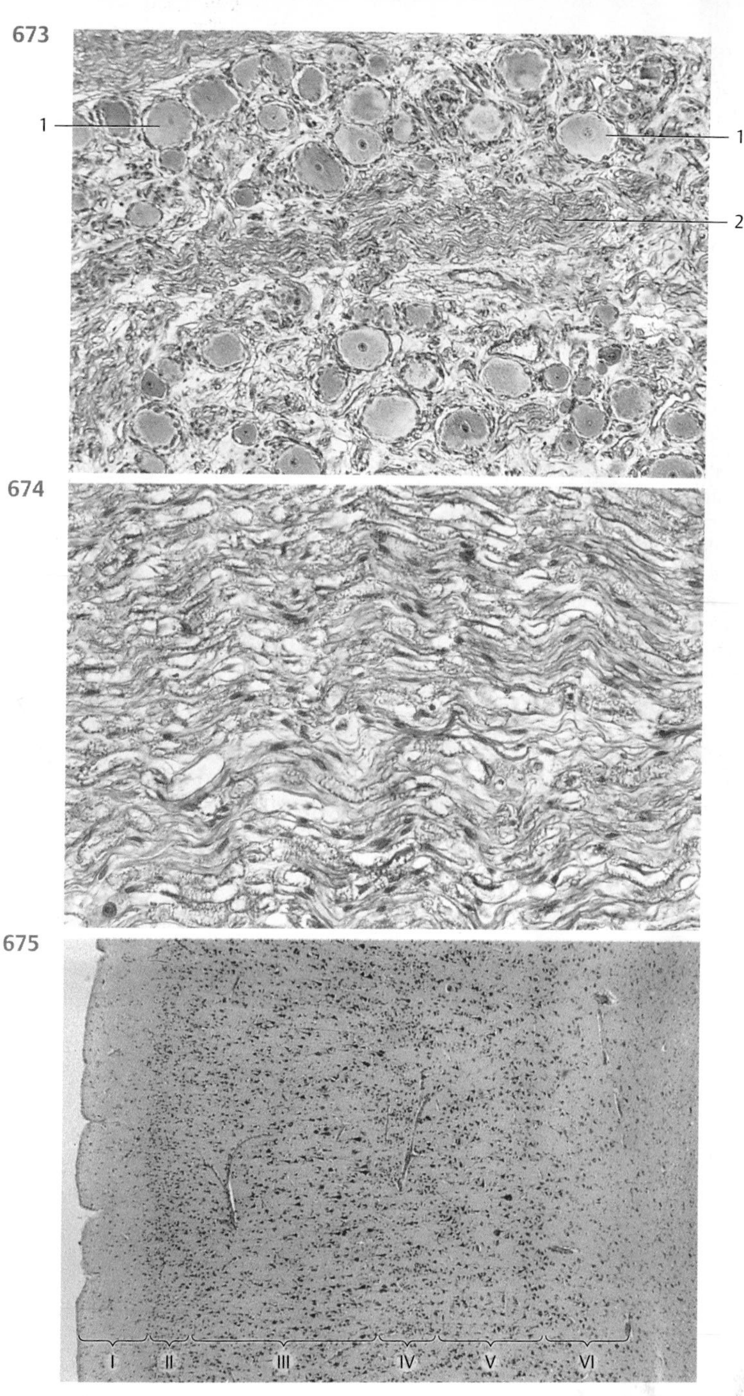
673
1
1
2
674
675
I
II
III
IV
V
VI

676 Cerebral Cortex

Detail from a vertical section of the *isocortex* with internal pyramidal layer (*lamina pyramidalis interna or ganglionaris*), layer V, and the internal granular layer (*lamina granularis interna*), layer VI. The pyramidal cells reach a height of 120 µm and a width of 80 µm. The cell bodies 1 are stained brown in this preparation. Pyramidal cells send out long ascending dendrites 2. A strong axon extends from the basal cytoplasm of the pyramidal cells. The axons of these *Betz giant cells* are part of the pyramidal tract (cf. Figs. 675, 677).

1 Cell bodies of pyramidal cells
2 Dendrites
Stain: Bielschowsky-Gros silver impregnation; magnification: × 300

677 Cerebral Cortex

Section of the *isocortex*, primary motor cortex, area 4 (precentral gyrus, Brodmann's area 4).
Pyramidal cells of the internal pyramidal cell layer (layer V) are stained using Golgi's silver impregnation technique. The cell bodies and all cell processes of the nerve cells are stained.
Pyramidal cells are *type 1 Golgi cells*. Axons, which end in extracortical tissue, are one of their characteristic features. The cell bodies of the pyramidal cells have diameters between 10 and 70 µm. The largest pyramidal cells are the Betz giant cells and the Meynert cells. The pyramidal cell owes its name to the roughly triangular faces of its cell body. The basis of the pyramid usually points toward the medulla. The branching apical dendrites run from the tip of the pyramid to the cortical surface. There are also dendrites at the basal plasma membrane. These run predominantly in a horizontal direction. The axon exits the pyramidal cell at the basal axon hillock and extends toward the medulla. Apical and basal dendrites are densely covered with spikes. Collaterals split from the axon shortly after it exits the pyramidal cell at the axon hillock. The collaterals either ascend or run in horizontal direction (cf. Figs. 2, 20, 248–253, 675, 676).

Stain: Golgi silver impregnation; magnification: × 500

676

677

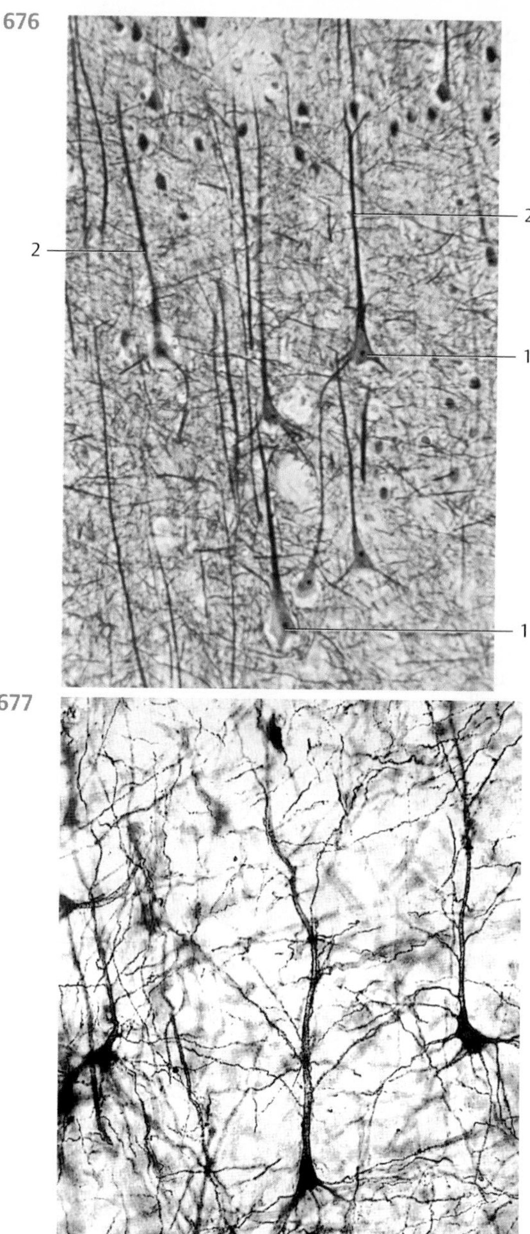

678 Cerebellar Cortex

Central sagittal section of the *cerebellar vermis*.
The cerebellar cortex is the about 1-mm thick folded layer of gray matter overlying the cerebellar surface. Grooves subdivide the gray matter in many small coils. The medullary layer of white matter consists of thin *medullary layers* [1]. In a medullary sheath preparation, the cerebellar cortex shows an outer molecular layer (*stratum moleculare*) (stained yellow) [2] and an inner granular layer (*stratum granulosum*) (stained brownish) [3]. The layer between the inner and outer layers is the wide *stratum ganglionare* (*stratum neuronorum piriformium gangliosum*) [3]. This layer is easily recognized. It consists of large *Purkinje cells (Purkinje cell layer)* (cf. Figs. 5, 254, 681, 682). Remnants of the soft pia mater [4] are visible on the surface of this section.

1 Medullary layer
2 Molecular layer
3 Stratum ganglionare, Purkinje cell layer
4 Pia mater
Stain: medullary sheath stain (modified Weigert hematoxylin stain); magnification: × 5

679 Cerebellar Cortex

Staining clearly differentiates between the *granular layer* [1] and the molecular layer [2], which contains few cells and appears pale. The molecular layer is 430 μm thick, the granular layer measures about 350 μm at the turn of the coils. The layer is clearly thinner in the grooves. Numerous densely packed cells form the granular layer [1]. The granular structure is based on the crowded presence of small cells. In general staining procedures, only the cell nuclei are clearly rendered (see Fig. 680). The Purkinje cells of the *stratum ganglionare* (*stratum neuronorum piriformium*) are located between the granular and molecular layers (see Figs. 5, 681, 682). The medullary layer [3] contains the myelinated nerve fibers of the cerebellar tracts.

1 Granular layer
2 Molecular layer
3 Medullary layer with laminae
4 Pia mater
Stain: Weigert medullary sheath staining; magnification: × 10

680 Cerebellar Cortex

Detail from a center sagittal section of the cerebellar vermis (cf. Figs. 678, 679). The figure shows the result of Nissl staining of the nerve and glial cells (*Nissl image*). The cell-rich granular layer [1] is rendered particularly well, while the molecular layer is only slightly tinged with a grayish blue hue. The laminae of the *medullary layer* [3] have remained unstained.

1 Granular layer
2 Molecular layer
3 Medullary layer, laminae
4 Pia mater
Stain: Nissl stain; magnification: × 10

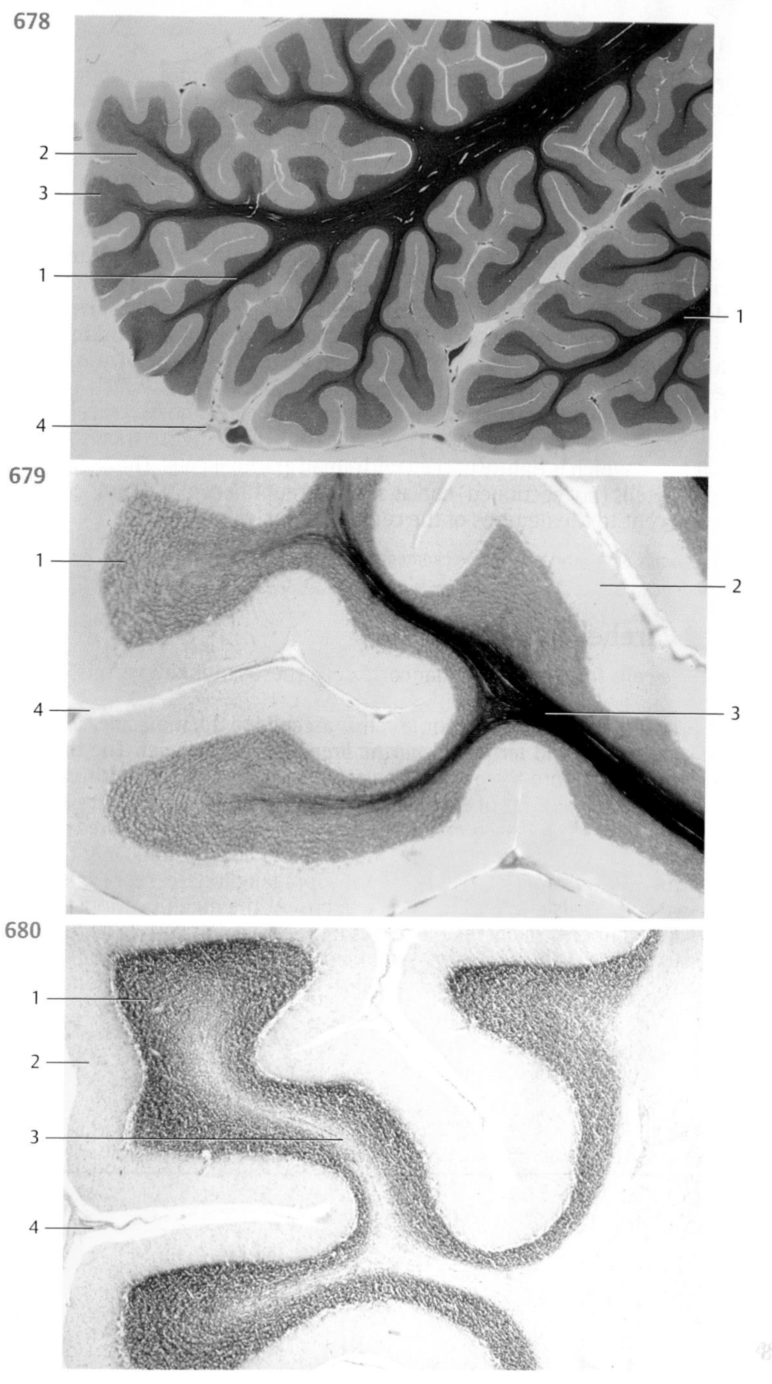
678
2
3
1
1
4
679
1
2
4
3
680
1
2
3
4

681 Cerebellar Cortex

The perikarya of the Purkinje cells in the *stratum ganglionare* are about 30 µm thick. They are arranged in a row. Purkinje cells appear striking even with general staining methods because they are by far the largest neurons of the cerebellum (cf. Fig. 254).
The round or rounded Purkinje cell bodies are darkly stained in this preparation. From their somata ascends an elaborately branched dendritic tree into the molecular layer and the *glial external limiting membrane*. The usually strong primary dendrites branch into secondary and tertiary dendrites. They form an espalier-like configuration in the molecular layer. The territories of individual Purkinje cells may overlap. There are fiber tracts in the lower third of the molecular layer immediately over the cell body of the Purkinje cells, which run parallel to the granular layer and vertical to the dendritic trees of the Purkinje cells. These fiber tracts are axons of *basket cells*, which are often called *tangential fibers*. There are many small *astrocytes* and *basket cells* in the molecular layer (stained black). The lower edge of the figure shows the *granular layer*, which is tightly packed with small granular cells. The axons of the Purkinje cells (not sectioned) end as sole efferent fibers of the cerebellar cortex adjacent to the neurons of the cerebellar nuclei.

Stain: Bielschowsky-Gros silver impregnation; magnification: × 200

682 Cerebellar Cortex

Purkinje cells from the cerebellar cortex of a rhesus monkey, vermis, lobulus II.
The primary dendrite of a Purkinje cell 1 ascends to the molecular layer and forms *secondary* and *tertiary dendritic branches* in this layer. The nuclei of *granular cells* 2 from the *granular layer* are located adjacent to the body of the Purkinje cell. A layer of cross-sectioned myelinated nerve fibers 3 in the lower third of the molecular layer follows. These are *myelinated parallel fibers*, which are abundant in some parts of the cerebellum. Only the very large myelinated fibers in the plexus supraganglionare represent retrogressive collaterals of the Purkinje cell axons. At the magnification, the very fine parallel fibers are not visible in this figure in the upper two thirds of the molecular layer. There is a cross-sectioned capillary at the lower edge of the figure. The oligodendrocyte 4 next to it was identified by its dense cytoplasm.

1 Cell body of a Purkinje cell
2 Nucleus of a granular cell
3 Myelinated axons
4 Oligodendrocyte
5 Capillary
Semi-thin section; stain: methylene blue-azure II; magnification: × 630

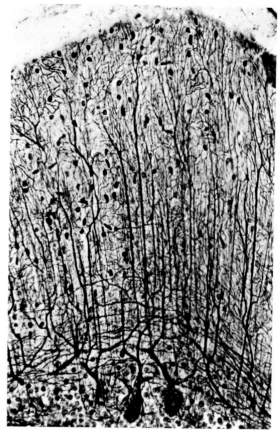

681

682

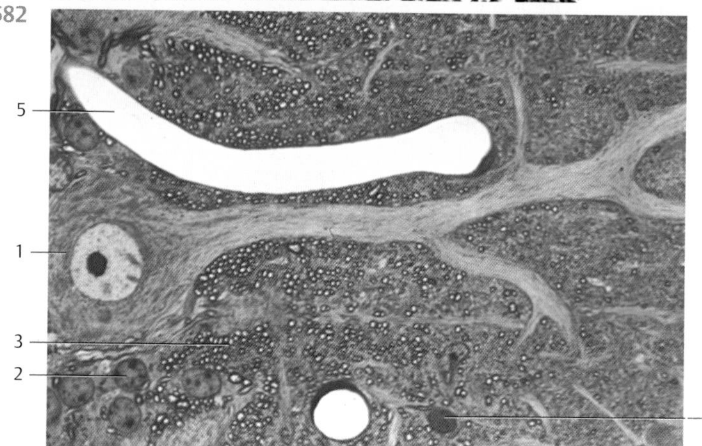

Table 1 Frequently used histological stains

Stain	Mayer HE	Heidenhain azan	Masson-Goldner trichrome
Staining agent	Hematoxylin-eosin or hemalum-erythrosin	Azocarmine-orange aniline blue G	Iron hematoxylin, Ponceau acid fuchsin or azophloxin-or G, acid green G
Cell nuclei	Blue	Red	Black-brown
Cytoplasm	Pale red	Reddish	Intense dark red
Connective tissue fibers			
Reticular	–	Blue	Pale green
Collagen	Red	Blue	Green
Elastic	Soft pink	Orange-red	–
Hyaline cartilage intercellular matrix	Pale blue, blue, violet	Pale blue(reddish)	Light green
Muscular tissue	Red	Red-orange	Orange-red (brown)
Erythrocytes	Orange-red	Orange-red	Orange-yellow
Lipids in adipocytes	Solubilized/removed	Solubilized/removed	Solubilized/removed

Table 2 Surface epithelia: classification

Epithelium	Examples
Single-layered (simple) squamous epithelium (including endothelium)	Mesothelium (serosal epithelium), endothelium (inner lining of the heart as well as blood and lymph vessels), posterior corneal epithelium, epithelial labyrinth, Bowman's capsule, amnion epithelium
Single-layered (simple) cuboidal epithelium (isoprismatic epithelium)	Secretory ducts, defined segments of the renal tubules, plexus choroideus, anterior lens epithelium, small bile ducts
Single-layered columnar epithelium (cylindrical epithelium)	
Without kinocilia	Stomach, small intestines, large intestines, gallbladder, hepatic ducts, papillary ducts
With kinocilia	Oviduct (uterine tube), uterus, ventricular ependyma
Multilayered pseudostratified epithelium (columnar epithelium)	
Without kinocilia	Segments of secretory ducts
With kinocilia	Nasal respiratory region, airways
With stereocilia	Epididymal duct, vas deferens
Multilayered stratified squamous epithelium	
Nonkeratinizing	Oral cavity, esophagus, anterior corneal epithelium, vocal fold, vagina, anus
Keratinizing	Epidermis, nasal vestibule, vermilion, filiform papilla
Transitional epithelium (urothelium)	Renal calyces, renal pelvis, ureter, urinary bladder

n Gieson	Heidenhain iron hematoxylin	Weigert elastica stain	Mann methyl blue-eosin	Romeis lipid stain
n hematoxylin-ric acid-acid chsin	Tanning with iron alum-hematoxylin	Orcein or resorcin-fuchsin-nuclear fast red	Eosin-methyl blue	Hematoxylin-Sudan III
ck-brown	Chromatin and nucleoli: black	Red	Blue, nucleoli: red	Blue
lowish brown	Slightly gray, gray	–	Violet, reddish	Pale gray-blue
 d low	Gray-green, yellowish Gray-green, yellowish Yellowish, gray	– – Brown-red or violet to black-blue	Blue Blue Orange-red	– – –
d and yellow	Gray-grayish blue	–	Violet, reddish blue	
ow	Black	–	Red	–
ow	Black	–	Red-orange	–
ubilized/removed	Solubilized/removed	Solubilized/removed	Solubilized/removed	Orange-red

Table 3 Salivary glands: attributes of serous and mucous acini in light microscopy (after O. Bucher and H. Wartenberg, 1989)

Salivary gland	Serous acinus	Mucous tubule
Total diameter	Smaller	Larger
Configuration	Acinus or serous demilunes	Tubulus
Lumen/clearance	Very narrow, stellate	Relatively wide, round
Configuration of the nucleus	Round	Flattened, sickle-shaped
Positioning of the nucleus	Basal	Basal, peripheral
Cytoplasm	Granulated apical region, secretory granules	Light, honeycomb structure
Cell borders	Diffuse	Clearly visible
Terminal bars (junctional complexes)	Rarely visible	Present, usually visible
Secretory ducts	Intercellular	Absent

Table 4 **Seromucous (mixed) salivary glands and lacrimal gland: morphological attributes**

Glands	Acini	Intermediary ducts	Secretory ducts	Other attributes
Parotid gland	Acinar, purely serous, narrow lumen	200–300 μm long, multiple levels of branching	Well-formed, intralobular, branched	Stroma often contains adipocytes, abundant nerves
Submandibular gland	Tubuloacinar, mixed seromucous, predominantly serous, mucous tubules with serous demilunes	Some ducts are short and unbranched, others are long and branched	Well-formed, intralobular, branched	Areas with purely serous acini
Sublingual gland	Tubuloacinar, mixed seromucous, predominantly mucous, branched mucous tubules with serous demilunes	Rarely present	Very short secretory ducts	Areas with purely mucous acini, lobed intermediary ducts filled with mucus
Pancreas	Acinar, purely serous with central acinar cells, small myoepithelial cells	Well-formed	Absent	Endocrine glands: Langerhans islets (may be absent in the pancreatic head), few adipocytes
Lacrimal gland	Serous, branched tubules, wide lumen	Absent	Absent	Abundant connective tissue stroma with many free cells (lymphocytes and plasma cells

Table 5 Connective tissue fibers: morphological attributes

Type of fiber	Collagen fibers	Elastic fibers	Reticular fibers
Arrangement	Fiber bundles, weaves of various types of networks, variable mesh sizes, thickness: 1–12 μm	Fiber networks, fenestrated membranes, isolated fibers, web lamellae. thickness: up to 18 μm	Very delicate webs, matrix fibers at interfaces—e.g., between parenchymal cells and connective tissue, basal membrane, thickness: 0.2–1.0 μm
Structure in light microscopy	Anisotropic fibers (no light refraction observed), with cross-striation, not argyrophilic	Isotropic (strongly light-refracting) fibers, homogeneous, anisotropic stretched fibers, not argyrophilic	Thinner fibers, weak anisotropy; thinner fibers are clearly visible only after silver impregnation (argyrophilic fibers); positive PAS reaction
Structure in electron microscopy	Fibrils—microfibril bundles, microfibrils built from primary filaments, cross-striation of the microfibrils with a periodicity of 64 nm	Microfibrils—diameters are 10–14 nm, or amorphous elastin; no periodicity	Same as collagen fibrils, reticular microfibrils are about 50 nm thick
Mechanical attributes	Fibers have tensile strength but do not stretch	Reversibly expandable by 100–150%	Moderately expandable
Chemical attributes			
Effect of weak acids	Swelling	No swelling	Slight swelling
Effect of weak alkali	Decomposition	Resistant	Low degree of decomposition
Effect of boiling water	Soluble, forms a glue	Insoluble	Insoluble

Table 6 Biological "fibers": nomenclature

Connective tissue fibers	specific structured constituents of the intercellular matrix
Collagen fibers	Collagen fibers are birefringent in polarized light. They form fascicles (fasciculi collagenosi). When boiled in water, they form glue, such as bone glue. Collagen fibers occur in all connective and supportive tissue
Reticular fibers	Structured constituents of the intercellular matrix in reticular connective tissue, positive PAS reaction
Argyrophilic fibers	Thinner reticular fibers, which can only be seen using the silver impregnation technique, delicate matrix fibers, for example
Elastic fibers	Shiny fibers, strongly refract light in unstained preparations; the fibers branch and form meshworks, web lamellae and elastic membranes, contain elastin and microfibrils about 12 nm thick
Sharpey fibers	Collagen fibers, which radiate from the periosteum into the bony tissue, they secure the attachment of tendons, bands and periosteum to the skeleton
Tomes fibers	Processes of odontoblasts that are located in the dentine canaliculi (dentine fibers), also cellular structures
Lens fibers	Lens epithelial cells that have grown longitudinally and lost their nuclei; lens fibers can be up to 10 mm long. They are the major components of the lens
Glial fibers	Processes of certain macroglial cells
Nerve fibers	Processes of nerve cells—i.e., axons and their sheaths (oligodendrocytes for central nervous system fibers, Schwann cells for peripheral nerve fibers)
Smooth muscle fibers	Muscle cells or bundles often are erroneously called muscle fibers
Striated muscle fibers (skeletal muscle fibers)	Smallest building units of the skeletal musculature, multinucleated tubular syncytia
Heart muscle fibers	Incorrect name for heart muscle cells; often also used for a strand (cord) of apposed heart muscle cells
Purkinje fibers	Subendocardial termini of the nervous system of the heart, specific muscle cells

Table 7 Exocrine glands: principles of classification (after Sobotta/Hammersen, 2000)

Morphological criteria	Classification	Examples
Number of secretory cells	Unicellular glands, multicellular glands	Goblet cells Salivary glands
Localization of the secretory cells	Intraepithelial (endoepithelial) glands – Unicellular glands – Multicellular glands – Extraepithelial (exoepithelial) glands	Goblet cells Olfactory glands All large exocrine glands
Mode of secretion	Eccrine Apocrine	Salivary gland, pancreas, lacrimal gland mammary gland, prostate gland, olfactory gland
Type of secretory product	Holocrine Serous – serous glands Mucous – mucous glands Mucoid – mucoid glands	sebaceous glands, parotid gland, pancreas, lacrimal gland, goblet cells, cardiac glands, pyloric glands, duodenal glands, vestibular gland, urethral glands
Shape of the acini	Tubular glands Acinar glands Alveolar glands Tubuloacinar glands Tubuloalveolar glands	Intestinal glands (mostly branched tubules), glands of the colon (colon crypts), uterine glands, eccrine and apocrine sweat glands (if the tubules are coiled: coiled glands) Parotid gland, pancreas Scent glands Lacrimal glands, submandibular glands, sublingual glands Mammary glands, prostate gland
Presence and morphology of secretory ducts	– Simple glands: each acinus ends separately on the epithelial surface – Branched glands: glands with several levels of branching; several acini connect to an unbranched secretory duct – Mixed (seromucous) glands: the elaborately branched secretory ducts end in one acinus	Sweat glands Pyloric glands All large salivary glands

Table 8 Muscle tissue: distinctive morphological features

Muscle tissue	Smooth musculature	Skeletal musculature		Heart musculature
Components	Thin, spindle-shaped single cells	Type I fibers (red fibers)	Type II fibers (white fibers)	Cell (cell territory between intercalated disks)
Nuclei per cell	One nucleus, length: 8–25 μm	Many hundred nuclei, length: 5–16 μm	Many hundred nuclei, length: 5–16 μm	One or two nuclei, length: 10 12 μm
Shape and position of nuclei	Oval, rod-shaped to elliptic, central	Long, flat, peripheral, underneath the sarcolemma	Long, flat, peripheral, underneath the sarcolemma	Plump, round to oval, often lentil-shaped nuclei, central with fibril-free cytocenter
Length of components	40–200 μm, up to 800 μm in the uterus during pregnancy	Up to 40 cm	Up to 40 cm	50–150 μm
Diameter of components	5–15 μm	10–50 μm	80–100 μm	10–120 μm
Other features	Longitudinal section: cells occur in slightly undulating bundles; cross-section: nuclei are not sectioned in every cell, no myofibril mosaics	Longitudinal section: striation; cross-section: myofibril mosaics, dense capillarization, many mitochondria, wide Z disks	Less capillarization, fewer mitochondria, thin Z disks	Components form web-like structures (heart muscle fibers); cross-section: myofibril mosaic, endoplasm, fibril-free cytocenters, lipofuscin inclusions

Table 9 Stomach: differential diagnosis of the various segments of the stomach. Gastric areas (raised areas) and foveolae of variable depth with uniform prismatic epithelial cells up to 40 μm high are found in all segments of the stomach. These epithelial cells produce the gastric mucus (not goblet cells). There are also smooth muscle layers with the form and organization that are characteristic of the intestinal canal. However, oblique fibers (inner face) are also present

Stomach segment	Cardiac portion with cardial glands	Body and fundus of the stomach with gastric glands	Pyloric portion of the stomach with pyloric glands
Gastric glands	Relatively deep foveolae, elaborately branched tubules with an irregular appearance, often distended to ampulla, loosely structured	Short foveolae: long, relatively stretched tubules, mostly unbranched, but bifurcated at the fundus, narrow lumen	Deep foveolae: short, winding tubules with wide lumina and branched termini, on average not quite so densely packed
Unicellular glands	Homocrine glands (one secretory product = mucus), sporadic endocrine cells	Homocrine glands (secreting mucus, exclusively) in the foveolae, heterocrine glands in the tubules, 3 different cell types: mucous neck cells, (chief) peptic cells and parietal cells	Homocrine, mucus-producing gland cells, sporadic endocrine cells
Special morphological features	Lamina propria recessed against the gastric glands, sporadic lymph follicles	Lymph follicles are absent, but many free cells between gland tubules	Cell-rich lamina propria in the upper two-thirds of the mucous membrane; between fundus and pylorus, there is an intermediary layer about 1 cm wide, with transitional forms of gastric and pyloric glands

Table 10 Intestines: differential diagnosis of the segments

Intestinal segment	Plicae circulares	Intestinal villi	Intestinal crypts	Goblet cells	Special morphological features
Duodenum	Tall, wide circular plicae (circular folds)	Dense, large plump villi	200–400 µm deep tubular epithelial cells (Lieberkühn crypts = intestinal glands	Present	Mucoid duodenal glands (Brunner glands) in the submucosal tissue, including plicae; there are small groups of Paneth cells at the fundus of the crypts.
Jejunum	High, slender, circular plicae	Long, slender villi	Same as for the duodenum	Present	Increased presence of Paneth cells
Ileum	Short circular plicae, may be absent	Short, less dense villi	Deep crypts	Present	Increased presence of Paneth cells at the fundus of crypts, lymphatic nodules opposite the adjoining mesentery branch (only visible in suitably cut preparations)
Colon	Rarely present, but semilunar plicae	Absent	Dense population of deep crypts (colon glands); their depth increases closer to the anus	Very abundant	Hardly any Paneth cells any more; mitotic cells at the fundus of the crypts. The outer external tunica muscularis forms three tenia in the colon, plicae semilunares. Solitary lymphatic nodes break through the lamina muscularis mucosae; subserous lipid inclusions
Vermiform appendix	Absent	Absent	Present, but absent in some areas	Abundant	Much smaller than the other intestinal segments, many lymphatic nodules (intestinal tonsils) in the tunica propria, which push through the lamina muscularis mucosae and often extend to the inner circular muscle layer; mesenteriolum
Rectum	Absent	Absent	400–800 µm, less dense population of deep crypts	Copious numbers	Many solitary lymphatic nodules; the peritoneal lining is usually absent, in its place there is a tunica adventitia

Table 11 Kidney: tubules and their light microscopic characteristics

Part of the duct	Diameter	Epithelial cells	Cell nucleus	Affinity to stains	Basal striation
Proximal tubule	50–60 µm	Pars convoluta: cuboidal, diffusely delimited surface, tall brush border, cell borders usually not visible pars recta: very tall brush border	Spherical, close to the basal part of the cell at different distances from the base	Strongly acidophilic, diffuse	Pars convoluta: well developed pars recta: well developed, decreases toward the intermediary tubules
Intermediary tubule, descending and ascending limbs	10–15 µm, relatively wide lumen	Extremely flat, cell nuclei bulge underneath the surface, cell borders not distinctly visible	Lentil-shaped, nuclei bulge into the lumen (more nuclei than in blood vessels)	Light, neutrophilic, sometimes lipofuscin inclusions	Absent
Distal tubule	Pars recta: 25–35 µm; pars convoluta: 40–45 µm	Lower than in the proximal tubules; no brush border, therefore surface sharply delimited. Note: macula densa	Pars recta: spherical to lentil-shaped; pars convoluta: nuclei in a more apical position	Clearly stained, acidophilic; however, lighter than in the proximal tubule	Well developed
Connecting tubule	Approx. 25µm	Cuboidal, surface is sharply delimited, sharp cell borders	Spherical	Light	Absent
…lecting tubule …ystem, cortical …nd medullary collecting ducts	40–200 µm	Ranging from cuboidal to columnar, often slightly convex, very distinct regular cell borders	Spherical	Light, neutrophilic	Absent
…apillary ducts	200–300 µm	Columnar, sharply delimited surface, distinct cell borders	Spherical	Light, neutrophilic	Absent

Table 12 Trachea and bronchial tree: morphological characteristics

Segment	Epithelial lining	Glands	Smooth musculature	Cartilage
Trachea (diameter: 16–21 mm) and principal bronchi (diameter: 12–14 mm)	Multilayered ciliated columnar epithelium with unicellular endoepithelial glands (= goblet cells)	Seromucous tracheal glands, predominantly between tracheal cartilage and in membranous walls (paries)	Tracheal muscle in the membranous wall	Horseshoe-shaped hyaline tracheal cartilage
Lobar bronchi (diameter: 8–12 mm) and segmental bronchi (diameter: 2–6 mm)	Multilayered ciliated columnar epithelium with many goblet cells	Seromucous bronchial glands, predominantly in the cartilaginous tunica muscularis	Cartilaginous tunica muscularis	At first residual hyaline cartilage of irregular appearance and organization, then cartilage; elastic cartilage in the smaller bronchi
Bronchioles (diameter: 0.3–0.6 mm)	Single-layered ciliated cuboidal epithelium without goblet cells	Still sporadic seromucous (mixed) glands	Tunica muscularis	Absent
Respiratory bronchioles (diameter: 0.25–0.5 mm)	Single-layered cuboidal epithelium without cilia; no goblet cells	Absent	Tunica muscularis	Absent
Alveolar ductules (diameter: 0.2–0.4 mm)	Single-layered cuboidal epithelium of gradually decreasing height	Absent	Smooth muscle cells in the basal rings around the alveolar opening	Absent
Alveoli	Single-layered squamous epithelium; alveolar epithelial cells type I and II, alveolar phagocytes	Absent	Absent (only elastic and reticular structures remain)	Absent

Table 13 Lymphatic organs: distinctive morphological features

Organ	Capsule and connective tissue septa	Parenchyma	Characteristic vessels	Other features
Lymph nodes	Well developed, clearly visible trabeculae	Lymphoreticular, compact cortex with lymph follicles, lighter medulla with medullary cords	Afferent vessel, marginal sinus, intermediary sinus, medullary sinus, efferent vessel; in the lumina of all sinuses: a bow-net (weir) system of reticular fibers and reticular cells, no blood cells	Surrounded by loosely organized connective tissue and adipose tissue; lymph vessels with valves often exist in the vicinity; no surface epithelium
Spleen	Very well developed, strong, strong trabeculae	Lymph nodes and lymphoreticular sheaths around the central artery = white pulp. The red pulp is not part of the lymphatic system	Characteristic blood vessels (laminar vessels, central artery, penicillary arteriolae, splenic sinus with gaps, muscle-free pulp and laminar veins); blood cells in the lumen of the splenic sinus	Single-layered flat peritoneal epithelium forms a sheath around the capsule
Tonsils				
Palatine tonsils	Well-developed, weak trabeculae	Lymphoreticular nodes (lymph follicles) surround 10–15 branched, narrow epithelial invaginations (fossulae tonsillares with tonsillar crypts)	–	Multilayered nonkeratinizing squamous epithelium, interspersed with lymphocytes inside the invaginations and crypts; in the vicinity, but outside the capsule, there are small mucous glands, which normally do not end in the epithelial invaginations;
Pharyngeal tonsils	Not well-developed, thin	Lymphoreticular nodes (lymph follicles) surround wide epithelial folds and epithelial invaginations	–	bulging shape, multilayered ciliated epithelium with goblet cells; mixed (seromucous) glands end in the epithelial invaginations;
Lingual tonsils (= all lingual follicles)	Not well developed, thin, no trabeculae	Lymphoreticular nodes (lymph follicles) surround solitary epithelial pits	–	multilayered nonkeratinizing squamous epithelium; mucous glands end in the epithelial invaginations; basic lingual tissue, striated lingual musculature
Thymus	Well-developed, partitioning into lobes by connective tissue septa	Lymphoepithelial; no lymph follicles; denser cortex, more loosely organized medulla with interspersed lymphocytes; epithelial Hassall bodies in the medulla	–	Involution after puberty; adipose tissue gradually replaces the parenchyma; in senescence: adipose tissue with parenchyma islets

Table 14 Hollow organs: differential diagnosis of hollow organs (ducts) with stellate or round openings

Organ	Epithelium	Glands	Musculature	Special features
Esophagus	Multilayered nonkeratinizing squamous epithelium	Branched, tubular mucous glands (esophageal glands) in the submucosal tissue	Lamina muscularis mucosae; tunica muscularis, defined by inner circular muscle fibers and outer longitudinal muscle fibers; striated muscle fibers in the upper third	Layered structure like in the entire intestinal tract; clearly defined lamina muscularis mucosae
Ureter	Transitional epithelium (urothelium)	None	Strong tunica muscularis, three-layered: inner and outer (weak) longitudinal muscle fibers and a medium layer of (strong) circular muscle fibers	Muscle layers often not clearly defined, less compact, copious interspersed connective tissue
Urethra	Female urethra: transitional epithelium, multilayered nonkeratinizing squamous epithelium toward the vestibular opening. Male urethra: transitional epithelium up to the pars prostatica, then multilayered, cuboidal epithelium; fossa navicularis with multilayered nonkeratinizing squamous epithelium	Urethral glands and urethral lacunae; endothelial mucous glands and goblet cells	Inner longitudinal and outer circular muscle fibers, in some cases, striated muscle fibers of the urethral pelvis	Female urethra: muscular stratum spongiosum urethrae. Male urethra: tunica muscularis connects with the smooth musculature of the prostate gland; wide, muscle-free veins of the lamina propria
Vas deferens	Two-layered columnar epithelium with stereocilia	None	Tunica muscularis with a diameter of 1.0–1.5 mm, particularly thick; three-layered helical structure: inner and outer longitudinal muscle layers, intermediary circular muscle layer	Lamina propria is rich i elastic fibers; often, t entire spermatic cor also sectioned
Oviduct	Single-layered columnar epithelium with brush border and goblet cells	None	Tunica muscularis is relatively thin, double-layered, outer longitudinal muscle fibers, stronger inner circular layer; often also a longitudinal inner layer of muscle fibers (cells)	Elaborate folding of t mucous membrane in the ampulla; strong muscle fibers in the isthmus, only flat resid mucous membrane fo
Vermiform appendix	Single-layered columnar epithelium with brush border and goblet cells	Crypts	Thin lamina muscularis mucosae; tunica muscularis with inner circular muscle layer and outer longitudinal muscle fibers	Many lymph follicles i the lamina propria push through the lamina muscularis mucosae; seros and meso-appendix
Gallbladder	Single-layered columnar epithelium with short rod-like microvilli and junctional complexes (terminal bars)	Goblet cells and mucous glands only after stimulation by inflammatory processes	Tunica muscularis is more loosely structured, web-like	Irregularly shaped mucous membrane folds, formation of Luschka's ducts
Bile duct	Single-layered columnar epithelium	Tubular coiled glands	Muscle cells arranged in a braid-like configuration, mostly circular muscles	Strong musculatu the opening clear the second p denum, sph Oddi

Table 15 Alveolar glands and "gland-like" organs: differential diagnosis

Organ	Formation of lobes	Acini – mucous membrane – epithelium – duct systems
Prostate gland	Marginally developed; outer periurethral zone, inner and outer zone	30–50 tubuloalveolar glands with wide lumina; raised epithelial areas and invaginations; cuboidal epithelium as well as single or double-layered columnar epithelium; 15–30 secretory ducts end on the seminal colliculus and in the surrounding urethra, prostatic ducts
Efferent ductules of the testis	8–12 efferent ductules form a conical lobe	Raised surface areas and pits create an undulating surface in the lumen; cuboidal epithelium in the base of the pits, multilayered columnar epithelium with kinocilia and/or microvilli (brush border) on the upper raised portions; the efferent ductules wind strongly and end in the vas deferens
Seminal vesicle	Only apparently partitioned into lobes	About 15 cm long coiled duct; bizarre relief of surface folds with primary, secondary and tertiary folds and invaginations (alveoli) with wide lumina; single or double-layered columnar epithelium; secretory duct
Bulbourethral glands(Cowper's glands)	Barely expressed	Branched tubular glands with invaginations, sometimes alveolar acini; single-layered cuboidal to columnar epithelium, secretory duct
Mammary gland	Very clearly discernible	15–20 single branched tubuloalveolar glands, alveolar acini of different size, epithelial cells of different height with lipid droplets; apical protrusions (apocrine extrusion); always visible: sections of large lactiferous ducts
Ampulla of the oviduct	–	Tunica mucosa with many folds, primary, secondary and tertiary folds; narrow slit-shaped lumina; single-layered columnar epithelium with secretory cells and ciliated cells
hyroid gland	Clearly discernible	Follicles (= "alveolar acini"), variable in shape and size (50–500 μm); single-layered epithelium, height varies with functional state; no secretory ducts, because it is an endocrine gland
bryonic lung	Clearly discernible	Acini often appear in the form of branched epithelial tubes or not quite developed alveoli; cuboidal epithelium; clearly discernible system of canals

Musculature	Special morphological characteristics
/lany smooth muscle cells in the interstitial connec-ive tissue ("fibromuscular stroma")	Capsule with smooth muscle cells, wide subcapsular venous plexuses; occasionally prostate stones in the gland chambers; elastic and collagenous fibers in the stroma, ganglia cells
mooth muscle cells in circular arrangement in the mina propria and outside it	Connective tissue lamina propria is cell-rich but small
:rong wall made of a meshwork of smooth muscle ells (= tunica muscularis)	Tunica adventitia becomes dense and forms a capsule on the surface
and tubules surrounded by smooth muscle cells; terspersed with striated muscle fibers of the deep ansverse perineal muscle	Noticeably light gland cells, clearly defined cell borders
	Poorly developed connective tissue; the secretory product in the gland lumina can be stained
nica muscularis: outer longitudinal layer, more pro-unced middle circular layer of smooth muscle cells, ier longitudinal layer (weakly developed)	Clearance with tall branched mucous membrane plicae that most fill the lumen; outer serosa
	Follicles filled with colloid; connective tissue capsule, trabecu lae; parafollicular cells (C-cells)
	Remarkably cell-rich mesenchymal connective tissue

Table 16 Skin areas: differential diagnosis

Skin area	Common characteristics	Epidermis
Palms of the hands and soles of the feet	Multilayered, keratinized squamous epithelium (epidermis), which is layered onto a connective tissue layer (corium) and subcutaneous connective tissue (subcutis)	Particularly thick, at 1.5–4.0 mm; thick stra- tum corneum
Fingertip		Thick; thick stratum corneum
Scalp		Thin
Abdominal skin		Thin
Skin of the axilla		Moderately thick, pigmented stratum basale
Skin of the scrotum		Thin, moderately keratinized epithelium; tensively pigmented stratum basale
Skin of the labium minor		thin, transition to nonkeratinized squamo epithelium; sparsely pigmented
Skin of the outer eyelid		Thin, scarcely keratinized, transition to no keratinized squamous epithelium of the p pebral tunica conjunctiva
[illegible]		Moderately thick, multilayered keratinize outer squamous epithelium; transitional zone: vermilion border, inner layer: high multilayered nonkeratinizing squamous e thelium
[illegible]a nasi		Moderately thick, transition to respirator epithelium in the nasal vestibule

Tables